Advance Praise for All About Eve:

"*All About Eve* is a welcome addition to the growing library available to women interested in their health. Tracy Chutorian Semler has given us a veritable encyclopedia that will be on my shelf for many years to come."

Senator Carol Moseley-Braun

"Tracy Chutorian Semler, a concerned and compassionate journalist, has written a book that every woman can use to maximize her health and well-being to the fullest. It is more than just informative. It is also lucid and comprehensive. By delving into normal physiology as well as stressing prevention, Chutorian Semler makes a significant contribution to the literature of women's health care."

Jill Maura Rabin, M. D.
Head, Urogynecology and Ambulatory Care
Long Island Jewish Medical Center

"We've learned the hard way over the years what it takes to be a smart consumer when it comes to women's health. In Tracy, you'll find that we have an advocate who's passionate about helping guide us through a system that does not always have our best interest at heart. *All About Eve* is a must-read if you want to make informed decisions about your health. I have worked with many bright, thorough, indefatigable and thoughtful producers throughout my career. Tracy's work stands alone."

Paula Zahn
Co-Anchor
CBS This Morning

"With nearly a decade of experience in the women's health genre, Tracy Chutorian Semler gives women the power to be strong advocates for their health and lives. *All About Eve* will help American women to stay up-to-date about the latest women's health news. This book is a must as a reference in any woman's personal library."

Congresswoman Patricia Schroeder (D-CO)

"Tracy Chutorian Semler has done an excellent job of presenting important health-related information to women in a relevant, understandable manner."

Robert C. Young, M. D.
President
Fox Chase Cancer Center, Philadelphia

ALL ABOUT EVE

THE COMPLETE GUIDE TO WOMEN'S HEALTH AND WELL-BEING

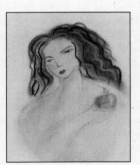

TRACY CHUTORIAN SEMLER

HarperCollins*Publishers*

HarperCollins books may be purchased for educational, business, or
sales promotional use. For information please write: Special Markets
Department, HarperCollins Publishers, Inc., 10 East 53rd Street,
New York, NY 10022.

Designed by Nancy Singer

Library of Congress Cataloging-in-Publication Data
Semler, Tracy Chutorian, 1964–
    All about eve / by Tracy Chutorian Semler.
      p.   cm.
    Includes index.
    ISBN 0-06-271577-1.—ISBN 0-06-273248-X (pbk.)
    1. Women—Health and hygiene. I. Title.
RA778.S517   1995
613'.04244—dc20   94-35236

95 96 97 98 99 ❖/RRD 10 9 8 7 6 5 4 3 2 1

Dedication

I dedicate this book to the three most important people in my life—all of whom lived patiently, in utter chaos, as the book came together:

My husband, H Eric Semler, the love of my life. Who pushes me *almost* as hard as he pushes himself (thereby knocking about 3 months off the delivery time of this book). Who squeezes every nanosecond out of a day, his tail wagging. Who at once flatters and exhausts me with the belief that I can do it all, and shouldn't settle for less. Who wows me with the size of his dreams, and his ability to realize them.

My mother, Helen Carol Chutorian, the most decent human being I have ever known, or will ever know. Who defines the word *parent*. Whose "tough love," as she proudly names it, has instilled in me the faith that with good old-fashioned hard work (and a mother with the remarkable energy to pick up the pieces) anything is possible.

My father, Dr. Abraham Milton Chutorian, a one-of-a-kind intellectual tough-guy with a conscience of steel. Who has dedicated his life to making sick children well, his family happy and advancing the field of pediatric neurology. Whose thirst for a mental challenge spurred my own interest in health and medicine. And who gave me a guiding principle I'll never forget: that you haven't found the right life's work until you'd rather do it than be at leisure.

Contents

Acknowledgments

I will always remember and deeply appreciate the contributions of the following friends, family and colleagues. Without their counsel, their belief in me and in this project, *All About Eve: The Complete Guide to Women's Health and Well-being* would never have come to be.

I thank soon-to-be-doctor Lisa Sanders, my former CBS colleague, for standing in my cubicle, listening to and liking my idea enough to urge me to write to her friend, the incomparable Kris Dahl—and for sticking her phone number in my hand immediately. I am indebted to Kris Dahl of ICM, who became my agent and positively floored me with her sharp, clearheaded intelligence, her competence and efficiency, and her certainty from square one that she could and would make this project happen. (I suspect there isn't much she *can't* make happen). I also sincerely thank Dorothea Herrey, Kris's right hand, another smart and enthusiastic woman who egged me on with her excitement about the book and made me believe, when my confidence flagged, that it would all come to pass.

Going back several years I thank Bob Shanks and Pete Bonventre, my first television mentors, for giving me the health beat and for trusting me, at such a young age, to write stories instead of answering telephones. You made it exciting to come to work every day. I was lucky to learn from both of you.

I am deeply grateful to Janet Goldstein, my editor at HarperCollins, who truly cares about books and about the people who write them. She manages to do sixteen things at once while making you feel like you're the only person on her agenda, and has the uncanny ability to draw out the essentials of a passage or chapter, making a jumbled section clear as a bell between bites of pizza or Indian food. And my heartfelt thanks to wonderful Betsy Thorpe, Janet's assistant editor, who tackled, clarified and offered terrific advice on hundreds of pages faster than a speeding bullet—and somehow always managed to smile while doing it. Her humorous notes with each chapter delivery kept me chugging along those tired last days.

As I know well from my years in television, there is always a team of talented and driven people whose names you don't hear and whose faces go unseen in assembling projects like this one. I wish to thank that team: Elaine Verriest, supervisor Reference production; Susan Kosko, production manager; Nancy Singer, designer; Joana Jebsen, marketing; and David Youngstrom, sales. And to the many others at HarperCollins who toiled along with me but I've never met or thanked: my gratitude extends to you, as well.

To all the women who shared their private and sometimes painful health experiences with me for this book and over the past eight years, I can never thank you enough. It was often hard to dredge up old memories and to put your difficult experiences into words. Your openness and generosity of time and spirit, no doubt will help other women who may someday find themselves in the same situations.

Thanks also to Ted Savaglio, former executive producer of "CBS This Morning," and to current e.p. Jim Murphy, who were supportive of this project from the minute I announced it, and gave me the precious time I needed to get it done properly at a time when their staff was already stretched to the limit. And thanks to Paula Zahn, co-anchor of "CBS This Morning," a joy to work with, for caring so much about women's health issues and committing herself to covering them frankly and frequently. And to the Health Unit, past and present: Bob, Howard, Susan, Gordon, et al., thanks for the education and the adventures.

My deep thanks also to bright, efficient and cheerful Dipak Kshatriya, who appeared on the scene like a savior in the eleventh hour to secure final interviews, locate statistics and get reprint permissions as he neared the end of his college career.

I am grateful to countless hospital personnel and public relations people, but can only name a few here. Stand-outs over the years and who also came through for this book include Myrna Manners of The New York Hospital, Eric Rosenthal of the Fox Chase Cancer Center, and Kate Rudden, formerly of the American College of Obstetricians and Gynecologists, whom I have never met in person but have talked to probably 50 times by phone over the past several years.

Thanks also to Dr. Vivian Pinn for her beautiful foreword and for her work on behalf of all women's health, and to her colleagues Mary Chunko and Ellen Pollack at the Office of Research on Women's Health at the NIH.

I can't overlook irreplaceable friends like Julie, Karin, Liz, Lori, Marion, Nancy, Jon, Lance and others who stick out in my mind for how heartily they shared my enthusiasm for the book from its inception to its completion, and for often forgiving my long periods of "Sorry, I can't talk on the phone" or just vanishing off the face of the earth to work. You all cheered me on almost daily, and I'll never forget it.

I will always be indebted to my big sister Leslie, who exhorted me from the day I could write a clear sentence to make a career out of writing, though she probably has no idea how big an impact her encouragement made on me. I knew that my brother-in-law Douglas, always brimming with bright ideas, would come up with a great title—and of course he did. My thanks to him are on the cover of this book forever. Thanks too to my loving sister Sandra and brother-in-law Greg for their faith and support. I also thank my wonderful parents-in-law Shirley and Dr. Herbert Semler, who knew this would come to pass and boosted me month after month with their cross-country faith and encouragement. Thanks too to my terrific Oregonian sisters and brothers-in-law, Deena, Gregg, Jill, Matthew, Rick and Shelli, for their support.

My angel J. Nicholas Chutorian Semler gestated alongside this book and was born just as hard labor and delivery of the manuscript began. As if he knew the value his cooperation would supply, he immediately became a most delightful child, and the joy he brings me is a new source of energy and creativity beyond compare.

Finally, I salute talented Arleen Frasca, whose lovely images at once capture the power and delicacy of the female body, celebrating the beauty of woman's form.

Foreword

In recent years, women's health has captured headlines and the national consciousness in what has been called a new—and long overdue—awakening.

Through the efforts of thousands of women across the country, members of Congress, physicians and other health professionals, scientists and prominent figures in the media, issues relating to women's health and well-being have come to the forefront of the public's and policymakers' attention. In fact, this movement has engendered a shift in consciousness with a new recognition that women's health deserves distinct attention from the scientific and health care policy communities. The result has been an unprecedented level of attention and resources directed toward improving medical research and health care services for women.

The new focus on women's health has developed, in part, from the changing role of women in our society, as well as changing demographics. Women currently make up 51 percent of the U.S. population and 45 percent of our nation's work force. Demographic projections suggest that, by the year 2000, a majority of new entrants into the work force will be women of all ethnic origins. Thus, women not only maintain their traditional roles in the home and in child rearing, they also contribute significantly to the economic productivity and security of our nation. Policymakers and health care providers alike recognize that in order to keep our economy robust, we must keep women healthy.

Yet, over the course of their lives, women suffer from a higher incidence of disease and debility than do men. Even when reproductive problems are eliminated from the calculations, women's activities are limited by health problems approximately 25 percent more days each year than are men's activities, and women are bedridden 35 percent more days than men.

Since the turn of the century, the average life expectancy for American women has increased by almost 30 years, and women constitute the majority of our nation's elderly. Yet too many women reap a bitter harvest during their later years of life: osteoporosis, heart disease, cancer, depression, frailty and social isolation. In the next century, elderly women will make up an even larger proportion of the U.S. population, and physicians, policymakers and women nationwide now recognize the importance of keeping women healthy and mentally and physically active throughout all the years of their lives.

Since they are living longer, women now also spend about one-third of their lives following menopause. This fact has altered the very meaning of the term "women's health," which used to imply women's reproductive health and was the exclusive purview of gynecologists and obstetricians. Traditionally, women's other health concerns—conditions like heart disease and cancer that affect both men and women—were studied and understood in terms of male models of prevention and treatment, without focusing on potential gender differences.

Today the medical and health care policy communities are beginning to realize that improving women's health requires the skills and efforts of talented men and women representing the full spectrum of medical specialties and scientific disciplines. Consequently, the focus now is for all physicians, in fact, all health care providers, male and female, to possess a full understanding of how to prevent and treat diseases and conditions in women, to recognize the symptoms of disease in women when these are different from the symptoms in men, and to know when treatments for women differ from the accepted treatments for men.

Unfortunately, past medical research has not provided an adequate understanding of a number of diseases and conditions that affect women and their optimum treatment interventions. For example, cardiovascular diseases are still not widely recognized as the leading causes of death in women, and women often do not receive optimum interventions for cardiovascular disease. Immunological disorders, such as lupus erythematosus and rheumatoid arthritis, afflict a much greater proportion of women than men. And cancers of the breast, lung, ovary and colon are still major contributors to the mortality of American women.

Fortunately, the long-standing failure to understand or to determine gender differences in health, disease and access to care has now been recognized and is being redressed through new policies and programs on the Federal and local levels.

In 1990, the National Institutes of Health (NIH) established the Office of Research on Women's Health to address gaps in the medical community's understanding of women's health through biomedical and behavioral research. The office has the mandate and resources to support basic and clinical research that will provide the scientific knowledge base needed to develop gender-appropriate techniques and efficacious treatments and interventions to improve the health of women. The office's research agenda encompasses the full spectrum of diseases and conditions that affect women from birth and childhood through menopause and the later years of life and also focuses on determining what constitutes normal growth and development in women. The agenda addresses not only conditions unique to women and their reproductive system, but also diseases and conditions that may affect both men and women and for which interventions have been defined using men as the research model. Another important element of the office's agenda requires ensuring that women are adequately represented as participants in all NIH-supported clinical research. This policy was given the force of law in the NIH Revitalization Act of 1993. And lastly, the office's mandate includes increasing the opportunities for women's participation and advancement in biomedical careers.

The efforts of the Office of Research on Women's Health are complemented by the NIH's Women's Health Initiative (WHI). The Women's Health Initiative, the largest preventive study ever undertaken in the United States, is a 15-year clinical study of the prevention of the major diseases and conditions that affect the health of women during their postmenopausal years: cardiovascular diseases, breast and colorectal cancers and osteoporosis. This nationwide study will examine the benefits and risks of long-term hormone replacement therapy, the role of low-fat diet modification using behavioral change and calcium and vitamin D supplementation in preventing disease. The WHI will include some 160,000 postmenopausal women in large and small communities nationwide.

Over the next decade, all of these research efforts should begin to provide much needed answers for many of the questions concerning disease prevention and treatment in women. Yet, even if the major gaps in medical knowledge of women's health are addressed through research during the 1990s, the fact that there will always be differences between men and women because of each gender's normal physiology and hormonal milieu, dictates a continuing need for women's health research. With women now demanding better care and increased understanding of their health concerns by all health professionals, women's health must continue to be a high priority for the scientific and health care communities.

Today, as never before in our nation's history, women have the opportunity to improve and protect their health. But the improvement of women's health must be a shared concern and a shared responsibility. While the medical community works to provide answers and guidance regarding health-promoting lifestyles and optimum treatments for illness, women themselves must take responsibility for safeguarding their own health. A first step is self-education to make the right choices.

Reading *All About Eve* can be that important first step toward making the right choices to stay healthy. With its emphasis on prevention, this book provides practical advice on a wide variety of health issues, ranging from pointers on how to select and talk to a physician to strategies for preserving bone strength, avoiding skin cancer and guarding against sexually transmitted diseases. In cases where the medical community still lacks hard-and-fast answers for women—such as the benefits and risks associated with hormone replacement therapy—the author summarizes medical knowledge and opinion to date in a way that may help women to make informed personal choices.

All About Eve can serve as a reliable guide for women seeking to learn more about their bodies and about the health care options available to them in the United States. With this increased knowledge, women can be empowered to take better care of themselves and to ensure that they receive the best available care from health care professionals.

Vivian W. Pinn, M.D.
Associate Director for Research on Women's Health
Director, Office of Research on Women's Health
National Institutes of Health

Introduction

Just by picking up this book, you have made an important decision: you want to be healthy. Whether it's because you want to feel better when you wake up each morning, get more out of every day of your life, battle a chronic health problem or pain, be strong for a pregnancy, live longer—whatever your personal health goals—you have decided that it is important to care for your body. It's a decision that millions of women are making today, as it becomes clear that many major women's health problems can be prevented, managed or cured. It is possible to live both longer and *well,* and this book will help you do that. This book will also help you come to understand that living *well* isn't any harder—and can actually be a lot more fun—than ignoring your health and settling for less than your personal potential for wellness.

For the last eight years, I have been researching, writing and producing health news stories for CBS News. Most of that time, I worked for "CBS This Morning," a national morning news program that places great emphasis on health topics (often airing seven health segments per five-day week). Because we have a disproportionately high number of women viewers, women's health issues have always been at the top of our agenda. We've tried to cover the issues that concern women most, as well as those that *should* be on women's minds because of their seriousness or prevalence. Over the years, I became increasingly frustrated by the fact that there is only *so* much you can explain in a four-minute television segment. You can briefly explain a problem, and even more briefly talk about new solutions or approaches to care. But there's precious little time to put stories in the greater context women need to make informed decisions about their health care, and almost no time at all to individualize advice to particular women's needs. Unfortunately, it's through television sound bites that many women get the bulk of their health news—which means that millions of women are getting only half the story at best, leaving them confused or frightened.

The result of our providing information piecemeal, I discovered over the years, was a flood of thousands of phone calls and letters from women of all ages and backgrounds, from around the country and even beyond our borders, asking us to fill in the blanks, connect the dots, and give answers where, in 240 seconds, we had only raised new questions. Our viewers were seeking further information on how to protect themselves or their loved ones from disease—or cure illnesses they already had. Sometimes I was able to take those calls, or respond to those letters, and refer women to sources of further information on their problem. But there was no way to respond to every person, or answer every question. Always I was plagued by the lack of time, and the ever-present "blanks" in the data.

It was from the need to flesh out those answers that this book was born. I've tried to deal with the topics about which women were most concerned, most confused, or most curious. You'll find in these pages specific, rather than generalized, advice (not just that you *should* get more calcium in your diet, but *how much* to get; not just that you *should* get a fast and complete workup for infertility, but *what the components* of that workup should be). No book contains all the answers, but this one attempts to give practical information wherever possible, to point you in the direction of the next appropriate step in seeking good health care, to raise the big questions and, where it can't answer them completely, to guide you to further information.

Too many women, because of a lack of information, bad luck, poor access to medical care, or other common obstacles, fail to obtain adequate health care—and the results can be devastating, as the following case shows. Several years ago, when producing a story on breast cancer for "CBS This Morning," I met a woman in her late 60s living in a sleepy town in rural New Hampshire. I'll call her Sally. Sally was thankful to be alive: She had survived breast cancer. However, she had *not* survived with her body intact. She had had one entire breast and part of her chest wall removed as treatment for her disease. For some women, this relatively extensive procedure, called a mastectomy, is the appropriate treatment for breast cancer—and for many of them, it's a small though painful price to pay for one's life. For Sally, however, the price was too high—and unnecessary. Sally learned too late that her breast cancer was so tiny, caught so early, and confined to her breast (not spread throughout her body) that the tumor alone could have been removed, *without* removing her entire breast.

While she certainly is happy to be alive, Sally continues to suffer a great deal with body image problems; talking about the lost breast brings her to tears many years after the procedure. Many women in Sally's situation opt for breast reconstruction, which can be both emotionally physically healing. Others live comfortably without a reconstructed breast. Sally chose *not* to have further surgery, but has never come to terms with her condition; she relives the pain of her ordeal every morning in the shower and every evening when she undresses for bed. Looking at the bare space on her chest, Sally is reminded of what could have been—had she been given the information she needed.

Why did Sally have "too much" surgery, and fall short of her own health potential? Because she just happened to see a physician who failed to offer her the less invasive alternative. She found out her "option" too late, when she went to a new physician for follow-up care. It never occurred to her, especially at a time when she was frightened and vulnerable, that her doctor might not give her state-of-the-art care. She put her life in his hands, and happily, she has her life to show for it. Still, what happened to Sally was *wrong*. She should have been able to *choose* her procedure; making choices about our own health management is not only empowering but a fundamental part of managing our lives as a whole. Some women in Sally's position might have *chosen* a mastectomy; others, a less invasive procedure. The point is, where there are options, where there are choices to be made in our health care, we should be informed about them—and WE should make them.

I hope that after reading this book, you'll have learned some easy lessons that Sally learned the hard way. No single doctor has all the answers, regardless of his or her intelligence or best intentions. When your problem is serious, you owe it to yourself to play an active role in the process of getting the best care possible. Learn about your options. Seek second opinions. Question an approach to care that makes you uncomfortable, or that doesn't fit with *your* philosophy of health and wellness. Always keep in mind that *you are the #1 expert on your body:* you live inside of it, feel it, experience its norms and its changes year in, year out. Certainly you can and should play an active and important role in its care. Good health care professionals will appreciate your playing that role; it makes their jobs easier by taking some of the mystery out of the diagnostic process and by creating a cooperative, interactive approach to your health management that is quietly becoming the new (and more effective) medicine of the future.

No single book or resource can answer all of your questions. And certainly a book is no substitute for actual medical care. This one, however, will empower you to take action to better your experience in the often confusing and conflicting world of health care. Above all else, by guiding you on effective ways to think and behave in the health care setting, this book will help you avoid the two kinds of mistakes that can cost people their health and sometimes even their lives: getting the wrong treatment, or missing out on the right one. This is especially vital for women, because there is such an enormous amount of contradictory information about women's health in the media today. You deserve some hard answers—but where hard answers simply don't exist in the medical literature, you deserve to know *that* truth as well . . . and to learn which factors should be weighed when making *personal, individual* decisions about your health.

This active role in your health care, in the way you receive medical "news" and the way in which you deal with health care professionals, will take some research and activism on your part. You will have to learn about your health risks—your family history of certain diseases, your behaviors and how they might be impacting your future risk of disease, and your current risk factors, including your blood pressure, your cholesterol level, the strength of your bones. These pieces of information will help you determine *your* risk of certain diseases, not your next door neighbor's, or that of the fictive "average American woman." You can only protect your body from illness if you are prepared to learn about and modify your risks. This book will help you to do so.

With so much health information flowing our way, it's hard to decipher the quackery from the legitimate information. Logic tells us not to get our health information from the tabloids. But many people would be surprised to know that even the leading "serious" media outlets are riddled with misinformation, sweeping advice garnered from questionable sources, and conflicting advice from week to week. The advice you'll find in this book was culled from scientific and clinical research by some of the best health care professionals in the world, and from hundreds of interviews with leading health experts who dedicate their lives to making people well. You'll find the information in these pages, while diverse in topic, to be quite complementary: The same diet that helps prevent bone loss can help keep fat down and protect you from heart disease; screening tests for various diseases often overlap, and can often be accomplished in one doctor visit each year. The fact is, it's easy to tend to your health! You don't have to be a "health nut," or become obsessed with staying well. You just have to decide that you deserve to be healthy, and seize this opportunity for yourself starting today.

A doctor once told me, sadly, that Americans spend more time shopping for a car than they do shopping for health care. Just as you wouldn't want to drive a lemon, don't let your body turn into one, either. Remember, you only *get* one body. To a certain extent, what you do *with* it and *to* it over your lifetime will help determine what it does to you in return. Treat it well, and with a blend of good fortune and good health care, it will treat you well in return.

PART ONE

Women's Health Care, Your Health Care

CHAPTER ONE

THE SECOND SEX

BIAS IN WOMEN'S HEALTH CARE TODAY

*The medical model is still male in many ways. Women have been
ignored far too much. This has gone on too long. It's traditionally been
that human chemistry and physiology were male until proven
otherwise. Women will make a revolution in health care.*

—Kathryn C. Bemmann, M.D., Past President,
American Medical Women's Association

Women have never been given a fair shake in the world of health care. One
of the many important reasons: almost all of the research on how to prevent and treat major diseases has been conducted *on* men and *by* men. As a
result, doctors have had to apply information gathered from male subjects
to female patients. If this seems at once silly and appalling to you, you're not
alone. Top researchers in science and health, as well as political leaders, have
cried out about this injustice—and they're being heard.

Trouble often starts at the top, and this was certainly true in the case of
women's health care. According to a June, 1990 report from the General
Accounting Office (GAO) of the House of Representatives, commissioned
by the Congressional Caucus for Women's Issues, our leading federal agency
for providing information on health promotion—the Department of
Health and Human Services—wasn't doing its job effectively. The report
charged that the department was doing a terrible job of developing a
women's health research and prevention agenda. Specifically, the report
found no overall strategy regarding what information about women's
health was needed, or how to get that information to the average woman.
During the research that led to the report, callers requesting women's

health-related advice from local public health service offices were turned away; instead of getting needed information, they were referred to local bookstores and hospitals for help. In one astonishing example, a public health employee asked the caller what osteoporosis was! It was this combination of inadequate information and poor communication of what we *did* know that left women in such a quandary.

In short order, something substantial was done to rectify the dearth of information and lack of direction in women's health. In September 1990, the Office of Research on Women's Health (ORWH) was created at the National Institutes of Health. The goal of the office was three-fold: to increase women's participation in health research studies, to insure that NIH-supported research pays due attention to women's health issues, and to promote the number of women in biomedical and biobehavioral careers. In April 1991, Dr. Bernadine Healy was named the first female director of the NIH; she launched a multimillion-dollar study of over 150,000 women at 45 clinical centers across the country to investigate the causes and potential prevention of major diseases of women—particularly heart disease, cancers of the breast, colon and rectum, and osteoporosis. Dr. Vivian Pinn became the first full-time director of the ORWH, and co-director of this massive study. Now underway, the Women's Health Initiative will provide, in about a decade's time, many hard answers about midlife women's health that we are forced to fudge on today.

What about the next decade, while we wait? Unfortunately, we now have far more questions than answers about women's health care. We therefore have to be extremely cautious in accepting treatment or prevention plans that are often suggested to women *without* the backup of good sound medical data. And we must be wary of inadequate information and bias against women in all areas of health and disease management. We must demand complete explanations for any and all procedures or other health management plans offered to us and, when complete explanations aren't available, we must ask *why?* What are the known benefits? What are the known risks? What are the potential unknowns?

There's nothing new about discrimination against women in health care—in fact, it starts at the level of the *provider* and only then trickles down to you, the patient or consumer. In eras past, women held positions of respect in surgery and other health professions: ancient Sumerian and Egyptian tombs more than five thousand years old show surgical tools belonging to renowned female surgeons; most obstetricians in first-century Italy were women; women attended medical schools alongside men in ancient Egypt; ancient Hebrew women were respected doctors. But in the Middle Ages, things took a serious turn for the worse that has yet to be reversed. Women were gradually excluded from both the study and practice of medicine (though a few brave and talented individuals continued their work) and it wasn't until the mid-to-late 1800s that women started making their move back into the formal ranks of the medical professions. Just as today women scientists, clinicians and other public leaders have had to seize the initiative in steering health care in a direction useful to women, so 100 years ago women bravely broke the largely male ranks of organized medicine by starting their *own* hospitals and their *own* schools. We must continue to look out for ourselves.

But decades of male-dominated medicine have taken a toll that will be long in reversing. According to the Society for the Advancement of Women's Health Research (SAWHR), 30 years ago women accounted for just 5–6% of American physicians and 10% or fewer of medical school enrollments. Today, their numbers have jumped to about 40% of new medical school classes—but by the year 2000, still only one in five American doctors will be women. A recent study from the Medical College of Pennsylvania reveals yet another insidious form of bias built into medical education: on average, illustrations in anatomy textbooks depict male bodies more than twice as often as female bodies. Not only does this pose the risk that students will develop incomplete knowledge of normal female anatomy, the authors report, but it also shows once again the troublesome view in health care that *men* reflect the *rule,* and *women* the *exception.* Furthermore, according to SAWHR, women in medicine and science are so far failing to reach senior ranks; only 4% of all medical school department heads are women, and women in science and medicine earn just 63 cents on the dollar compared to men in the same fields. Is it any wonder that women's health issues have been on the back burner for so long?

LOCATING AND RESISTING BIAS IN WOMEN'S HEALTH CARE

As we know only too well, generic discrimination against women is old news. It was only 70 years ago that we got the vote, after all. We're still paid less for comparable work, and sexual harassment is a part of life in many workplaces. But the fact that it's common doesn't make it acceptable. This book will help you sidestep or confront the many biases toward women that exist in doctors' offices and hospitals everywhere. More than half the battle is recognizing it, especially when it's subtle.

Discrimination comes in many forms. Sometimes it's blatant: for instance, a woman will come into the doctor's office complaining about dizziness and chest pain and she'll be told she's under stress, it's all in her head; she may be given a tranquilizer, told to calm down and go home. A man comes in with similar symptoms and is thoroughly tested for heart disease. Sound outrageous? It's not uncommon. This might be more understandable if heart disease was uncommon in women. In fact, it's the *leading killer of women!* Every time a woman reports faintness, shortness of breath, chest pain or other related symptoms, heart disease should be *one* of the things that jumps into the clinician's mind. The hackneyed image of the perspiring damsel in distress should have no place in the doctor's office. But those stereotypes won't die unless *you* insist that they do.

Sometimes, bias is less obvious. For example, many studies have shown that women are less likely to receive aggressive diagnostic procedures and treatments for heart disease than are men. As a patient, and not an expert, you may not even realize you're missing out on valuable health care options. To make matters even more complicated, when women *are* given some of these options, their health outcomes are often worse than men's. One of the reasons is that delays and oversights in treatment mean that women come under the knife in the operating room in far worse shape than men do. As clinicians become increasingly aware of these significant gender differences in quality of care and health outcomes, more attention is being paid to giving women the same standard of care that men receive. But the fact that most diagnostic tools and treatments were designed for men in the first place makes it hard even for the best-intentioned clinicians to even the long-tipped scales.

Sometimes, bias in the health care setting is age-related. When ageism and sexism intersect, women are in big trouble in the doctor's office. An older woman with vaginal bleeding may be advised to have her uterus removed (a hysterectomy) because "she doesn't *need* it anymore." A younger woman, on the other hand, might still put her uterus to "good use." Sound like a conversation from the Dark Ages? Unfortunately it isn't. Who's to determine in what ways, beyond childbearing, we *need* our body parts? What could possibly be more personal, more individual, than that *need?* Yet health care providers often jump to prejudicial conclusions on the basis of a patient's advanced age. Older women can be particularly vulnerable to health care bias because they were more likely raised in a time when clinicians—usually male—were treated as authorities with the last word. Doctors' words are to be heeded, not challenged, many older women believe. Younger women may be more likely to challenge authority in whatever form it appears—but they too are certainly not immune to bias. Remember, if it *sounds* discriminatory to you, it very well might be. Trust your instincts, and, using the information in this book and elsewhere, sniff out inappropriate care wherever it lurks.

Regional bias is yet another problem within women's health care. One study in a top medical journal showed that the kind of treatment you receive for breast cancer will differ dramat-ically depending on where you live. Women in the south and middle portions of the country were found to receive less up-to-date surgical and radiation treatment than did women on the U.S. coasts. I visited Hattiesburg, Mississippi, where older, more radical treatment for breast cancer is still quite common, even among women with early stage disease. Many of the doctors I interviewed blamed patient preference for the preponderance of radical procedures. Patients didn't always agree. One might stop to question how patients *form* their preferences in the first place. One notably frank physician acknowledged that many doctors in his region give health advice in the form of "well, if it were my mother or daughter, I'd do *this*—but you're free to do *that.*" Does it sound to you like these women were making free, unbiased choices?

Race and socioeconomic status also play important roles in women's health discrimination. Study after study shows that women of color are more likely than Caucasian women to receive substandard health care, and to have poorer outcomes as a result. Minority women are less likely to get *preventive* care than are Caucasian women, which is particularly tragic in that it perpetuates chronic health problems that are rampant in minority populations, such as hypertension, obesity, diabetes and other major heart disease and early death risk factors. Sometimes, access to care due to poverty or lack of insurance is the problem. But many feel that biases in health care for women of color step *over* economic lines. And as revealed in a 1993 report on women's health from the Commonwealth Fund (a New York-based philanthropic organization dedicated to bettering health care for groups in need) even *having* insurance fails to guarantee adequate care for women: one-fifth of women who *are* insured are *not covered* for *preventive* care, the report states.

The cumulative effect of these biases is *mammoth:* being excluded from major research studies; poor funding for diseases that disproportionately affect women; regional, racial and age bias and pure gender discrimination create tragic endings. Unnecessary disease, disability and death are the results. The only way to get around these biases is to note them when they occur and take the opportunity to *uncover your options* before submitting to substandard care. In a medical crisis, this kind of aggressive consumerism won't be possible. But in most situations where elective procedures or nonemergency treatment for disease are concerned, you can and must play a role in demanding better. This book will help you to do so.

WOMEN'S USE OF HEALTH CARE

It's ironic that women have gotten such short shrift in health care considering the fact that we *use* health care more than men do. We live longer (79 vs. 72.3 years), have more chronic diseases and spend more money and time on health care than men do. And as Dr. Suzanne Oparil, president of the American Heart Association, points out, "Women are responsible for the health of the nation because women take care of themselves, the boys and the men." Because we are often still the caretakers in our families and communities, health needs and concerns fall under our jurisdiction. Whether it's through preventive care and family "habits" (being responsible for our families' diets, arranging outings that might or might not involve physical activity) or by facilitating medical treatment (getting our spouses to take their pills, dragging children to the pediatrician's office) women are often in charge of family, and thus population, health. Unfortunately, we too often subsume our health needs to those of others in our families—sick children, partners or parents.

The result of putting our health needs last? We're at considerable risk of falling prey to *detectable* and *preventable* diseases. The Commonwealth Fund report found that 44% of women over 50 failed to get mammograms to detect breast cancer in the last year; one in three women failed to have Pap tests for cancer of the cervix, general pelvic exams for gynecological health or clinical breast exams by a doctor. Of course, not all of this is our own "fault" for failing to seek medical care. The same report found that one in four of the women who failed to get mammograms said they were never instructed to do so by their doctors!

Another important result of inadequate health care and research for women is wasted dollars. According to the Society for the Advancement of Women's Health Research, we spend 6 billion dollars a year on breast cancer, 10 billion dollars a year on osteoporosis, another 10 billion on incontinence, and a staggering 237 billion dollars a year on depression (which affects women twice as often as men). Most experts agree that we'd spend only a *fraction* of this kind of money if we understood more about how to prevent these conditions, instead of waiting for the high costs of severe disability and critical care once medical problems have become advanced. But without adequate information on how to reduce our risk of, or even *prevent* major diseases, we're at a terrible disadvantage, especially as we age.

What are the solutions? There are many, but I've grouped them into several manageable *categories* of response—on the level of health care providers, the dissemination of health news and information, and your own *personal* actions in the health care setting. I urge you, in your frustration with the many problems in women's health care, not to abandon mainstream medicine in favor of unproven or alternative care. For some women, alternative care often has a place alongside traditional medicine or, in rare instances, as a substitution for certain aspects of it. But mainstream medicine has a tremendous amount to offer the woman who uses it wisely. Learn to access the best of it, so it will work for you.

HEALTH CARE PROVIDERS: A WOMEN'S HEALTH SPECIALTY?

Some leading authorities on women's health are calling for a separate specialty for women's health within medicine. They argue that only if women's health receives special, independent status as an area of study and practice will women get the attention we deserve. Proponents of a separate women's health specialty are concerned that women's health management currently falls under the auspices of gynecology alone—reducing women to their breasts and their reproductive organs below the belt. A separate women's health specialty, which might fall under the heading of general internal medicine, could broaden women's health care to include more attention to our risk of heart disease, diabetes, and many other *general* health problems.

Other experts sharply criticize this approach as a way of further isolating women and women's health issues from the mainstream,

worsening many of the problems that have existed to this day. Why should *basic* health care be health care for *men*, they ask, while *women's* health care is relegated to some kind of special, isolated status?

Should women see gynecological specialists, or primary care generalists? We'll discuss this briefly in the next chapter. But as these healthy debates are played out in the medical community, *you* are more concerned with your *personal* solutions to the absence of needed health information for women. Throughout this book, I'll discuss ways that you can derive information about your *own* health needs and risks given the information that's out there already—by finding the right kinds of authorities on your problem, discovering your options as they are best understood by medicine today, and so on.

YOUR HEALTH CARE AND THE MEDIA: THE IMPORTANCE OF BECOMING A SAVVY AUDIENCE

Another vital solution to health care confusion, bias and misinformation is to become a more savvy consumer of health care information. Too often, we're quick to accept the latest headline, the latest promise of a cure or relief if it's on the front page of our favorite paper or television program. Try to keep in mind that these stories are prepared by human beings, and that human beings are fallible. Their employers also have a bottom line *business* driving their actions, no matter how strong their journalistic integrity. The fact is, big headlines sell papers; they catch *your* eye, and they attract advertisers. The line between health news and health entertainment is thinning (as it seems to be in many areas of news). If you take a close look at the headlines, you'll find that they are often laden with contradictions, misinformation or *missing* information—all designed to pull you in.

Become a more aggressive critic of health news. For starters, consider who's doing the reporting. Is the reporter a health news specialist or a generalist? Who did the original research that's being cited? Was it reported in a top-notch medical journal (ask your doctor) or a second-rank version? Have you heard of the medical center from which the information originated, and is it reputable? If you don't know, have you asked your doctor about it? Does this piece of news fit into the pattern of information you've heard on this topic in the past, or does it seem to come from left field? The more you scrutinize health news, the more you'll find holes and contradictions that will help you become a better judge of its value.

Beware of promises, hype, hope and despair in medical reporting. Don't get sucked into believing that a cure-all suddenly exists for your complicated problem, and that your doctor is the last to hear about it. Perhaps there *is* an important piece of new research—but you need to find out what, if anything, it means to *you* before you get your hopes too high. I was appalled to see an article on the front page of a major newspaper extolling the virtues of a treatment for an incurable disease. While the study had only looked at six patients, the article talked about a remarkable cure rate and gave inappropriate hope to thousands of sick people. The doctors who had been interviewed for the story were terribly distraught that the context of their remarks had been skewed, and the meaning distorted, to create a *major story.*

PLAYING AN ACTIVE, PERSONAL ROLE IN BETTERING YOUR CARE

Perhaps the most useful way to avert discrimination and boost the quality of your health care is to improve your skills in interacting with the health care community. The doctor-patient relationship lies at the heart of any health management strategy; it is the bottom line that results in the kind of care *you* are going to receive. In the next section, we'll focus on ways that you can get more out of your relationship with your health care providers—by choosing them wisely in the first place, and by taking an active role in bringing your care to a new, higher standard.

CHAPTER TWO

YOUR HEALTH CARE VISIT

CHOOSING AND RELATING TO HEALTH CARE PROVIDERS

Doctors are trained to look at diseases. The focus is narrow, as if through a microscope. They're not looking at the whole patient. People seek *medical care. Broken arms don't. Livers don't.*

—Richard Frankel, Ph.D., expert on the doctor-patient relationship

If we forget that the doctor-patient relationship is one of human beings interacting with one another; if we forget that on both ends of medical care—both the giving and the receiving—basic human needs and desires are at stake—then we risk a total failure of the caring process. At that point, medicine is reduced to its technical aspects, and in this increasingly high-tech age, with every minute on the clock at a premium, we risk getting ever closer to an inversion of what health care is *supposed* to be all about.

With this in mind, it's essential to have a clear sense of what you can expect from your health care provider. You must know how to select that *person* in the first place, and how to enhance your interaction once you've entered into a caregiving relationship. The bottom line: the best care is two-way care. Do your part and the effectiveness of the medical attention you receive will increase. This may be even more imperative for women than for anyone else, because of the classical power imbalance between doctor and patient, male and female, that has for so long hindered equality for women patients in the worlds of science and medicine.

How to Choose the Right Clinician for You

Selecting the person or team that will manage your health, whether in wellness or in sickness, is one of the most important and life-affirming decisions you can make. It can help determine both your future well-being, and the quality of your life in the present. It's a decision that requires a tremendous amount of trust: putting your health management in someone's hands, you're entrusting them with by far your most valuable asset. Why then do we often make this decision hastily, with so little thought or research?

One reason is we often look for doctors when we're having a medical *crisis*—a symptom or problem that's worrying us and needs attention. It's so easy to forget about medical care when we're feeling well: health care appointments are often inconvenient, can be uncomfortable depending on the kinds of tests we might be given, and they're often costly. Why bother, if you don't have to, many people say. This is mistake #1. A second reason we choose our health care providers hastily is often we simply don't *know* a better way to select them. We take the first person or plan we stumble upon, because we wouldn't know how to proceed otherwise. While there are no hard and fast rules about how to choose a health practitioner, following are some useful approaches.

Word of Mouth

When seeking a health care provider, word of mouth may be your best guide. Whose word? Just about anyone you trust would be valuable, but there are some who are better than others.

Listen to friends and neighbors who highly recommend a particular caregiver—but keep in mind that this might tell you more about a clinician's personality than their clinical skill. If the doctor in question detected and resolved a long-overlooked problem in your friend, that's a better clue to their effectiveness. Word of mouth from other health professionals is the best kind. A nurse you trust in the labor and delivery room, for example, might be a good person to ask about a good general internist for women at that same hospital. If she doesn't know the name of one offhand, she may be able to ask her colleagues in the hospital for a doctor with a great reputation. "Inside" information is always best.

Contact Medical Specialty Boards

Once you're given some specialists' names, you might want to check out their credentials. Calling your local medical specialty board to confirm that they are board-certified in the area they claim is a good start. I know someone who made this call and discovered that their surgeon wasn't board-certified after all. Sometimes, a generalist is all you need. But someone who is passing themselves off as having had more training than they've actually completed should raise a red flag. Depending on where you live, some of these specialty groups will provide the names of doctors who focus on your problem and offer care in your region.

Begin with a Reputable Medical Center and Go from There

If there is a reputable hospital or medical center in your area, you may want to start your search there. Teaching hospitals (that is, hospitals affiliated with medical schools, where doctors are trained) are often good places to begin, since they should be more attuned to the latest advances in research and treatment.

CONTACT SUPPORT OR EDUCATIONAL GROUPS FOR YOUR PARTICULAR PROBLEM

If you are looking for a specialist in a given health problem, start by talking to other women who live in your area and have the same problem, says Cindy Pearson, program director for the National Women's Health Network. Support or advocacy groups, educational clearinghouses and other disease-specific groups can provide you the opportunity to meet others in your situation and learn about potentially good (and bad!) practitioners in your area. These are often listed in your phone book, or under toll-free information. Throughout this book you'll find "information boxes" with the names, addresses and phone numbers of some of the major support and information groups for different health problems.

The fact is, any one practitioner can get a rave review from one woman and a pan from the next. But by talking to groups of women you'll start to pick up on the more general reputations of specialists in your problem. Many groups also provide written information and other important background material on your disease, so that you can become more informed *before* selecting a doctor. This will not only enhance your ability to choose the right kind of practitioner, but it will improve your interaction with that person once you enter his/her office (more on this below in the discussion of the doctor-patient relationship).

FIND THE RIGHT DOCTOR FOR YOUR PRIMARY CARE

There is considerable disagreement on the issue of what kind of doctor, or specialist, should be caring for women. In the previous chapter I briefly mentioned the question of creating a women's health specialty; this gets passionate support and equally passionate rejection from intelligent people in the health care fields. While that battle is being waged, what should *you* do now? Many women get *all* of their health care from their gynecologist, and there's considerable disagreement about whether this is a good or bad thing. Dr. Marcia Angell, executive editor of the prestigious *New England Journal of Medicine,* feels it's a terrible thing: Women are more than just their reproductive organs, she says, so our only caregiver should not be one who focuses only on the reproductive organs. She would like to see women with good primary-care physicians, generalists who look at the body and health as a whole.

Dr. Florence Haseltine, director of the Center for Population Research at the National Institute of Child Health and Human Development and senior editor of the *Journal for Women's Health,* has a different take on the issue. She feels that as long as gynecologists are doing (or referring you to) the needed general screening tests for women—that is, blood pressure, cholesterol and weight screening, in addition to the standard screening tests of reproductive organs (the Pap smear, mammogram, etc.)—it's perfectly fine for women to get their health care from these specialists until about age 50. At that point, she feels a general internist should enter the picture.

So the question you have to ask is, *Is your*

gynecologist referring you for all the tests you need? At the end of this book you'll find a complete list of the recommended screening tests at different life stages. Go through these tests with your doctor, whatever his or her background, and make sure that you're getting the overall preventive care you need.

KEEP AN OPEN MIND ABOUT DIFFERENT KINDS OF HEALTH CARE PROVIDERS

When searching for the best care, don't get hooked on the idea that you have to have one particular kind of provider. While you may want a medical doctor (particularly if you have a known medical problem that requires treatment by an M.D.) there are other terrific categories of health care providers who give special attention to women's health, and to preventive/wellness care in general. An example would be the nurse practitioner. More and more nurse practitioners are offering wellness-based primary care for women in group settings, or in team efforts with medical doctors. For example, nurse practitioners are more likely than your traditional OB-GYN to address your non-gynecological needs, such as chronic colds or flus, or even problems managing family or work-related stress. They ask broad-based health questions that medical doctors might not ask, and if your problem falls outside of their expertise, they often refer you to appropriate medical care or peer support.

Your local hospital or a nearby women's health clinic or center can likely point you to one or more nurse practitioner groups, or nurse-doctor teams. Some women like combined practitioner teams because nurses—who

often take more time and focus on the needs of the "whole person"—handle the bulk of wellness care, while doctors are always available for sickness care.

CONSIDER WOMAN-CENTERED CARE

Health care by women and for women is growing by leaps and bounds in this country. More women's health centers are opening all the time, and the network of so-called feminist health centers is expanding in some areas as well. Women's health centers are often, although not always, affiliated with major medical centers and focus on a wide variety of women's health needs. There is no single model of what a women's health center does or should provide, so you may need to shop around a little to find the one best suited for you. You'll want to keep your eyes peeled for centers that are using the timely "women's health" shingle on their door just to get you inside: Ask questions about what makes this center particularly geared toward women's health (the qualifications of the staff, the availability of women's health-oriented equipment like state-of-the-art mammography machines, the focus on female-gender risk factors, etc.). You're probably at greater risk of being caught in a marketing gimmick with the "women's health center" than you are with the "feminist health center," although there are examples of superb (and less superb) care in both settings.

Feminist health centers—which are related to women's health centers but unique in several ways I'll discuss—focus both on women's health and, above all, the *empowerment* of female patients in relation to health care professionals. Feminist centers are run by women;

both the caregivers and the administrators are women. Some of the advantages of care exclusively by women and for women are quite clear: Who can better empathize with your female health needs than a team of caregivers who have many of the same needs and concerns themselves? Feminist care is especially useful for reproductive services (abortion, sexually transmitted disease counseling, and so on) and related issues that can be hard to discuss with someone of the opposite sex—or hard to discuss period. Lesbian women often favor feminist health care because it is likely to be more familiar with and less biased against their particular health needs. Feminist health centers often value and carefully protect patients' privacy in an effort to give the best confidential care to women of all ages. For teenagers who want to keep their reproductive health care private from parents or other family members, this kind of care can be quite reassuring. Dr. Florence Haseltine of the National Institutes of Health says that while feminist health centers certainly don't guarantee the very best care available in your region (some are excellent, some aren't, like any other type of program) feminist health centers *do* guarantee some of the best *intentions* for women's health care— and that too is worth a lot. As one feminist health care provider said dryly, there aren't too many charlatans in "feminist health" since the term "feminist" has lately come under disfavor, so those who say they practice feminist medicine usually do so quite faithfully.

Feminist health centers make a great effort to provide the kind of equality-based, affordable, empathetic, patient-centered care that so many women have been denied. "I've been there before," says Christina Malongo, a family nurse practitioner at the Feminist Women's Health Center in Portland, Oregon. "I know what it's like to have a Pap smear. In the medical setting, women are often treated roughly, their questions not answered. I try to do an empowering kind of health care that educates a woman, and involves her in decision-making and includes her as a partner in the process".

CHOOSE DOCTORS WHEN YOU'RE HEALTHY, NOT WHEN YOU'RE SICK

This is one point on which *everyone* I interviewed concurred: ideally, we should find our doctors when we're feeling *well*, and we have time to interview them, to investigate their skills and personality. If you have a good primary care clinician—that is, someone who cares for you when you are well, monitoring your blood pressure, your cholesterol level, your gynecological health, and so on—*that person* can refer you to expert care should it be needed for a particular problem. There may be no better recommendation than that of a health care provider you already trust and admire. Chances are, they've referred other patients to these specialists, and have gotten feedback on their performance over time.

Having a primary health care provider helps insure that any problems you develop will be caught *early* through regular screening tests and attention to your body as it ages and changes. If your weight or blood pressure go up considerably one year, someone will be there to catch it before you reach the trouble zone. And if you've carefully chosen that primary caregiver when you're feeling your best, your strongest and most confident, chances are better that if you hit a rough spot in your physical or mental health, you'll have someone you know you can count on to guide you through the process of getting well.

INTERVIEW YOUR POTENTIAL PROVIDER, CONSIDERING PHILOSOPHY AND RESPONSIVENESS

Health care providers don't *deserve* your business: they should *earn* it. Dr. Susan Skochelak, associate professor of family medicine at the University of Wisconsin and an expert on the doctor-patient relationship, recommends an initial introductory visit with a potential caregiver during which you can screen them for the qualities that matter to you most. Some doctors will charge less for this kind of appointment; others will even provide a brief introductory session free of charge—but this is not the rule. In this meeting, be direct in questioning the clinician about his/her approach to health care (Is prevention important to them?) and take note of whether she is giving you time to talk, listening to your questions and answering them directly. Chemistry is important in the doctor-patient relationship. Is this practitioner respectful, focused, attuned to your particular needs?

Dr. Irwin H. Kaiser, professor emeritus at the Albert Einstein College of Medicine, warns *women* patients in particular to watch for doctors who speak to them as if they were children. The "don't-worry-your-little-head-I'll-take-care-of-it" syndrome is rampant in the care of women, he says. Listen for inappropriate language like "honey" or "little girl," and don't accept it. And always be attuned to extra, inappropriate attention that could border on, or cross the line, into sexual harassment, he urges.

This initial meeting with a potential health care provider will give you an idea of whether your personality, philosophy and needs about health care are likely to be met by this particular person—in short, if the two of you are an appropriate "match." If not, you've lost a little time and hopefully just a small amount of money, and you can continue your search. On the plus side, you found out what you needed to know with your clothes *on*—and for that you may be grateful.

What if you're part of a health care plan, such as an HMO, in which your choice of health care provider is strictly limited? Even in the most tightly-regulated plans, there is some room for maneuvering. You may not be able to choose among 15 health care providers, but you could be given a choice (or demand a choice) among 2 or 3. Some HMO settings limit your time with the practitioner, which could rush your initial interview. Talk to a scheduling secretary and see if you can schedule your first appointment at a less busy time of day, or on a day when your assigned provider has fewer patients. Remember that HMO's are businesses and they wouldn't be around if people like you walked out. So within reason, demand some consumer attention.

A MAJOR ISSUE IN WOMEN'S HEALTH CARE: HOW IMPORTANT IS YOUR DOCTOR'S GENDER?

In a phrase, it's up to you. This is an issue of highly personal preference on which no one can adequately advise you. We all know that there are good female clinicians, and bad ones—good male clinicians, and bad ones. Still, many women's health experts and advocates have a gut feeling that female physicians are better, on the whole, for female patients. Cindy Pearson of the National Women's Health Network in Washington, D.C., notes that because they share the same body and many of the same health experiences, women physicians are less likely to think about *changing* your body in order to cure it (that is, taking parts out or putting them on or inside of you), and adds that because women doctors are often younger, they may have been exposed to less *openly* sexist training in medical school and to more patient-centered, whole-person care. Dr. Marcia Angell, of the *New England Journal of Medicine,* says that all things being equal, she would choose a female physician because there is great inherent value in sharing the same basic life experience with your doctor. However, both Angell and Pearson (and just about every other person I interviewed) were quick to qualify these personal preferences with the fact that it isn't fair to judge all female doctors as good, or all male ones as bad. There are plenty of sensitive and insensitive, talented and untalented physicians in both gender groups.

Several positive factors about the relationship between female patients and female doctors must be considered, however, as important studies have borne them out. Deborah Roter, a leading researcher on physician and patient gender relationships at the Johns Hopkins School of Hygiene and Public Health, has found in her own studies that female doctors are more warm, more engaged and more intimate in their handling of the medical interview than are male doctors. They exhibit more positive facial expressions than male doctors do, including more smiles, more "uh huhs," "yeahs," and "I sees"— all of which constitute positive feedback for the patient. Roter also finds that female doctors are

more likely to disclose their own feelings than are male doctors; this openness may be conducive to patients' opening up as well, and more information being exchanged during the doctor visit.

Dr. Aaron Lazare, Chancellor/Dean of the University of Massachusetts Medical Center at Worcester, points to studies showing that female doctors are better listeners and are less apt to try to control the interview than are male doctors. Female doctors are repeatedly found to be more compassionate, empathetic and attentive to patient's feelings as well as to their physical symptoms. Again, there are certainly exceptions in both genders, but studies lean heavily in this direction.

Other studies show that when you pair the female doctor and the female patient, you get the most effective health care relationship of all. Female patients ask more questions and offer more information to female doctors, and female doctors draw more out and offer more themselves, studies show. Sherrie Kaplan, senior scientist and co-director of the primary care Outcomes Research Institute at the New England Medical Center, notes that in the average 15-minute office visit, female patients ask about 6 to 8 questions, while male patients ask .1 (that's point-one!).

Cynics have questioned whether the alleged "information" exchanged between female doctors and female patients is more chitchat than anything else (a typical sexist analysis). In fact, Roter says, if you divide the doctor-patient visit into three classic parts—the patient's medical history, the middle of the visit (physical exam, for example) and the counseling portion at the end—you find that it's during the *history* portion of the interview that female doctors and patients spend extra time and draw out more information. This is extremely important, since the saying goes that the medical history is 99% of the diagnosis. Rather than "schmoozing," the female doctor-female patient duo is doing a better job of getting to the substance of the matter early in the visit.

Clearly there are certain advantages to female physicians across the board. But "across the board" may have nothing to do with your personal experience, preference or with the doctors available to you in your area. Your best approach would be to find the best *person* to care for you, regardless of gender. If it's a 50–50 toss-up between two physicians you admire, one male and one female, we've seen some good reasons to select the woman. If you for some reason just prefer one gender over the other to give you health care, then skew your practitioner screening interviews to that gender and subject them to whatever standards of skill and communicative ability are important to you.

THE DOCTOR-PATIENT RELATIONSHIP: GETTING THE MOST FROM YOUR DOCTOR VISITS AND OVERALL CARE

The doctor-patient relationship is failing, and we have to do something about it to protect ourselves from inadequate and unsatisfying care. Patient surveys and other measures of consumer satisfaction are carrying the message loud and clear: patients are unhappy with their interaction with doctors. According to Richard Frankel, an expert on the doctor-patient relationship at the Rochester School of Medicine and Dentistry, 70% of malpractice cases concern not just medical negligence, but also patients' displeasure with their doctors' failure to communicate with them. Patients feel abandoned—their emotional needs unmet, Frankel says. Considering the fact that in 51% of doctor visits there turns out to be no disease present, doctors *must* become attuned to other reasons patients may be turning up in their offices. Someone who has chronic aches and pains, or fears or depression, may feel terribly disenfranchised when sent home with the non-diagnosis of "you *don't* have this, that or the other." They may be seeking attention for an intangible problem, and if care is to improve, doctors will have to start addressing those intangibles. Later in this section we'll discuss ways that *you* can help draw out your doctor's attention to your nondisease concerns.

Dr. Ian McWhinney, professor emeritus of family medicine at the University of Western Ontario, has written extensively on this subject and complains that doctors too often deal in abstractions rather than concrete human needs. For example, he says, they focus on a given disease rather than on the impact of that disease on a patient. So while the doctor's narrow view centers on how to manage multiple sclerosis, for example, the patient's real concern is what it feels like to not be able to walk without assistance, or not be able to control their urination. These are the tangible, real-life issues that concern patients, and they are the issues that should concern doctors, he asserts.

The biggest problem may be that doctors are failing to adequately communicate even the information they *do* try to give. Cindy Pearson reports that a substantial number of women call her organization to say, "I got a diagnosis and a prescription—now can you tell me what this means?" This is especially true where sexual issues are concerned, she notes, where patients find that doctors often get "white-knuckle syndrome." It's quite scary to consider that a woman can be given a physical exam and other tests, a diagnosis of her problem and a slip of paper with a treatment regimen on it without an adequate explanation of what's going on in her body and how it might be managed. But it's not surprising given the number of women who, for example, walk around with prescriptions for hormone replacement burning a hole in their pockets because the doctor who prescribed it in the first place never covered the significant risks and benefits of the regimen. Yet because women have read countless media reports on both sides of the coin, they're scared—and may take no action whatsoever given a lack of concrete or at least individualized advice.

Moira Stewart, another leader in the field of doctor-patient communication at the Center for Studies in Family Medicine at the University of Western Ontario, reports similar problems. Patients who complain to licensing bodies (which is Canada's "malpractice" route) are more often unhappy with their doctors' communication skills than their diagnostic or therapeutic abilities. Patients in Canada complain, as they do in the U.S., that doctors just don't listen enough or take the time to explain complicated issues.

WHY AREN'T WE COMMUNICATING? WHOSE FAULT IS IT, ANYWAY?

An increasing number of studies are looking at the specific dynamics of the doctor-patient relationship and they're turning up answers to the question of where communication falls

short. One study found that, on average, doctors are interrupting patients after about 18 seconds of conversation. Before the patient can get all of her points on the table, she is steered in another direction by the doctor-interviewer. Instead of having a mutual conversation, the doctor is driving the discussion, and the result is the patient gets cut off. Sound familiar? Certainly, to some degree the "expert" must keep the conversation on course and use the available time to get to the essence of a patient's problem. But that's exactly what *isn't* happening. By interrupting patients too soon, doctors are stopping them from ever getting their worries or problems out in the open.

Interruptions, lack of empathy for emotional needs and a disease-focused rather than patient-centered approach to health care add up to poor doctor-patient communication and, more important, poor health outcomes. For the remainder of this chapter, we'll look at advice from some leaders in the field of the doctor-patient interaction on how you can get more from your health care provider and boost your chance of staying well and getting well faster.

YOUR DOCTOR VISITS: WHAT YOU—AND YOUR DOCTOR—CAN DO TO MAKE THEM MORE PRODUCTIVE AND SATISFYING

In several locations around the country, changes are being made in the way medical education is conducted, particularly in regard to teaching new doctors how to relate better to patients. Many doctors who are being trained today are more likely (but certainly not guaranteed) to have a more "patient-centered" approach to care—one in which patients are taken as whole human beings, not just carriers of disease. Interestingly, the mirror image of much of the same advice that's being given to doctors is what experts are recommending to *you*—the patient. We'll take a look at the doctor's obligations first.

YOUR DOCTOR'S END OF THE BARGAIN: WHAT YOU SHOULD DEMAND FROM PHYSICIANS NOWADAYS

Dr. Aaron Lazare is teaching doctors to hold their tongues while patients finish their initial stories. Getting a patient's definition and explanation of the problem is key to bettering the doctor-patient relationship. Allowing patients to participate in choosing their treatment is also expected to help improve health outcomes (patient compliance with taking medication, coming for follow-up visits, improving preventive health habits, and so on). If your doctor interrupts you before you've made important points, or foists treatment plans on you without consulting you in any meaningful way, he is failing to hold up his end of the bargain. You can and should demand better.

Dr. Susan Skochelak teaches new doctors to let patients express their feelings about their disease—how it affects their daily life, how emotionally painful it may be to live with a given symptom, their hopes and dreams for recovery, etc. She also emphasizes the importance of negotiating a treatment plan, urging new doctors to avoid the traditional authoritative approach to care ("you will take *this* medicine at *these* times"). Most important, she says, is teaching new doctors to tailor treatment to patients' individual life circumstances. A patient

who works an overnight shift will obviously need to be put on a different medical regimen than one who works days. Unfortunately, as obvious as this seems, it isn't always taken into consideration in the current doctor-patient meeting. You must demand this kind of sensitive, personalized care from *all* health care providers.

Moira Stewart wants the "new doctor" to consider patients in the context of their life cycles and support systems—are they adolescent, middle-aged or older? Do they have significant others who are involved in their care and support? Do they accept a treatment plan in what she calls a "win-win situation?": that is, both doctor and patient are pleased with the result, rather than both feeling like they gave up something significant. Think about whether your health care providers pay attention to these important issues. Have they ever asked you about your relationships with family and friends, or if you have the support you need to care for your health adequately and consistently? If not, and if you have concerns in this area (perhaps you're older and have no one to help bring you to the doctor), discuss your feelings openly and ask for help. Your doctor can't read your mind.

One of the most powerful arguments against this kind of patient-centered, empathetic, humane health care is that it will simply take too long. In an era of health care reform and managed care in which our minutes in the doctor's office are increasingly sliced, time is unfortunately more and more of the essence. But you may be surprised to learn that patient-centered care takes far *less* additional time than critics believe. Stewart's own research revealed that an effective, compassionate and attentive doctor visit takes on average just two more minutes than the traditional clipped, doctor-dominated visit! And talk about bang for your buck: those additional two minutes result in significant patient satisfaction and "calmness" about their health conditions ten days after the medical encounter. It's all about sharing power, finding common ground between two individuals, Stewart says.

YOUR ROLE: WHAT YOU CAN DO TO GET MORE OUT OF YOUR CARE AND YOUR RELATIONSHIP WITH YOUR DOCTOR

It's time you started playing a more active role in the doctor-patient relationship. The bonus for your assertiveness will be better care and better health, studies show. Sherrie Kaplan and colleagues have shown that the so-called "activated patient" has better health outcomes (and that includes major chronic diseases like diabetes) than the passive patient. Here are some practical ways in which you can start to play a central, active role in your care.

1. **Schedule the appropriate length appointment for your concerns.** Your physician's time may be hard to come by, so if you expect to need more of it than usual, book it ahead of time, advises Dr. Norman Jensen of the University of Wisconsin at Madison. Dr. Jensen teaches new doctors and patients how to improve the doctor-patient relationship, and how to get the most out of a given office visit. If your doctor is pressed for time, and you're trying to squeeze more of it than he or she can provide, you're going to start getting negative feedback and you'll both feel frustrated and unfulfilled by the visit. On the other hand, if you book the appropriate length appointment, you'll allow your doctor to do the best job possible in a reasonable time frame. Remember, Dr. Jensen adds, this is *not* a social appointment—it should be a humanistic business appointment, with goals both you and your doctor need to meet.

A scheduling nurse or other contact in your physician's office may be able to help you determine how much time you'll need to discuss a particular problem. If you're not comfortable discussing your concerns with anyone but your doctor, book 3 minutes with your physician for a telephone conversation to determine how much time you're likely to need in person. Dr. Jensen warns that a 30-minute office visit is likely to cost more than a 15-minute visit; find out about this ahead of time, and determine if it's worth it to you. If he were made czar of health care, Jensen says, he would make one firm rule: no office visits shorter than 20 minutes. Why? Because the more time spent with patients, the more information is gained and *possibly* fewer unnecessary tests, procedures and drugs will be used, he believes. Consider this possibility when booking time with your doctor. *Talking* may be the best medicine in some cases.

If you find that your questions haven't been answered and your physician is out of time at the end of your office visit, try to respect that reality—that is, unless he/she *always* seems to be running late and not meeting your needs. Sometimes, the best approach is to make a follow-up appointment before you leave the office, choosing a time of day (perhaps early or late) when your doctor is less pressed for time. Or schedule a telephone conversation for the end of the day to complete your questions or list of concerns.

2. **Write down what you want to discuss.** How many times have you left the doctor's office, made it halfway down the hall and remembered something really important you had intended to discuss? Partly because patients are interrupted so early and so often, we get sidetracked and often don't get to discuss at least one issue of importance to us. If you write down the top three issues you want to discuss, this is less likely to happen. Then, if you start to discuss a topic and your doctor interrupts you, you can either say "let me first get through two other things I wanted to mention," or you can let the conversation take a left turn—but look at your list before leaving the doctor's office to remind yourself of the topic that got left behind.

3. **Ask absolutely every question that comes to your mind about a given treatment plan: Don't be shy.** As we've seen, one of patients' biggest complaints is that doctors just aren't explaining things fully before they leave the office. Kaplan urges women to demand those explanations: ask for details on follow-through of care ("Exactly when is the best time to take this medication; are there any foods to avoid; should I expect any side effects; when should my symptoms abate"; and so on); request more material to read or a place to go for further information and/or counseling, etc. Do not be embarrassed to ask questions; you cannot be expected to be an authority.

To some extent, the doctor-patient relationship should resemble the teacher-student relationship. Dr. Skochelak says one of her most important obligations as a doctor is to teach patients about their bodies and their overall health. The word "doctor," she reminds us, derives from the Latin word for "teacher." The more you ask of your doctor, and the more information she imparts to you, the greater the chance you'll learn to care for your *own* body better—in addition to getting more from your medical care.

4. **Prepare for doctor visits in the waiting room.** Many of us pass the tedious minutes in a doctor's waiting room reading junk magazines or chewing our fingernails. This is a time when you could be preparing for your visit. For example, run through your most important questions and issues in your mind. Check your list of topics, or remember the three most important issues you want to cover during this visit. If you're embarrassed to raise a given issue, such as your concern that you may have been exposed to a sexually transmitted disease, plan how you might be able to do it the least painfully. Being direct is the best approach. Remember there's almost nothing your doctor hasn't heard a hundred times before.

5. **Be as specific as you can be when describing symptoms or problems.** Whenever possible, make your practitioner aware of the important details of your problem. How should you define "important"? Consider the where's, when's and how's, for starters. Where are you when the symptom appears (only at work? sitting in a certain position?

in bed? outdoors? indoors?); when does it most often occur (when exercising? early in the morning, or late at night? before or after meals?); how does it feel, exactly (a sharp pain? a dull pulsing pain? a sensation that moves from one part of your body to another? a shivery feeling? does it come and go, or do you feel it pretty steadily?). The more information of this kind you can give to your clinician, the better the chance your problem will be deciphered quickly—or at least the appropriate tests will be done promptly.

6. **Be as steady, calm and professional as possible when discussing your symptoms.** It can be difficult to remain calm when you're afraid of a symptom or disease. But a very interesting study recently found that the way you present your symptoms may have a strong impact on the way doctors interpret your problem. For instance, hysterical or relatively histrionic presenters were less likely to have their symptoms taken seriously than those who described symptoms in a more steady, matter-of-fact manner. You don't have to be an actress in your doctor's office—your personality is worth a lot in letting the clinician know who you are and how you feel both emotionally and physically. But when you're describing your symptoms, a steady and controlled manner may just boost the chance that your problem will be taken seriously.

    Of course, there's always the flip side of the coin, too. If you tend to be stoic, not wanting to complain about aches or pains or to appear frail in the face of illness, you too may be failing to hold up your end of the doctor-patient communication—and that can lead to misdiagnoses or missed diagnoses. By explaining your feelings openly and calmly, you will more likely have your needs met and no reasonable health care provider will find you to be unduly fearful or frail.

7. **Have all major discussions with your clinician when you're fully clothed.** When you're naked, you're vulnerable. Sherrie Kaplan urges women to ask to speak with their doctors either before they undress for the physical exam, or afterwards when they are clothed once again. Do *not* have a discussion about your health in general, the next step of your treatment, or your fears about a particular problem when you're in the buff. If the doctor can't wait for you to dress, then tell him/her that you'd prefer to call later to ask questions or to discuss the details of your treatment program.

8. **Lay out your health concerns immediately.** Do not wait for your deepest worries about your health to be teased out of you, Moira Stewart warns. If you wait, they might never be addressed. If you are talking to your doctor about the occasional pain you feel in your left shoulder, but what you're really thinking is that you're terrified you're going to die of a heart attack like your mother did and that the shoulder pain is an early sign, *express that fear.* Your doctor cannot read your mind. He/she might be able to assuage your fears with appropriate tests, or relieve you with just some calm reassurance. If you don't make your emotional needs known, they cannot be tended to.

9. **Let your doctor know how you feel about him/her.** Dr. Thomas Inui, chairman of the department of ambulatory care and prevention at Harvard Medical School and at the Harvard Community Health Plan, tells patients to *let doctors know* what's good and what's bad about their treatment style. He's amazed at the number of patients who complain about doctors to friends, but never in fact confront the clinicians with their negative feelings. Without feedback, doctors aren't going to change. If you like many things about your doctor, but are unhappy with a certain aspect of your care, speak up! For instance, don't hestitate to tell a doctor that you're unhappy with the fact that your last two appointments have been rushed. Perhaps there is a better day of the week, or a better time of day on which to schedule appointments. Or maybe you don't like the fact that the doctor didn't consult you about your treatment plan. In a positive way, let him/her know! As with any other relationship, you cannot expect your doctor to change if you don't provide information on where the problems lie. The key is to find the right balance between expressing disappointment and placing blame. If you are generally satisfied with your health care provider, but dissatisfied with a particular interchange or experience, frame your criticism in a constructive, supportive manner: "You've always been very clear and direct with me about my treatment regimen, so I'm disappointed that in this case, with the discovery of my high blood pressure, you're being evasive about how dangerous this is and what I should do about it."

If it's just too hard for you to be this open with your clinician in a one-on-one situation, consider bringing a support person with you for this purpose (your spouse, partner, sister, friend, parent). Often this can make all the difference between feeling empowered and feeling cowed in the doctor's office—especially when you're frightened about a symptom or a diagnosis. A good friend of mine was given an equivocal diagnosis of endometriosis after enduring years of chronic pelvic pain. The more pain she had, and the fewer answers she was getting from her doctor, the more intimidated she became by the process of talking to him about her discomfort and her fears. Though she is a competent adult living on her own, she decided to bring her mother with her to subsequent doctor visits. She discovered that just having her mother there helped take the edge off of her fear and her discomfort about asking multiple questions. Furthermore, she found that her mother asked questions and demanded answers that she had been too distraught to ask herself. Bringing a support person does *not* indicate weakness; it speaks to your resourcefulness in calling upon the support systems available to you.

Remember, there's a greater purpose to this frankness: be open with your doctor not just for your own sake, but also on behalf of the many other women who will come into this clinician's office after you.

10. **Give information, but don't try to diagnose your own problem.** Dr. Inui points out that women patients have a tendency to self-blame in diagnosing their own health problems. Far more often than men do, he says,

women are apt to attribute their symptoms to something they did wrong. In painting a problem as their own fault, they play into an already problematic tradition in which doctors blame women for their symptoms, or tell them "It's all in your head." One example he gives is the woman who comes into his office and says that she has had chronic headaches as of late. She suggests that her headaches are caused by tension she created in the workplace by getting on her boss's nerves. Don't plant those self-deprecating concepts in your doctor's mind, Inui urges. Report your symptoms, how you feel and how long you've felt that way, when the symptoms get worse and how it's all affecting you emotionally. But leave the diagnosis to the doctor. Don't add to the already rife problems of the doctor-female patient relationship with inappropriate self-blame.

11. **Ask for a complete explanation of everything that's given to you or done to your body.** Judith LaRosa, former deputy director of the office of research on women's health at the NIH, notes this as the single most important thing a woman can do to insure that her own health care is appropriate. Become every bit as informed as you can become, she urges. Find out not just *what's* being done, but *why* it's being done. LaRosa points out that the only way to effectively get this information is to ask questions of your entire team of health care providers. While your doctor should be able to give you an overview of all aspects of your care, other health professionals can often give more detailed explanations of your treatment. For example, if you're working with nurses, physical therapists, pharmacists, nutritionists or any other category of caregiver, take the opportunity to ask all about their contribution to your care. Don't make the mistake of assuming that no one's credibility is as good as your doctor's. Different health care providers specialize in different areas, and you should capitalize on the diversity of their talents and information.

Of course, ask for complete information from your doctor as well as your other caregivers. Women in general, and older women in particular, have a tendency to not want to "burden" their physicians, LaRosa adds. If you forget something that was explained during your office visit, don't hesitate to call and ask for a refresher. Sometimes, a nurse will be able to provide the information. Sometimes, you'll have to demand to speak to the doctor when he or she is available.

It's especially important to get information from all of your health care providers because sometimes their care for you can conflict. For example, if you see more than one physician, you may be prescribed multiple medications with troublesome interactions. If you don't have a clear idea of everything you're taking and why, you can't inform each practitioner of the other's actions. Ideally, your overall care should be orchestrated by one central physician—but this isn't always the case. Older women in particular may be vulnerable to the cumulative effects of several medications. In fact, some alleged dementia is nothing more than overmedication. Get all the information about your care, and keep it on paper so that each new provider will have the needed information about your condition and its management to this point.

12. **Avoid the "Father knows best" attitude to medicine.** Even if you're feeling vulnerable, resist the temptation to say, "Just take care of me," becoming the passive, childlike patient in the doctor's fatherly hands. Approach each visit with the assumption that you are on an equal playing ground, and that your input will be essential to getting the best care and getting well faster.

13. **Educate yourself about your general health and/or particular medical condition:** The more you know, the more empowered you will be in the doctor's office. Arm yourself with the kind of information that all doctors need in order to give you the best care. Learn everything you can about your family history of various diseases, including when your parents or grandparents suffered major health problems (that is, the age at which your grandmother developed ovarian cancer, the age at which your mother first noticed her blood pressure was high, the age at which your father's sister got breast cancer, etc.). Remember that both your maternal and paternal family histories are important; just because you're a woman doesn't mean you can't inherit diseases from your father's side of the family. Often, women overlook this fact.

If you already have a health problem, read everything you can on the subject so that you can better understand your doctor's comments and advice. Support and education groups often give free reading materials on diseases; these are loaded with issues of importance to you, the consumer of health care. Talk to others who have similar problems, and learn the specifics of what works for them so you can discuss it with your doctor intelligently.

If you're going to bring information to your doctor about your particular health problem, make sure it's as complete as possible. For example, don't tell your doctor that you want to know more about "that article in the *Washington Post* on a new treatment for infertility." You cannot expect that your doctor reads everything you read, or watches every program you watch. Bring the article with you, or write down the relevant details: the name of the drug or procedure, the names of the hospitals or physicians quoted as using the technique, and so on. Often, health information in the lay media is based on a study or report from another source, such as a medical journal or health conference. If you can provide your doctor with this information as well, you'll help him/her locate more information on the subject.

Above all, advises Dr. Marcia Angell, women must cultivate a healthy dose of skepticism about new medical research. As Americans, she complains, we have a tendency to go off in one direction, trend or fad based on the "latest study." In fact, individual studies in science and medicine are parts of a long, cumulative process—steps toward answers rather than answers in and of themselves. Each study should be looked at as tentative—as a lead, Dr. Angell advises. Certainly ask your doctor about anything interesting or promising you read or hear about, but understand that trends are what you're looking for, rather than the latest hottest piece of trivia about your disease and its management.

14. **Admit it if you're just plain scared.** This kind of confession can be hard to make, especially if your doctor seems "tough" on the outside. But by expressing your emotional needs, you may draw out a side of your doctor that you didn't know existed. If you don't admit that you're frightened, you'll never get support for those feelings. Whether you're afraid to have a procedure done, anxious about going on medication for the first time, afraid of dying from your illness, or worried about being ostracized because of it, all of your feelings are valid and important. Part of getting physically well is getting emotionally well, so until those butterflies in your stomach are calmed, you're expending energy working against your own body's defenses. Reach out for support and you may be surprised at how much you get. Perhaps your doctor will refer you to other patients with the same problem, or a formal support group where you can vent your fears. If your doctor is totally unreceptive and disrespectful of your vulnerable emotions, you're in the wrong hands.

15. **Ask what you can do for yourself.** Many physicians focus on their role in making you well (medication, procedures, etc.), giving short shrift to what *you* can do to improve your condition. One reason for this is that the efficacy of self-help techniques is often anecdotal, not proven by scientific study—and many doctors are uncomfortable in the realm of the anecdote! If your doctor doesn't tend to be forthcoming about the role of self-help, ask about it directly. Would changing your diet make a difference in your condition? Would exercise—taking it up or changing what you already do—be useful? You may get an equivocal answer, such as "some patients say this helps but it's never been proven." That's better than no self-help advice at all. Some open-minded practitioners will refer you to self-help groups or reading materials for more "lay" advice. If your doctor says a given self-help approach isn't harmful (an apple a day?) you'd serve yourself well to try it in addition to your more formal medical regimen.

THE TWO-WAY STREET APPROACH TO MEDICAL CARE

In sum, what you get out of your health care relationship will be, to some degree, commensurate with what you put into it. There are exceptions: The most activated patient can get few results from an ungiving and unreceptive physician. For the most part, however, when you provide information, when you are direct and honest about your physical and emotional feelings, when you work with your doctor to create the best possible plan for your future health and speak up when that plan isn't working for you, when you demand the kind of care that you know you deserve and seek new expertise when your needs aren't met, your health care rises to a higher level.

Making demands, of course, means putting yourself first once in a while. Women in general don't have a great track record in this regard—particularly when it comes to our health. Once our partners, our children, and our parents and even grandparents' health has been accounted for, we *sometimes* turn to our own health and give it a little attention (for some of us, it's too little, too late). But putting our own health first may have its costs, too, warns Dr. Beth Alexander, editorial board member for the journal *Women's Health Forum* and an expert in family medicine. She has seen the unfortunate outcome when women who have long subjugated their needs to others step forward and assert themselves on their own behalf. In some families, she says, men push back; they may become hostile, and even harm women who start to assert their own value and importance. These intrafamily conflicts are not isolated from your general health; they are very much a part of it. If you feel squeezed into denying yourself care, this in itself is an issue to discuss with a health care professional.

Becoming a demanding but realistic and cooperative consumer of health care is the most important thing you can do for yourself and your future. As a woman, you must keep in mind that while tradition may have placed control of your body and health in someone else's hands, starting today, you hold the reins. Steer them in the right direction and you *and* those around you will be healthier for it.

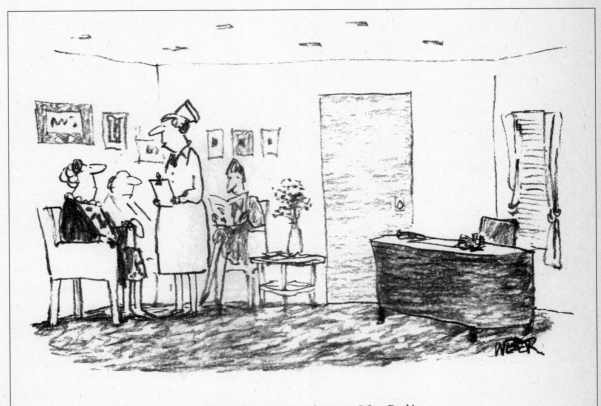

"The doctor will see you now, Mrs. Perkins.
Please try not to upset him."

PART TWO

Your Body, Inside and Out

CHAPTER THREE

YOUR REPRODUCTIVE ANATOMY

I'd the upbringing a nun would envy and that's the truth. Until I was 15 I was more familiar with Africa than my own body.

—Joe Orton, *Entertaining Mr. Sloane, I*

We like to think of ourselves as living in liberated times, times in which just about any topic, sexual or otherwise, is fodder for talk-show hosts or even dinner table conversation. Times in which it takes a *lot* to make us blush—if we're capable of blushing at all. Why, then, if we're so open about *other* people's sexuality, are we so very closed about our own sexual parts? I'm astounded at the lack of knowledge women possess about their own bodies, and the implications that may hold for our sexual and general health.

A college graduate tells me sheepishly that she isn't aware that tampons go in a different opening than the one urine comes out of. A health news reporter asks me where her cervix is located. These cases may surprise you, but they're far from unusual. Even today, many women lack basic information about their bodies. For centuries it was considered taboo to look at, touch or otherwise investigate ourselves, particularly below the waist. Women were to keep themselves clean and chaste, but not ask about—nor certainly look for—anything usual. Biology probably plays a part in the mystery of female anatomy. While male genitalia is out in the open and easy to see, female genitalia is largely hidden—between the legs, parts *inside* the body. It takes a concerted effort for us to become familiar with our sexual parts. And according to Dr. Eboo Versi, associate professor of OB-GYN and reproductive biology at the Harvard Medical School, the fact that we have no comfortable lay language with which to discuss our genitalia makes it even harder to become open and informed. There is medical jargon, and there is profanity or slang, Dr. Versi points out, but nothing useful and comfortable in between. The lack of an easy vocabulary further distances us from the topic of our body parts and makes asking even simple questions much more awkward. Finally, a long history of negative stereotypes about female sexual and reproductive function has had an impact especially on older women; if you grew up thinking that your period killed plants, you weren't exactly empowered to learn more about your wonderful body.

Let's now take the first steps to learning about our reproductive health. Step by step, we'll explore our genitalia; what's where, what it looks like, what it might feel like, and how to watch for changes. The essential take-home message in this section is that if you don't know what your body looks like *normally,* you won't know what it looks like when something goes wrong with it. On the other hand, if you are familiar with your vaginal parts, for example, just as you are with that chicken pox scar on your nose, you can be the first to alert your doctor to a sign of change.

EXTERNAL GENITAL ANATOMY

Let's start by looking in the mirror at the visible structures of your genitals. You'll need a good light and a mirror—unless you're an acrobat! Open your legs, set up the mirror where you can see your vulva—the outside of your vagina—and start to investigate. It's best to use a mirror that you don't have to hold, so you can use your

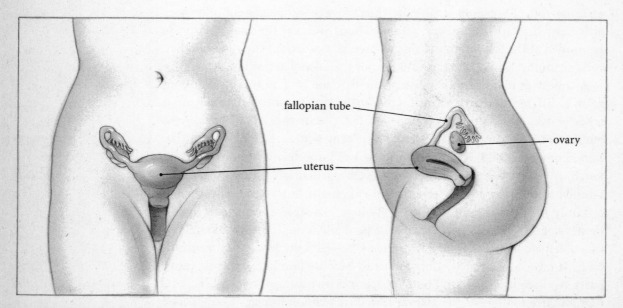

Front and side views, female reproductive system

fingers to get a better look at your genital parts.

Without pulling anything aside, you should be able to see the following:

First, you'll see the opening to your vagina, called the vaginal orifice, and if you have never had sexual intercourse, often you'll see a sheath of skin called the hymen stretched partially across the opening. Normally, you'll also see a small space where the hymen doesn't cover the entire vaginal opening; that's so your menstrual blood can flow out and not get trapped inside. You can also see the labia majora, the large, outer lips of the vagina. These lips are thick and fleshy, have the same type of skin that's on your arms and legs, and usually have pubic hair on them. If you gently pull the large vaginal lips aside, you'll discover more interesting structures.

First, you'll see the labia minora, the small, inner vaginal lips. These are made of mucous membrane skin, much more delicate than the skin of the outer vaginal lips. The inner lips meet to form the hood of your clitoris, which is named for the Greek word for "key" and is often the key to sexual pleasure in women. Delicate as these inner lips are, they help protect the highly sensitive clitoris from excessive stimulation. Most sexual orgasms occur when the clitoris is stimulated, although there are other types of orgasms as well. If you are not sexually aroused, you'll see only the hood of the clitoris, formed of loose skin. If you gently pull back the hood, you'll see the clitoris itself underneath. Dr. Versi notes that while many women know they have something called a clitoris, few are familiar with exactly where it is, and therefore fail to inform sexual partners

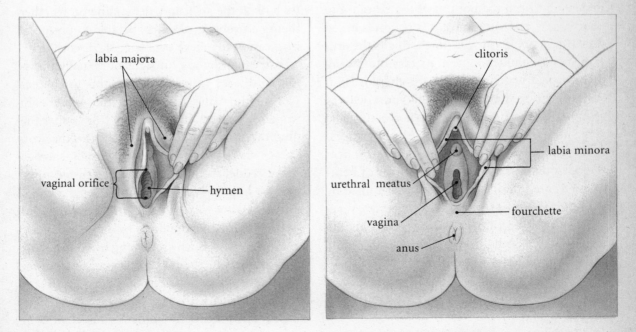

External view of female genitalia

Internal view of female genitalia

about its potential for sexual pleasure.

Moving along with your investigation, you will also see the external urethral meatus, a fancy name for the opening through which urine exits the body. Clearly, you can see that the opening through which you menstruate— the vaginal opening—is *not* the same as the opening for urine.

Collectively, this external vaginal area (everything you've seen above) is known as the vulva. When your doctor speaks of vulvar irritation, for example, she is talking about irritation of these outer vaginal structures. Once you're accustomed to examining your vulva when it's *healthy,* you'll be better able to recognize changes or problems should they arise in this region. Read on for more information on common signs of vulvar problems.

Continuing with your viewing, take a look at the area between the bottom of the entrance to your vagina and your anus: this region is called the fourchette. If you give birth, this is the area where you would be given an episiotomy (an incision that widens the area for childbirth), if you choose to have one, or if your delivery requires it. Further down, you'll see the anal verge and anal canal, where many women discover hemorrhoids (painful, tender lumps near the opening of the anus). Other forms of hemorrhoids are internal and must be examined by your doctor with a scope. Taken together, everything from your clitoris to your anus plus the area *between* both inner thighs in this same region, comprises your perineum.

RECOGNIZING PROBLEMS

Any swelling, redness, irritation, discharge, change of color, lump, bump, mole or other unusual mark in the vulvar area should be examined by a doctor. It may be nothing at all, but better safe than sorry. Once you are aware of your anatomy and can precisely describe to your doctor what you're feeling or what you're worried about, you can be a tremendous help in getting to the bottom of a problem. In the past, you may have told your gynecologist, "I feel some pain in my vagina." After reading this section, you're now aware that that was a lot like saying, "I have a pain in my leg"; it gives your doctor very little information. Being able to say exactly where the pain, or the source of worry, is ("I have a sore spot on the right side of the inner lip of my vagina") adds a lot to the diagnostic process. Sometimes, your doctor will take a biopsy—a sample of tissue from the troublesome spot—and have it examined in a laboratory. In other cases she'll just take a careful look at the area, and, depending on whether there's a problem, she may be able to prescribe medication to relieve your specific discomfort.

You can also look for signs of sexually transmitted disease (much more on this in chapter 13). While many cases are symptom-free in women, you may find discharge from either the urethral or the vaginal openings (now that you know where those are!). Sometimes sores— either reddened bumps or actual crusted pimple-like lesions—will be visible. Some vaginal warts are easy to see—they may be white and large or consist of tiny little bumps. Others are invisible, which is why screening by your doctor is so important. She may put a vinegar solution on your vulva or inside your vagina and reexamine the area with a microscope: the vinegar "lights up" potentially hidden trouble spots in cases like human papillomavirus (the virus that causes genital warts).

INTERNAL GENITAL ANATOMY

Now let's take a look inside: You won't be able to do this in the mirror by yourself, but you *can* do it with a mirror at your doctor's office, when a speculum—a tool used to open your vagina so the doctor can get a better look—is inserted.

Your vagina is like a tunnel, in some respects: the illustration below shows the inside of the vaginal walls, which are formed of mucous membrane—very delicate tissue. At the "end" of the vagina on the inside is your cervix—the gateway between your vagina and your uterus. Some call it the neck of the uterus, others, the mouth of the uterus. Not everyone's cervix looks alike—there are variations, like those in the illustration at top right.

Beyond the cervix, neither you nor your doctor can see from the outside. Your reproductive organs are tucked inside your pelvis; the only access to them is through the vagina and cervix. So at this point, follow along with the illustrations and you'll get a good idea of what's going on inside your body.

After the cervix, the entrance to the uterus, is the body of the uterus itself.

While it can expand to hold a fairly hefty baby, in fact the uterus is usually quite small—weighing only about four ounces. The lining of the uterus is called the endometrium; you probably recognize the term from diseases like endometriosis (where the uterine lining grows outside the uterus) or endometrial cancer (cancer of the lining of the uterus). An illustration

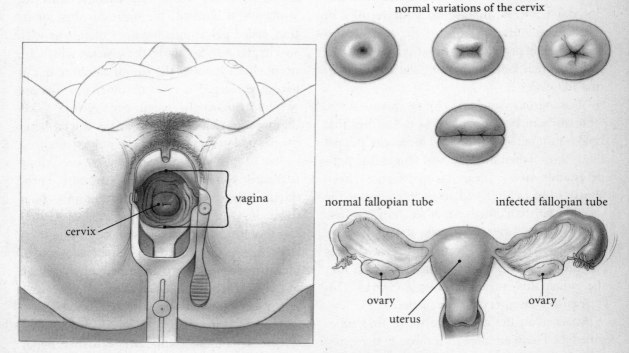

normal variations of the cervix

External view of cervix

normal fallopian tube   infected fallopian tube

ovary   ovary

uterus

Female reproductive tract

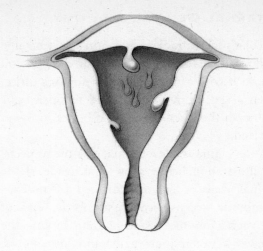

on the previous page shows the uterus in the most common "normal" position. (I put "normal" in quotation marks because there are normal variations on this position as well.) In about 85% of cases, the uterus is "anteverted", or tipped forward. In about 15% of cases, it is "retroverted", or tipped back. In rare cases, it is "axial", or centered. In the old days, doctors believed that a retroverted uterus was a *disorder* in need of treatment—that it caused miscarriages, emotional lability and other problems. In fact, it's usually harmless. The reason you might want to find out the natural position of your uterus is if that position *changes*—for instance, if your doctor notes that a once-anteverted uterus is now tipped backward—it could be a sign that an adhesion, infection or some other problem has developed. There are other variations on the body of the uterus that can, but don't always, impact on your fertility or other issues. One variation is the uterine septum or wall protruding into the body of the uterus, which looks something like the illustration following .

Your uterus is supported by ligaments—these "threads" can be thought of as the strings that hold a puppet: when they are loose, the puppet flops down; when they are held taught, the puppet stands erect. These ligaments come from above, from behind and from the sides of the uterus. With childbirth or other stresses, these ligaments can begin to stretch; if they become weak through a loss of tone and elasticity, they can drop, in which case the uterus can fall into the vagina: this is called a prolapsed uterus. This is discussed in more detail in chapter 7.

Attached to the uterus are small, thin tubes called the fallopian tubes; it is through these tiny tunnels that the egg comes down, released from the ovaries, to be fertilized. You can't feel your own tubes or ovaries, but certainly your doctor can, and this is one of the things she's feeling for during your pelvic exam. The tubes, which are normally quite small, can become infected, swollen and blocked (for more on this condition, called pelvic inflammatory disease or PID, *see* chapter 13). Similarly, the ovaries, which are normally each about the size of an almond, can become enlarged if cysts or other growths are present. Amazingly, when comedienne Gilda Radner's ovarian cancer was finally detected, her ovaries had grown to the size of grapefruits.

Just to give you an idea of where everything is placed, you can see that below your reproductive organs sits your bladder, and behind them is your colon. Everything fits closely together inside your pelvis, so it's easy to understand how a given disorder—such as a cancer, for example—can have an impact on any or all of these structures. It's also clear, when you see how everything is positioned, how hard it is to tell exactly where pain is coming from, since discomfort in the colon can seem like pelvic pain, and vice versa. In the pelvis, there is often

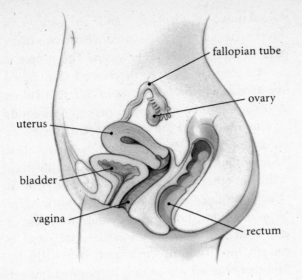

Side view of internal organs

fallopian tube

ovary

uterus

bladder

vagina

rectum

a problem with so-called referred pain, or pain that originates in one area but reverberates to another, nearby region. Through a variety of tests, your doctor can help you sort out where a given pain originates.

YOUR BREASTS

There are certain basic myths about breast health that must be dispelled.

First, size is not a factor of health. There are perfectly healthy large breasts, and perfectly healthy small breasts. Some breasts are "perky" and seem to defy gravity by sitting high on the woman's chest. Others are "saggy," and hang down against the chest. Both are normal. Breasts are almost never exactly the same size, just as our hands and feet aren't exactly the same size.

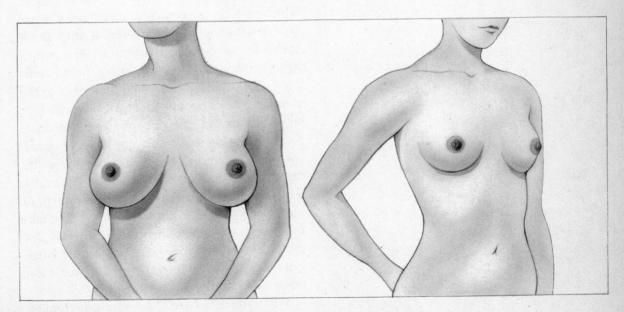

Two normal variations on breast size and shape

Some women are concerned about a dramatic difference in the size of their two breasts; if this is the case, surgery can bring them closer in size. Breasts can also be surgically enlarged or reduced, if you are dissatisfied with their size (*see* breast health in chapter 6).

There is no such thing as "normal" nipples, any more than there is such a thing as a "normal" face. Nipples come in pale pink (usually in fair-skinned Caucasians) and in very dark brown (usually in African-American women), and in many colors in between. The nipple is surrounded by an area of colored skin called the areola, which also comes in different colors and sizes. On the areola you may find all kinds of tiny lumps and bumps and often tiny hairs: some of these normal bumps are called Montgomery's glands; others are simply hair follicles; others are normal sebaceous glands which produce a fatty or oily lubrication. Nipples are most commonly external—sticking out—but can also be inverted—pointing in toward the inside of the breast. It used to be said that women whose nipples pointed inward could not breast-feed: this is a myth, and the condition can usually be corrected with breast shells and pumping (*see* breast-feeding, page 298).

Let's take a look inside the breast:

The breasts sit on a surface of chest muscle, which rests on the clavicle and rib bones. There is a fascinating matrix of vessels and tissue inside the breast. There are milk ducts, which bring milk to the nipple during breast-feeding—these ducts lead through the nipple to the outside, where the milk emerges; there are lobules throughout the breasts where milk is formed; and there are different kinds of tissue, including tougher connective tissue and softer fatty tissue, throughout the breast. Generally, when lots of the hormone estrogen is present in your body (before menopause or if you're taking hormone replacement), the breasts are more dense and firm; when there is little estrogen in the body, the breasts tend to become less dense and easier to feel and image with X rays.

When you understand how internally complex your breasts are, it's easier to understand why

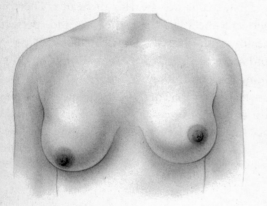

Asymmetrical breasts

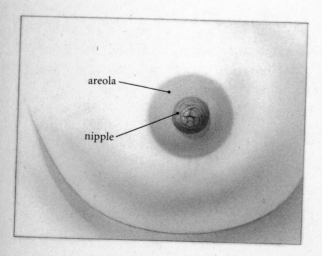

areola

nipple

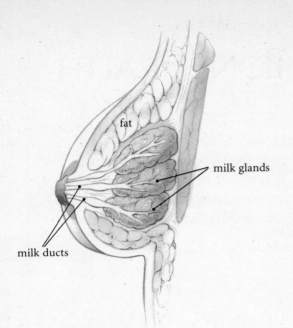

fat

milk glands

milk ducts

to the touch, and can develop lumps that aren't present at other times of the month. After menstruation, they often revert to a smaller, less lumpy state. The key value in getting to know *your* breasts is to distinguish normal monthly changes that occur at identical points in your cycle from unusual, lasting breast changes. For instance, if a new or unusual lump appears *after* your period and doesn't go away, you'll want to take note of it and show it to your doctor. We'll go into this in more detail when we discuss the breast self-exam in chapter 6. But just for starters, gently get to know how your breasts look and feel at different times of the month.

Above all else, learn to appreciate your body for its uniqueness—struggle against the stereotypes foisted on us by swimsuit ads and bra commercials. As there is beauty in every kind of face, regardless of color or shape or size, so there is beauty in every shape of body, heavy or lean, short or tall, big or small. And as every nose or pair of eyes is different from another, so your sexual organs are very much your own, and to be celebrated, not shamed, for their individuality.

mushy or loose, in others, more firm or lumpy inside. Knowing the complexity of the inside of your breasts can also help you to comprehend the many different locations and characteristics of potential breast *problems;* for instance, breast cysts, infections or cancers can occur at any of the sites shown, and their location will help determine the best way to treat them (*see* the breast cancer discussion in chapter 25).

As you become more familiar with your breasts, you'll discover that they are *not* static; they change in size and character throughout your monthly hormonal cycle. Before menstruation, breasts often swell, become more tender

....

FOR MORE INFORMATION ON PROBLEMS WITH YOUR REPRODUCTIVE ANATOMY, SEE THE SOURCES AT THE END OF THE CHAPTER ON GYNECOLOGICAL HEALTH, PAGE 126

....

Chapter Four

Your Bone Health

I knew a woman, lovely in her bones
   When small birds sighed, she would sigh back at
      them;
And when she moved more ways than one
   The shapes a bright container can contain!

—Theodore Roethke, "I Knew a Woman"

Your skeleton makes up as much as 15% of your total body mass. It is the foundation on which the rest of your body is formed. Its strength is essential for the general well-being and placement of your major body organs, your posture, and your overall feeling of health and vitality. Why is a structure so large and vital so easy to ignore? "Out of sight, out of mind" may have something to do with it. Or maybe it's because we're so accustomed to the image of a dry, clackety-clack halloween skeleton that many of us think of our bones as static entities, always there for us but not deserving special care.

In fact, our bones are anything but static. They're living, evolving structures, constantly remodeling themselves in a process of bone deposition and removal. With some urging from the National Osteoporosis Foundation, the experts' favorite analogy is to look at bone as a bank account. During our childhood, teens and some say up until our mid-30s, we make more deposits to our bone bank account than withdrawals. These deposits build up to our "peak bone mass"—the most bone we're likely to accumulate in our lifetime. From that point until menopause, when our menstrual periods stop, our bone bank account approaches a balance in which bone deposits equal bone withdrawals. Finally, at the time of menopause and the few years that follow, our bone bank account takes a dangerous dip, during which withdrawals greatly exceed deposits. The bone bank account gets poorer each year. The result? For many women, the potential for osteoporosis. In this chapter, we'll discuss ways of protecting our bones so *they* may protect *us* well into old age.

In many mundane ways, we neglect our skeletal and muscular health. With heavy purses, briefcases and baby snugglies, we tax our shoulders and backs; with ill-fitting shoes we damage our feet. Later in this chapter, you'll find expert advice on reversing these chronic abuses and making your body feel better from head to toe.

Osteoporosis: What It Is

Osteoporosis is *not* a "normal part of aging", as some uninformed health care workers might tell you. It is a disorder often *associated* with aging and related medical conditions, but it can often be prevented and/or treated to a significant degree. Osteoporosis is a condition of bone loss in which the bones become weak, porous and vulnerable to fracture at various places throughout the body. The spine, hip and wrist bones are especially hard hit by this disorder, since they have a large amount of what's called trabecular bone—that is, a spongy, interior portion of bone that's more prevalent in certain parts of the body. A frightening statistic: The average woman will lose half of her spongy-type bone and a third of her outer, hard bone over the course of her lifetime.

The Hard Facts

Osteoporosis affects 25 million Americans, mostly (8 out of 10) women. Experts believe that as many as one-fourth of all women between the ages of 60 and 70 have osteoporosis. Many of these cases can be prevented if we start taking proper care of our bones. The disease can cause extreme pain, or—in some instances—it can remain silent until a fracture occurs. Even these fractures can be painless at first.

The fracture rate due to osteoporosis is staggering. One in four women will fracture a bone at some point in her lifetime as a direct result of osteoporosis. Hard as it is to believe, the disease causes over a million fractures a year, including half a million spinal fractures and 300,000 hip fractures. The cost in pain and suffering is immense, and so is the cost in dollars. We spend six billion dollars a year treating hip fracture alone. Despite all the money and resources we're pouring into treating these fractures, half of all women who fracture a hip will never walk again without assistance, experts say.

You might think that because fractures are usually dramatic events, osteoporosis would be hard to miss. Unfortunately, the opposite is true. Osteoporosis is an insidious disease. First, the fractures don't always occur with accidents or falls. Osteoporotic fractures can occur in completely unexpected ways—for instance, when you lift a bag of groceries. The bones are so weak that even a light load can be the straw that breaks the camel's back. You may not even *feel* these fractures when they occur. A deformed posture might clue you in to the possibility of disease. You may seem to be shrinking, or stooped, or your stomach may seem to protrude more than normal. At this stage, notes Deborah Gold, senior fellow in the Aging Center at Duke University Medical Center, with your rib cage practically sitting on your pelvis, it can be difficult to lean forward, look behind you when you're driving, or pull a shirt over your head without assistance, especially if other health problems like arthritis have also set in. On top of the physical problems, Gold stresses, the emotional consequences of this disease are quite serious, including depression, feelings of isolation, and loneliness—particularly for those who become homebound as a result of their condition.

For many women, hip fractures are far more complicated than just broken bones. According to Dr. Paul Hirsch, chairman of the committee on public education for the American Academy of Orthopedic Surgeons, hip fractures significantly increase a woman's chance of dying due to complications including infection, blood clots, shock, pneumonia (if she is bed-ridden), and many other associated problems. According to the National Osteoporosis Foundation, nearly 50,000 women die each year from complications of hip and other fractures.

OSTEOPOROSIS: WHAT YOU HAD TO SAY ABOUT IT

Greta, 74 years old
Luckily I had my bone density measured, and I'm 25% below the norm for my age. Very serious. I'm at serious risk of fractures. I take an exercise class two times a week to stabilize my muscles, I'm much stronger. I did a lot of dance all my life and the idea of losing my mobility was very real to me. We do a program designed for people with bone density loss. I'm taking Premarin and I'm taking a lot of calcium and vitamin D. I was very terrified, it really is demoralizing; before I enrolled in the program I was terrified to get out of bed and start the day! It had not occurred to me, you see people with humps on their backs, but even when you're 70 you don't identify with it. My advice is whatever stage you're at, stabilize it, take charge of it.

Maggie, 80 years old
People don't take it seriously enough. I know they don't because I didn't, either. I don't know how long I've had osteoporosis, a lot longer than I was diagnosed. I fell down our steps, and I broke my elbow and collar bone. [Later] they said "you have advanced osteoporosis," I guess the first thing that came to mind probably was being dependent, having always been a pretty independent soul.

I could see ahead of time that I wasn't going to be able to do lots of things that I had done. They just said "get a cane." They said you've got it very serious and it can only get worse. I'm having a bad time right now. My back has had too many fractures, I'm not even sure how many, there's nothing you can do about it. I didn't believe in pain pills, but I've never been in pain like this ever, including childbirth, so I had to take pain pills, which contributed to my constipation. My rib cage sits on my pelvis, it's gotten progressively worse, my floating ribs as I call them are literally pressed inward and I can't straighten up without a lot of pain, and that pain doesn't respond to treatment. It's hard to breathe. I am lying down now, resting so that when [my aide] gets here I'll have enough energy to take a bath. About the only thing I can do is switch my weight from one foot to another. I hope to use the stationary bike again. Trying to put panty hose on is impossible.

I'm thinking about what I can do to prevent getting worse. I'm back on the calcitonin, I was taken off the etidronate. We've been going to the support group, I'm very lucky, I have a husband who not only can but *does* everything with a lot of TLC. Without that I'd have to be in some kind of long-term care I guess. The support group means so much to me, I can't give it up, it's been a life-line to me.

Adele, 85 years old
In '91 I fell and my back hurt, I didn't know I had compressed a few vertebrae. And when my back didn't stop hurting with rest and ice and heat my doctor suggested I have an X ray.

I hadn't really heard much about osteoporosis but he said right away it looks like osteoporosis. I thought it's part of growing old, something I had to live with. I hadn't heard much about it. I knew I had to be careful and not fall.

The doctor put me on [the drug] Didronel, but he also suggested I go to his exercise class and there's a special therapist who knows what seniors should be doing especially if they've had fractures. The therapist keeps us aware of how we should sit and stand and bend and all our exercises are to strengthen our muscles and joints, and a good 20 minutes of getting our heartbeats up. I have shrunk of course, a good three inches, and after a year on this medication and exercise my bone density in my spine went up 11% and with the exercise I stretched out an inch! I can reach my cupboards two and a half inches higher than I could after my injury. I don't have to ask people to help me get things, or get a stool.

After I had my accident I couldn't play with my grandkids, even catch—I was afraid I'd hurt my back. I'm 85 years old and I feel a lot better—I do play catch now but I'm very careful. There are times when I do too much kitchen work and the backs of my hips hurt. I have myself a pretty good program, I do get on the floor almost every morning. I have a good tape and I just do it before

breakfast. You really need to do it every day and walking is especially good.

WHO'S AT RISK?

The following list of risk factors comes from the work of many osteoporosis experts. If you fit even a few of these categories, talk to your doctor about your potential risk of osteoporosis. Sadly, a Gallup poll found that seven out of ten women who are at risk for serious bone loss fail to discuss the problem with their doctors, and therefore miss out on vital information about prevention and treatment. The best time to talk to your doctor is NOW—whatever your age. While osteoporosis usually sets in after menopause, the problems that lead up to it are created many years before that. The sooner you establish your risk factors and start to reverse them, the better the chances your bones will stay healthy. Also note, however, that if you don't fit any of the risk factors listed here, you're not immune to osteoporosis. According to Betsy Love, associate director of the Center for Metabolic Bone Disorders at Providence Medical Center in Portland, Oregon, *far* more women have low bone mass than you'd expect, and develop osteoporosis even though they had no known risk factors to begin with.

RISK FACTORS FOR OSTEOPOROSIS

- female sex
- Caucasian or Asian race (but please note: some researchers are reporting finding more osteoporosis than previously thought in African-American women of smaller, thinner build)
- family history of osteoporosis

- fair skin and freckles
- blond or reddish hair (of course, dark-haired women are also at risk, but fairer women are considered to be a higher risk group)
- early natural menopause *or* surgical menopause (your ovaries were removed) *or* your periods have stopped due to other conditions, such as anorexia nervosa or an extremely vigorous exercise regimen
- smoking
- never having biological children
- eating few dairy foods/little dietary calcium
- consuming foods with little vitamin D and/or little exposure to sunlight for vitamin D synthesis
- chronic dieting or fasting
- short or thin build
- older age
- sedentary lifestyle
- excessive exercise
- heavy alcohol intake
- heavy caffeine intake

The following medical problems and/or medications you might take to treat them have also been associated with an increased risk of osteoporosis:

Illness

- kidney or liver disease
- chronic diarrhea
- diabetes
- celiac disease
- jejunal bypass
- hyperthyroidism
- primary hyperparathyroidism
- prolactinomas
- hypercalciuria

- primary biliary or alcoholic cirrhosis
- certain rheumatologic disorders
- certain connective tissue disorders
- postgastrectomy

Medication

- Dilantin and other anticonvulsant medications
- heparin
- methotrexate
- glucocorticoids (prednisone and cortisone)
- thyroid hormone
- GnRH (gonadotropin releasing hormone) agonists
- lithium
- aluminum-based antacids (Remember! Antacids with no aluminum, such as Tums, can help *prevent* osteoporosis, so don't confuse the two)

Prevention of Bone Loss

It's obvious from the bank account analogy that the more bone you have in the bank to start out with, the more you can afford to lose without suffering serious consequences. So the goal for all women, regardless of their age, is to try to maximize bone-building (that is, bone absorption) and minimize bone loss (bone resorption). Here's how to do that:

CALCIUM

Let's start with what you eat. The main building block for bone is calcium. Without adequate calcium as a foundation, no other bone-building strategy will work. On page 404, you'll find the

RDAs *and* the newer National Institutes of Health recommendations for calcium intake. While the RDAs are low—and the newer recommendations probably much wiser—most American women get only *half* of the RDAs to begin with!

The best way to get calcium is in the diet, where it appears along with other nutrients—many of which also promote bone health. For instance, foods that contain both calcium *and* vitamin D are especially good for your bones, since vitamin D helps your body absorb and use the calcium you take in (fortified milk is a good example of a calcium- and vitamin D-rich food). Dairy foods—including milk, yogurt, cheese, and other milk-based foods—are the best source. There is a terrible misunderstanding among many American women that dairy foods are all high-fat and therefore bad for the heart. In fact, there are many low-fat or nonfat versions of all types of dairy foods, and they have at least as much and sometimes more calcium in them than the high-fat versions. If you are lactose intolerant—that is, if you become ill when you eat dairy foods because you are sensitive to lactose—you might want to try one of several lact*ase*-based liquid products that can be added to dairy foods to counteract the lactose problem. There are also many calcium-rich nondairy foods, including a number of highly nutritious vegetables. (*See* the chapter 20, "Nutrition," for a long list of calcium-rich foods and food combinations.)

If you have tried and failed to get enough calcium through diet—as many women have—you should consider calcium supplements. (Again, for a list of the different supplement types, *see* chapter 20, page 403.) While experts do not recommend getting *all* of your calcium from pills, it's not a bad idea to get some supplementation from these commonly used tablets, especially if you are pregnant, lactating or near or after menopause. You should carefully consider the different absorbancy rates of the various supplements, as well as the cost—which varies tremendously.

EXERCISE

The most overlooked factor affecting bone integrity is exercise. Weight-bearing exercise—that is, exercise in which you have to work against gravity, bearing the weight of your entire body—protects against bone loss. There is nothing high-tech required here; some think that the best weight-bearing exercise of all is walking. Other exercises that fall into this category are jogging, stair-climbing, cross-country skiing, dancing and playing tennis or squash or basketball. If you're carrying your weight, you're doing the right thing. Don't be misled by exercises such as swimming, or even most cycling; while these sports are great for your heart, lungs and muscle tone, they don't do much for your bones.

Many of us want to know how much—or, too often, how little—weight-bearing exercise it takes to protect our bones. The experts disagree slightly on this one, but a minimum range to shoot for is three to four exercise sessions a week, for about 30 minutes each outing. If you're a real couch potato right now, try setting a simple goal—just to do a little more than you're doing already. Build up slowly. Start walking when you would otherwise take the bus or car. Do some of your own housework if you normally have someone else do it. Whoever said "use it or lose it" was right when it comes to bones. Just as when we don't use our muscles, they sag, so when we don't use our bones, they thin out and weaken. A terrible cycle then begins, in which we feel we've become too weak to exercise at all. So get out there and start doing *something*. Even standing up while talking on the phone is better than sitting down. Set small goals and move from there. You *can* do it. Enlisting the company of friends, a neighbor or a spouse can make it harder to quit. If you're fit enough to begin vigorous regular weight-bearing exercise, Dr. William Robb of Evanston Hospital in Illinois urges you to give your bones a day off every other day or so to avoid stress fractures—at least in the first several months of your new activity program. A note for older women, women who live alone, and women who live in dangerous neighborhoods: Surveys show that many of you miss out on regular exercise because you cannot afford indoor fitness clubs and are afraid to exercise outside alone. If you are in that position, consider going out in groups of friends or neighbors, if possible—or, if you simply aren't comfortable doing that, try walking up and down the stairs in your apartment building or home, or pacing up and down the halls. The effect on your bones will be just as good as a fancy treadmill or stair machine.

CIGARETTES AND ALCOHOL

In case heart disease and lung cancer are not strong enough reasons for you to stop smoking, add bone disease to the list. Smoking is strongly associated with osteoporosis on two fronts: first, it promotes actual loss of bone, and second, it impairs the healing of fractures. The more you smoke, the worse off your bones will be—but even minimal smoking has a deleterious effect on bone.

Alcohol is another bone poison. Excessive alcohol intake leads to decreased bone density in part by boosting the amount of calcium you lose through urine and stool. Alcohol *also* makes you more vulnerable to falls—which can lead to fractures. Alcoholics have reduced bone density and are at high risk of osteoporosis.

(For information on how to quit smoking, and for information on the unique issues in curing alcohol problems among women, *see* chapter 19.)

Caffeine in large quantities (some experts say five or more caffeinated drinks per day) impairs the quality of bone. Try switching from coffee to milk in the morning, for a double bonus to your bones. If you can't drop coffee that quickly, or don't like milk, at least try watering your coffee down to decrease your caffeine intake and add lots of skim milk to the brew. Calcium-fortified juice is another good bone-healthy morning choice.

HORMONE REPLACEMENT

One of the most powerful ways to prevent bone loss is with hormone replacement therapy: that is, taking the hormone estrogen alone, or estrogen plus progesterone, close to the time of menopause. This is the time when the body's own estrogen levels drop, and bone loss accelerates. Ideally, hormone replacement should be started when your periods start to fall off, in what's called the perimenopausal period. But there is still a window of opportunity within the first several years *after* menopause in which hormone replacement seems to offer significant bone protection. We need more information on the benefit of starting hormone replacement many years after menopause; some data suggests there is a slight benefit, but this is yet to be confirmed.

As you have no doubt heard, there are both significant risks and benefits to taking hormone replacement—beyond the issue of bone loss. *See* chapter 10, "Menopausal Health," for a more complete discussion of the pros and cons of hormone replacement therapy.

DIAGNOSIS: DO YOU HAVE A PROBLEM, AND IF SO, HOW BAD IS IT?

There are now widely available screening tests for bone loss. The good news is the newest machines are highly effective, quick and give only *tiny* doses of radiation. The bad news is that for screening purposes, insurance doesn't always cover the cost—which runs anywhere from about a hundred to several hundred dollars. If your doctor recommends the test to diagnose a problem, such as a fracture, insurance usually will cover the cost of the test. Here are your main options:

SPA (single photon absorptiometry): is used for screening the wrist bones—not the spine or hip.

DPA (dual photon absorptiometry): can be used to screen the hip and the spine, which most experts think is the best way to go for osteoporosis screening since these bones are vulnerable to fracture.

SXA (single energy X-ray absorptiometry): tests the bones of the wrist and heel.

DEXA (dual energy X-ray absorptiometry): tests the spine and hip and is considered by many experts to be the gold standard test for bone loss.

QCT (quantitative computed tomography): tests the bone of the spine, and is used experimentally to test the hip as well. The downside of this test is it gives more radiation than the others (This test gives a range of about 60 to 600 REM of radiation, with older machines giving the most, and newer ones the least. The other bone tests listed above give only a few (or less) REM per scan. To give you a means of comparison, a chest X ray gives about 20–50 REM, and a full dental X ray gives about 300 REM.) This test also costs more than the others—about $300 per scan. The other tests are all about even at $100–150 per scan.

Some experts are trying to use ultrasound or sound wave tests to detect bone problems, but this method has not been proven effective. Also, regular X-ray exams are thought to be inadequate tests for osteoporosis.

WHEN TO HAVE YOUR BONES TESTED

There is some disagreement over when, and how often, you should have your bones tested. The National Osteoporosis Foundation (NOF) urges testing for all women approximately six months after menopause or after menstruation stops due to having the ovaries removed or for any other reason. These experts argue that if women were tested at this time, we would find out who has low bone density and is at risk for fractures; then early, preventive treatments could be started. This is a costly ideal, however. Each woman should consider her own risk and discuss it with her doctor. The NOF also recommends testing for the following groups: patients who are on long-term glucocorticoid therapy, those with asymptomatic hyperparathyroidism, and those with abnormalities in the bones of the spine or a spinal disease called roentgenographic osteopenia. If you fall into any of these groups, talk to your doctor about screening. Keep in mind that depending on your situation, you might have to pay for the screening test yourself.

EFFECTIVENESS OF SCREENING

In general, the screening tests listed earlier are quite reliable, but for a variety of reasons, experts feel that bone density measurements are less effective in women who are many years past menopause. First, these women are more likely to have other diseases present that can interfere with screening. Second, they are more likely to have fractures and other deformities caused by more advanced osteoporosis, which can throw off bone measurements. In addition, the bone marrow of postmenopausal women and even their cardiovascular structure can impair screening. Ask your doctor about the reliability of screening for *your* particular case, and if you have already been screened, ask how clear the results actually are.

TREATMENT FOR BONE LOSS

STEP ONE: FIND OUT THE CAUSE OF YOUR BONE LOSS

Osteoporosis is *not* a single, isolated problem. It has many different causes. As a result, the only way to treat it properly is to figure out which *source* of osteoporosis you're dealing with and go from there. So if, for instance, your bone loss is caused or accelerated by a particular medication you're taking, like steroids, you might be able to vary the dose or regimen to reduce the adverse effect on your bone. If your bone loss is caused by a lack of estrogen after menopause, then hormone replacement might be the right answer for you. If poor diet and lack of exercise are causing your bone loss, your problem might be solved with simple adjustments in these areas. If your bone loss is due to hyperparathyroidism, then a parathyroidectomy (removal of the parathyroid gland) or other solution short of surgery can be tried. Figuring out the cause or causes of your particular bone problem is the first step in designing the right treatment program.

STEP TWO: FOCUS ON BOTH TREATMENT AND PREVENTION OF BONE LOSS

It's worth noting that "prevention" and "treatment" of osteoporosis are closely related, so many of the methods I have already suggested for preventing bone loss—such as getting adequate calcium in your diet, and doing weight-bearing exercise several times per week—will also help *treat* osteoporosis if you have it. No single drug or other bone-preserving regimen will work without these basic building blocks of healthy strong bone.

PREVENTING FALLS

One of the best ways to protect your bones, especially once they've become porous, is to avoid traumatizing them. Many women are now learning to avoid the bone-threatening falls that leave so many of us home-bound or dependent on 24-hour, long-term care. Ninety percent of hip fractures result from falls, and nearly four in ten people over the age of 65 have at *least* one fall per year.

There are several approaches to preventing falls, but the three main categories to think about are (1) medications or beverages that upset your balance, (2) obstacles in your home or greater environment and (3) basic health problems that make you vulnerable to falls.

For the first category, alcohol is high on the list—when you're drunk, you're far more likely to lose your balance than when you're sober. Also in this category are medications that affect your thinking or balance, such as long-acting hypnotic drugs, some antidepressants and antipsychotics, and sleeping pills (especially those that remain in your body for longer periods of time—known as having a "long half-life"). Talk to your doctor or pharmacist about the possibility of timing your medication so that you are least affected in the daytime when you're up and around—and also discuss the possibility of switching to an alternative medication with fewer mental side effects or a shorter half-life.

Within the second category, home obstacles, there is a *lot* you can do to reduce your risk of falling. Experts suggest putting strips on your bathtub to prevent slipping, adding handles or support bars in various parts of the bathroom and elsewhere in the home where you think you might need them, securing all loose rugs, getting proper lighting in all areas of your home and keeping key lights on at night if you tend to get up and walk around. You should also wear supportive shoes with low heels and a moderate grip, and use supports such as canes or walkers when you feel unsteady on your feet. You'd be surprised how much you can do to protect yourself without

spending too much money. Some experts note that physical therapy, appropriate exercise and "gait training" (learning how to walk more safely) can also reduce both the incidence and the severity of falls.

Finally, your overall health will affect your chances of falling. If your vision or hearing is impaired, if you are generally weak from lack of exercise, you are more likely to fall. Have regular checkups so that your vision, hearing and balance can be corrected if need be, and talk to a general physician about your overall body strength and fitness. Sometimes minor changes in your lifestyle can help build strength, flexibility and greater body control. Some believe that low estrogen levels after menopause not only contribute to bone loss, but also impair our sense of balance, predisposing us to falls. This is still controversial, but estrogen replacement, which we discuss in further detail in chapter 10, can be a good bone protector nonetheless.

STEP THREE: CONSIDER THE PROS AND CONS OF THE DRUG OPTIONS

If diagnostic tests show that you have significant bone loss and your doctors feel that lifestyle changes will *not* bring adequate protection, you should consider medication. As with all drugs, you will have to weigh the benefits of treatment against the risks, and determine if the regimen is right for you. Most likely the first option your doctor will discuss is hormone replacement, which is discussed above and in chapter 10. Following is a list of other medications currently being used, both in general practice and experimentally, for the treatment of bone loss:

Calcitonin.

Besides hormone replacement, calcitonin is the only other approved drug for the treatment of osteoporosis in the U.S. This drug is in fact a synthetic version of a hormone we make in our own thyroid gland. It has been approved to be given by injection only, which makes some patients leery about it—but scientists are studying a nasal spray form of the drug which is already available in Europe. In addition to *reducing* bone loss, calcitonin has been shown to reduce some of the *pain* associated with osteoporotic fractures in some patients, according to Dr. C. Conrad Johnston, Jr., former director of the division of endocrinology and metabolism at the Indiana University School of Medicine. This is an important and desirable side effect of the drug. Calcitonin is considered a good choice for women with osteoporosis who are fifteen or more years past menopause, as well as for those who have a strong family history of osteoporosis.

On the down side, about one in six patients on calcitonin suffer from nausea (which sometimes disappears) and others report flushing of the skin while taking the drug. Calcitonin is costly—about two to three thousand dollars per year, which insurance won't always cover. Finally, there is some early evidence that the effectiveness of calcitonin might wear off after a few years in some patients. Dr. Johnston reports that in some cases, varying the dose of your treatment, or trying cycled therapy—that is, several months on and several months off treatment—can help offset this problem. The research in this area is still relatively new, but it's worth discussing with your health care team.

Bisphosphonates.

These drugs, with names like etidronate, alendronate, residronate and others, are still in *experimental* use for osteoporosis. This means that the Food and Drug Administration (FDA) requires you to enroll in a formal clinical study in order to use them. The bisphosphonates have been shown to slow bone loss. Etidronate has been widely used in the treatment of other bone diseases such as Paget's disease. For this reason, many doctors prescribe it for osteoporosis without FDA approval.

On the down side, because etidronate is poorly absorbed by the intestine, you must take the drug after complete fasting for several hours; experts feel that drinking even a small beverage before taking the medication can impede its absorption. Some patients experience mild stomach upset and/or nausea while taking the drug, but other side effects are rare or insignificant. We will have to wait years for the long-term safety and side effect record on these drugs.

A controversy arose over etidronate when, after showing a *decrease* in the bone fracture rate after two years on the drug, scientists found an unexplained *increase* in fractures the following year. It is now believed that this latter finding was the result of statistical errors, and many leaders in the field of osteoporosis treatment feel that the "grandchildren" of etidronate—that is, the newer generations of bisphosphonates—hold strong potential for the treatment of bone loss.

Sodium Fluoride.

Also under experimental study for bone loss (and therefore available only through formal research programs), sodium fluoride once held great promise as a bone *promoter*. The trouble is, some scientists think this drug, particularly in high doses, promotes brittle bone, not healthy bone, and may therefore contribute to fractures of the hip even as it reduces fractures of the spine. Dr. Susan Allen, associate professor of medicine at the University of Missouri School of Medicine in Columbia, points to newer evidence that the drug is more effective at a lower dose, and when given in a slow-release fashion—but this remains to be seen. The side effects of this treatment include stomach upset and some pain in the legs and feet. Again, researchers are considering whether a slower-release formula of this drug would cause fewer adverse side effects.

FURTHER DOWN THE ROAD

Antiestrogen Compounds.

You may have heard of a drug called tamoxifen which has received lots of media attention as a treatment and even preventive for breast cancer. Tamoxifen is known as an "antiestrogen" compound, and some experts believe that this kind of drug holds promise for bone preservation. This may sound strange, since we just discussed the fact that estrogen protects bone, but antiestrogen drugs work differently in selected parts of the body. The Eli Lilly company received some attention at a 1993 osteoporosis meeting for their antiestrogen drug, raloxifene. According to Lilly's executive director of skeletal disease research, Dr. John Termine, early studies suggest that this drug might bring some of the benefits of estrogen replacement therapy, but *without* the risks of breast cancer promotion—a concern with estrogen therapy. Other experts I interviewed were excited about the potential for this type of drug. Large studies with several thousand patients began in 1993, but it will be several years before we have solid answers on this drug's effectiveness and safety.

Vitamin D Analogs.

Not to be confused with the vitamin D that's found in your regular supplement tablets, vitamin D analog is a potent drug that reduced spinal fractures in studies of post-menopausal women.

Parathyroid Hormone.

Parathyroid hormone has been studied for many years and still interests many researchers as a possible treatment for bone loss. When given by injection daily along with oral vitamin D, parathyroid hormone increases bone density. The problems center around the fact that there is a very narrow safe dose range for the drug, so it must be given by injection and patients closely monitored. It's thought that too *much* of this drug would *harm* bone, not help it.

Growth Factors.

Scientists are aggressively looking at the potential role of growth factors, which are similar to growth hormones, in treating a wide variety of problems, and bone loss is high on that list. The goal is to stimulate bone production, a more aggressive approach than slowing bone loss. Results are several years down the road. According to Dr. Gregory Mundy, head of the division of endocrinology and metabolism at the University of Texas Health Science Center at

San Antonio, the challenge will be to grow bone cells but *not* to stimulate excessive growth of other cells in the body (which could promote cancers). Dr. Mundy believes that growth factors will be at the forefront of bone preservation *and* fracture healing in the future.

STEP FOUR: MANAGE THE PAIN

If fractures from osteoporosis have caused pain, immobility or trouble doing everyday tasks, you should consider physical therapy. This step can and should be integrated into other forms of treatment, whether you choose hormone replacement, other medication or just lifestyle changes. By retraining you to use your body for things as simple as driving your car, cooking, or lifting your grandchildren, physical and occupational therapists can make your mental and physical life easier. Believe it or not, exercise progams prescribed by physical therapists have been known to give back an inch of height, increase flexibility and reduce pain for women with even the most severe cases of osteoporosis. The exercises aim to stretch and strengthen the back muscles. For women with additional pain from arthritis or osteoarthritis, physical therapy can be even more important. Experts find that those who continue their therapists' regimens at home have the best results.

You should also discuss pain medication with your health care team. Sometimes occasional over-the-counter preparations are adequate, but for more severe pain, you might need prescription medications. Whatever you use, be sure never to take more than your doctor advises—despite what you may think when you're in pain, more is *not* necessarily better. If you aren't getting relief from the drug you're using, you'd be better off finding a different option than taking more and more of the unhelpful drug. Also, nondrug therapies like massage, heat or icing therapy and other pain-relief regimens could make an important contribution.

YOUR ACHING FEET

Go to a region where no one wears shoes—that of certain African tribespeople, or some fishing boat workers in Hong Kong, for example—and you will not find foot problems of the sort that affect Western women in epidemic proportions. Most foot problems are a product of modern civilization and the vanity we pour into foot-constraining fashion. In fact, Japanese women, who used to wear nice, open, foot-friendly sandals before World War II and had no foot ailments to speak of, started getting serious foot problems after they were exposed to Western footwear following the war. When we lock our feet into narrow, pointy, high-heeled, stiff-soled or otherwise ill-fitting shoes, we're performing a modern version of ancient Chinese foot-binding, with the same effect: destruction of the normal shape and growth of bones and other foot structures—and a lot of pain. The foot takes on the shape of the shoe, rather than the shoe being fit to the shape of the foot!

Women are hard-hit by foot problems because we're more likely than men to wear the kinds of tight, narrow, high-heeled shoes that cause problems. Even flat shoes can damage the feet if they're stiff and narrow. In addition, our bones are more flexible than men's, so we're more vulnerable to damage. While men do have problems with the bones of their feet, they're much more rare, thanks to the low-heeled, more vulnerable to damage. While men do have problems with the bones of their feet, they're much more rare, thanks to the low-heeled, wider shoes they're more likely to wear.

If you want to know what *normal* feet look like, says orthopedic surgeon Carol Frey, director of the Orthopedic Foot and Ankle Center in Los Angeles, take a look at a healthy baby's feet. You'll find that they are pretty squared off at the toe, there aren't any lumps and bumps on or around the toes, corns and calluses are absent, and so on. Your feet could look that way too, if you stuck to wide, flat, flexible shoes or athletic shoes *or* better yet, if you ran around barefoot some of the time. Here are some of the common problems that arise—and some solutions for them—when we abuse our feet:

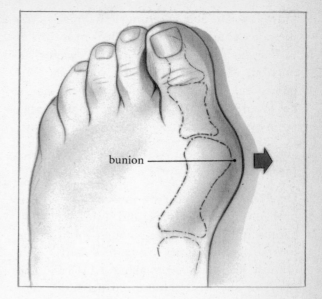

bunion

BUNIONS

Those big, tender bumps on the sides of your big toes, the drift of your big toes toward your other toes—those are bunions, among the most common foot problems in women. The bunion, which refers to the bump itself and comes from the Latin word for turnip, affects 54% of American women, according to Dr. Frey's research. Only 10% of men have the problem. Not all bunions hurt, but some can be extremely painful. They can also grow so large it's almost impossible to find shoes that fit. To blame are shoes that are tight and narrow in the toe box. High heels worsen the pressure.

Solutions: If your bunions don't hurt and aren't making life difficult in any way, there's no need for invasive procedures. Switch to shoes with a wide instep, ample room in the toe area—width is the key—and, if you have a bit of discomfort, pads inside your shoes may help.

Exercises can also help, Dr. Frey finds: stretch your big toe in the *opposite* direction from where it's drifting—that is, away from the other toes. These stretches probably won't reverse pain or deformity, but they can help you if your bunions are in an early stage.

If you're having a lot of pain, or if your bunions are enormous and it's hard to find shoes that fit, you may be a candidate for surgery. Warm foot baths may soothe the pain temporarily, but they don't cure the underlying problem. To get rid of bunions, your surgeon will actually break the affected big toe(s), remove the bunion and restore normal shape to the foot. Ask to see before and after pictures to give you an idea of the possible outcome of your surgery. Expect to spend several weeks in something called a postoperative shoe—not exactly a fashion statement, but then again, that's probably what got you into this situation in the first place. You won't be able to run or work out competitively using your feet for a few months, but you will be able to resume low-impact activities after about eight weeks. You'll miss time at work, which can be costly in more ways than one, but when you're back on your feet, your pain should be relieved. Now your goal should be to prevent the problem from happening again by wearing proper-fitting shoes every day.

HAMMERTOE

Here's #2 on the list of most-common foot problems among women, and it's easy to spot: because they aren't given enough room in the toes of pointy shoes, your toes curl under (almost like your feet making a fist) and the knuckles of your toes bump up, becoming very prominent and exposing the bones to the tops of your tight shoes. Because they're crunched, the tendons on these toes tend to contract, making the problem worse.

Solutions: As with bunions, if the problem is painless and isn't getting in the way of wearing

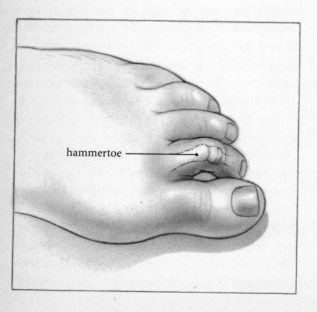

hammertoe

shoes, you should be able to avoid surgery—if you start wearing shoes and stockings with plenty of toe room, that is (width and height). But you may get a related problem on *top* of the protruding joints: corns. As the toe knuckles rub against the top of too-tight, narrow-toed shoes, corns (which are like thick calluses) often develop. You may be able to shave the corns down with an emery board or pumice stone after a shower or bath—mineral oil or rich emollient creams can help. Over-the-counter corn remedies contain acids that may be helpful, and shoe pads can also offer relief, but neither cures the underlying cause: that is, the protruding bone under the corn. If you can't wear corns down yourself, your doctor can do it with a scalpel or other tool. This may sound gruesome, but actually doesn't hurt because we're talking about dead thick skin.

Only if hammertoes become so prominent that they hurt, or they're getting in the way of normal activities, should you consider surgery. In this procedure the protruding bones will be shaved down.

BONE SPURS

These are knobby bony growths on various parts of the feet where tendons and ligaments are so tight they actually pull the bone, causing it to grow out of its proper alignment. Most bone spurs develop on the heel (and are called heel spurs). They usually *don't* cause pain or any other problems.

Solutions: Heel spur surgery is very *overperformed.* Many women are referred for an operation on these common and harmless protrusions. Certain stretches, such as leaning against a wall and stretching the Achilles tendon in

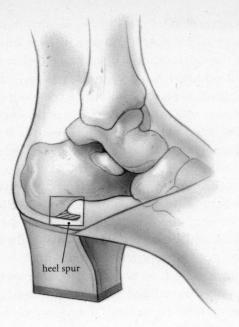

heel spur

stretches for the tightened tissues in your feet. Another nice foot stretch involves rolling your feet back and forth on a small can of juice on the floor until your feel your foot loosening up.

Heel pads or cups can also help promote comfort, as can wearing low-heeled shoes with a proper arch.

If you're having pain with a bone spur, surgery may be appropriate. First try removing any corns or other skin problems that may have developed on top of the spur; if your pain remains, consider surgery to shave down the bone.

ABOUT SHOES

BUYING SHOES

Dr. Frey advises women to shop for shoes late in the day, when feet are at their largest. Fit the shoe to your larger foot (about two-thirds of women have one foot larger than the other). Don't get hooked on one shoe size for life: most women's feet grow larger over the years: it's best to have your foot resized every few years or so, especially after pregnancy. Choose shoe fabrics that stretch and breathe, like soft leather (*not* patent leather). These fabrics may be more costly but they'll save you money down the line when you don't have problems with your feet. Choose shoes with a rounded, wide toe box and make sure there's about a half inch of room between the tip of your longest toe and the end of your shoe. You should be able to wiggle all of your toes when you're wearing the shoe. Do *not* listen to shoe salespeople who tell you "the shoe will stretch." Shoes only stretch when your feet force them to do so; that is, when the shoe is too tight! Shoes should fit comfortably when you walk out of the store in them. Remember, wearing the right shoes will prevent the vast majority of foot ailments.

If you insist on wearing high heels, Dr. Frey adds, stick to two and one-quarter inches or *less*, for no more than three hours at a stretch. That means slip the shoes off under your desk at work, under the table at dinner, and so on.

There are some shoes on the market now that blend fashion with comfort. Try them on carefully before you buy them—but in general, if they're wide, more flexible and relatively low-heeled, they're probably better than the fashionable shoes you've been wearing in the past.

How to Wash and Groom Your Feet.

Instead of just letting the shower water pour over your feet, clean them gently with whatever cleanser you're using, rinse them off thoroughly and, most importantly, dry them completely afterwards. Leaving feet damp promotes fungal infections. Trim your toenails every couple of months, but don't try to curve them; cut them straight across, to avoid ingrown toenails. If you have pedicures, *do not* let them trim your cuticles; they are meant to be there to protect you from bacterial and fungal infections. If you insist on doing something about large cuticles, push them back gently with a proper tool such as a Hindu stick. Finally, whenever possible, walk around barefoot for a while. It's very good exercise for your feet, which weren't designed by nature to wear shoes in the first place!

Note: If you have diabetes or another health problem that promotes problems with your feet, talk to your doctor about specialized foot care. Walking barefoot may *not* be appropriate for you. Athletic shoes could be a good alternative.

Painful Shoulders and Back

Shoes do it to our feet; too-heavy pocketbooks, briefcases, babies on our hips and phones in the crook of our necks do it to our shoulders and back. "Overuse syndrome" is the catchall phrase that orthopedic surgeons use to describe the musculoskeletal problems so common in all of us—but especially women. In fact, the muscles are more often the problem than the bones, but we often *think* of these pains as bone pain. Women may be vulnerable to upper body aches and pains because we tend to be weaker on top than men. When was the last time you did 30 push-ups without feeling like you were going to collapse? This was required of many men in gym class, but fewer women. We are *not* inherently weak in our upper bodies: on the contrary, trained women athletes develop excellent upper body strength, tone and flexibility and do *not* have the problems so many of us have with overuse injury. But for the rest of us, even if we're in good cardiovascular shape, our upper body strength leaves a lot to be desired—and puts us at risk.

According to Dr. Jo A. Hannafin of the Hospital for Special Surgery in New York, one of the most common offending activities is carrying a heavy bag *on one side* year in, year out. We tend to make a habit of carrying our purses on one side, or toting a baby under the same arm or on the same hip. The result is that the muscles in our shoulders shorten and tighten in response to chronic overuse. The solution is to switch your carrying side day to day or week to week, and do a range of motion exercises for your head and neck: tip your head to the right slowly and gently, resting it on your right shoulder; then tip your chin to your chest; then rest your left cheek on your left shoulder; then look up at the ceiling, tipping your head back. Repeat this several times until you feel the area loosening up.

Holding the phone in the crook of the same side of your neck is also a bad idea. Try switching sides if your neck and shoulders ache—or better yet, get a headset that doesn't require any neck acrobatics at all!

Another common way to get shoulder overuse problems, Dr. Hannafin adds, is to use a computer keyboard that's too high up, so your elbows are lifted all day long. When your elbows are lifted, your shoulder muscles become strained. Drop your hands into your lap and see how much better your shoulders feel. Then either raise your chair or lower your keyboard to a point where your shoulders are completely relaxed.

If you have deep, aching pain inside your shoulders that flares up when you comb your hair or perform similar activities, you may have developed chronic problems from overhead lifting (such as putting things on a high shelf repeatedly). What may be going on is that your big outer shoulder muscles, called the deltoids, are developing an imbalance with your deep inner muscles, called the rotator cuff muscles. Often the inner muscles aren't strong enough to keep up with the outer ones. A little fluid-filled sac called the bursa that sits inside this region can become inflamed and painful; this is called bursitis. This problem is especially common in women in their 50s and 60s. The solution: strengthen and stretch your rotator cuff muscles.

The best way to protect your upper body musculoskeletal health *in general* is to work out the area regularly, building both strength and flexibility. This doesn't necessarily mean going to the gym, although that's one good option. Weightlifting and other so-called resistance exercises are terrific for women since they not only make the muscles more fit, they also help protect against bone loss, as discussed earlier. You can also do stretching and toning exercises in your home (try squeezing your shoulder blades together behind your back and doing a couple of push-ups each day until you build up to a higher level: these are two exercises women don't do often enough). In addition to formal workouts, physical activities that work the upper body—like kneading bread, working in the garden, and so on—are terrific too. (Of course, if you have been diagnosed with osteoporosis and are prone to fractures, don't do *any* stress-bearing exercise without your doctor's approval and, ideally, the advice of a physical therapist trained in helping osteoporosis patients. As you may already have learned the hard way, even minor stressors can cause fractures in porous or brittle bones.)

If you find yourself with chronic aches or pains anywhere in your body, you probably can't tell if they're caused by bone, muscle or other problems. See your regular doctor, an internist with training in musculoskeletal problems or an orthopedic surgeon to be fully examined.

TEETH

Because teeth are anchored in bone, some experts believe they too are vulnerable when bone problems develop. When osteoporosis weakens the jaw bones that anchor the teeth and a lack of calcium in the diet reduces tooth strength, some say teeth can loosen and, in extreme cases, fall out. The data on this is controversial, but there's enough evidence that dentists and other oral health experts urge women with significant bone loss to be even more vigilant about oral hygiene, including regular brushing, flossing and visits to the dentist. Increasingly, experts are coming to believe that dental health—or lack of it—is yet another important sign of overall bone health as we age.

Women are also prone to gum (gingival) problems at times of hormonal change. During puberty, menstruation, pregnancy and menopause, for example, women may experience dental problems as a result of severe gingivitis (inflammation of the gums that can cause bleeding, pain and swelling, and can weaken the teeth). The most common symptom women will notice when hormones are changing is bleeding gums brought on by little or no pressure. This can be scary, especially if there is lots of blood; but it's rarely a big problem. Usually, according to Howard Glazer, president-elect of the Academy of General Dentistry, it's simply a matter of the gums becoming increasingly sensitive to plaque and other dental irritants—not a fundamental change in gum or tooth health.

You certainly *don't* want to start having

unnecessary invasive tests or X rays during pregnancy. If your gums bleed heavily during pregnancy or at other times of hormonal change, experts recommend more frequent visits to the dentist (more than the general twice-a-year regimen) and more vigilant oral hygiene to prevent irritants from building up in the teeth. The old saying, "For every baby, lose a tooth," is pure myth. When you eliminate irritants with good oral hygiene, bleeding problems usually improve. Throughout pregnancy, however, even with excellent brushing and flossing care, *some* bleeding may continue. After delivery your oral health should return to normal. If it doesn't, talk to your dentist; this is a better time to do a more thorough investigation.

Another gender-specific dental risk: Barbara Steinberg, professor of dental medicine at the Medical College of Pennsylvania, warns that some women taking oral contraceptives (the Pill) are at greater risk of developing painful "dry sockets" after oral surgery to remove wisdom or other teeth. Dry sockets are areas with poor clot formation that can cause excruciating pain and can lead to infection. If you're taking the Pill and having invasive oral surgery, discuss this risk with your dentist and be sure that he/she monitors you closely for the first sign of a problem. The sooner you're treated (possibly with preventive antibiotics) the less pain and risk you'll have to endure.

FOR MORE INFORMATION ON BONE HEALTH

NATIONAL OSTEOPOROSIS FOUNDATION
1150 17th St. NW, Suite 500
Washington, DC 20036
202-223-2226

AMERICAN ORTHOPEDIC FOOT AND ANKLE SOCIETY, INC.
701 16th Ave.
Seattle, WA 98122-4525
800-235-4855

AMERICAN ACADEMY OF ORTHOPEDIC SURGEONS
6300 North River Rd.
Rosemont, IL 60018-4262
800-346-2267
708-823-7186

AMERICAN PODIATRIC MEDICAL ASSOCIATION
9312 Old Georgetown Rd.
Bethesda, MD 20814
800-ASK-APMA
301-571-9200

AMERICAN DENTAL ASSOCIATION
211 East Chicago Ave.
Chicago, IL 60611
312-440-2500

ACADEMY OF GENERAL DENTISTRY
211 East Chicago Ave.
Suite 1200
Chicago, IL 60611
312-440-4300

AMERICAN ASSOCIATION OF ORAL AND MAXILLOFACIAL SURGEONS
9700 West Bryn Mawr Ave.
Rosemont, IL 60018
800-822-6637

CHAPTER FIVE

YOUR SKIN, HAIR AND NAIL HEALTH

With her skin deeply tanned by constant exposure to the sun, she had the shriveled appearance of a wind-dried shrimp.

—Li Ang, *The Butcher's Wife*

For those of us bound by the constraints of hurried modern life, tending to our skin, hair and nails is a luxury that quickly goes by the wayside. At best, we give a few spare moments to improving their cosmetic appearance. But their health gets short shrift. The fact is, you can use those same few minutes each day not just to make your skin, hair and nails presentable, but also healthy and durable for the long haul. And despite what the person behind the cosmetics counter tells you, you DON'T have to spend a lot of money accomplishing either goal. Read on.

WHAT IS SKIN AND WHY SHOULD YOU TAKE CARE OF IT?

Your skin is the place where the environment meets your body, the interface between everything healthful—as well as everything toxic—that the environment has to throw at you. Nature has prepared the skin for this "gateway" role in several ways. First, the outer layers of skin, called the epidermis, form a barrier of sorts to protect the inner layers. The most outer layer, called the stratum corneum, is made up of dead cells which shield the underlying, living skin cells. The deepest layer, called the dermis, consists of protein substances called collagen and elastin which make the skin pliable, toned, resilient and healthy looking. Women's skin is thicker and consists of more loosely packed fibers than men's—and we have fewer androgens (hormones), so our skin tends to get drier than men's.

Every day, our skin is assaulted by a series of toxins, from pollution to allergens. The biggest offender to the skin, no doubt, is the sun. Most of us have heard this warning so many times it goes in one ear and out the other. But it's time to listen up. There's a lot you don't know about sun damage and your skin . . . and what you don't know can kill you.

THE HARD FACTS ABOUT SKIN DISEASE

There are countless important skin diseases that affect women, but the one we'll focus on for the moment is skin cancer. Skin cancer rates are exploding in this country: nearly a half million people will get basal cell skin cancer this year, and 32,000 will get malignant melanoma, the deadliest skin cancer (in some areas, this disease is thought to be quite *under*reported). Six thousand eight hundred will die of it. One in five Americans will get some form of skin cancer in her or his lifetime, and that number is growing by a few percent a year. The American Academy of Dermatology estimates that we lose between 220 million and 1 billion dollars a year to skin disease treatment and lost productivity. The vast majority of skin cancer cases *and* deaths could be prevented through proper skin protection, avoiding the sun, and early detection of pre-malignant changes in the skin.

Less dire but perhaps no less traumatic for some women, other skin diseases like psoriasis, severe acne, lupus-related skin problems, and allergic reactions to cosmetics, affect millions of women and are also, in many cases, preventable

and treatable. Our culture is so preoccupied with what we can do to make our skin look "prettier," spending billions of dollars on questionable potions and promises, that we neglect many of the steps we could take to make our skin healthier.

DAILY CARE OF YOUR SKIN

A stroll through the cosmetics section at your local shopping center would suggest that daily skin care is a complex, multistep process that costs an arm and a leg. Remember, there are dozens of skin-care and cosmetics companies making a fortune on that premise. It's a very expensive myth, and you don't have to fall prey to it. Every dermatologist I have interviewed feels that women are being taken for a ride by false claims on everything from toners and scrubs to antiaging creams. Here's their consensus on how to properly care for your skin, every day:

Wash skin daily with a nonsoap cleanser. Especially avoid deodorant soaps on your face. If your skin is very dry, or if you live in an area with little pollution, one wash a day is sufficient—perhaps at night to wash away dirt and/or makeup. If your skin is oily, or if you live in a filthy city, two or even three washes a day may be preferable, as long as you're washing gently and not using too harsh a cleanser. Be your own judge—if your skin feels dry, your cleanser is too harsh. A cleanser with a pH between 5 and 7 is good. Some of the cleansers dermatologists recommended are: Neutragena, Cetaphil, Unscented Dove, Basis and Purpose.

Don't rub your skin to dry it. Pat it gently with tissue or a soft clean towel. Rubbing not only abrades the skin, making it more vulnerable, but also tugs on the skin's elasticity, over time making it more prone to sagging.

Believe it or not, sunscreen is part of the *daily* skin care regimen of most dermatologists. About 80% of your lifetime sun exposure is from day-to-day exposure, not from intentional tanning. Even if you don't actively seek a tan, you're exposed to skin-damaging sun just by being outside, walking from place to place. Your face and hands are most often exposed. If you think that aging causes the wrinkling and discolored spots on your face and hands, you're wrong. It's the sun. If you're not a nude sunbather, just take a look at the skin on your bottom; chances are it looks a *lot* more youthful than the skin on your face, hands, or neck. Protect yourself from the sun and your skin will, for the most part, maintain its even color and smoothness as you grow older.

SUNSCREEN

Use a sunscreen with an SPF (sun protection factor) of 15 or greater. Apply the sunscreen evenly to avoid a streaky, partial sunburn. If you have acne or are prone to oily skin, you might prefer a gel-form sunscreen, but these need to be reapplied more often than creams if you're perspiring or going into water. Look for a full-spectrum sunscreen, one that filters out both UVA and UVB rays, as both cause wrinkling and sunburn. If you're sensitive to the ingredient PABA (Para-aminobenzoic acid, which absorbs UV rays), just look for a PABA-free lotion.

Even those who know to use sunscreen often use it incorrectly. The two biggest mistakes: #1: We don't use enough of it. A full fluid ounce is what you need to cover your body. Measure out this amount and take a good look at it: chances are, it's a *lot* more than you usually put on your body. Mistake #2: We don't cover our entire bodies with sunscreen. Oft-overlooked body parts include the ears, the back of the neck and other easy-to-forget or hard-to-reach places. Have a friend help you.

What to do about SPFs? Even though this guideline has been around for *years,* many people still don't understand what it means. An SPF of 15 means that if it would take you 10 minutes to get a sunburn *without* protection, this lotion will multiply that time by 15 (10 minutes × 15 SPF = 150 minutes or two and a half hours before you burn). Is a higher SPF always better? Up to a point, yes. But keep in mind that there's no such thing as a *total* sunblock. While sunscreens with an SPF of 15 block 93% of the sun's rays, one with an SPF of 35 blocks just 97%—an improvement, but certainly not doubly good. Because you get so little bang for your buck once you're over the 15 SPF level, there are some who think the highest SPF lotions—now at 50 SPF—can be a bit of overkill. Finally, remember to choose sunscreen that filters both UVA and UVB rays, since scientists now know that *both* kinds of ultraviolet rays cause cancer and premature aging.

OTHER TIPS FOR PROPER SUNSCREEN USE

- Apply it 20–30 minutes *before* going into sunlight.
- Reapply it after swimming or lots of sweating.
- Apply to places you might not ordinarily think of, like your lips. They burn too.

Moisturizers. Most dermatologists recommend a daily moisturizer. You *can* simply use a sunscreen with a built-in moisturizer to avoid using multiple products. Be careful, however, to check the SPF (sun protection factor) level if you use a combination product. An SPF of 15 and over is good. And make sure it has both UVA and UVB protection. If you're going to use a regular, nonsunscreen moisturizer, look for a "noncomedogenic" kind—that is, one that doesn't promote clogged pores or acne. Light, oil-free moisturizers are often the least offensive to the skin. Of course there are plenty of dry-skinned women who swear by heavy, creamy lotions, too—so use what works for you. During the summer, you might need less moisturizer (unless you're swimming and sunning) since your skin will be more moist. In winter, you might want to apply moisturizer both morning and night, after cleansing. While some skin doctors recommend that you leave your skin a bit damp after washing and use moisturizer to seal that dampness into your skin, Dr. Rachelle Scott of The New York Hospital recommends a different approach. To avoid overuse of moisturizers, she advises, try waiting 30 minutes *after* washing before using your moisturizer. Then, look in the mirror: those parts of your face that are already producing oil *don't* need additional moisturizing. Experiment and find the best balance for you.

FOR VERY DRY SKIN. Apart from genetics, the external environment is usually the cause of excessively dry skin. Artificial heat and a lack of humidity can sap skin of moisture and leave it cracked and uncomfortable. If moisturizers aren't doing the trick for you, hydrometers are a great solution—but few people have these in their homes. Humidifiers

are more common, and they're helpful, too. Keep the humidity at about 40% in your home. According to Dr. Jerome Litt, author of *Your Skin: From Acne to Zits,* if your plants wilt, your furniture cracks, and your doors shrink, you can be sure your skin is suffering too—and it's time for more moisture in your home or apartment.

And that's it. That's all there is to it: cleaning, protecting and moisturizing. Your daily skin regimen: three steps, your choice of two or three products.

COMMON MISTAKES IN DAILY SKIN-CARE REGIMEN

1. **Overscrubbing.** People with blemishes often are the worst culprits of overscrubbing their faces, as they're trying to "clean away" the problem. In fact, rubbing aggravates the problem. Gentle cleaning and drying is the best approach. Remember, we're talking about your face, not a table surface!

2. **Overwashing hands.** Dr. Diane Bihova of the NYU Medical Center finds that women wash their hands too frequently and remove the protective lipid layer from the surface of the skin, making the skin on the hands more vulnerable to damage. Wash when you're dirty!

3. **Using too many products or too much of a single product.** Remember, cosmetics and other skincare products are often made up of dozens of chemicals. When you put several on your face at once, you're conducting a chemical experiment! Sometimes the chemicals interact in ways that are harmful to the skin. Keep it simple and you'll be better off.

4. **Too much exfoliation.** Women are urged to constantly abrade their skin through facial scrubs and beauty-salon facials. In moderation, it's okay to remove the dead surface skin cells from your face, revealing fresh skin underneath. But when overdone, exfoliation can cause permanently dilated blood vessels and acne mechanica—that is, acne brought on by excessive manipulation of the skin.

5. **Not using sunscreen.** This one's on almost every dermatologist's mistake list. Yes, it's hard to remember to put sunscreen on your face and hands *every day*. Put it next to your toothbrush and you may remember. There's no immediate payoff but 20 years from now when your face is still recognizable, you'll be glad you did it.

6. **Taking too-hot baths.** They may feel great, but they're hard on your skin. Try to avoid piping hot baths; warm is okay.

7. **Fad diets.** The skin, like the rest of your organs, needs a balance of many food types, vitamins, minerals, and fluids. Eating only grapefruit or living on diet pills will show up soon enough in colorless, lifeless skin.

8. **Lack of sleep.** Deprive yourself—and your skin—of sleep, and you'll see the consequences in the mirror. There's no ideal length of time to sleep—whatever makes you feel refreshed when you wake up is adequate.

9. **Sharing makeup.** Sharing cosmetics means sharing the bacteria and other critters that are on others' faces. That can lead to infections, blemishes, and so on. Also, keep your own cosmetics containers tightly sealed.

10. **Using oily makeup.** Cosmetics that are loaded with grease or creams can clog your pores and promote eruptions on your skin. Sometimes creams are hidden in products that *look dry*. Try some on your hand and see if it's greasy before purchasing it.

"ARTIFICIAL" TANNING

A WORD ABOUT TANNING SALONS

Anyone who tells you there's a "safe" way to tan is lying. There's nothing safe about getting ultraviolet rays on your skin, and that's exactly what happens in a tanning salon—just like it happens on the beach. Astonishingly, even with the abundant information we have about the dangers of the sun, we make about a *million* indoor tanning visits a day in the U.S. From health clubs to beauty salons, they promise everything from "safe" tanning to cures from skin diseases.

First, you should know that if you have a skin condition that requires light or heat treatment, the procedure can often be done in a hospital setting with proper control over the amount of light, the timing, and other safety precautions for your skin. As for safe tanning, there's no such thing. The most popular type of sunlamp used in tanning salons today gives off *more* ultraviolet radiation than natural sunlight! Also, the American Academy of Dermatology finds that many salons fail to comply with safety regulations—not using proper timers, for example. Don't subject yourself to needless risk.

SUNLESS TANNING PRODUCTS

Ideally, we will all come to appreciate the beauty of a wide spectrum of skin colors, from the darkest to the palest. But if you're not there yet, and are bothered by the paleness of your skin, you might want to try the so-called "sunless tanning products" that are on the market. Usually in the form of creams and lotions, these products promise to turn your skin darker *without* sunlight. In the past, what they often did was turn you orangy-yellow or orangy-brown—seldom the golden or brown color most tanners seek. Now, there are products containing DHA—short for dihydroxyacetone—an FDA-approved substance that some say turns the skin a fairly realistic tanned shade. Some experts recommend applying the product two to four times per day, and then tapering off to once every few days when you have achieved your desired shade. You might also try washing your skin and gently buffing it afterwards so it's smooth before you apply the lotion.

POTIONS AND LOTIONS

What about all of the toners, scrubs, astringents, strengtheners, pore-minimizers and so on that pack supermarket shelves, are promoted aggressively by manufacturers and promise childlike skin in a matter of weeks? A couple of dermatologists said that if you're *really* feeling greasy even after a thorough cleansing, you might try a nonalcohol "toner" on just the oily parts of your face (if these are your forehead, nose and chin, they're collectively called the T-Zone). But toners are certainly *not* necessary items.

As for scrubs and other exfoliators, not a single dermatologist I spoke with (other than those who are actively employed by cosmetics companies) felt that there was any *need* for these products. If you absolutely insist on using them—whether it's because you believe they work or because you like to have extra bottles in

your cabinet—use them only once a week and keep the following in mind:

Overly abrasive scrubs, such as those made from the pits of apricots or other fruits, can cause hemorrhages and broken blood vessels in the skin, can abrade the skin, and can even cause clogged pores (the opposite of what they're intended to do) by creating little cysts on the skin.

The least abrasive scrubs are made with tetraborate decahydrate granules. They're easier on the skin.

You've probably heard quite a lot lately about **alpha-hydroxy acids, or** AHAs. These are fruit acids which help smooth the look and feel of your skin by removing some its rough surface, and they're found in increasing numbers of moisturizing products. The acids are derived from different sources, such as apples, grapes, citrus fruits, and sour milk (AHAs) and sugar cane (glycolic acid), and they're thought to be safe and nontoxic. Some studies suggest that when applied to the skin, these products reduce fine wrinkling by promoting "shedding" of surface skin cells—one of American women's obsessions—but some dermatologists are still skeptical about how big a difference these products really make. Some of these products contain bleaching agents as well, to fight brown spots. Dr. D'Anne Kleinsmith of West Bloomfield, Michigan finds that they cause less redness and peeling than Retin-A, which promises some of the same kinds of results. Keep in mind that AHAs are available over-the-counter as well as by prescription, and that there is no way to confirm which products will be more or less effective than others. While it's generally thought that products containing higher concentrations of these acids will be more effective at smoothing the skin, in fact some formulations containing a *lower* concentration are better than those with a higher one because of their chemical compositions. Many over-the-counter preparations have between 3% and 7% concentrations of AHA, while prescription forms have higher concentrations. Rather than remaining at the mercy of advertisers, ask a dermatologist for a list of products that he or she finds effective.

As for alleged pore-minimizers, experts say there is no way to permanently reduce the size of your pores. Changes in temperature and certain home remedies like applying fluffy egg whites to your face do just as good a job of *temporarily* minimizing the size of your pores as more costly potions. The key word, however, is *temporarily*. These "remedies" last a couple of hours at best.

ANTIAGING CREAMS

Notice that the wording on antiaging creams claims only that the product "Reduces the 'visible' signs of aging," as an example. Take note of the fact that advertisers *cannot* tell you without being sued that their product actually reverses aging in skin. Sure, products can moisten and plump up your skin, giving the *appearance* of fewer fine wrinkles. But the actual structure of your skin remains pretty much the same. (This may *not* be the case with certain products containing fruit acids, as discussed above. These acids—as well as Retin-A [*see* more below]—have been shown to actually reduce fine wrinkling and other minor signs of aging. But keep in mind that the changes are minimal; there is to date no cream that can significantly turn back the clock. You can be sure when it arrives, you'll be hearing about it.)

Retin-A.

Alternately touted as a miracle antiaging cream and slammed as a potential carcinogen, Retin-A cream has received more press, both glowing and negative, than most any other skin product. In fact, it has been around for many years and is considered quite safe; if anything, it may *reverse* early, precancerous skin changes, rather than causing them. A miracle cream, however, it's not. If you're using the cream to try to take decades off of your skin, forget it.

Retin-A, or retinoic acid, smooths the skin and helps reduce the very *fine* skin wrinkling and discoloration associated with sun exposure and aging. Early results can often be seen after just a few weeks. Retin-A certainly does *not* eliminate deep wrinkles, or create a chemical face-lift. But it does make a difference, for some patients, in the overall quality of the skin, both color and texture, over time by plumping up skin cells that have become flattened with damage. Some dermatologists recommend use of Retin-A for a lifetime, since skin discoloration and signs of aging resume when you stop using the product. But even though the safety record for the product is good, many women don't like the idea of putting what is essentially a medication on their skin for decades. Discuss the issue with your doctor.

Some women, especially those with sensitive skin, report initial reddening or irritation of the skin while using Retin-A. This can be reduced by trying a much more diluted form of the cream and moving up quite gradually to more potent doses. Another complaint about Retin-A is that it makes the skin more sun-sensitive: Dr.

Nia Terezakis, clinical professor of dermatology at Tulane Medical School, says that this is only a temporary problem as the surface skin sheds early in Retin-A use. After a short while, the skin strengthens, and sun sensitivity should disappear.

Note: The pill form of Retin-A, which is used to treat acne, can be quite dangerous for pregnant women; it is known to cause birth defects in fetuses of women taking the drug. The cream form is not known to cause the same problems, but most practitioners prefer to err on the safe side and tell their pregnant patients to avoid the drug completely until after delivery.

PROCEDURES FOR THE SKIN

There are almost as many skin-improving procedures as there are shades of skin. Some are quite beneficial, others useless or even dangerous. How do you decide if any are for you? Here is a brief guide . . . but your best bet is to talk to a dermatologist. These days, many doctors can show you, by means of a computer image, the potential outcome, *for your skin,* of the treatment in question.

Dermabrasion.
A rotating object, like a sanding device, abrades the skin to eliminate tattoos, sun-damaged skin, or mild scarring from acne. This technique can be extremely effective for more surface skin problems. It is not the best choice for deep pitting from severe acne, however.

Peels—Chemical and Other.
It seems like every dermatologist has *some* type of peel these days, using everything from mild to severe fruit acids to chemical compounds like TCA (trichloroacetic acid) and others. Peels differ so dramatically in their ingredients and in their effects that it's important to talk to your doctor about what she or he is using, and why. Your best bet is to try the peel on a tiny area of skin to see what kind of effect it has on *you*—everyone's different. That way, if the effect is harmful in any way, the damage will be minimal. There are both superficial and deep peels. Superficial peels can help eliminate brown spots and other minor discolorations of the skin. Deep peels can be used for more substantial facial lines, but there's a caveat: the stronger the peel, the greater the chance you'll end up with uneven pigmentation.

Collagen Injections.
Originally all the rage for cosmetic procedures like lip-plumping, collagen is actually not a great choice for enhancing skin that has lots of mucous membranes. Collagen *is* useful for wrinkles and scars, minor contour defects and other shallow dips in the skin. Some people are irritated by or allergic to collagen; for them, fat injections might be more desirable.

Fat Injections.
Called "autologous" fat injections, this procedure involves taking fat from elsewhere in the body and injecting it where you desire more fullness or plumpness—such as the lips or the fine wrinkles around the mouth. While the advantage of fat injections over other related procedures is that you're unlikely to reject the fatty substance (after all, this is your *own* fat, from your own body) some complain that this procedure makes only a minor difference and doesn't last all that long. Some patients are pleased with the results, however, and opt for

replumping every couple of months using fat cells harvested and stored by their doctors.

Sclerotherapy.

This is a common procedure in which bloated veins, called varicose veins, are stripped or treated in such a way as to make them collapse and become invisible. Sclerotherapy, as well as saline injection treatments for more minor "spider veins," are safe and effective treatments when done by qualified people. The results are instant: I once watched a treatment that eliminated an enormous patch of purple-blue veins from a woman's leg in about five seconds. It's not painless—there is some stinging from the injection and the saline entering your blood—but it is a quick outpatient procedure. For tiny but visible blood vessels on the face, a different technique is usually used, called electrodesiccation (in which an electric needle is inserted in the vessel, which immediately vanishes). Lasers are also being used on the face and body for removal of birthmarks, other visible conditions involving blood vessels, tattoos, scars and many other problems.

"Cosmetic" Skin Procedures.

There was a time when dermatologists invariably would tell women to stay away from facials and steams at all costs. All of that prodding and squeezing and heat could only bring infection, scald or otherwise damage delicate skin, and widen pores, they said. Today, I am surprised to hear much more support for these treatments—within limits—from medical doctors. One reason is that many salons have taken lessons from the medical community, upgrading their hygiene, using gentler products and less abrasive equipment, and offering noninva-sive, relaxing facials. Dr. Nia Terezakis says that facials—minus the deep squeezing—are just fine for people with *normal* skin. They're like a wonderful massage, she says—and, if you don't expect any miracles from them, "it's your money." If, however, you have skin problems, such as acne, and the facialist wants to do lots of picking and squeezing of your skin—forget it, Terezakis warns. It takes quite a bit of training to empty a pore; the pore goes down about a quarter of an inch into the skin, making proper extraction quite difficult (without damage to the surface skin cells).

Of course, while most facials are perfectly harmless, there are exceptions. One dermatologist told me of a patient whose facialist squeezed warts, not pimples—and spread those warts around the patient's face! Just another reason why squeezing the skin isn't a great idea.

Steams are a different story, Terezakis says. Contrary to what most people believe, steams do not open the pores: They actually swell up the corneal or dead surface layer of skin cells, hydrate them, and tend to have more of a plugging-up than an emptying-out effect.

If you do opt for skin treatment in a salon, make sure that the environment is spotless, that the equipment used is absolutely sanitary (find out how thorough their cleaning process is), and that no strong abrasives or extreme temperatures will be used on your skin.

A FEW WORDS ABOUT PLASTIC SURGERY

It is nothing short of miraculous how much can be done to change our skin, our faces and other parts of our bodies with the use of plastic and reconstructive surgery. Whether you're hoping to repair a congenital abnormality, make yourself more "attractive" on your own terms, or turn back the clock a bit, plastic surgery can create a remarkable array of changes today.

One of the most common procedures—the face-lift—has grown up quite a bit since its early years. In the past, surgeons simply cut (behind the hairline, the ear, the neck, and so on, to disguise the scar) and lifted the outer layer of drooping skin to create a less wrinkled, dowdy appearance. Today, surgeons go deeper under the skin, lifting the tissue (fascia) that lies over the muscles in the face to create a better overall lift and support effect for the skin that sits on top of it. Some surgeons go even deeper than this, lifting facial *muscle*—but this can, in some cases, create a taut, unnatural appearance, says Dr. Petra Schneider, a plastic and reconstructive surgeon in Melbourne, Florida.

Having realistic expectations is the most important thing you, as a patient, can bring to the plastic surgery process. First, you must learn your terminology, and know exactly what it is about your face (for example) you want changed. For instance, a "face-lift" formally means a lift of the skin along the jawline, the neck and a portion of the cheeks. Many patients asking for a face-lift actually want their eyes or their foreheads lifted; these are different procedures that *can* be done in addition to or instead of a traditional face-lift. Other procedures mentioned earlier, such as dermabrasion, chemical peels, and collagen and fat injections can sometimes be combined with face-lifts as well. Liposuction, which we'll discuss more below, can also be combined with face-lifts these days.

Your surgeon should be able to help you determine what improvements can be made in your appearance and what procedures are available to make those improvements. Some surgeons use computer images to show you how *your* face can be altered with surgery. But many of those I interviewed felt that computer images give too glossy and perfect a picture of potential surgical results. Because individuals scar differently and heal differently, it's unrealistic to try to gauge your outcome by means of a computer image. Far more realistic, says Dr. Diane Gerber, a surgeon based in Chicago, are actual "before and after" photographs of patients who had corrections similar to the ones you're considering. Most surgeons can provide these. Sometimes former patients will talk to you about their experiences as well. Ask your doctor for names.

If you're worried about the risks of facial surgery, the good news is that things are better than they were in the past. Recovery time is still a few weeks; this hasn't changed over the years (and you may have symptoms of numbness, swelling and bruising for up to six months after that). But patients often go home the day after surgery, thanks to improved drainage systems, and stitches usually come out after about ten days. Perfections in surgical technique have reduced, but certainly haven't eliminated, the incidence of major complications. Rarely, patients will have permanent numbness in parts of their face, or even a crooked smile, as a result of nerve damage. Severe bleeding under the skin may have to be corrected with follow-up surgery. And of course the risks of anesthesia and infection are always present with a surgical procedure. Ask your surgeon if your procedure can be done under local, rather than general, anesthesia; many minor procedures are done this way today.

It's important to keep in mind that plastic

surgery, while it can turn back the clock, cannot *stop* the clock. The natural aging process and other behaviors that accelerate it will affect your newly taut skin just as it affected your loose skin. Dr. Gerber notes that while well-performed, well-cared-for face-lifts normally hold their shape for about eight to ten years, exposure to excessive sun and smoking can shorten your face-lift's life span to just a couple of years! So don't consider your newly youthful visage immune to the elements. Significant changes in your weight can also take a toll on face-lifts, stretching the skin and leaving it lax once again. Caring for your newly tightened skin with gentle cleansing (as discussed earlier in this chapter), using sunblock, and treating yourself to a well-balanced diet will go a long way to preserving your new younger looks.

LIPOSUCTION

When liposuction (or fat suction) first appeared on the plastic surgery scene, millions of people believed, or hoped, that the magic bullet for toning and weight loss had arrived. Empty the ice cream container, be a couch potato, and just have your fat sucked out occasionally, many daydreamed. Quickly, however, those fantasies were replaced with horror stories about infections and other complications, terrible cosmetic results and even death from liposuction procedures. Many shied away from the procedure or forgot about it altogether.

Today, the truth about liposuction lies somewhere in between fairy tale and horror story. Tremendous improvements have been made in liposuction technique. The three main areas of improvement include replacement of blood lost during surgery, taking out less fat in the first place (2–3 liters is about right), and *not* combining liposuction with other surgeries that predispose the patient to infection (such as bowel surgery, in which lots of bacteria is released). These three changes have significantly reduced the risk of both infection and poor results.

Essentially, liposuction is just what it sounds like: sucking fat out from under the skin, using either traditional vacuum tubing or, more recently, a long syringe-type instrument. Dr. Petra Schneider urges women to look at it not as a weight-loss procedure, but as a contouring procedure. The best results are had when you're at your ideal weight at the time of surgery, since weight gain or loss can throw off your appearance afterwards. Liposuction can be done on many parts of the body, including the thighs, knees, abdomen, hips, even under the arms. The fat can be stored and used for other procedures, such as fat injections (discussed above) or in larger amounts to build up sunken areas like deep scars. In the past, liposuction was recommended only for younger people, since their skin is more elastic and therefore "bounces back" to a tighter position after fat is removed. But today, older patients are having it done as well, with the caveat that they keep their expectations realistic. Liposuction cannot make 70-year-old thighs look like 20-year-old thighs, no matter how skilled the surgeon. As with any cosmetic procedure, approach liposuction with as realistic an idea of your potential result as possible. Look at "before-and-after" pictures of women who have had similar procedures done. Don't imagine that after surgery your body is going to look like a swimsuit model's—unless it was almost there to begin with. Liposuction can be helpful for particular fatty pocket areas, such as the sides of the thighs or hips where dimply fat can resist even faithful dieting and exercise. But if you don't expect miracles, you're less likely to be disappointed.

SKIN CANCER

WHO'S AT RISK FOR SKIN CANCER?

Everyone is at risk for skin cancer. But you're at higher risk if you have a family history of skin cancer, if you have fair skin and light eyes, burn easily when in the sun, work outside or spend lots of time outdoors, have had severe sunburns as a child, have lots of moles on your body naturally (particularly if you have unusual moles), or live in hot, sunny parts of the country. Keep in mind that while you're being exposed to lots of sunlight, your risk of getting skin cancer doesn't immediately jump. Most often, skin cancer appears a decade or two after you've been exposed to the sun. So the problem is deceptive. You think you're doing fine and then discover a problem later.

With many cancers, there are multiple causes—often unknown. Skin cancer is an easier case. The sun is usually the culprit—and it's a powerful one. Not only does the sun burn your skin, but it's also been found to impair the skin's disease-fighting immune system and to damage the nuclei or central controllers of surface skin cells. It also damages the elastic fibers that rest deeper in the skin, robbing it of its springy, youthful quality. If you ever have the chance, Dr. D'Anne Kleinsmith suggests, take a look at the skin on the buttocks of a 90-year-old person and compare it to her face. Far fewer wrinkles, discolored spots, and roughness is what you'll find—unless they've been hanging out on nude beaches. It's amazing that people are willing to trade a fleeting tan for wrinkles and cancer.

Because we know what causes skin cancer, there's a very simple message about preventing it. The vast majority of cases simply would not occur if people (a) avoided the sun, (b) covered themselves with clothing when in the sun, or (c) wore an adequate amount of sunscreen. Few Americans follow these guidelines and, as a result, skin cancer rates are climbing. One Kentucky-based dermatologist told me that 95% of his patients have been overexposed to the sun by the time they reach his office.

DETECTING SKIN CANCER

As we've discussed, the best way to prevent skin cancer is to avoid the sun. The next best thing to prevention, as with many cancers, is early detection. Since many of us were exposed to too much sun as children, even if we're being careful today, we're still at risk of getting skin cancer. Every blistering sunburn of childhood doubles your risk of developing melanoma later in life. You must be vigilant about screening your body for early signs of skin cancer. One approach is to become familiar with your skin in its normal condition with the help of a dermatologist or your family doctor. The best way to do that is to use a bright light and a mirror (or two, for examining hard-to-reach body parts) and slowly examine the entire surface of your skin. Then, once you know potential trouble spots to watch for—for instance, unusual moles, or areas that clearly have had sun damage in the past—you can do self-examinations on a regular basis—perhaps at the same time as do your monthly breast self-exam. Once you're used to doing it, examining your skin will take just a few minutes. The good news is women are better than men at detecting skin cancer in its early stages.

The American Academy of Dermatology has developed an excellent tool to guide you as you examine your skin: it's called the "ABCD" rule for examining moles. First, "A" for asymmetric: If one side of your growth doesn't match the other, have it examined by a doctor. "B" for borders: if the borders or edges of the growth are irregular, "ragged, notched or blurred," have it checked out. "C" for color: If the growth isn't one uniform color, but rather is mottled or speckled, show it to your doctor. Finally, "D" for diameter: A mole greater than 6 millimeters in diameter (which is about the size of the eraser on a pencil), should be examined. Finally, beyond the ABCD's, anything *new* or unusual about the mole—changes in size or color, scaliness or oozing, pain, itchiness or tenderness, or if it spreads into the surrounding skin area—should put you on alert, says the AAD.

What's so great about early detection? For most skin cancers, including the most deadly form, malignant melanoma, very early detection gives a strong chance for cure. The longer you let a suspicious growth or patch of skin remain unexamined, the greater the chance your skin cancer will become untreatable or at least require more drastic treatment, perhaps creating a disfiguring scar or requiring long-term, uncomfortable therapies. People in the health care field know that many of us practice "denial"—that is, we don't like to look for problems on our bodies for fear we'll actually find something serious. Keep in mind that denial can kill you. Taking fast and aggressive action can save your life.

TREATING SKIN CANCER

The most important factor in choosing a treatment for skin cancer is to determine (1) what kind of skin cancer you have, and (2) how advanced the cancer is. Most early cancers that affect only surface cells on the skin can be cured on a quick, outpatient basis with freezing (cryosurgery, using liquid nitrogen) or other techniques, such as an electric current to the skin. Sometimes classical excision is the treatment of choice: that is, cutting the diseased skin out, plus a small margin of healthy skin around the cancer. Radiation, as well as drugs (both applied directly to the skin and taken by mouth) are also in the arsenal of weapons against skin cancer. Two important factors that will come into play in choosing your treatment are the type of cancer you have, the degree of spread (if any), and the type of treatment center you're attending. Some treatment centers have a strong team in a particular treatment area and weak resources for other types, and will therefore push a given method. Your best bet, regardless of what kind of cancer you have, is to visit an NIH-designated cancer center with a variety of options. At the end of this chapter you'll find information on how to contact these organizations.

If your cancer has spread deeper into the skin, you may need a relatively large portion of skin and tissue removed. If you are bothered by the scar that remains after the procedure, you may be eligible for reconstructive surgery in which surgeons take healthy skin and tissue from elsewhere on your body and use it to reshape the damaged area.

The most serious form of skin cancer, called malignant melanoma, has the ability to spread to distant parts of your body. This process is called metastasis—the same term used to describe other cancers when they move from their original site to other parts of the body. The longer you wait to be diagnosed and treated, the more time cancers have to travel. This is why early detection is so very important. If you are diagnosed with malignant melanoma that has spread to other parts of your body, talk to your doctor about how widespread the disease is. Your chance of survival has a great deal to do with the extent of the spread. You also should talk about the different treatment options for metastatic malignant melanoma.

After a certain degree of spread around the body, there is no cure for malignant melanoma. That does *not*, however, mean that you should lose hope if you have this diagnosis. The goal is to control the disease as best as possible, fighting the stray cancer cells with every tool available. It is up to you and your doctor to decide how much discomfort you are willing to endure in treating your cancer. This is true for any disease; there are risks, benefits and side effects for most so-called "systemic" treatments. Systemic treatments are those that target stray cancer cells that are moving throughout your body. Because the cancer is no longer in one site, it's not possible to target a specific area for treatment. Instead, through use of several cancer-fighting tools, including drugs (known as chemotherapy), radiation therapy, conventional surgery, and other promising experimental treatments, doctors can aggressively battle your cancer as it tries to take over more healthy cells.

COSMETICS: COMMON IRRITATIONS AND ALLERGIES

High on the list of common women's skin complaints are reactions to cosmetics. From mascara to moisturizers, from lipstick to nail lengtheners, the products we use to enhance beauty or conceal flaws can cause skin problems for many women.

There are two main kinds of skin reactions: true-blue allergic reactions, and irritations. Irritations usually occur at the site where the product was used (the cheeks for blush, for example) or at a site that comes into contact with the product (such as the eyes after being touched with fresh nail polish). Allergies, on the other hand, can show up in places that were not touched by the product. In addition, they appear not during the *first* use of the product, but in response to a *repeat* use of the product. This is very important, because many people assume they can't be allergic to a product if they had no problems with it in the past. What happens, in fact, is the body becomes sensitized to an ingredient in the product and reacts when it next "sees" that chemical.

What irritation looks and feels like: burning, stinging, itching, red area on the skin. Products that commonly cause irritations include bath soaps, detergents, antiperspirants, eye makeup, moisturizers, permanent solutions, and shampoos.

What an allergic skin reaction looks and feels like: redness, swelling, itching, fluid-filled blisters—generally more severe than an irritation. A list of products that commonly cause allergic reactions and irritations follows.

THE WORST OFFENDERS

Fragrances.
Fragrances are found in just about every type of cosmetic (and household) product, and they can cause allergic reactions—the more serious kind of skin reaction—in many women. There

are over 5000 fragrances out there, and single products often contain more than 300 of them! This means it can be tough to figure out exactly to which fragrance(s) you're reacting.

What to do: You might think that a label "unscented" is a good way to avoid fragrances altogether. That's *not* the case. Products marked "unscented" may in fact contain so-called "masking fragrances" that are used to *block* scent, but can themselves cause skin reactions. Look instead for the label "fragrance free."

Preservatives.

Perhaps culprit #2, preservatives are next on the list of skin-aggravating products. A common cause of skin reactions are the parabens, which can be found in a vast array of products, and can cause a red rash, scaly skin, and swollen eyelids. Manufacturers are responding to people's problems with parabens (a common type of preservative), however; there are now products on the market that are paraben-free.

Lanolin.

Found in many moisturizers, lanolin is usually not too bothersome to healthy skin but some people get irritation reactions from it—such as red, itchy eyes.

Propylene Glycol.

This chemical is commonly found in moisturizers. It causes about 5% of all cosmetic reactions—usually in the form of skin irritations or contact dermatitis.

Assorted Others.

Some ingredients that promise to *help* the skin, such as aloe and vitamin E, can also cause skin problems. The fact is, you don't even get enough aloe in most of these products to do

you any good (the concentration in the plant is about 20%, in the products, 3–5%). So experts' best advice is to keep it simple—the more fancy ingredients, the greater your chance of having a problem with one of them. You may also react to unexpected items like elastic hair bands, or nickel in earrings, for example. Let your dermatologist look at your irritation and help you figure out the cause. Other products that cause irritation more often than allergic reactions are antiperspirants and deodorants. Sometimes friction in the armpit combined with the aluminum salts many of these products contain can cause irritation. Also, the fragrances in some of these products can cause irritations.

HAIR: BASIC CARE

There is nothing wrong with washing your hair daily—the old belief that you'll ruin your hair is just a myth. Because hair is an insoluble protein, it does not dissolve in soap or water. You *can* ruin your hair, however, by treating it improperly while it's wet. Never brush your hair while it's wet—remove tangles with a wide-toothed comb, never stretching or tugging your hair. The worst possible thing you can do to your hair is to "tease" it or "backbrush" it, tugging against the hair's natural direction. Here's why: Hair is like a cable with many wires inside. The outer hair, called the cortex, is like a film of shingles laid down carefully on the hair. Hair normally has luster because the shingles lie flat. If you disturb that normal position, through perms, curling, teasing and so on, you cause those shingles to stand up, making it easier to break or harm the hair.

There's also nothing wrong with brushing your hair every day, but the old myth that you need a hundred strokes a day is just that—a myth. Overbrushing, even when the hair is dry, pulls out hairs that would have stayed in the head for several weeks longer.

Like shampoo, conditioners rarely cause anything more serious than irritation to the skin. In general, they are a *good* thing to use because they encourage the hair "shingles" to lie flat, thereby keeping the hair shiny. They also reduce static electricity in the hair. Some say that protein conditioners are best (they're made with emulsified, ground-up animal proteins) because they stick to the hair better. Dr. Joseph Bark, chairman of dermatology at St. Joseph Hospital in Lexington, Kentucky, likens conditioners to reglueing roof shingles on your home. However, like glue on your roof, conditioners can build up and become heavy and mucky, clogging the area, if you use too much of them. Bark recommends using a conditioner every second or third washing.

HAIR PRODUCTS AND PROCEDURES THAT CAN CAUSE SKIN REACTIONS

While shampoos seldom cause anything more serious than irritation to the skin (on the eyelids, tops of the ears, or forehead) other hair products and procedures can be far more damaging. Here are the most prominent examples:

Permanent Hair Dyes.
Long-lasting hair dyes can cause severe allergic reactions that show up as redness and itching on the scalp, and severe swelling of the face and eyelids. The offending agent is called PPD—standing for paraphenylene diamene. Some people react so badly their heads swell up like balloons and they need emergency medical attention. If you have *ever* had a serious reaction to a perma-

nent hair dye, you should completely abstain from using them. There are safer alternatives, such as metallic dyes, and vegetable dyes, which are far less likely to cause skin problems. Some dermatologists recommend having a skin patch test either before using permanent dyes the first time around or if you've had even a suspected allergic reaction to one in the past, since repeat exposures can be more severe.

Permanent Waves.
"Perms," as most of us call them, usually involve one of two chemicals: For older "alkaline" perms, the chemical is Ammonium Thioglycolate; for newer "acid" perms, it's glyceryl thioglycolate. Both can cause irritations and even burns to the skin if left on too long.

NAIL PRODUCTS AND PROCEDURES THAT CAN CAUSE SKIN REACTIONS

Several products and procedures can harm your nails, usually by blocking the nail's own well-designed defense system. Considering the fact that it takes several months to grow a full nail, we're pretty hard on our nails. As a bottom line message, remember that there's a reason our nails are designed as they are—and we need all of the regular parts! For instance, the cuticle is an important protective device that helps keep bacteria and yeast out of the nail fold, and should *not* be torn or pushed or clipped away. Just pressing on that part of the nail is unhealthy. Beyond trimming and clipping, however, are the procedures that can seriously damage or destroy your nails *and* cause irritations or full-blown allergic reactions on your skin. Here are a few common troublemakers:

Fake Nails.

Bacteria and fungi thrive underneath fake nails. If you insist on using them, be sure to remove them every three months at the very least. Swelling, redness and/or darkness on your own nails are signs of trouble. If you don't treat the nails and remove the offending product, you run the risk of *permanently* losing your nails! Furthermore, press-on nails often contain resins or acrylic glues (epoxy resin or mephacrylic acid) that may also cause allergic reactions.

Nail Enamels.

The chemical toluene sulfonamide, found in nail enamels, can cause allergic reactions.

Nail Wraps.

Both the enamel in nail wraps and the acrylic adhesives that some contain can cause both irritations and allergic reactions. Sometimes the problem appears on the eyes, after you touch them with the chemical.

Nail Polish.

While these products seldom cause skin reactions, the red and rust-colored polishes can stain your nails a yellowish color until they grow out.

Nail Polish Remover.

This is an extremely drying product that can cause your nails to split. Try touching up your nail polish instead of completely removing it and repainting all the time.

A FINAL WORD ABOUT NAILS

Your nails *can* reflect your general health. If you find that your nails are extremely flat, or that they have prominent transverse lines on them, they might be alerting you to lung or kidney disease. Don't confuse this with typical lines and ridges that develop with age (or if you have the habit of pressing on the moon-shaped portion of your nails). If you're concerned, or if your nails have changed a great deal, show them to your doctor.

TREATING SKIN REACTIONS

Treatments for both skin irritations *and* allergies are usually based upon prescribed topical steroid creams—that is, steroids in a cream form that is applied to the affected area. For severe allergic reactions, oral steroids or even injected antihistamines may be necessary—but this is quite rare. Of course, in addition to medicating the affected skin, you should abstain from using the product (and others that your dermatologist says resemble the offending item), and try to keep the area clean and dry while the skin repairs itself.

After you've healed from a skin reaction, it's a good idea *not* to rush back into using a wide variety of products, since you might not yet know which one caused you the problem. A better approach is to use one product at a time—starting with soap, for instance—and if that's okay, moving on to shampoo, a single item of makeup, and so on.

You should find out as quickly as possible what ingredient(s) caused your problem so you can avoid a repeat episode. Remember that second and third allergic reactions can be far worse than initial reactions. The best detective work is done in your dermatologist's office, where she can develop skin tests using *your* products to locate the offending item.

FOR MORE INFORMATION ON SKIN

FACIAL PLASTIC SURGERY
   INFORMATION SERVICE

AMERICAN ACADEMY OF FACIAL
   PLASTIC AND RECONSTRUCTIVE
   SURGERY, INC.
1110 Vermont Ave. NW, Suite 220
Washington, DC 20005-3522
800-332-FACE (in Canada, 800-523-FACE)

AMERICAN ACADEMY OF
   DERMATOLOGY
930 N. Mecham Rd.
Schaumburg, IL 60173-4965
708-330-0230

THE SKIN CANCER FOUNDATION
245 5th Ave., Suite 2402
New York, NY 10016
212-725-5176

AMERICAN SOCIETY FOR
   DERMATOLOGICAL SURGERY
930 N. Mecham Rd.
Schaumburg, IL 60173-4965
800-441-2737

AMERICAN SOCIETY OF PLASTIC AND
   RECONSTRUCTIVE SURGEONS
Att'n: Plastic Surgery Information Service
444 E. Algonquin Rd.
Arlington Heights, IL 60005
800-635-0635

PLASTIC SURGERY INFORMATION
SERVICE
800-635-0635

Call for a list of board certified plastic surgeons
in your area.

CHAPTER SIX

YOUR BREAST HEALTH

The nakedness of woman is the work of God.

—William Blake, "The Marriage of Heaven and Hell"

You, and not just your health care providers, can make a *major* contribution in maintaining your breast health. By monitoring your breasts as they change throughout your menstrual cycle and over the course of your lifetime, becoming intimately acquainted with them in the same way you're acquainted with the beauty mark on the left side of your nose that you see in the mirror every day, you can play an active role in keeping your breasts healthy and alerting medical experts when you think their health is threatened. Instead of fearing breast problems, take an aggressive approach: decide to head them off in the first place. Many women have, and continue to do so, and have saved their own lives as a result.

MONITORING YOUR BREAST HEALTH: WHAT YOU MUST DO

The three tools that *every* woman should make regular use of include: (1) a regular physical examination of the breasts by a health practitioner—ideally, once a year; (2) your own monthly breast self-exam (called the BSE); and (3) mammography—the breast X ray that can detect cancerous tumors often long before they can be felt. If you follow all three guidelines *properly,* some experts say, (that is, keeping track of your doctor appointments, performing the BSE correctly, going to an accredited mammography center) you will end up with a 98% chance of at least a five-year survival if a breast cancer is found (five years is the first major marker for cancer survival: if you can pass that point, your chances are *better,* but not guaranteed, that you're cured).

How You Can Get the Best Results from the Breast Self-exam (BSE)

Getting to Know Your Breasts

Dr. Yvonne Thornton of Morristown Memorial Hospital in New Jersey bemoans the fact that the medical community has turned the breast self-exam into something women *fear,* rather than cherish, because doctors have set women up to fear either doing the exam *wrong* or discovering something frightening in our bodies. Instead of telling her patients to search for lumps in their breasts, Dr. Thornton tells them to simply learn what their breasts are like! Are they firm, soft, large, small, bumpy, smooth, or thick in certain places? Just as if you walked outside with your eyes closed you'd feel pebbles under your feet, so, Dr. Thornton says, if you close your eyes and feel your breasts you'll automatically get to know the map of their bumps and lumps. You don't need a special degree to do this! Bend over with your hands on your hips and see how your breasts fall—are they dimpling, or do they look different from how they looked a couple of months ago? Stand straight and look at them in the mirror. Run your hands over them in the shower when they're soapy and easy to feel. Dr. Thornton also recommends a proper breast self-exam (we'll outline one method in just a moment). But above all else, she urges women to just plain become acquainted with their breasts in a natural, unthreatening way.

Doing the Breast Self-exam Right

There is value in doing the breast self-exam correctly; it won't do you much good to do it wrong, which is unfortunately what many women do. First of all, since most breasts are somewhat lumpy, if you don't do the exam systematically you're likely to be scared by just about everything you feel. Second, if you're "feeling" the breast incorrectly, you're more likely to miss the kinds of lumps that matter. But don't worry: it's not hard to do breast self-exams properly—you just have to be taught. Nothing's better than learning from an experienced teacher in person, but try to follow the pattern below and you'll greatly improve your technique.

One of the best breast self-exam techniques—and the one we'll focus on—is the Mammacare method, which is illustrated below. A favorite saying of Henry Pennypacker, a behavioral psychologist who developed the Mammacare method, is "if you can teach fingers to read braille, you can teach them to read small breast lumps." He was proved right when a woman in Hershey, Pennsylvania set the record for finding the smallest two tumors ever caught with this method: both lumps were two millimeters in size! Two millimeters looks something like that shown on the following page. She was promptly cured with minimal surgery and follow-up radiation. Nancy Toth, coordinator of the breast care center at Hershey Medical Center, taught this woman how to do the BSE. She attributes her patient's success to the strip search method, which as you'll see in a moment, covers much more breast tissue than the circular method. The traditional circular BSE method often misses lumps in the nipple and under the armpit, Toth explains.

Here's how the Mammacare technique works; there are two keys to getting it right. The first is to use three levels of pressure when examining your breasts—checking close under the skin, deeper into the breast, and very deep into the breast. (Extremely large breasts may

2 millimeters ————→ ●

require a fourth degree of pressure to get to the bottom of the breast.) Use the pads of your fingers to do the feeling. Ideally, to learn the Mammacare method properly, you should practice on one of the company's breast models which contain hidden lumps. The information box at the end of the chapter gives information on how to obtain one. Since they're not cheap (about $60 for a breast model and video), you might want to see if friends or neighbors want to go in on it with you; you'll only be using it once a month each, so it's easy to share.

The second key to doing this right is being sure to cover *all* of the breast tissue—and that means covering a larger area than most people realize contains breast tissue. Note how you have to get well under the breast, way over to the armpit, up to your collar bone, and so on to cover all of your breast. The Mammacare method suggests that to increase your chance of covering all of the important breast tissue, you lie on your side, then twist slightly so that the breast that normally would hang down to your side is flattened across your chest and easier to palpate. (*See* illustration on next page.) Pennypacker notes that if someone were to tell you to count the number of chocolate chips in a pile of cookie dough, the first thing you'd do is roll the dough out flat. It's the same idea with your breast: the flatter you can get it, the better your chance of feeling something hidden inside. Don't do it standing up, when gravity pulls your breasts downward.

Another way of examining the breast which you may have heard about—going in concentric

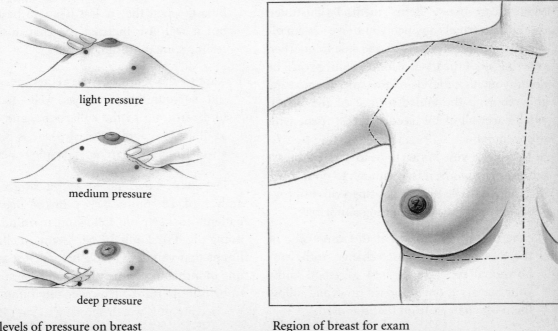

light pressure

medium pressure

deep pressure

Three levels of pressure on breast

Region of breast for exam

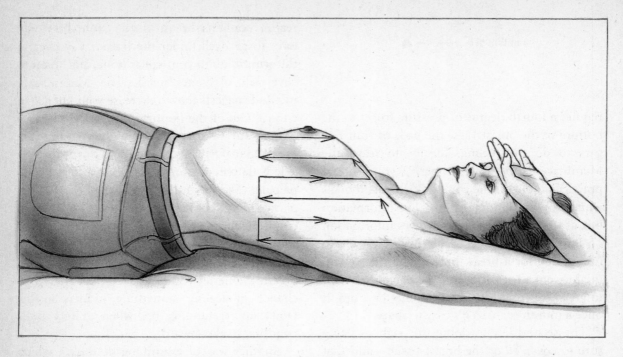

circles, covering a larger and larger circle of breast tissue as you go—often results in missing whole strips of breast, including the nipple. Mammacare uses a "strip" method (illustrated on the next page) in which you move systematically across the breast from one side to another, covering all of the tissue carefully. Since you'll be doing your three levels of pressure at each site, and covering the entire surface of the breast, you'll cover all of the needed breast tissue with this technique.

Now that you know how to do the breast self-exam properly, it isn't enough to do it "once in a while." The following tips will improve your odds of finding something abnormal:

Do the BSE every month, at the same time of the month. Your breasts change with your hormonal cycle, so it's best to get to know your breasts at one standard time, and follow them for changes from that standard.

Do the BSE during the week *after* your period, when your breasts are least swollen or lumpy. Not only will it feel better to handle your breasts when they're less likely to be tender, but it will also increase the chance of your feeling something abnormal.

Be sure to check not just the actual breast itself but surrounding areas as well—near the underarm, up to the collarbone, and so on, as illustrated above. Breast tissue is found at a wider margin than most people realize.

Dr. Susan Love, noted breast surgeon and author of *Dr. Susan Love's Breast Book,* tells patients to keep the following in mind when doing the BSE: Look for persistent, unchanging lumps that you didn't have before (if it appears one month and is gone the next, it's more likely to be unimportant.) However, any lump you're worried about is worth showing to your doctor;

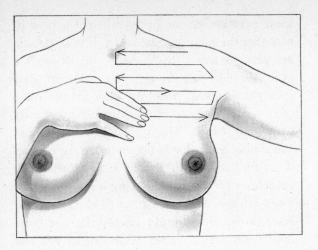

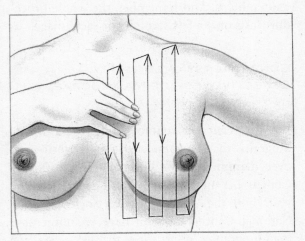

your instincts are good, especially if you have learned to do the BSE properly.

OTHER SIGNS OF BREAST PROBLEMS THAT YOU CAN LOOK FOR YOURSELF

- A change in the appearance of one or both nipples
- Discharge from the nipples, particularly if it's bloody, comes from just one nipple, and comes out without your applying pressure to your breast

- Dimpling of the skin on your breast or breasts
- Persistent eczema-like rash on your nipple that you haven't had before
- A change in the color of your nipples or prominent veins in your breast (both of which *can* be perfectly normal during or after pregnancy)

SOME SIGNS OF UNUSUAL BREAST PROBLEMS

Certain types of breast cancers and other problems are more visible than others, and are therefore much easier to detect. Dr. Love urges women to be aware of the signs of these diseases—for example, inflammatory breast cancer can show up as a red, warm breast; Paget's disease presents with itchiness and scaliness on the breast that is often confused with eczema. So if your breast(s) looks or feels unusual and doesn't seem to go back to normal, see your doctor.

MAMMOGRAPHY: BREAST X RAYS

According to Dr. Marc Lippman, director of the Lombardi Cancer Center at the Georgetown University Medical Center, most women do not get mammograms regularly, despite the exhaustive efforts of some health professionals to promote this lifesaving screening tool. Only 60% of women have had even *one* mammogram, Lippman says; and only ⅓ of women have them regularly, as is recommended. There are as many reasons why women avoid mammography as there are women. Cost is one barrier. The test can cost about $150, and is not always covered by insurance. Poor women are less likely to have mammography screening than more affluent women. Other groups less likely to be screened include women over 65 (only ¼ of women in this age group are screened, which is disturbing, since they're at high risk for breast cancer); Hispanic women; those with lower education levels; and those who live in rural areas. Dr. Mary Jane Houlihan, a surgical oncologist at the Beth Israel BreastCare Center in Boston, cites another important (and astonishing) barrier to mammography. In some western and southern parts of the U.S., studies show that general internists are steering their patients *away* from mammography. Dr. Houlihan urges women to protect themselves and follow the recommended screening guidelines (see page 86 and Appendix I) for mammography.

Women who can afford and have access to mammography but don't get it have all kinds of excuses. Some are afraid that the test itself is risky, since it involves radiation. This is *not* a concern with modern equipment. (In the old days, when a technique called xeromammography was used, women got significantly more radiation per mammogram than we get today. The newer so-called "film screen" mammograms give less radiation and are also more effective than the older kind. The Radiological Society of North America equates the radiation you get from one film-screen mammogram to the same exposure as daily living in your regular environment for several months.) Other women are just lazy and don't get around to scheduling the test, or forget to arrange for it, or simply don't realize that it needs to be done annually to be effective.

Some women are afraid that mammography is painful—or perhaps they've had a mammogram done once, and it hurt. The test should *not* hurt at all. Certainly there is a feeling of some pressure on the breast when it is held in place for the picture to be taken. If your breasts are very sensitive, this pressure might seem a little more like pain. To give you an idea of what it might feel like, rest your bare breasts on a table top and press on them firmly but gently with your hands. That's the most discomfort you should feel—that is, an amount most women don't find uncomfortable at all. Following the guidelines for *your* role during a mammogram listed later in this section will help you avoid discomfort; for example, having the test done *after* your period, when your breasts are less tender, helps. And remember, the whole procedure lasts only a few seconds for each image!

CONTROVERSY OVER THE EFFECTIVENESS OF MAMMOGRAPHY IN YOUNGER WOMEN

A more recent deterrent to getting regular mammograms may be connected to the controversy over mammography's effectiveness in *younger* women. Let me bring you up to date. For many years, both the American Cancer Society and the National Cancer Institute have recommended mammography every one to two years for women aged 40–49, and every year for women 50 and over. Recently, the National Cancer Institute *removed* its recommendation for the 40–49 age group, saying that there was not conclusive evidence that mammography was useful in these younger women. The NCI does *not* now say that women 40–49 should *not* have the test: it just stopped saying they *should* have the test (which was enough to make major headlines, and stir lots of confusion among women of all ages). This change in recommendations from a large, respected organization—and the fact that the same change was *not* endorsed by other highly regarded groups—was terribly confusing for women. The American Cancer Society, the American College of Radiologists (ACR) and other high-profile groups stuck by the *older* recommendation to screen women aged 40–49 every one to two years—leaving women wondering whom to believe. Part of this was an issue of philosophy: The NCI felt that it could not *issue* recommendations on the basis of the test's uncertain value; other organizations argued that they could not *repeal* recommendations just because we aren't *sure* of the value. It depends how you approach the issue.

Why did the NCI change its guidelines? First, after reviewing all of the studies on mammography for younger women, they announced that these reports have *not* shown that screening mammography brings about *decreased mortality* for women aged 40–49. Since decreased mortality is the goal of any screening test, mammography for younger women was deemed a failure (at least as far as current evidence was concerned). Dr. Suzanne Fletcher, professor of ambulatory care and prevention at Harvard Medical School and chair of the NCI international workshop on screening for breast cancer, argues that not only is mammography for younger women of unproven benefit, but it also can bring about a good deal of personal *harm* to younger women. She points to the extremely large number of younger women who will be sent for unnecessary invasive procedures, such as needle biopsies of the breast, due to inconclusive mammograms (a more common problem in younger women than in older women). She also points to studies showing the extreme emotional distress experienced by women who were told they *might* have breast cancer, even if the disease was later ruled out by further testing. The fact is, she says, women hear breast cancer, and they worry.

But a large number of leading scientists and researchers are outraged by the NCI's backing off of the mammography recommendation for younger women. They say that several of the major studies cited by the NCI have serious flaws. Dr. Steven Feig, director of the breast imaging center at Philadelphia's Thomas Jefferson University Hospital and a major proponent of mammography, was an adviser to one of these questionable studies, which was carried out in Canada. The study used less-than-optimal mammography machines and techniques, he argues, and may also have been designed poorly in the first place. While members of the Canadian study have acknowledged that there were problems early in the study, they claim that those problems were eliminated later on. But Dr. Feig's analysis of the data *late* in the study found that 75% of the mammograms were of inadequate quality. How can we possibly tell women aged 40–49, he asks, that mammography won't save their lives, when the data we're basing it on has serious problems?

A number of other top experts in mammography have echoed his concerns, expressing anger over the fact that the NCI would base its decision on flawed studies. Part of the trouble stems from the fact that there are no so-called randomized studies (the most rigorous kind) to support the value of screening mammography in younger women. The best data supporting mammography for this age group comes from so-called *non*randomized studies, which are less scientifically rigorous. Dr. Daniel Kopans, director of the breast imaging division at Harvard's Massachusetts General Hospital, charges the NCI with playing politics and engaging in the inappropriate role of setting health policy. He calls the NCI's concern over unnecessary biopsies and anxiety in young women "paternalistic": if you want to avoid unnecessary biopsies and anxiety, he says, then you might as well keep women away from their breasts altogether, since manual breast exams reveal questionable masses, too. Let all women decide for themselves if they want biopsies, he urges—and let them have mammograms on which to base their decisions, regardless of their age.

One thing the experts on *both* sides of this argument agree on is that *all* of the data on this topic is inadequate. We have imperfect data on *both* sides: imperfect studies showing mammography *does* work for younger women, and imperfect studies showing it *doesn't*. Unfortunately, it would probably take over a half million women, many years, and still more dollars to do the proper study. In the meanwhile, women must make immediate decisions about how to manage their health.

The controversy is equally frustrating in Canada, where each province has a slightly different recommendation about mammography for younger women; some parts of the country endorse and pay for it, some don't. Dr. Linda Warren, executive director of the screening mammography program for British Columbia, also argues that the studies on this subject have been seriously flawed, and that the best information we can go on is the work being done in screening centers that catch early cancers in young women—thus saving their lives—every day.

So what's an intelligent woman to do—let alone believe? One survey showed that a large percentage of women would continue having mammography at a young age "just to be safe"

regardless of a change in official recommendations. But for those who aren't sure, let's look at some data.

About one-quarter of the breast cancers found at a given breast imaging center will be in women aged 40–49—so we know this population is at risk, albeit at lower risk than women over 50. We also know that most—about three-fourths—of breast cancers occur in women with no identifiable risk factors—in other words, they're a mystery, and could not have been anticipated. Finally, the death rate from breast cancer has been going down in women aged 40–49 partly in response to mammography screening.

Few would argue that there are some difficulties in screening younger women with mammography—the most important of which is they have more dense (that is, less fatty) breasts which are harder to read on X ray. Dr. Mary Jane Houlihan, a surgical oncologist at the Beth Israel BreastCare Center in Boston, explains the problem well when she likens looking for breast cancer in a young woman to "looking for a polar bear in a snowstorm." Since younger breast tissue contains lots of glandular tissue which comes up white on X ray, and since cancers come up white on X ray as well, you can see how it would be hard to make these cancers out: looking for white on white. Older women have fattier breasts, and since fat shows up grayish or black on X ray, it's much easier to see white cancers hidden in it. Dr. Houlihan and many other mammography experts insist, however, that with good machinery, proper compression of the breast and keen eyes reading the result, it is more than possible to find early cancers in young women. They argue that these three quality control issues have not been in place in some of the studies on mammography for young women, skewing the results.

Another factor that makes mammography screening *seem* less useful in younger women is that there are fewer cancers in this age group on the whole, so you need to screen a relatively large number of women to catch a large number of cancers. Some researchers argue that studies haven't included enough women over enough time to prove effectiveness.

At this point, given the paucity of solid data on either side of the argument, the American Cancer Society and the American College of Radiologists still support screening mammography for women aged 40–49. They are convinced that screening younger women will save lives. Until more solid data comes along on either side of the issue, I will stick with these more inclusive recommendations throughout this book.

GETTING THE BEST RESULTS FROM YOUR MAMMOGRAM

Not all mammography centers are alike, and unfortunately there are bad ones as well as good. A number of factors can make a center less reliable, including everything from the quality of the machinery used to the technician performing the test to the person who reads the test result. The patient herself can make a difference in getting a good picture of the breast, which we'll discuss in a moment.

Recently, the U.S. government issued several guidelines for quality control in mammography centers, including the requirement, for example, that the mammography machines are used *solely* for the purpose of breast screening—that is, the requirement that centers use "dedicated" mammography machines. But many feel the

government's guidelines don't go far enough, even though several thousand U.S. mammography centers will have to upgrade to meet their requirement. More complete quality assurance comes from voluntary accreditation by the American College of Radiologists. Centers do not *have* to become accredited, but those that choose to do so must meet certain standards; a few of those requirements are listed below.

SOME OF THE REQUIREMENTS FOR ACR ACCREDITED MAMMOGRAPHY CENTERS

1. The physician supervising and/or interpreting the mammograms must either be certified by the American Board of Radiology, the American Osteopathic Board of Radiology or the Royal College of Physicians and Surgeons of Canada *or* must have certain documented minimum training in mammography and certain related areas.

2. The physician must read a minimum of 480 mammograms per year *and* must maintain records on the results.

3. The radiation technologists who perform the tests must be certified by the American Registry of Radiologic Technology or have the equivalent state license, plus continuing education.

There are more requirements for ACR accreditation, including restrictions on the type of equipment to be used, quality control and dosing. Overall, while the requirements do not guarantee safety and effectiveness, they certainly help increase your chance of getting a good result. You can ask your mammography center to show proof of accreditation—or, if you're more comfortable this way, call the ACR at (703) 648-8900 and ask for the name of an accredited center near you.

How you Personally Can Improve the Quality of Your Mammogram

According to Dr. Debra Monticciolo, director of the division of breast imaging at the Emory University School of Medicine, there are several steps you can take to help insure that your breast image is as clear as possible, upping the chance that a tiny cancer will be spotted, and not obscured. This is *not* to suggest that if a cancer is missed, it's your fault. It simply means there are a few things you can do to help the odds of a good result.

Go regularly, as recommended, for your age group (*see* the guidelines in the next section). Skipping a couple of years here or there can mean missing an early cancer.

Try to relax during the exam: if you tense up, you may put your breast in a less-than-optimal position for the test.

Do not schedule a mammogram for the week *before* your period: ideally, schedule it for the week *after* your period, when the breast is easiest to visualize clearly.

Stay absolutely still during the test. It only lasts several seconds per image (they'll take several views of your breast).

Don't fight the technician as she attempts to position your breast properly. Even if you feel a bit uncomfortable, trust that it's necessary to get the best image.

Avoid deodorants and powders on the day of the test—they can obscure the X-ray image.

Make sure the person reading the mammogram has all the necessary information about you—for instance, if you are postmenopausal but taking estrogen replacement therapy, your breasts might be more dense than those of the average woman your age. If the reader knows this, she can make the right assumptions and take the right precautions when scanning your picture for abnormalities.

When to Have a Mammogram: American Cancer Society Guidelines

(*Note:* As discussed earlier, the National Cancer Institute has eliminated the recommendation for women under 50; but because other groups and experts are keeping it in place, I have chosen to include it here.)

Have a "baseline" mammogram at age 40. This is a mammogram to be used for the purpose of comparison—and although it is of questionable value if your breasts change dramatically between age 35 and 40, it still provides basic information about your breast tissue that can be referred to later if a suspicious lesion appears.

Between age 40 and 49, have a mammogram every one to two years. If you are considered to be at high risk of breast cancer, your clinician may favor every year; if not, every two years may be fine for you.

Age 50-plus, have a mammogram every year. Don't forget! Schedule it on the same day each year, if that's an easy way to remember. How about your birthday, to celebrate life?

IF THE MAMMOGRAM FINDS SOMETHING SUSPICIOUS

Mammography is a screening tool, but it can't tell you for sure if you have cancer or not. It can alert your doctor to an unusual lump or change, which then must be examined more directly, through a biopsy. With a biopsy, the surgeon takes out some cells from the suspicious mass to see if it is cancerous. Dr. Monticciolo says that even with *good* mammographers, 80% of the biopsies will be benign; only 20% will show cancer.

There are several kinds of biopsies; different practitioners tend to have their favorites, and sometimes this has to do with the technique available at their particular center. Biopsies vary in two key ways: first, in the technique used for getting the cells out of the lump; and second, in the amount of tissue or cells removed. A biopsy that takes out *most* of a lump is really more like a lumpectomy than a biopsy, for example, while another type of biopsy might just take a few cells from the mass. According to Dr. Rebecca Zuurbier, director of breast imaging at the Georgetown University Medical Center, the so-called fine needle biopsy, which is less invasive for the patient, can miss cancerous cells because its range is so small (in this procedure, a tiny needle is inserted in the breast to get cells from the mass, rather than opening up the breast or taking lots of tissue out). Both she and Dr. Monticcciolo prefer the core biopsy, which is less common around the country, but involves removing more tissue and therefore getting a bigger sample of cells. The core biopsy can be done under the guidance of an X ray, MRI or ultrasound. Patients need to be followed every six months for a few years after core biopsies, since the procedure is still relatively new. Dr. Marc Lippman of the Lombardi Cancer Center at Georgetown University Medical Center recommends the stereotactic breast biopsy, which allows patients to avoid much of the pain and cost of conventional surgery. The stereotactic biopsy is guided by X-ray images of the breast; a core of tissue is removed from the suspicious lump with a *relatively* painless split-second procedure by means of a spring-loaded "gun." A little local anesthesia is used. The most invasive biopsy procedure (still the old standard), involving conventional surgery, may still be needed in some cases. Dr. Mary Jane Houlihan says to choose the kind of biopsy best suited to your particular problem. Fine needle aspiration can be useful for lumps in the lymph glands, for example; stereotactic core biopsies for clusters of small masses or microcalcifications; and so on. These are decisions your doctor will make, but the more you know about the options, the better you'll be at understanding and influencing your care.

OTHER IMAGING TECHNIQUES FOR THE BREAST

Mammography is and probably will remain for a long time the gold standard screening test for breast cancer. But there are other tests, some available now and others on the horizon, that may be useful as well.

Available today in some centers is the MRI—magnetic resonance imaging. The MRI is a sophisticated and costly scanning tool that can be extremely helpful in diagnosing a wide variety of problems throughout the body, including cancer spread. It is *not* now recommended for widespread breast cancer screening. In the next couple of years, however, it may be used for so-called high-risk patients—that is, women for whom mammography might not be as effective. Dr. Richard Patt, chief of MRI at the Georgetown University Medical Center, says possible candidates include younger women with very dense breasts that are hard to examine with mammography; older women on estrogen replacement therapy, again because their breasts may become relatively dense; women who have had prior breast surgery or radiation to the breast, whose scarring or other changes make them harder to image; and women with silicone breast implants, in whom mammography might miss a small, blocked region of the breast.

In the future, you can expect to see variations on mammography as we know it; for instance, computerized "eyes" will help read mammograms to increase the chance of catching a tiny lesion. Also coming down the pike is digital mammography, in which superb, sharper images are created through computer enhancement of the X-ray image. According to Georgetown experts who are refining the technique, digital mammography will detect lesions half the size of those currently visible on mammography.

Another tool sometimes used for breast cancer detection is the ultrasound, which creates images by means of sound waves. This tool is definitely *not* appropriate as a sole method for breast cancer screening, but can be helpful, especially in younger women, to determine if a suspicious lump merits further screening.

SOME NONCANCEROUS BREAST PROBLEMS AND WHAT TO DO ABOUT THEM

There are a great many breast problems that are not life-threatening but can be bothersome and scary for women who believe that something more serious is developing. Here are some of the more common problems—and some solutions.

BREAST PAIN

Dr. Mary Jane Houlihan of the BreastCare Center at Boston's Beth Israel Hospital, says that 70% to 100% of women over age 30 suffer some breast pain. Women often associate pain with cancer—even though this association doesn't usually exist—and panic. In fact, most breast pain is cyclical and related to hormone changes in the body. The most common time for breast swelling and pain is before the menstrual period. But even noncyclical breast pain is rarely cancer, and shouldn't be too worrying. The key is to figure out how to relieve the discomfort so you can live your life more fully—and to see a doctor to rule out any treatable problems.

PAINFUL BREASTS: WHAT YOU HAD TO SAY ABOUT IT

Kate, 30 years old
I went to the doctor about three years ago for it. I think it [the pain] was sort of in general, but especially around my period, my breasts got very sore. When I took my bra off it hurt, I could feel hard areas in them especially around the sides. I also felt pain under my arms, in my armpits, because there are glands there too. When my arms were down I felt like there was something in there. And my nipples hurt. It was incredibly uncomfortable, an ache. More like a heaviness. I didn't know what it was, I thought, "I hope I don't have breast cancer." I was thinking it probably was *not,* but the earlier you get things checked the better.

One doctor said I have cystic breasts, but the other laughed and said everyone does. The (second) doctor asked if I ate caffeine and drank diet soda, and at the time I was eating and drinking a lot more of it—a few brownies a week, and diet soda at least one can a day, and I was drinking lots of coffee because I was staying up late. She said to cut down. I asked, "Do I have to eliminate it?" and she said, "You have to find the right balance for yourself." She also suggested I take 400–800mg of vitamin E. It was way above the RDA so I asked about it and she said they haven't found that it's hazardous, and it also helps prevent heart disease.

So I started taking vitamin E every day, 400 mg. I didn't stop caffeine or diet drinks completely, but I really cut back—maybe three sodas a week and once a week a piece of chocolate. It stopped. It's gone, that's it—it's not painful anymore. It's nice not to have to worry, it's not a fear anymore, and not having pain is nice. I can drink decaf coffee—and I was never a person who *had* to have coffee in the morning.

I really think the vitamin E is good, if I do have caffeine and take the vitamin E, I still feel it helps. If there are times when I do have more caffeine, I do feel it again. Diet drinks I haven't had in two years. Still (my breasts) get a little enlarged when my period is coming, and my nipples get sore, but not like before.

....

Breast surgeon Dr. Susan Love finds that oral contraceptives can help reduce breast pain, and that the more potent menopause-causing hormone regimens—with the cost of side effects—relieve it for some women. Wearing a proper-fitting and supportive bra can help, as can avoiding excess fluid buildup in the body (avoiding salt and sometimes using diuretics, within limits, can help). Over-the-counter painkillers help some women, too. Cutting caffeine and taking vitamin E relieve pain for some women, but these, like most "remedies" for breast pain, have not been well studied, says Dr. Houlihan.

Obviously, avoid the things that irritate your breasts; for some women, sexual stimulation of the breasts should be avoided during bouts of pain. Try soothing, relaxing activities for your whole body, such as taking a warm bath or applying something to the breasts that make them less sore—for some, ice packs might help; for others, a heating pad could do the trick.

BENIGN MASSES AND CYSTS

Most breast lumps aren't cancer, but your doctor has to make sure. She will insert a needle into a mysterious lump to try to drain it of fluid and determine if it's solid or fluid-filled (the latter is characteristic of a benign cyst). You may have heard of something called fibrocystic disease, a problem allegedly caused when breasts develop lots of cysts, lumps or bumps of unknown cause or origin. Houlihan and other breast specialists feel that the term "fibrocystic disease" is not only overused but has no real meaning at all! It's used as a catchall phrase to refer to all lumpy, bumpy, painful breasts, and is still on insurance forms as a real diagnosis—but it just means that you have some benign masses in your breast. The most common benign lump is called the fibroadenoma; it often must be removed from your breast because the diagnosis is made by a pathologist who studies the tissue under a microscope. The fact that it must be removed does *not* mean the mass is cancerous, however, and women should not be led to think that they have a breast "disease" just because they have a generous helping of benign lumps and bumps.

Breast cysts often appear in women in their 30s through their 50s, and can appear overnight. The perimenopausal period—those years shortly before, during and after menopause sets in when hormones sometimes wreak havoc on the female body—is a time when breast pain and cysts often occur.

LUMPS, BUMPS AND PRECANCEROUS CONDITIONS

Certain breast tissue that is not cancer may be somewhat dangerous in that it has a tendency to progress into cancer. One such entity, called atypical hyperplasia, should be removed because it is predictive of later breast cancer. Atypical hyperplasia belongs on the list that loosely makes up the questionable diagnosis "fibrocystic disease," and since this particular problem *is* associated with potential cancer, lots of people panic and put *all* "fibrocystic disease" diagnoses in the precancerous category! This is how rumors get started. It makes for a lot of unfounded fear that doctors are still trying to dispel.

BREAST REDUCTION SURGERY

Many women are unhappy with the appearance of their breasts. They want them to be bigger or smaller, more symmetrical, less pendulous. Part of this stems from our obsession with an unrealistic standard of beauty; the bare breasts we see in *Vogue* are usually perky, rounded and seem to defy gravity. But the fact is, most women point to something "wrong" on their breasts, complaining that they sag, have stretch

marks on them or "unsightly" bits of hair, or nipples too big or too small. These variations on the "perfection" of high-fashion photos is simple reality; the best thing we can do is stop thinking of them as "flaws," and start to see beauty in all colors, sizes and shapes of breasts.

However—and this is a big however—there are some women who are so bothered by the appearance or feeling of their breasts that it begins to negatively affect their behavior. Often, women with extremely large breasts suffer from this problem. They hide under large shirts, won't wear bathing suits without a T-shirt over them, avoid sports like jogging or golf where very large breasts can get in the way or even cause pain. Women with extremely large breasts may suffer from shoulder grooves when their bras dig into their shoulders, says plastic surgeon Dr. Diane Gerber, and significant back pain or pain in the breasts themselves is quite common for these women. Dr. Gerber also finds that the emotional toll of having and hating enormous breasts can be devastating for some women; they may feel that others stare at their breasts when they walk down the street, or look into their chests, not their eyes, during conversations.

BREAST REDUCTION: WHAT YOU HAD TO SAY ABOUT IT

Lucy, 53 years old
I'd been thinking about it for years. I was 8 years into menopause and started taking estrogen: I gained 15 pounds, two dress sizes and five bra sizes! Can you imagine? I was a 32 C, I went to a 34 double D. I'm a petite five feet two inches! Is that remarkable? All of a sudden I gained a size a year for five years.

At that point I felt grotesque, they hung down. I

hated doing anything without a bra, like going to the doctor and putting on a gown and sitting in a waiting room. Picture carrying watermelons on your body. I had severe back trouble aggravated by it. I thought part of being a woman was having big grooves in your shoulders—the weight, they hung down so low.

Now I'm a size 34 B. You should see what (my surgeon) did! I didn't look this good at 16! They're just adorable. I wear lacy, thin-strapped bras. It looks cute as anything. My daughter is 27 and borrows my bras. I feel like a young lady. I'm 53, I'm dating a 48-year-old man who thinks I'm 48! I bought a new bathing suit, a bikini. I don't have to pin my shirts closed anymore. My chest is so much more in proportion with my body.

It's the best thing, no more aching shoulders. I can do things I couldn't do before, I got out of breath, I couldn't run. I was so worried about the pain, but there was never pain. Minimal discomfort. I would recommend this to anyone. I was back to work, back in my office in 6 days. If I'd known I'd have done it ten years ago! It's the best thing I ever did. I feel like a million dollars, it's just wonderful what modern medicine can do.

....

If you have these kinds of physical and emotional problems with your large breasts, you may be a good candidate for breast reduction surgery. There are several ways to do the operation, which is actually done in two parts, during one surgical session: reducing the breasts themselves, and then moving the nipples to the correct new spot. The difference in procedures normally involves the placement of the scar: most traditionally, the scar is done in *T*-shape, going down the midline of the nipple and across under the breast—plus a circle around the nipple and areola itself. Depending on how

well you heal, the scar may be barely visible or quite prominent after the surgery.

The challenge for the surgeon who performs breast reductions is to keep blood supply to the breast ample, so that you will have sensation in the breasts after they are reduced in size. Rarely, nerve damage or lack of blood supply can make this impossible—but in cases where nerves are cut but not severed, the sensation of numbness can subside over a period of time. A worst-case scenario occurs when blood supply to the nipple is completely lost, and the nipple cannot be replaced—but this isn't common. Should it happen, nipples can be re-created from skin grafts as is done with breast reconstruction surgery (discussed in the section on breast cancer, page 520). A much happier and not uncommon result is that the nipple is not only preserved but, if you and your surgeon plan it this way, your ability to breast-feed in the future is fully retained.

Breast reduction surgery is usually done under general anesthesia and carries the same basic surgical risks of infection that other major surgery entails. If your reduction is quite minor, you may be able to have it done under local anesthesia.

Proper timing of your breast reduction surgery is critical. First, says Dr. Gerber, don't have the procedure done if your breasts are still growing. If your bra size has changed over the past year, wait awhile until you're sure your breasts have stopped growing before having the surgery—that is, unless you're willing to risk having a second operation when your breasts regrow. Also be aware that weight loss and, more important, weight gain will affect your surgical outcome. If you gain, say, ten pounds after having the surgery performed, your breasts will likely get bigger. Another caveat: Birth control pills often put weight on the breasts—not just water, but actual breast tissue, Dr. Gerber notes. Consider all of these lifestyle factors before you have surgery done so you can more appropriately plan for the size of your new breasts.

Choosing a new breast size can be tricky. If you've always hated extremely large breasts, you may be tempted to go for the other end of the scale and ask for a dramatic reduction. Keep in mind that tiny breasts may not look proportional on your body. If your hips are wide, or your stomach protrudes, an A-cup might look just as displeasing to you as your double D-cup looked before surgery. Look at before-and-after pictures of women who have had the procedure done, talk to your doctor about your goals for breast reduction (feeling less pain, participating in a sport, wearing a certain type of clothing, avoiding ridicule, or whatever else) and try to make a decision based on reason rather than on passion.

BREAST AUGMENTATION SURGERY

The French have a saying, *chaqu'un à son gout* ("to each his own taste"), and millions of women have decided that their taste points to larger, rounder, fuller breasts than nature gave them in the first place. Breast augmentation surgery, or breast enlargement, should not be confused with breast reconstruction (discussed in the cancer chapter, page 520). Breast reconstruction involves building completely new breasts where they have been removed by mastectomy for breast disease. With breast augmentation, your own healthy breasts are left in place, but given a boost in size by means of some kind of implant.

Until recently, you could choose between two main types of implants: silicone gel-filled, and saline (saltwater)-filled. But a major controversy over the safety of silicone-filled implants and a potential risk of autoimmune disease (discussed further on page 521) led to the FDA banning use of silicone gel-filled implants for any use other than breast reconstruction after cancer surgery. Hence, so-called "cosmetic" use of silicone-filled implants became a thing of the past. Millions of women still have the gel-filled implants in place, and most are doing just fine with them. But others have had a confusing complex of symptoms that have piqued researchers' attention, led to mammoth lawsuits and have resulted in significant ongoing research into the possibility that for *some* women, silicone-filled implants may cause significant harm. At this point, we really don't have all the answers.

So let's focus on the use of saline-filled implants. These implants are actually made of silicone shells filled with saltwater. They aren't as resilient as the gel-filled implants were—they're more prone to breakage on impact (in an auto accident, for example), which can not only be frightening but also quite inconvenient and uncomfortable, since you'd need repeat surgery to remove the damaged implant and replace it with another. The good news is that the release of saltwater into your system is thought to be perfectly harmless, in contrast to the concerns about silicone gel leakage into the body systems. Researchers are divided over the issue of whether the silicone casing around the saline implants poses any harm; it's thought that since the silicone shell is relatively hard and not gelatinous, only minute amounts break away and get into the body. But this is still under study.

If you choose to have breast enlargement surgery, you'll have to decide, with your doctor, *where* to put the implant. Your two choices are in front of the chest muscle or behind it (*see illustration* on page 522). Some surgeons, including Dr. Roxanne Guy of the Holmes Regional Medical Center in Melbourne, Florida, prefer to put the implant *behind* the chest muscle in order to reduce the chance that the implant will block your natural breast tissue during an annual mammogram or breast X ray. When placed *behind* the chest muscle, the implant pushes your natural breast forward, making it easier for you or your doctor to feel for breast lumps, or to aspirate breast tissue in the event that something suspicious is found. Furthermore, from a cosmetic standpoint, Dr. Guy points out that because saline implants have a tendency to ripple a bit, putting them behind the chest muscle reduces the chance that rippling will interfere with the natural look of your enlarged breasts.

BREAST AUGMENTATION: WHAT YOU HAD TO SAY ABOUT IT

Shelley, 35 years of age
I'd been thinking about it probably for a year and a half. I'm quite healthy, I work out all the time, lift weights and do the Stairmaster four to five times a week. But I'd never get much "up there." That's the first place I'd lose weight. It didn't run in my family. I have pretty low body fat and never had much size on my chest. I just wanted a more voluptuous figure. Just trying to get that perfect figure.

My doctor was very open, wanted me to ask a lot of questions. She brought out the points negative as well as positive. I didn't want to be sagging in the next 20 years, so she thought it was best to put it (the saline implant) behind the chest muscle. A person has to pretty much have it in mind that you really wanna do it, because it's major surgery. I never had an operation of any kind, I've always been healthy.

I'm happily married, this is my second marriage. He could care less about it, but he knew I wanted it so bad he said, "Do whatever you want." He's not really a chest man, he's more of a butt man. I haven't told my family. They're in Michigan and I'm in Florida. I'm sure it'll be obvious. They're from the old school, and this is pretty big stuff—I didn't want to shock them. I feel great. I'd do it again in a second.

One of the most common risks associated with breast enlargement surgery is a problem called capsular contracture, in which the scar tissue around the implant hardens significantly and can alter the feeling and appearance of the entire breast. You may have read about those terrible surgical outcomes in which patients are left with rock-hard breasts, rather than natural-looking or -feeling ones. This is usually due to capsular contracture, not to the implant itself getting hard. In about 1–2% of implant cases, capsular contracture is severe enough to require repeat surgery to free the implant. In another 2–3% of cases, contracture is mild and doesn't require further invasive surgery. Most women do just fine with the implants. Other risks of breast augmentation include bleeding, infection (rarely), a change in breast sensation or significant scarring. Some surgeons believe that when the incision is made near the armpit or around the areola (see breast illustration on page 38), scarring is less noticeable than when the incision is made underneath the breast, where the breast meets the chest wall. You *might* expect just the opposite, since the breast, should it sag a little as most breasts do, could cover up a scar underneath it. But most women who have breast augmentation have very small breasts that *don't* sag, and since augmented breasts tend to be high and "perky," these under-breast scars are often in fact visible.

You may have heard that with breast *reconstruction,* the surgeon needs to stretch the chest tissue for a period of time using a special device *before* implants can be placed inside. This is because there is no loose breast tissue left to work with after a mastectomy. In the case of breast augmentation, however, your natural breast tissue is still present, so preoperative skin stretching is not necessary. The one exception: in the rare case when a woman wants *extremely* large breasts, surgeons can do a brief preoperative skin stretch at the same time as the main operation, adding about 30 minutes to one hour to the entire procedure, and creating enough room for a very large implant.

FROM BREAST HEALTH TO BREAST CANCER

Just one tiny step, over a nearly invisible line, can take us from breast health to the earliest (and most treatable) breast cancer. One of the main purposes of the screening techniques discussed in this chapter is to help you become so knowledgeable about your breasts that the "line" becomes more visible, so that you and/or your doctor will be attuned to the small change from health to disease. Only when you become comfortable with your body as a whole, and your breasts in particular, will you increase your chance of detecting that change. Don't fear it; detection can save your life. The only thing you have to fear is *ignoring* your breasts altogether. Should the day ever come when you find something suspicious, and that something turns out to be cancer, you can thank *yourself* for finding it early and greatly boosting your chance of survival. We'll discuss breast cancer in more detail in chapter 25.

FOR MORE INFORMATION ON BREAST HEALTH

FOR RESOURCES ON BREAST CANCER, SEE PAGE 548

MAMMOGRAPHY ACCREDITATION
AMERICAN COLLEGE OF RADIOLOGY
1891 Preston White Drive
Reston, VA 22091
703-648-8900

BREAST SELF-EXAM:
MAMMATECH CORPORATION
P.O. Box 15748
Gainsville, Florida 32604
800-MAM-CARE

CHAPTER SEVEN

YOUR GYNECOLOGICAL HEALTH

We should always presume the disease to be curable
until its own nature prove it otherwise.

—Peter Mere Latham, *Collected Works,* Book 1, ch. 174

Of the vast number of health problems that affect women solely or disproportionately, I have selected several that I consider important for at least one of the following reasons: (1) the disorder is extremely common; (2) it is often misdiagnosed or undiagnosed, but easily cured if recognized; (3) it causes a great deal of pain or chronic discomfort—often unnecessarily. In other words, these are female problems that cause a fair share of misery and could be handled both by the health care community and by *us* much more effectively.

CHRONICALLY IRRITATED VULVA (OUTER VAGINA)

Sometimes called vaginitis, vulvovaginitis and a variety of other names, you're familiar with this problem if you have chronic itching, stinging, burning, or other discomfort on the outer part of your vagina. Sometimes swelling and/or redness accompanies the stinging; sometimes it doesn't. Perhaps you make it worse with chronic scratching, or by wearing tight clothing that aggravates the problem. Some women suffer with this kind of discomfort for weeks, months, and years without relief—in some cases because they don't alert their doctors, and in others because they keep receiving inadequate treatment visit after visit. The key to ending this kind of discomfort is to determine the cause—or often, the causes—and treating each cause appropriately. The most common scenario for women who suffer for years with this problem is they treat one culprit (let's say, a yeast infection) but not another (say, sexually transmitted bacteria). Following are some common causes of outer vaginal irritation, and what should be done in each case.

YEAST INFECTIONS (ALSO CALLED MONILIA VAGINITIS, CANDIDA VAGINITIS, CANDIDA ALBICANS, AND MONILIA ALBICANS)

If you're a woman, consider yourself lucky—and quite unique—if you've never had a yeast infection. Yeast, like many other organisms, grows normally in most vaginas and rectums, causing no trouble most of the time. It is kept under control by the normally acidic environment in the vagina. However, when the vagina loses some of that acidity for any reason (some common reasons include pregnancy, taking antibiotics and eating lots of junky, sugary foods), the yeast seizes the opportunity and thrives. There's nothing dangerous about this situation; you could walk around with a so-called yeast infection forever and not have serious health consequences. But it can be extremely uncomfortable. The burning and itching of a yeast infection can be painful and distracting, and the vaginal discharge often associated with it unpleasant. Yeast discharge is usually white, and many doctors call it "cottage-cheesy" because of its white, curdlike character. It's possible to have a yeast infection with lots of discharge, or with minimal discharge—in both cases, it feels crummy. Your doctor may find that there's a lot of yeast inside your vagina where you can't see it. Other symptoms of a

yeast infection include the feeling that you need to urinate often, and pain with sexual intercourse.

A bigger concern than yeast infections themselves is their misdiagnosis. Dr. Connie Jackson, a vulvovaginal specialist at Boston's Beth Israel Hospital, notes that about half of women who *think* they have a yeast infection really do not. The most common problem confused with yeast infections is called Doderlein's cytolysis—a condition in which the lactobacillus, a bacterium that's part of our normal natural flora, overgrows and causes a watery white discharge, burning and itching that can easily be mistaken for a yeast infection. While baking soda douches and sometimes antibiotics can help with *this* problem, yeast medication won't help at all.

Dr. Eileen Hilton and colleagues came up with even more disturbing news about alleged yeast infections during a study at the Albert Einstein College of Medicine. They found that women who were actually examined by physicians and treated for so-called chronic yeast infections did *not* have any problem with yeast, but rather had a whole range of problems from gonorrhea to chlamydia—infections that can cause serious long-term problems with fertility and general health. Dr. Hilton fears that lots of women are living with what they *believe* is a benign irritation, but could in fact be something far more serious masquerading as yeast.

It has been estimated that one-fourth of cases of vulvovaginitis are caused by yeast. The key is to have a good diagnosis of a yeast infection; don't just assume you have one, or let your doctor make that assumption with nothing more than a glance at your discharge. You should be given both a culture test and a "wet prep" test to be sure yeast is the offending organism. Ideally, you should also be periodically screened for other infections with a similar appearance as well.

Because yeast medications are now available over the counter, doctors are concerned that women will just assume they have yeast infections and self-treat. Obviously, if the infection isn't caused by yeast, the medicine will be useless, and your real problem will persist. If you have been diagnosed with chronic yeast infections and know the signs well—and you have recently been screened by your doctor for *other* vaginal infections and found clear—it's probably okay to act on your own. In some cases, though, there may be an underlying problem in *addition* to yeast that was masked by the yeast cream—or perhaps was exacerbated by some yeast in the vagina—so you've only temporarily solved your problem. A little more detective work on your doctor's part might go a long way to relieving your discomfort.

YEAST INFECTION: WHAT YOU HAD TO SAY ABOUT IT

Joy, 41 Years old
I get them when I take penicillin, or if I spend a lot of time in a wet bathing suit. Even four hours, five hours in a wet bathing suit and I'll get one. It starts a couple of days later. It's itchy, kind of like a whitish, yellowish discharge. Uncomfortable, itchy—I go insane. They're so painful, so annoying. Sex is really painful when you have a yeast infection.

You don't need a prescription for the medicine anymore. You can get it over the counter. I got the same kind that was always prescribed for me. In two days my symptoms are gone, then you take

it another couple of days—I don't want to risk it coming back! When I was younger I had more of them.

How to Avoid a Yeast Infection.
There's a lot you can do to avoid getting a yeast infection in the first place. Here are several things to consider:

Clothing: Certain fabrics will trap moisture and heat in the vagina, creating a friendlier environment for yeast. Tight nylon is a good example. Try to wear more pure cotton—especially in underpants—and when possible, avoid airtight panty hose. Tightness, as well as fabric, affects yeast in the vagina. Skintight pants or underwear that cuts into your crotch will help trap yeast by preventing the vagina from "breathing." The ideal antiyeast outfit for warm climates: loose, all-cotton underwear, a loose-fitting cotton skirt or dress, and bare legs. For colder climates, try loose layers of natural fabrics from the waist down.

Dampness: Avoid chronic dampness in the vagina. If you're finished swimming, take off your bathing suit rather than sitting around in it for an hour. After a bath or shower, pat your vagina dry, gently, and if you have time, take a few minutes before putting on underwear so the vagina will dry out more completely.

Diet: The better balanced your diet, the poorer the chance yeast will take hold. For example, if you eat plenty of fresh fruits and vegetables (with a couple of possible exceptions to be mentioned below) and get the right amount of protein, calcium and other nutrients in your diet, the acidity of your vagina is more likely to stay close to normal, and yeast will be kept in check. Drinking excessive alcohol and eating lots of sugary junk foods like candy bars and refined sugar pastries may help promote a terrific feeding ground for yeast in your vagina, says Dr. David Sherman of New York's Mt. Sinai Medical Center. There is a correlation between high blood sugar and yeast infections, he notes, which is why women with diabetes often have a particularly hard time controlling these infections. He says that the skin of certain fruits, such as grapes and raisins, can promote yeast infections in some women—in fact, some bakers actually isolate yeast from raisins! Dr. Sherman advises women who have chronic yeast infections to limit their intake of leavened and fermented foods and beverages, including alcohol (beer, vinegar, etc.). If you notice *any* association between the foods you eat and yeast infections, take action! You may not have to eliminate the food altogether, but cutting back—especially if you're eating lots of it—might help. It's an easy enough experiment to stop eating a certain way for a few weeks and see if your symptoms abate.

Some experts believe that eating lots of plain (no sugar) live-culture yogurt will reduce your chance of getting a yeast infection. In Dr. Eileen Hilton's study, women eating a cup of yogurt a day cut their chance of yeast infections threefold. The theory is that by cutting the amount of yeast in the gut, you'll have less of a chance to spread yeast from your rectum to your vagina. Others, like dermatologist Dr. Jerome Litt of the Case Western Reserve School of Medicine,

advocate a more direct approach: putting small amounts of plain, live-culture yogurt *in* the vagina to nip an early yeast infection in the bud. It could be a bit messy, unless you do it at bedtime. See what works for you.

Antibiotics: Don't rush to your medicine cabinet for antibiotics every time you feel a sore throat. People tend to overuse antibiotics, often "treating" problems that wouldn't respond to an antibiotic at all—let alone the right kind in the right dose. Most colds and flus are caused by viruses, which can't be helped with antibiotics. The more you take unnecessary antibiotics, the greater your chance of getting yeast infections. Furthermore, you may build up a resistance to these important drugs that could help you when you really *do* need an antibiotic.

Other yeast infection triggers (like pregnancy, diabetes, a suppressed immune system, or taking needed antibiotics for a diagnosed infection) can't be avoided. If you have been fully screened for other vaginal irritants and chronic yeast infections continue to plague you, you might be a candidate for yeast medication *along with* any antibiotic you're taking, for example. Talk to your doctor about this possibility. Of course, if you're pregnant, don't take *any* medication without your doctor's okay. For most people, however, keeping the vagina clean and dry, keeping your diet in check, and avoiding the fabrics and tightness that yeast love will greatly reduce the incidence of yeast infections.

How to Treat a Yeast Infection.
As I mentioned, there are several over-the-counter remedies for yeast infections—such as Monistat and Gyne Lotrimin. These have the

same ingredients as some prescription treatments, at a reduced cost. But Dr. Connie Jackson warns that insurance doesn't cover the over-the-counter drugs, slapping women with the cost of treatment. Over-the counter preparations are helpful for generally benign, rare-to-occasional yeast infections. They may not be strong enough for more potent yeast infections, however, in which case a tougher prescription yeast medicine could be necessary. Terazol is a favorite of some clinicians because of its excellent coverage of several strains of yeast.

Be sure to take your yeast medication for the full length of time—and amount—prescribed. If you stop as soon as you feel better but before you've finished your dose, the yeast is more likely to grow back—stronger! It's the old survival of the fittest rule come back to haunt you. Almost always, you'll be given a cream or suppository that you insert with an applicator once or twice a day for several days. The applicator is similar to the one used for inserting contraceptive jelly. (There is even a potent one-time-use cream available by prescription.) Be sure to clean and dry the applicator properly after each insertion—it only takes a few seconds, and reduces the chance you'll put old yeast and other unclean items into your vagina.

Some women find that boric acid suppositories or vinegar help cure early yeast infections. The idea is to change the pH of the vagina and thereby discourage yeast from proliferating. According to Dr. Robert Sassoon of the New York Hospital/Cornell Medical Center, these are usually just palliative measures that help a bit with minor yeast infections. For full-blown infections, anti-yeast medication should be used, he says.

If your yeast infections are so recalcitrant that you cannot control them with creams and the preventive measures discussed above, you might be a candidate for oral medication. Ask your doctor about this possibility, but keep in mind that if you're one of the few people prone to chronic yeast infections no matter what you do right, it's possible that even oral treatment won't permanently solve your problem. It should, however, dramatically reduce your discomfort.

A Word About Douching.
You might be tempted to resort to using a douche to soothe your irritated vagina and flush out discharge caused by yeast or other infections. *Don't do it.* Unless specifically advised by your doctor, douches are not the best solution for vaginal irritations. The reason: while rinsing away abnormal bacteria or other organisms, they also rinse away *needed* vaginal flora—that is, the organisms that normally live in your vagina and keep it healthy and balanced. Furthermore, some products contain deodorants or other chemicals that can irritate the vulva themselves! Find out what's causing your irritation and treat the problem properly, whether with yeast medication, antibiotics or whatever your doctor determines is appropriate. After that, regular cleaning in the bath or shower is sufficient.

ALLERGIC VULVOVAGINITIS

Another common cause of chronic burning and itching in the vagina is an allergy to something in your environment. Perhaps it's a product you use, like a detergent in the laundry, a soap in the shower, spermicide, a douche or so-called "feminine hygiene spray." Or maybe you're allergic to a food you're eating, or a medication you're taking. Dr. Connie Jackson notes that this is yet another category of irritation often confused with yeast.

Figure out if there are times that the problem is worse or better, and if it's connected to anything in your lifestyle or behavior. Talk to your doctor about ways to eliminate potential allergens one at a time to try to detect the culprit. If you have ruled out every possible infection, from yeast to sexually transmitted diseases and on down the line, you might want to explore the possibility of an allergy more closely. Your OB-GYN might refer you to an allergist so you can learn more about your skin's sensitivity to various chemicals.

Sometimes, a one-time irritant can set up a chronic problem of itching, burning and scratching that prevents the vagina from healing. Add another problem on top of that—let's say, a low-grade yeast infection—and you can feel pretty miserable. If you have cleared any known infection and still have chronic redness and itching, your doctor may recommend a topical anti-inflammatory agent (like a corticosteroid cream). Sometimes halting the cycle of irritation and pain will cure your problem once and for all. What you *don't* want to do is scratch and irritate the area constantly, as you can predispose yourself to much more serious problems, including malignancies.

For truly mysterious, chronic vulvovaginal irritation that your doctor can't figure out, consider seeing a vulvovaginal specialist who has done special training in disorders of the vulva. They can be hard to find, but your doctor or hospital should be able to refer you to at least one near your area.

BACTERIAL VAGINOSIS, ALSO CALLED GARDNERELLA VAGINITIS, "GARDEN VARIETY" VAGINITIS, HEMOPHILUS VAGINITIS, NONSPECIFIC VAGINITIS, GARDNERELLA, GARDNERELLA VAGINALIS, AND OTHER NAMES

Perhaps *half* of cases of irritated vulvas are caused by this common infection. It goes by a number of related names, partly because for many years doctors weren't sure what organism was actually causing the discomfort. In fact, even today, rather than actually doing a culture to see what organism is bothering you, some health care professionals will settle for the generic "nonspecific vaginitis" theory and give you nonspecific, generic treatment. While generally this isn't a great plan of action against an organism in your reproductive tract, with this problem, there are certain clues that your doctor can hardly miss—such as the strong, fishy odor caused by this infection, and the yellowish, thin discharge that is usually associated with it.

While some women have no symptoms with Gardnerella, some feel itching and burning not unlike that caused by yeast infections. Also, like yeast, the hemophilus bacterium thrives in a warm, damp arena, so an overheated vagina with trapped moisture is more prone to the problem. Where do you get the infection in the first place? Sex is one route—and you *can* pass it back and forth between yourself and your partner. Other routes (from the toilet seat to the bathtub) are plausible, but certainly not as "efficient" a route of transmission.

With bacterial vaginosis, the amount of lactobacilli (that normal vaginal flora mentioned earlier) drops significantly and no longer protects us from other bacteria that are normally around our vaginas—but well controlled. The goal of treatment is to restore the normal bacterial balance in the vagina.

Preventing and Treating Bacterial Vaginosis.

Many of the same precautions that deter yeast will also deter this organism—*see* page 97 for how to keep the vagina dry and clean. But once you have an infection, treatment is quite different. The quickest and best medication is metronidazole, which can be placed into the vagina as a cream, with an applicator. Generally, it's not necessary to treat male partners, because the penis isn't nearly as pleasant a breeding ground for these bugs as the vagina is. If it would give you peace of mind, however, ask your doctor about providing cream for your partner, too.

TRICHOMONIASIS

Another common vaginal irritant—and another in the long list of infections that can be mistaken for yeast—is trichomoniasis—commonly known as "trich." For more information on this and other sexually transmitted infections that can irritate the vulva, *see* chapter 13, "Sexually Transmitted Diseases."

CYSTITIS

You may have heard it called "honeymoon cystitis"—but if you've had it, you know that cystitis is *no* honeymoon. The name cystitis is commonly used to refer to an infection somewhere along the bladder system—from the urethra that leads urine out of your body, to the ureter, to the bladder itself. More accurately, when doctors know exactly where the infection lies, they give it a more specific name—like urethritis if the infection is in the urethra. The symptoms include stinging or burning with urination (or even without it), and a feeling of urgency (like you absolutely *have* to go) and then little or no urine comes out. If the infection travels to your kidneys, you may feel an ache in your lower back, toward the sides. Most women who have had cystitis in the past recognize it quickly when it recurs, but a first bout can be alarming, especially if you develop blood in your urine. If treated quickly (before the infection gathers momentum and moves to the kidneys) cystitis is usually no big deal to treat and resolves quickly.

The reason it's been called "honeymoon cystitis" is that this problem can be aggravated by either rough or newly frequent sexual intercourse. It's *not* a sexually transmitted disease, however. Here's how it often happens (you might want to consult chapter 3 on your reproductive anatomy): A normal bacterium that lives in the gut and therefore appears in bowel movements and in and around the rectum, called *E. coli* (Escherichia coli), can be moved by a number of means to the vaginal area (one common route is when you wipe yourself back to front, dragging some bacteria from the rectum toward the vagina). With sex or some other form of abrasion to the sensitive tissues around the urethra, the skin becomes raw and sensitive—and vulnerable to unwelcome bacteria. While *E. coli* is normal and not bothersome in the gut, it has *no* place in the vaginal area or urinary system. There, it multiplies, building up in the bladder and causing infection and discomfort. The less you drink, and the less often you empty your bladder, the longer the bugs have to multiply in your still bladder.

URINARY TRACT INFECTION: WHAT YOU HAD TO SAY ABOUT IT

Nancy, age 30
It was at its worst between age 18 and 22, I have no idea why. I felt really bad, it was awful and totally ruled my life. I have no idea why it was so bad then but I can speculate it was my diaphragm. The diaphragm would rub against my bladder. It's like burning, you feel like you have to urinate so badly and you go and nothing comes out. It's like a screaming burning pain. I had fevers, chills and you start feeling sick from drinking water.

I took one antibiotic so long I became immune to it. I had this gynecologist who told me to take it as a preventive measure, once or twice a day, and I became immune to it and got a virulent strain of infection. My next doctor put me on a new antibiotic. It's a miracle, it's incredible. You have to take the antibiotics immediately, nothing else works. And sit down with two gigantic pitchers of water and drink them. You'd have to drink cranberry juice like a river until you floated away for it to do anything!

Now I'm on the Pill. I've had just one (infection) in the last year. It's like a godsend not to get them. They're the worst, they're the plague. It's the kind of thing you're thankful for all the time, not getting them all the time. Thank God I passed beyond that.

TREATMENT

Immediately upon feeling the symptoms of a urinary tract infection, talk to your doctor. If you're a regular, chances are you'll be treated by phone. If you aren't sure what the problem is, make an immediate appointment (you'll probably feel crummy enough that you'll insist on being seen fast) to have your urine examined for infection. If you have cystitis, you'll be put on an appropriate antibiotic to kill the bug. Be sure to take your medication for as long as your doctor recommends. Stopping early can cause the infection to become far more potent and harder to treat. For your miserable symptoms, your doctor might prescribe Pyridium—a little red pill that turns your urine bright orange and anesthetizes only the area that's stinging, bringing relief while you wait for the antibiotics to take effect. For some women, Pyridium eliminates symptoms completely; for others, it's not quite as effective. You also should drink large quantities of fluid—water is best—until your infection has cleared up. Some recommend two quarts of water a day, which is a sure way to keep yourself in the bathroom most of the time, but it goes a long way toward getting those nasty bugs out of your bladder and urinary tract. Some recommend drinking cranberry juice, because of its acidity, to help cure cystitis. There's nothing wrong with giving it a try, so long as you keep in mind that it's not a cure, just an additional protective measure. Studies vary on how much more effective cranberry juice is than plain old water, but there's some evidence it may help some women. Careful not to have too many sugared drinks, though, since the combination of taking antibiotics and eating lots of simple sugars could set you up for a yeast infection.

PREVENTING CYSTITIS

A few simple measures can dramatically reduce your chance of getting cystitis. These are known by health care professionals as "good bladder hygiene" methods.
• Drink lots of fluids all the time—not just when you have an infection. At *least* six 8-ounce

glasses of fluid a day should be your routine—especially if you're prone to bladder infections. Dr. Tamara Bavendam of the University of Washington in Seattle recommends getting enough fluid that you urinate every three to four hours. You don't want to drink so much that urinating takes up the greater portion of your day! She also recommends that at least half of the water you drink be noncarbonated.

• Always wipe yourself from front (vagina) to back (rectum) when using the toilet.

• When you *do* have an infection, take your antibiotic for the full length of time prescribed, even if you feel better sooner. Otherwise, a tougher line of bacteria will set up shop and you'll be hit with *worse* symptoms in a short period of time.

• Urinate frequently. Experts find that particularly women who work tend to put off urinating for hour after hour. Forgetting the toll this takes on your kidneys, infrequent urination sets you up for infections by letting bacteria build up in the bladder and elsewhere in the system.

• When you haven't had sex for a while—or if you're having relatively rough sex—be sure to lubricate properly, so you don't abrade your skin excessively (if you don't have natural lubrication, try one of the gels listed on pages 255–256). Don't make the mistake of using sticky or goopy lubricants that can clog your pores and cause further irritation, however.

• Ideally, have sex when both your own and your partner's genitals are clean.

• Try to urinate *after* intercourse. It helps clear away any unwanted *E. coli* bugs that might be trying to get hold. Dr. Bavendam says it's not necessary to jump right up after sex and go to the bathroom; waiting an hour or so is fine. Just try not to go to sleep for the night without emptying your bladder. Obviously, if you have intercourse on an empty bladder, you won't be able to urinate afterwards. If you need to urinate *before* intercourse, Dr. Bavendam suggests trying to keep a little urine in your bladder—although this can be a bit uncomfortable.

• Take note if the form of contraception you use seems to trigger urinary tract infections. Some women find that spermicidal jellies and/or the diaphragm can help promote cystitis. If this is true for you, try switching to another form of contraception and see if you have fewer episodes.

• If you are doing everything right and can't seem to prevent urinary tract infections, talk to your regular doctor or to a urologist. It's not good for your kidneys to endure chronic infections in the urinary tract. You may be a candidate for preventive antibiotic therapy, in which you'll take an antibiotic whenever you have sex—or on some other regular schedule. Because there are risks to taking antibiotics over the long term, *don't* initiate this treatment on your own with leftover antibiotics in your medicine cabinet. Ask your doctor for advice . . . and supervision.

IRRITABLE BLADDER SYNDROME

Irritable bladder syndrome differs from cystitis in that it is more chronic, and the discomfort centers around the time *before* you urinate and *after* you urinate, as opposed to *during* urination, which is more characteristic of bladder infections. Of course, these are generalizations, and your symptoms may differ. It is important to have both a urinalysis and a urine culture to diagnose this problem. The solution is to follow the bladder hygiene advice listed above; patients who have lived with this discomfort for decades have found relief in these simple lifestyle adjustments. Also, carbonated water, coffee, tea, chocolate and tomato-based foods can be both-ersome if you have irritable bladder syndrome. The syndrome may act up at times of hormonal change in the body, but it isn't completely understood when or why it occurs. Some experts feel that irritable bowel syndrome is really just a catchall, nonspecific diagnosis used when there is no clear indication of what's *really* causing the unpleasant bladder symptoms. For instance, experts on interstitial cystitis (IC), discussed immediately below, feel that some patients who are told they have "irritable bowel syndrome" actually have IC. However, while IC is often extremely difficult to treat with medication or behavior change, the more generalized "irritable bowel syndrome" does seem to respond to lifestyle changes.

INTERSTITIAL CYSTITIS

Interstitial cystitis consists of inflammation in the bladder wall, frequent urination, tremendous pelvic pain, burning, pressure and feelings of urgency (the need to urinate immediately.) Dr. Vicki Ratner, president of the Interstitial Cystitis Association and a patient herself, notes that in severe cases patients feel chained to the bathroom, sensing that their bladders are going to burst even when empty. In these extreme cases, patients may feel the need to urinate every few minutes throughout the day. The major difference between interstitial cystitis and a bladder infection is that the urine is generally *free* of bacteria, or sterile, with IC, whereas traditional bladder infections are caused by bacteria. Often, IC patients are given antibiotics, but don't get better; this isn't surprising considering there's no "bug" present for the antibiotic to kill.

When they don't recover with standard bladder infection treatments, IC patients are often sent home with the classic "it's all in your head" or "you must be under stress" diagnosis. Dr. Ratner herself saw 14 doctors before she, through some research of her own, was properly diagnosed. There may be lots of women walking around with these terrible symptoms, not getting the help they need, Dr. Ratner worries. After her appearance on a major morning talk show, she received ten thousand letters from women with identical histories.

While a history of symptoms is really the best means of diagnosis at this point, sometimes cystoscopy (looking into the bladder) reveals pencil-thin, pinpoint hemorrhages in the wall of the bladder, indicating bleeding spots from chronic inflammation, Dr. Ratner says.

There is no cure for IC, but there are treatments to relieve pain. One is surgical, called bladder hydrodistention. Under general anesthesia, the bladder is stretched with water. This relieves symptoms, possibly by loosening scar tissue. Several drugs have been used to treat the problem with varying degrees of success. For example, the tricyclic antidepressant Elavil seems to have an antipain effect when given in small doses. A potent drug with anti-inflammatory properties called DMSO helps some patients. Another drug, Elmiron, not yet approved, is believed to coat the bladder and possibly protect it from an unidentified irritant in the urine—but this is still speculative. Some women are helped by dietary changes (avoiding spicy or citrus foods, chocolate and alcohol) but many find *no* relief from these changes. Interestingly, unlike the case with bladder infections, drinking more fluid can worsen the problem.

Other self-help methods include placing

either hot-water bottles or cold compresses against the perineum (*see* chapter 3, page 33), using lubricants before intercourse to relieve irritation (*see* list of safe lubricants on pages 255–256), reducing stress, and replacing high-impact exercise with lower-impact activities.

Deborah Slade, executive director of the Intersitial Cystitis Association, notes that some women report changes in their symptoms during pregnancy—some for the worse, more for the better. There have been cases of dramatic remission during pregnancy and lactation, suggesting some hormonal component to the problem. But more research needs to be done in this area.

LASER TREATMENT FOR INFECTIONS

Sometimes, when extensive laser treatment is used to clear an infection—such as human papillomavirus or HPV, the virus that causes genital warts—the sensitive cells of the vulva can be permanently damaged. The result: a chronically itching, burning outer vagina. There was a time not long ago, in the early and mid-1980s, when doctors believed that the best way to treat an HPV infection was to give extensive laser treatments to skin that didn't even have obvious genital warts. Using the laser this way causes extensive burns to the skin of the inner and outer vagina. The scabs heal and the skin usually looks normal, but for many women, it doesn't *feel* normal. Most experts now accept that this kind of treatment was overkill, and that it probably didn't make any difference in the recurrence of the virus (which lives in cells forever anyway).

According to Dr. Thomas Sedlacek, chief of the gynecology department at Graduate Hospital in Philadelphia, there are several treatments to help the chronically impaired vulva. These include anesthetic gels, the drug Elavil (which reduces the strength of neuron firing, thereby lessening pain) and, in certain specific cases, even the use of a different kind of laser called the pulsed dye laser. It's also vital, he notes, to treat any other causes of irritation—at least eliminating the easily-managed problems that could compound the chronic pain these women suffer.

SEXUAL ABUSE

As we discuss briefly in chapter 14, past sexual abuse can have a dramatic impact on how our sexual organs feel—particularly in response to a potential sexual act. Some women feel such extreme, chronic irritation or pain in and outside the vagina that sex becomes almost impossible. Many experts believe that a large proportion of women for whom all other possible causes of vaginal pain have been ruled out by an experienced physician may have a psychological problem with sex caused by a past damaging experience. These women *do* in fact feel pain and irritation—it is *not* all in their heads. But what's happening is they're getting what psychiatrists call a "secondary gain" from the pain—that is, an excuse not to have sex. If you have been tested and retested for STDs, yeast, allergies, every and any potential cause of vaginal irritation and you still have serious vaginal or vulvar pain that's putting a wall between you and any sexual relationship—and if you've tried soothing creams, the best lubricants for sex, and so on with no success—you might want to give therapy a chance.

. . . .

So far, we've been talking about problems

that irritate the vagina or vulva. Another set of problems cause pelvic or abdominal pain—or other so-called "lower quadrant" pain. Let's take a look at some of the most common causes for this type of pain (for more on pelvic inflammatory disease, or PID, *see* chapter 13, "Sexually Transmitted Diseases").

FIBROID TUMORS (ALSO CALLED UTERINE LEIOMYOMAS)

About one in five women of childbearing age suffers from uterine fibroids—that is, usually benign growths that develop in, on or near the uterus. Fibroids are extremely uncommon in pre- or postmenopausal women, for a simple reason: They thrive on estrogen, the hormone that's present in large quantities during our menstruating years. Because of the estrogen present during pregnancy, long-hidden small fibroids sometimes seize the opportunity to grow wildly, causing severe pain and occasionally compromising delivery.

Often, fibroids cause no symptoms at all; in fact, many women find out about them accidentally during some unrelated gynecological exam. In other cases, fibroids can cause extreme pelvic pain, vaginal bleeding and even infertility, depending on their size and placement. If they grow big enough, they can even cause distention of the belly that's visible from the outside. Certainly, your doctor should be able to feel them during a routine pelvic exam.

FIBROIDS: WHAT YOU HAD TO SAY ABOUT THEM

Liz, 39 years old
I didn't have any symptoms. I had seen the same gynecologist for years and years and years and I went in one time and (he found it). I had no idea whatsoever what it was, he said a tumor and said it might affect whether I can have children. It was a really bad experience. He said, "I don't know, it's way too early to talk about what to do." Then he shut the door and left and I was hysterical. I remember leaving and bursting into tears.

I said I have to do some research. Besides him I saw three other people. I started reading, it was bad news—you get more frightened. They can grow. You may need to have a hysterectomy. A woman I talked to was 46 years old and had three kids and the doctor told her it's just easier to have a hysterectomy than the myomectomy (surgery to remove the fibroid and preserve the uterus). It's important for older women to have the option to have the myomectomy, too!

After a year and a half, finally I found a doctor who was informative, he told me all about what fibroids do, and said I could go on a drug to shrink them, or have surgery. I found a woman who had had the myomectomy, and it was fine for her. The more women I talked to who'd had it, the better I felt.

It was my first surgery. Not a ton of fun but exactly as they described it. Four to six weeks you can't drive or go to work. But it was easy, one of the quickest ones he had done—he said it popped right out. (The surgeon) joked a couple of months later, "You can go and get pregnant now." Oh, I'm so glad I did the research and kept my uterus. It taught me a good lesson—to see more than one person. You should feel good about this kind of decision.

Sadly, even though fibroids are often harmless, they are one of the most common reasons for unnecessary hysterectomies. As we'll discuss later in this chapter, the hysterectomy (removal of the uterus) is one of the more overperformed surgeries. These days, with media publicity *against* hysterectomies, more doctors are thinking twice—and giving information—before going ahead and recommending a hysterectomy. But there was a time when just having a couple of harmless fibroids in the uterus was a good enough excuse to take out an otherwise perfectly healthy uterus.

Treating Fibroids

When fibroids are causing pain or interfering with your ability to get pregnant, there are other options for treating them. Drug treatment always involves shutting down the hormone estrogen, thereby depriving the fibroid of the "food" on which it grows. To block estrogen, you need to temporarily halt the function of the ovaries, causing a temporary menopause. One group of medications that do this are the GnRH (gonadotropin releasing hormone) agonists.

Remember, estrogen is an important protector of our circulatory systems, our bones and other body systems. There are risks to cutting it off; one example is loss of calcium from the bones, the beginning of osteoporosis. So most experts say it's a bad idea to keep a young woman on these drugs for too long. It's believed that the bones rebound after short-term antiestrogen treatment, but it's not known whether they do as well after long-term treatment. There are other unpleasant side effects that go along with antiestrogen treatment, such as hot flashes (the same kind many women have with menopause). Basically, since antiestrogenic drugs cause a temporary menopause in the body, most of the symptoms or changes that occur with menopause are caused by these drugs as well.

There are great advantages to short-term drug treatment for fibroids, however. One benefit is that you may be able to shrink the fibroid sufficiently so that it can be removed surgically with better success and *without* a hysterectomy.

Surgery for Fibroids

Beyond a hysterectomy, which many women want to avoid, there is a surgical procedure for removing fibroids, called myomectomy. A small but significant number of women will have fibroid recurrences after this procedure, and there is also a long list of major complications associated with it, such as internal adhesions, scarring and pain. As mentioned above, sometimes shrinking the tumor with drugs before surgery can improve your chance of a successful outcome. In the hands of a skilled surgeon, the myomectomy *can* be an effective option.

If you have tried everything else or have been told by *more than one expert* that a hysterectomy is your only option because of the size or placement of the fibroid(s), be sure to have the most minimally invasive form of hysterectomy possible. Vaginal hysterectomy, in which the operation is done through the vagina (as opposed to abdominal surgery), often results in a faster recovery. Sometimes, though, vaginal hysterectomy is not an option. In addition, several centers around the country are having success with laparoscopically assisted vaginal hysterectomy, in which a much smaller incision can be made than with the traditional open-abdomen surgery.

Abnormal Vaginal Bleeding

Abnormal vaginal bleeding is any unexpected bleeding outside of the normal menstrual cycle.

You know your own body best, and if you have an extremely irregular cycle with unpredictable blood flow, what's abnormal for another woman might be perfectly normal for you. However, it's a good idea to have one thorough workup to be sure that your irregular cycle isn't caused by a problem, hormonal or otherwise. (For more on menstruation and bleeding, *see* chapter 8.)

Abnormal vaginal bleeding, sometimes accompanied by cramping or pelvic pain, can be a sign of a threatened abortion or miscarriage (even if you don't know you're pregnant), or some other complication of pregnancy. It can also be a result of problems as diverse as thyroid or liver disease, clotting trouble, benign or malignant tumors of the genital or reproductive tracts, or a hormonal imbalance. For this reason, it's vital that your doctor gives you a complete workup until the answer is uncovered. This might mean blood and urine tests, a physical examination and perhaps other screening tests. Sometimes your regular doctor or obstetrician/gynecologist will do the complete workup. In other cases, you might want to see a reproductive endocrinologist, who specializes in hormone disorders, or a general internist, who has a good overview of the body systems and how they interact. Sometimes, the cause of vaginal bleeding is easy to determine and treat. In other cases, some good detective work is warranted, and more than one type of expert might need to get involved, often working together as a team.

It's important to be absolutely sure that your bleeding is coming from your vagina, and not from a nearby area like your rectum or urinary tract. Sometimes when blood appears on toilet paper or underwear, it's hard to be sure where it originated. Blotting with a tissue can sometimes give you the answer, sometimes not. That's why it's a good idea to have a physical examination by your doctor, to see if you might have a urinary tract infection or hemorrhoids or some other nonvaginal problem that can cause bleeding. Don't panic, and don't assume the worst, until you've been examined. Often vaginal bleeding is benign or manageable.

Treatment for abnormal vaginal bleeding depends entirely on its cause. If you have a growth, you might need to have it removed. If your problem is hormonal, you might be put on a hormone-modifying regimen. If it's a thyroid problem, medication again might be the answer. For this reason, the correct diagnosis is absolutely essential.

ENDOMETRIOSIS

Estimated to affect about five million American women, endometriosis can cause significant physical and emotional pain and can interfere with fertility. It affects women in their reproductive years—after menstruation has begun and before menopause has set in. That's because it's driven in part by the hormone estrogen, which is in good supply during these years. Endometriosis develops when tissue that lines the uterus, called endometrial tissue, migrates out of the uterus to other sites in the pelvis. This wandering tissue can latch onto other pelvic organs, and can cause adhesions that cause a great deal of pain or discomfort. Sometimes, endometriosis is invisible to the surgeon's eye, but lies underneath visible tissue, mysteriously causing pain.

Some cases of endometriosis are quite benign in that they cause little or no discomfort and are only discovered accidentally during other procedures. Others are quite disabling, and require one of several treatments, both surgical and hormonal. Some women find that their endometriosis symptoms wax and wane depending on the time of the month or at different periods in their lives.

Symptoms of endometriosis include general pelvic pain and pain with intercourse, menstrual periods, bowel movements or urination. For some women, though, endometriosis pain is *not* cyclical. Like any chronic pain, the discomfort of endometriosis can rob young women of their energy and enthusiasm for life, and can make sexual intercourse and most exercise unpleasant if not impossible. If this is your case, it is imperative that you attempt at least one, and ideally more, of the therapies available for treating endometriosis. First, though, you need a proper diagnosis.

DIAGNOSING ENDOMETRIOSIS

Dr. David Olive, chief of the section on reproductive endocrinology at the Yale University School of Medicine, points out that because many of the symptoms of endometriosis mimic other gynecological problems, it's vital to get a definitive diagnosis *before* starting treatment. The only way to do that is with a laparoscopy, in which a small incision is made (rather than a large opening as in traditional surgery), and your physician inserts a tiny camera with which to look inside your pelvic cavity. Often, at least *some* endometrial tissue will be visible, even if a good deal of your disease is hidden. Sometimes, additional screening tests are needed to find hidden disease—the MRI (magnetic resonance imaging) can be helpful in these cases. Ideally, at the same time that your doctor discovers the lesions, he/she will perform a procedure to remove them—which makes

more sense than doing one procedure to look, and another to take action. Make sure your practitioner is trained to do both.

Dr. David Adamson of Stanford University Medical Center does not like to do laparoscopy on adolescent patients if he can avoid it. When an adolescent comes in with unexplainable pelvic pain, he begins by treating her with minor painkillers (nonsteroidal anti-inflammatory drugs) and then tries oral contraceptives. Many of these young women simply have higher-than-normal prostaglandin levels, which causes some cramping and pain he finds. If the patients don't respond to these treatments, however, then endometriosis becomes a more distinct possibility—and he'll move on to laparoscopy.

If, on the other hand, a women in her late 30s shows up with suspected endometriosis, and wants to get pregnant right away, Dr. Adamson recommends going straight to laparoscopy and immediate removal if lesions are found, because surgical treatment is the best way to avoid infertility caused by endometriosis. (One caveat, however, is that surgery itself sometimes causes scar tissue that can impede fertility.)

ENDOMETRIOSIS: WHAT YOU HAD TO SAY ABOUT IT

Karin, 30 years old
The first sensations were during sex, I would have a stomachache afterwards. The gynecologist said there could be bits of endometrium floating around. It meant nothing to me, I thought it would go away. The next doctor firmly believed it *wasn't* endometriosis. As time went on I realized he wasn't really concerned. In 1987 and 1988 the pain was kind of manageable. In 1989 and 1990 it was unbearable.

By the time I started seeing specialists, it was completely affecting my life, every morning for 20 minutes I couldn't move. The first time I knew it was actually endometriosis was when I had [laparoscopic] surgery in 1991. At the point the pain was at its worst, there were so many pains— a pushing pushing pushing pain, and a pain that built to a peak and then would slowly, slowly go away—that was the worst.

I would not say my husband was 100% supportive. He loved me and hugged me and said this is "our" problem but he got kind of cranky, sometimes I felt why should I have to say "I'm not feeling well," when he knew I'd had the worst day, and why did he ask for sex, why did I have to say "no"? I know he was frustrated and trying to keep it to himself but little things come through.

It was a couple more years before I took medication, because they had so many hormonal side effects—I was like, "What am I putting in my body?" I took a GnRH agonist, which wasn't even approved when I first had the pain. There was immediate pain relief, in a week. The doctors said it would take a few weeks. It was such a gift. I could run and feel happy and giddy again. I could bend and pick up things again. If the light was blinking I could run across the street—I couldn't do that before. I could have sex, but the drug made me so dry it still really hurt. I also started acupuncture at the same time, which I think helped me mentally and helped me with the side effects of the drug. The doctors were shocked that I didn't get hot flashes from the drug.

The worst thing with this disease is that it will never really go away, I'll always have to have drugs, surgery, or pregnancy. I don't believe there will be a cure before I reach menopause, when I should be better anyway. And nobody really wants to hear about it. Doctors don't take the time to listen.

TREATING ENDOMETRIOSIS

There is no cure for endometriosis, but treatments can help a great deal in relieving pain and eliminating lesions. Surgery is usually the first step—to remove as many lesions and adhesions as possible and eliminate pain at least for now. As mentioned above, it's the best way to restore fertility to women with endometriosis, although not guaranteed.

Often, though, lesions will recur after surgery. That's where hormonal therapy comes in. There are several drug choices, all of which affect your hormones in some way. Danazol, which is FDA-approved for the treatment of endometriosis, keeps you from ovulating by preventing the surge of luteinizing hormone (*see* chapter 8, "Menstrual Health") and inhibiting the enzyme receptors in the endometrial lesions. The drug works pretty well, but has significant unpleasant side effects, primarily causing masculinization: for example, hair growth on the face, a lowered voice, weight gain and increased muscle mass. Some women will not risk enduring these side effects. Another group of drugs used for endometriosis include progestins, the most common of which in the U.S. is Provera. These are *not* approved by the FDA for endometriosis, but Dr. Olive finds that they help some women and have much milder side effects and cost less than some other therapies. Recently approved by the FDA for endometriosis treatment are the GnRH agonists, a group of relatively costly drugs like Lupron, Synarel and others that produce a medical menopause by cutting out estrogen in the body. The side effects are the same as during menopause, when estrogen is depleted from the body: everything from hot flashes to bone loss. These side effects are thought to be reversible, however, when the drugs are stopped (they should only be taken for six months). All of the above-mentioned drugs reduce both pain *and* the number and size of endometrial lesions.

Finally, a cheap option is the oral contraceptives: these have never been approved for endometriosis and do not help reduce lesions, but they can help many women with pain, are widely available and relatively inexpensive. Dr. Olive likes to start with the cheaper medications with the lowest side effect profile (oral contraceptives, progestins) and only if they fail does he move on to the "bigger guns," the GnRH agonists and the danazol. Again, there are no cures; relief is the goal—or, with surgery, restoration of fertility.

For some women, at least a little bit of pain relief comes from anti-inflammatory drugs, both prescribed and over-the-counter. Don't overrely on these drugs, however, as they have side effects and risks of their own, and do *not* solve the underlying problem.

Often, endometriosis patients go through one physician after another looking for a proper diagnosis, let alone a decent treatment. Many are told that they're imagining their problem, that they're depressed, or that they're trying to avoid sex. Remember that there's a chicken-and-egg issue here: chronic pain does contribute to depression. While more information has emerged in recent years, many physicians are still inclined to call all mysterious "female" pain "imaginary." Mary Lou Ballweg, president and executive director of the Endometriosis Association in Milwaukee, Wisconsin, urges women to locate not only experienced physicians, but also compassionate ones. Many women with this disease go undiagnosed for fifteen years, she points out, and are ultimately forced to choose among treatments that can't guarantee relief, and may be unpleasant in and of themselves. Ballweg urges women to contact the Endometriosis Association for written information on endometriosis, as well as to locate experienced physicians in their area, and other women with whom to talk about this often difficult disorder.

For more information, call the Endometriosis Association at 1-800-992-3636.

OTHER UNEXPLAINED PELVIC PAIN

If you have been extensively examined by experienced doctors for all known causes of pelvic pain—from fibroids to endometriosis to pelvic inflammatory disease and on down the line—if you're been screened and scanned and poked and examined more times than you can count, and still haven't found relief—you may want to visit a coordinated, multidisciplinary pain clinic. These centers, which are more often found in university hospital settings, have experts from a variety of specialties who work in concert to determine and treat mysterious causes of pain. Dr. Margaret Punch, who treats pelvic pain at such a center at the University of Michigan, notes that there are often non-gynecological explanations for chronic pelvic pain that gynecologists and general physicians may overlook. Other kinds of practitioners whom you might not ordinarily think of, like physical therapists, can detect unexpected causes of pelvic pain, like problems in the abdominal wall muscles; neurologists or pain specialists may discover nerve problems; a gastroenerologist might discover that the pain originates in the bowel; a urologist might find a cause in the bladder.

Sometimes a cause will never be found, which is terribly frustrating for doctors and patients alike. In certain unsolved cases, Dr. Punch notes, antidepressant medication can be used to relieve pelvic pain of unknown cause. The idea is *not* that depression caused the pain. Rather, the same system of neurotransmitters (brain chemicals) that affect mood also affect the pain system. Sometimes, old-line antidepressant drugs called tricyclic antidepressants have helped patients who have tried just about everything else for pelvic pain. These drugs do have side effects (*see* the chapter on mental health, page 348, for more details), but they may be worth the price if there is less pain. Dr. Punch expects more study to be done on newer antidepressant drugs with lower side effect profiles, to see if they work against pain as well.

Other more sophisticated methods of pain management are also being used at pain centers—such as nerve blocks and other techniques that can reduce pain in specific areas of the body. Don't give up until you've given everything a try. Even if you can't completely eliminate your pain, you may be able to reduce it sufficiently that you can regain a sense of pleasure in life, and resume both the functions and activities that you enjoy and that you're required to do each day.

LUPUS (SYSTEMIC LUPUS ERYTHEMATOSUS)

While it isn't a gynecological problem, nor is it solely a women's disease, I have included it here because lupus affects women disproportionately. There are about nine cases of lupus among women to every one case among men; African-American women have about three times the number of cases as Caucasian women, and younger women (from the teens to the mid-thirties) are more often affected than older ones. No one knows the cause of this disorder, but it is a so-called autoimmune condition in which the body's own disease-fighting system turns and acts upon its own healthy cells. Dr. Robert Lahita, chairman of the board of directors for the Lupus Foundation of America, describes lupus as the opposite of AIDS, in which the immune system totally fails. With lupus, the immune system goes into overdrive.

Lupus causes a wide range of symptoms, from the more mild—including skin roughness and rashes, joint swelling and pain, sun sensitivity, oral ulcers and abnormal blood measurements of certain immune factors—to serious kidney and other organ damage, and problems with the nervous system. Patients can experience vastly different extremes of the problem, notes Dr. Sara Walker, chief of the rheumatology section at the Harry S. Truman Memorial Veterans' Hospital in Columbia, Missouri. One woman might be bothered by occasional skin rashes and minor joint pain, while another has severe or even life-threatening kidney failure. Others will have occasional "flares" of bothersome symptoms, feeling fine most of the time (remissions that can last for years) but occasionally suffering more difficult bouts with the disease. Dr. Walker says that about two-thirds of patients have the milder form of lupus, while the other third suffers from more serious disease. Most women experience some degree of ups and downs with this disease—and while it cannot be cured, symptoms can often be at least relieved when they're at their worst. Some find that symptoms abate after menopause, which fits with a recent theory that sex hormones, like estrogen, may play a role in exacerbating the disorder.

....

LUPUS: WHAT YOU HAD TO SAY ABOUT IT

Susan, 47 years old
I first got sick 25 years ago. It took two years to be diagnosed! When I first became sick, they supposed I'd had an allergic reaction to penicillin. I became sicker and sicker, had a 106 fever. I had a rash across the bridge of my nose and cheeks. No one ever stopped to think lupus. No one tested me for lupus. I was screaming in joint pain. And it took two years. They packed me in ice and tried to bring down the fever. They gave me massive amounts of cortisone. By morning I was sitting on the end of my bed. Then it was a long process of getting better. I was in a wheelchair. They took me to every doctor in the book. I'm a young woman, in the prime of my life, married 6 months! I'd lost my hair, my face was a moonface from the cortisone. And nobody knows what's wrong with me. (I eventually got better and) about a year later I went to the Swiss Alps. In the bright light of the mountains I got sicker and sicker. I couldn't move my side, my arm, my shoulder, my knee. The doctor said, "You haven't been in the sun or anything have you?" I said, "Of course I've been in the sun, I'm in the Alps!"

They wired me cortisone to Europe. The cortisone gave me false energy, the sense I could do anything. When I got back I went directly to the hospital and spent 2 weeks there. It was at this point that the doctor began to suspect systemic lupus erythematosis. I said, "You're telling me I have a disease I can't pronounce? A disease no one else has?" I was newly married, which came to a rapid end. Often it's difficult for a spouse. I remember a holiday season my knees hurt so much I couldn't walk, but there was no way I could say "No presents." I got a car service and went!

There is a way to do anything. There are ways to make a positive from a negative, constructive from destructive. I'm currently very happily married, for 18 years. He knew I was sick when we got married. I don't want you to think it's all fun. It hurts. When my joints hurt, it's bad. I have bad hands in the winter—you can't touch them. I use tremendous amounts of medication, I take a hanful of pills every morning and every night. Cortisone, Imuran, corticosteroids, Xantac, a diuretic, mega doses of calcium. Immunosuppressants. The purpose is to suppress your immune system so we don't have an immune system—we have to be careful because if we get sick it can flare the lupus. But I have been given an opportunity to know how valuable life is. I'm full of energy.

You have to decide to go about living rather than dying. Become educated. If you seem to have symptoms of lupus, look lupus up in the phone book, ask for a doctor who might be able to give you a good test. Ask your own doctor. Don't write it off, "Oh well I might have the flu." It may not be nothing. You're not neurotic. Become educated. Find support from other people, it can help to live life to the fullest.

....

Typical lupus flares appear in the form of red, tender, swollen joints, especially on the hands; a facial rash; sensitivity to sun exposure that can result in skin and fever reactions; chronic fatigue; and chest pain with coughing. Experts should not, but often do, rely on subjective symptoms to make a diagnosis. Dr. Lahita urges clinicians to use the official diagnostic tool (covering certain symptoms and laboratory tests) before labelling anyone as having lupus, since many women panic with the news and in turn label themselves invalids. Lupus is a serious problem, but not a death sentence, Dr. Lahita insists. Too many women think they've reached the end of the line when they get the diagnosis, he says, and often for no reason. With proper management, watching for and catching serious symptoms early, the vast majority of patients can be well managed. But since many lupus symptoms resemble other problems (arthritis, for example, or Lyme disease) it's easy to be misdiagnosed if doctors don't run the right tests—including one for a telltale protein in the blood.

Because lupus is an autoimmune disease, and because it results in inflammatory processes throughout the body, the usual line of treatment involves anti-inflammatory and immune-suppressant drugs. From the most benign anti-inflammatory agents that you can buy over-the-counter to the more powerful corticosteroid and other drugs, there is a wide range of options. Those with the most severe, organ-threatening forms of the disease are treated with powerful chemotherapeutic drugs, similar to those used for cancer patients. Lots of research is going on in the area of drug treatment, with several new drug trials underway around the country and others in the planning stages.

Unfortunately, while control of the disease is possible, a cure is not—at least for now. If you are self-treating with over-the-counter pain medicine, be sure your doctor is aware of what you're taking, how much of it, and how often, since there are side effects and risks to even the most common and harmless-seeming agents.

In addition to drug treatment for lupus,

some experts recommend staying out of the sun, since sunlight triggers symptoms in many patients. You can determine for yourself if sunlight is a problem, and talk to your doctor about how—and how completely—you can avoid it. Dr. Lahita urges his patients whose symptoms are under control to get regular aerobic exercise and to rest adequately and eat well. But for those who are experiencing symptoms, he advises *avoiding* vigorous exercise, since it can further tax the immune system and weaken the body as it tries to fight the disorder.

URINARY INCONTINENCE

One of the most common, quality-of-life-impairing problems to affect women is urinary incontinence. It's estimated that about ten to twelve million Americans are incontinent, with two women enduring the problem for every one man. Because there is such a stigma attached to the problem, and people are embarrassed to talk about it, incontinence may be vastly underreported. Contrary to what most people believe, incontinence knows no age barriers; half or more of those who are incontinent are *under* age 65. Half of all women will be incontinent at some point in their lives, either temporarily or long-term. The stereotypical image we have of a wheelchair-bound, cognitively impaired incontinent person actually pertains to only 5% of the total population of incontinent people. Over 90% are mobile, outside the nursing home, and probably standing next to you on the grocery line. Urinary incontinence is also a major issue in health care facilities; 35% of hospitalized older people and 40–60% of patients in long-term care have the problem. The dollar figures are just as staggering:

we spend about 15 *billion* dollars a year—yes, that's *billion*—on incontinence.

To make matters worse, many doctors overlook the problem, often because they don't ask the right questions, and patients are too ashamed to raise the issue without prompting. This is especially tragic considering the powerful and devastating impact incontinence has on the quality of life for so many women. Kathryn Burgio, director of the University of Alabama at Birmingham continence program and author of *Staying Dry: A Practical Guide to Bladder Control*, finds that many incontinent women lead hermitlike existences, refusing to travel or attend engagements at which they might possibly be humiliated. The sex lives of incontinent people often become nonexistent. Burgio finds that 50% of women refuse to mention their incontinence even to their doctors!

The reason we *must* speak up and speak out about incontinence is that it can be treated successfully in the vast majority of cases. Sometimes, success means cure. In other cases, it means significant improvement of symptoms (that is, fewer urinary accidents—better bladder control). *Incontinence is not a normal part of aging.* It is a treatable disorder. If your doctor isn't comfortable with the issue or knowledgeable about it, seek the help of someone who is. There are incontinence programs within many hospitals, plus many obstetrician/gynecologists, gerontologists, urologists and some general internists are adept at treating the problem. Avail yourself of the kind of excellent care so many other people with incontinence have gotten. It may free you from what has turned into a very depressing, embarrassing and isolating experience.

INCONTINENCE: WHAT YOU HAD TO SAY ABOUT IT

Nancy, 46 years old

It started after I started having children. It was a gradual thing. I'd notice during exercise, jumping jacks, that there would be leaking. I didn't let it get too much in my way. I'd use a pad during exercise. This went on until ten years ago, it got *much* worse. Laughing, coughing, any activity other than moderate or slow walking would cause a problem. It got *really* bad in the fall of 1990. I developed asthmatic bronchitis, and with that kind of coughing, really explosive, I could absolutely empty my entire bladder. I'd go to sleep with a bath towel between my legs, and *that* didn't do it!

I had little stitches put in my bladder, they told me the only other option was major surgery. It helped for six months, then I probably blew out my stitches. My husband and I went to southern California on vacation, we went to Disneyland, and drove up the coast of California. I had awakened the second morning with bronchitis and I coughed and peed all the way up the coast of California while my dear sweet husband saw the scenery by himself. I wet the rental car, I wet my girlfriend's sofa. She's like a sister, so I could talk freely—I was in tears.

My doctor had me doing Kegel exercises, but it was hopeless at this point, like the proverbial putting the thumb in the dike. I was so distraught, the quality of my life was suffering so much. I tried to be lighthearted about it, my three teenage sons would joke, "Don't pick mom up, you'll get a puddle at your feet," or "Don't make mom laugh." My husband never acted disgusted, he knew the pain I was in. I could wear two, three super absorbent pads but it had such force it wouldn't have a chance to be absorbed. Here I am a professional woman, going to employee meetings in front of people. I was so freaked that once I knew I had bronchitis I was armed with a supply of heavy duty pads. If I laughed I'd start heading to the bathroom. I did wet my chair at work once.

I went to the urogynecologist. She did heavy duty testing, and the result of the tests was I'd be a perfect candidate for the surgery. I could walk a mile a week after surgery, I stopped at a picnic on the way home from the hospital! I'm happy to say that to this point I've had no problems. I'm still careful, if I drink a lot and I get to a bathroom, I go to it. Emotionally, just talking about it brings back that time, the way things were—I say oh my God, that problem's gone; not better, gone! What can I say? I can't find the words. It's like owning your life again, I can make choices and decisions again without saying, "What do I need to do, what do I need to bring?" The day goes by and I don't think about it anymore. I can't imagine anyone who was worse than I am—and I have not had a pad between my legs since the surgery.

MAIN TYPES OF INCONTINENCE

There are two main types of incontinence, with variations and combinations of the two as well. These are (1) stress incontinence and (2) urge incontinence. When you have both kinds of incontinence, it's usually called mixed incontinence.

The main symptoms of stress incontinence include a tendency to lose urine when your body is stressed in some way—either when you cough, sneeze or perhaps lift something heavy. Sometimes stress incontinence occurs when you stand up suddenly, walk or exercise. This type of incontinence is associated with a decrease in the strength of the muscles on your so-called "pelvic floor," which is made up of the muscles that support organs like your bladder and uterus. Sometimes damage during childbirth or simply bearing multiple children will wear these muscles down, as well as tiring out the ligaments that support the bladder. Therefore, small amounts of stress can result in leakage of urine—or a full-fledged accident.

The symptoms of urge incontinence are quite different. In this case, you don't need any pressure or strain on your body to lose urine. With urge incontinence, you might lose urine as soon as you feel the "urge" to urinate—wherever you are. Kathryn Burgio calls this the "key-in-lock" syndrome, in which a muscle in your bladder called the detrusor goes into spasm and pushes your urine out unexpectedly—when you reach the door to your house, for example, and not the toilet. You might be trying to make it to the toilet, but not get there. Or perhaps you haven't even started to try to go when the urge hits you. Urge incontinence can also cause you to lose urine when you hear running water, or when you drink small amounts. Accidents may happen by day or by night, in bed or when you're up and around. There are a large number of potential causes of urge incontinence, including both neurological impairment (from a stroke or chronic disease) or an infection or injury. Sometimes the cause is unknown.

Finally, there is another type of incontinence called overflow incontinence. With this problem, you may have the sense that you cannot empty your bladder completely even if you feel like you still have to "go." You may lose urine at any time of day, even without a feeling of fullness in your bladder.

Dr. Andrew Fantl, director of the continence program for women at the Medical College of Virginia, reports that from 10 to 30% of incontinent women have mixed incontinence: that is, a combination of the different types listed above. For these women, successful treatment must address each separate cause and form of incontinence. Even if treatment is only successful for one type, however, the woman's symptoms will be lessened, and her quality of life improved.

TREATMENT FOR URINARY INCONTINENCE

There are generally three main approaches to treating urinary incontinence: lifestyle changes (called behavioral treatment), medication and surgery. Ideally, your doctor will want to start with the least invasive option (behavior changes) and move up slowly and conservatively to the most invasive (surgery).

The key to success in treatment is to have a proper diagnosis of your type of bladder problem. Most say the best way to help your doctor accomplish this is to keep a record of your urinary habits, noting the kinds of situations that lead to accidents. Think about the symptoms mentioned earlier: for instance, does activity of some kind make you urinate, or do you have accidents as soon as you have the urge to urinate? Treatment for the different kinds of urinary incontinence vary considerably, since there are different causes for each type of problem. Your doctor might recommend a whole battery of tests, from blood and urine tests to scopes and other techniques for visualizing the urinary tract system, to figure out the cause of your problem. It may even turn out that your incontinence is caused by something completely unrelated to your bladder, such as severe constipation, a medication you're taking or a neurological disorder.

Behavioral Treatment.

The following lifestyle changes are useful for all types of urinary incontinence:

1. Learn pelvic exercises called Kegel exercises. This technique has been around for a long time, and has helped a lot of people when they do it properly. The trouble, Dr. Burgio says, is too many people do these exercises *improperly* and therefore get no benefit. What you're trying to do with these exercises is strengthen the pelvic muscles that help control bladder function. It may be hard to figure out which muscles to work on, but Burgio and her colleagues have a good suggestion: put a clean finger inside your vagina gently and try to squeeze your muscles in such a way that your vagina closes more tightly around your finger. Don't strain your buttocks, or legs; work on just those vaginal muscles. Another way to work on finding the right muscles for Kegel exercises is to sit on the toilet and begin to urinate. After you've started urinating, try to bear down and stop the flow. If you can do this, even briefly, you're working the right muscles. At regular intervals throughout the day, try squeezing these muscles tight for a few seconds, then let go. You can do it at your desk, or at lunch, or while you're walking—no one will know! Over time, you'll be amazed at the improvement in your bladder control, especially if you have stress incontinence.

2. Develop a urination schedule, and stick to it. Don't let yourself get too desperate to urinate—that's when accidents are more likely to happen. Try urinating every two or three hours—see what intervals work best for you to prevent accidents in between.

3. Learn to concentrate on other things when you feel the urge to urinate. Take your mind and put it somewhere else, perhaps on something important you have to attend to—business, a friend's needs, whatever—steering your thinking *away* from your bladder.

4. Talk to your doctor about how much you're drinking every day. While drinking lots of fluids is sometimes a good thing, you can be overdoing it—especially in the evening hours before bed. (Believe it or not, sometimes you'll need to drink *more* fluids to help your bladder problem. Your doctor will help you determine your particular situation.) In general, it's a good idea to avoid diuretic beverages, like caffeinated drinks and alcohol, especially in the evening.

Medication.

Depending on the type of problem you have, there are several drugs available for treating incontinence. If your bladder contracts automatically, forcing urine out, you can take a drug to stop that action. If your sphincter muscles are loose and don't squeeze urine out, you can try a medication to tighten them. If you have a bladder infection that causes incontinence, you might need an antibiotic to clear it up. Or, if you're postmenopausal and having bladder problems related to a lack of estrogen in your body, estrogen replacement might be

worth considering. Demand that your doctor give you a clear explanation of why he or she is choosing a particular drug—that is, what exactly the drug is being used to correct, and what the side effects and associated risks of the drug is. Some common side effects of incontinence medication include a fast heart rate, dizziness and/or headache, and constipation. More often than not, drugs are used for urge incontinence or mixed incontinence. Some common drugs for urge incontinence include the anticholinergics, such as oxybutinin; certain antidepressants, like imipramine, are used for several types of incontinence; phenylpropanolamine is used for stress incontinence; and there are many others.

Surgery.

There are several types of surgery for incontinence in women. Some focus on lifting the bladder back into its normal position if it has "fallen" out of place due to weakened ligaments. Others focus on bolstering the pelvic muscles that sit under and support the bladder. Most often, surgery for incontinence is useful for stress incontinence, in which there is some weakening or displacement of the bladder and its supporting muscles. Different surgeons tend to prefer and stick with particular techniques—and while there are similarities among many of the options, they tend to differ by means of where the incision is made (the vagina or the abdomen or both). Some well-known surgeries for incontinence include the Kelly procedure, the Marshall-Marchetti-Krantz procedure, and the Stamey procedure. There are many others. Depending on who you talk to, you'll get different advice on which choice is "best." The key is to find a surgeon who does lots of these procedures and can give you a good explanation (with a diagram) of how *your* problem matches *this* particular technique.

The most important thing to find out about surgery for urinary incontinence is, *What does your doctor expect the best possible results to be.* Your expectations before surgery are extremely important, because these procedures are not often cure-alls, and carry risks of their own. If you go into surgery expecting a complete cure, you may be disappointed. If, on the other hand, you expect some reasonable amount of improvement, which you may have to bolster with lifestyle changes, you're more likely to be pleased with your result. Your doctor should be able to give you a reasonable estimate of success (though certainly you could do better or worse than she estimates) based on your current condition.

In addition to repairing or readjusting the damaged parts of your bladder system or pelvic musculature, some doctors recommend inserting internal support devices—such as a hammocklike structure that helps hold your pelvic organs in place. Sometimes putting a pessary or looplike device in the vagina to support the uterus can help (if the uterus has fallen or prolapsed in the vagina), but usually this isn't a long-term or final solution.

"Transient" Incontinence

One excellent reason for getting treatment for incontinence is you might discover you're one of the lucky ones whose problem is temporary and quite easy to reverse *without* special treatment of any kind. Dr. Neil Resnick, a leader in the treatment of incontinence and chief of gerontology at the Brigham and Women's Hospital in Boston, remembers that when he first entered this field everyone said that bladder or sphincter problems were *always* the cause of incontinence. He has since learned—and taught others—that there are many other relatively minor, reversible causes of incontinence that must be ruled out before you jump to the conclusion that the situation is more serious.

Dr. Resnick created the following mnemonic for the causes of so-called "transient incontinence": DIAPPERS. The letters stand for Delirium, Infection, Atrophic vaginitis/urethritis, Pharmaceuticals, Psychology, Excess urine output, Restricted mobility, and Stool impaction. As you can see, most of these conditions are quickly reversible: delirium can be treated if there is a known cause; infection can be cured; vaginitis can be relieved; pharmaceuticals (medication) can be changed or sometimes stopped; psychological problems like depression can be treated; excess urine output, often caused by diuretics or excessive fluid intake, can be controlled; restricted mobility can be at least ameliorated; and stool impaction can be eliminated. With temporary or transient incontinence, patients can have normal continence restored within days or weeks, if not immediately.

Still, Dr. Resnick laments, even with multiple remedies at hand, we are afraid to talk about incontinence. When he and his colleagues tried to locate a celebrity spokesperson to get on the airwaves and talk about the many reversible causes and treatments for this common problem ("the Mary Tyler Moore of incontinence", as he puts it) they were threatened with lawsuits by every celebrity they approached. Not one would consider having their previous incontinence problem exposed, as if it were the dirtiest crime imaginable.

ENVIRONMENTAL CAUSES OF INCONTINENCE

Jane Marks, clinical coordinator of the continence program at the Johns Hopkins Geriatric Center, finds that often a person's home environment can be a central contributor to her incontinence. When she does home visits for patients, for instance—particularly older, less mobile patients—she often discovers that the toilet is difficult to access (perhaps it's on the second floor, and it takes so long for the patient to reach it, she has an accident). Or maybe the size or height of the toilet doesn't meet the patient's needs, especially when she has hip problems, chronic pain, or lack of mobility. Some solutions Marks recommends include the portable toilet or commode, which patients can use anywhere in the house if they need to; the so-called "female urinal" which has a wide lip and may be easier to use than a toilet for those who have trouble sitting; and sometimes a "lift chair" in the patient's main sitting room, which helps push the patient to her feet so she can start walking and make it to the bathroom with much less delay.

PADS, "DIAPERS," AND CATHETERS

Most experts on urinary incontinence feel strongly that people should not depend on padded undergarments, condomlike devices to catch urine, or so-called "in-dwelling" catheters—unless of course they are a last resort after thorough medical evaluation and treatment. These devices, which certainly add a sense of confidence to someone prone to public accidents, do not solve the underlying problem. In fact, overreliance on pads, for example,

might delay your seeking permanent help for your problem. It's fine to use these objects for added reassurance as you're working through incontinence, but by no means consider them an answer to your problem until all permanent solutions have been attempted.

HYSTERECTOMY

High on the list of overperformed surgeries—ranking number 2 overall on the most-common-operation list—is hysterectomy. Nearly one in three American women will have a hysterectomy by age 60, which gives us the dubious distinction of world leader in this arena. The problem of too many unnecessary hysterectomies has received a great deal of media attention in recent years, which is thought to have helped stem the problem to a limited degree. In the late '70s, about 700,000 hysterectomies were done per year in the U.S. Today, the number is down to fewer than 600,000 per year; certainly not a small number, but going in the right direction. In certain parts of the country, you're more likely to be given a hysterectomy than in others. For instance, the hysterectomy rate is five times greater in the southern U.S. than in the Northeast.

If you're having a hysterectomy you want to be sure that you're having it for a good reason. According to Dr. David Chapin, senior obstetrician and gynecologist at Boston's Beth Israel Hospital, about 80–90% of women are satisfied after the procedure and would do it again if given the option: another 10–20%, not an insignificant number, would *not* repeat the procedure if given the chance to turn back the clock. One way to help insure satisfaction *after* the fact is to have a good reason for the procedure—and a good attitude about it—going *in*. Some *appropriate* reasons for a hysterectomy include:

1. Invasive cancer of the cervix, or cancer of the uterus.

2. Severe, debilitating endometriosis that does not respond to repeated attempts at other treatment, including both drugs and surgery.

3. Severe prolapse of the uterus that cannot be repaired surgically.

4. Uncontrollable nonmenstrual vaginal bleeding—"uncontrollable" meaning that hormone therapy, dilation and curettage (D & C), minor surgery, and other less invasive options have been unsuccessful.

5. Certain fibroid tumors, because of their size, position, painfulness, recurrence or total failure to respond to other treatment.

Some *inappropriate* reasons for a hysterectomy are:

1. A pre-cancerous condition of the cervix, cervical intraepithelial neoplasia (which can be treated with laser, freezing or burning techniques).

2. Minor prolapse of the uterus (which can be repaired by lifting the ligaments that hold the uterus in place, or, in the short term, by putting some sort of support below the uterus).

3. Small fibroid tumors that cause no pain, bleeding or other problems—"just because they're there."

4. Moderate vaginal bleeding, before other treatment methods have been attempted (this may be one of the reasons for the most over-performed hysterectomies).

5. Mild endometriosis that does not cause pain or obstruction or any other problems.

Of course, there are going to be trickier situations where the appropriateness of a hysterectomy is not clear-cut; in these instances (in fact, in *any* case where a hysterectomy or other major surgery is recommended) second and third opinions from doctors who do *not* work together are a great idea. Dr. Chapin feels that most uses of hysterectomy, other than for treatment of invasive cancer, are "elective" in the sense that they are done to improve quality of life, not to save life. That means *you* are one of the key players in determining if the surgery is appropriate. You will have to decide if the symptoms you are living with—such as chronic heavy bleeding or pain—are bad enough that you're willing to have your uterus removed; and most important, if there are no other options to hysterectomy that you are willing to attempt.

Dr. Barbara Levy of the University of Washington worries that many unnecessary hysterectomies are done because of what she calls "fuzzy thinking" by doctors. That is, when a woman has many different minor complaints—*some* bleeding, *some* pain, *some* irregular cells on her cervix—the doctor recommends a hysterectomy to "simpilfy" things and deal with every problem at once. Instead, Dr. Levy stresses, women should demand alternate solutions to each individual problem—short of hysterectomy. Levy is particularly concerned about hysterectomies that are done to relieve chronic pain. Often, pelvic pain is caused by bowel, bladder or other problems that have nothing to do with the uterus. In these cases, hysterectomy is not just *excessive* treatment—it's also *useless*.

....

HYSTERECTOMY: WHAT YOU HAD TO SAY ABOUT IT

Patricia, 41 years old
This was five or six years ago, I was 34 when it happened. After they removed the ovaries they didn't tell me the repercussions like osteoporosis. It was a raw deal. I lost 20 pounds and I weighed 104 to begin with. I was 84 pounds. My bones, my joints started hurting. It was terrible. I had a laparoscopy, and he said I had endometriosis and irritation of the fallopian tubes and I had a vaginal discharge that led me to believe it was a disease process, and they told me I had to have it (my uterus) out. There was absolutely no reason to have it! My pathology was clear! I had a yeast infection! They scared me into it. Once a doctor renders an opinion it's hard to get it out of your mind.

I had a loss of desire, you lose interest in the simple things in life. It was the loss of pleasure in general. My husband said, "Where do you want to go for dinner?"—I didn't care. There's this spark that's lost. Only 60% came back. I still have the migraines and the pains. I sued and it took five years but I prevailed. The judge said all the doctors who cared for me lied. Follow your own instincts, if you think something's wrong. Don't rush into it unless it's a life-and-death situation.

Judith, 50 years old
I was bleeding off and on, I couldn't go on trips, I would have to take a suitcase of Kotex pads and tampons. We would plan trips around when I had my period. I tried not to have a hysterectomy. I was sick. I had a lot of cramping, I was up and down. I went to lots of doctors, I read almost every book on *not* to have a hysterectomy. It's hard, you don't know what the outcome will be.

I decided to take a chance, have a good emotional outlook. You need a doctor who is on your side. You'll feel a lot better about the decision. You need to be able to talk to him. I gave him a lot of problems, I pushed him a little bit, I asked about his medical record. A less secure doctor would have gone off the wall with the questions. He listened to what I had to say and he had a very compassionate nature. I had really good support. I felt we were partners in this. Find a good technical surgeon and someone with a heart. You need both.

It's a year and a half now (since the surgery). I feel 100% better. It's like a miracle. I feel much more level. Prehysterectomy I had lots of ups and downs. I was afraid I'd go from being a young woman within 24 hours to an old woman. It didn't happen! People tell you a lot of crazy tales. I'd never recommend a hysterectomy, but if you need it, have a good attitude about it, and have a good surgeon with good experience.

Penny, 50 years old
It's been going on since '87. Horrible. Totally altered my life and I consider it totally unnecessary. My gynecologist enjoyed an excellent reputation. He'd been my doctor since 1969. He didn't do proper tests beforehand. I was going to be 43. I had fibroids. He told me they could become malignant. Afterwards I found out that very rarely happens. The only complication he told me I could have was gaining weight. This was the only side effect I *didn't* get.

I come from a history of heart disease and osteoporosis, which would make it even stupider to have the ovaries removed. He did a D & C to "buy time." All hell broke loose after that. I was bleeding almost constantly, he gave me pain medicine. When I had the surgery I expressed concern on the table. I told him I was frightened. He kidded me out of it and changed the subject. I woke up on the table in excruciating pain. I had leaking from a blood vessel into my pelvis. My blood pressure was so low they couldn't give me pain medication. My fever spiked. He should've reopened the wound, I wouldn't have the adhesions I got. I developed anemia, had to have a blood transfusion. I had fatigue, aches and pains. Terrible pain when moving my bowels. I lost my sex drive, I had pain during intercourse, when I could finally have intercourse. If I have intercourse for five minutes I have cracking of the vaginal skin. I got breast lumps, joint pains, anxiety, mood swings. I had bone loss, I have atrophy of the vagina. It took me 15 minutes to walk a block, 15 minutes to get from the bed to the bathroom. It's devastated my marriage. My doctor never protected me with hormone replacement, even though I had this history of heart disease and osteoporosis.

I would give anything to have a Kotex pad back in my life. Take every kind of alternative method instead of a hysterectomy. The doctor is just walking around scot-free. If I could kill him . . . My life will absolutely never be the same again.

Vicki, 44 years old

I had the hysterectomy when I was 35. I am beyond happy. I am thrilled. It's the best thing I ever did. Getting my period was the worst thing—two weeks every month, the most unbearable cramps, I would almost faint from the pain. You can't control it. I was terrified when it was coming, scared to drive too far from home. It was the easiest decision of my life.

Psychologically, there's no difference. Anxiety I had before has diminished. It had no physical impact, no loss of physical pleasure. Sex I think is actually *better* because I'm not afraid of getting pregnant. I had two children—if I was losing that (ability), it would've been different. I still have my ovaries so I didn't go through the change. It's fabulous. I went everywhere, tried lots of other things—I didn't want chemical tinkering with my system, that seemed more artificial than the hysterectomy. I cannot think of any problem with not having a uterus. I feel fine and in control. I've had absolutely zero problems with it.

OPTIONS TO HYSTERECTOMY

There are options to hysterectomy that often resolve the problems listed above. To name just a few. Medication, usually hormone therapy, can be used to control or regulate abnormal vaginal bleeding in some cases. (Always find out the root cause of the bleeding, of course.) Sometimes simple birth control pills can put erratic or heavy bleeding back on a more normal cycle. Endometrial ablation is another technique that can be used to stop uterine bleeding; with this procedure, an electric current is run with a special device to clear away the uterine lining, making the uterus nonfunctional *but* leaving the physical body of the uterus in place—which some women find preferable to a hysterectomy. This procedure cures bleeding about half the time, while another quarter of patients are somewhat relieved, and the final quarter continue to bleed heavily. A traditional D & C (dilation and curettage) can be used to treat emergency vaginal bleeding, though it is not used for routine control of bleeding. Sometimes it only works for a short period of time, but it can be repeated, and preserves the uterus. Hysteroscopy (to find an anatomic abnormality like a polyp or fibroid) is often appropriate and helpful. For a prolapsed uterus, surgery to lift the uterus back into place is sometimes an option, as is the use of a pessary or other device to support the drooping organ (but this latter is a short-term solution). Finally, there are ways to remove fibroid tumors without a hysterectomy—depending on their position and size. At most hospitals, for example, surgeons are using an electrical cutting loop to remove small fibroids through the cervix—with no incision necessary. This preserves your ability to bear children. Other centers around the country have various methods of removing fibroids short of hysterectomy—the procedures are all variations of myomectomy or removal of the growth itself.

MAKING YOUR INFORMED CHOICE

Beware of people who are too rabid on either side of the hysterectomy issue. The fact is, the procedure is neither all bad nor all good. Some women say they wish they never considered it; others say it was the best thing they ever did, and wish they had done it sooner. If you have a physician who considers hysterectomy a simple cure-all that shouldn't have any emotional consequences for you, that's a bad sign. If, on the other hand, you're being told that *all* hysterectomies are bad, that's equally misleading. As with most things, there is a gray area. You must weigh the risks and benefits of the procedure along with your personal feelings about keeping your uterus in your body and the possibility of future childbearing. It's a highly personal decision but one that must be made with solid medical information on the likelihood of symptoms and problems both with and without the

procedure.

One important feature of your decision-making process should be learning more about your anatomy. You should understand the difference between your uterus and your ovaries, for instance. Having your uterus removed will not significantly affect the hormone balance in your body. Having your ovaries removed, however, puts you into an artificial menopause, as we'll discuss in a moment. Talk to your doctor about whether he or she is planning to remove your uterus alone, or along with your ovaries; it makes a very big difference in what you can expect afterwards.

TYPES OF HYSTERECTOMY

If you elect to have a hysterectomy—or if you have no choice—talk to your physician about the different types of surgery available and see if the least invasive forms are appropriate for you. About ¾ of hysterectomies are done with an incision in the abdomen. This results in the longest hospital stay and the highest cost, but might be your only option—especially if your surgeon is planning to do other exploratory surgery in addition to the hysterectomy. One-fourth of hysterectomies are done vaginally, either with an incision in the vagina or, in the case of laparoscopically assisted vaginal hysterectomy (LAVH), with a tiny incision in the abdomen—and then removal of the uterus through the vagina. These are shorter procedures with shorter hospital stays.

It's also extremely important that you talk to your doctor about how extensive your hysterectomy will be. Just as there are various degrees of surgery for breast cancer (ranging from the removal of the lump to removal of the entire breast with surrounding lymph nodes), so there are different degrees of hysterectomies. With a supracervical hysterectomy, your uterus is removed and your cervix is left in place. With a total hysterectomy, your uterus and cervix are both removed, and your ovaries left intact. With a total hysterectomy with bilateral salpingo-oophorectomy, your uterus and cervix will be removed *along with* your fallopian tubes and ovaries. With a radical hysterectomy, all of the above will be removed *along with* the upper third of the vagina, the ligaments that hold the uterus in place, and nearby lymph nodes.

The reason it's so important for you to discuss the extent of your surgery is twofold. First, the more you know *before* your surgery, studies show, the greater your satisfaction will be afterward. Second, having your ovaries removed means going into artificial menopause—that is, you will no longer have high levels of estrogen in your body. The result: all of the changes of menopause, from hot flashes to bone loss to increased risk of heart disease and sometimes serious mood changes. If you *don't* have to have your ovaries removed for any medical reason, make sure your doctor isn't one to remove them "just because he's already in there." If you need to have your ovaries removed in addition to your uterus, then you should discuss the option of HRT (hormone replacement therapy) with your doctor beforehand, and have a plan of action. (*See* chapter 10 for more on the risks and benefits of hormone replacement.)

WHAT YOU CAN EXPECT AFTER A HYSTERECTOMY

There is great disagreement over the degree of psychological and sexual impact of hysterec-tomy. That's because different studies have had dramatically different results—naturally, because women's responses differ. There is conflicting data on whether the uterus has any role in sexual pleasure. Many OB-GYNs point to data showing that the uterus (and cervix at its neck) are *not* needed for orgasm. They argue that it is the loss of the ovaries and the estrogen that they produce that can lead to sexual problems (since the vagina becomes dry, and other menopausal changes set in), and that most female sexual response is centered around the lower third of the vagina—the clitoris, vulva, and so on. (*See* chapter 3, "Your Reproductive Anatomy," page 33). Others say that the uterine contractions that sometimes occur during orgasm are sorely missed after hysterectomy. Nora Coffey of Hysterectomy Educational Resources and Services (HERS) has data to support this latter perspective. HERS data shows that an extremely large number of women suffer significant feelings of loss after a hysterectomy, along with both physical feelings of exhaustion and pain, and emotional symptoms of depression, lack of sexual desire and satisfaction.

Some would say that because the women with the most severe problems after hysterectomy are the ones who contact support groups like HERS, their data could be quite on the pessimistic side. After all, there are some positive aspects to hysterectomy: for those who no longer want children but do want a sex life, removal of the uterus erases all concerns about contraception, leaving them more free to enjoy sex unencumbered by contraceptive devices. Or, for the woman with cancer of the uterus, or chronic uterine problems, hysterectomy can signal a time of great relief and the sense that once again she can move on with a more care-free existence. Experts caution, however, that women who go into the procedure with less certainty about their desire to bear children in the future—or who believe that the uterus is an important symbol of femininity or sexuality— are more likely to suffer adverse psychological consequences of hysterectomy.

Dr. Thomas Sedlacek of Graduate Hospital in Philadelphia urges women who have the *choice* of hysterectomy (i.e., elective hysterec-tomy) to sit down and evaluate their personal feelings about their uterus. It's something we rarely do about *any* body part until we run the risk of losing it. If, he says, you feel that the uterus is nothing but a bunch of tissues that performed a function no longer needed by your body, you're more likely to do great after its removal. If, on the other hand, you realize that you have a strong attachment to the very *idea* of having your uterus in your body, you might prefer to live with bothersome symptoms rather than having it out.

Dr. Chapin agrees. "Preoperative attitude is everything," he insists. He asks women to deter-mine if they place an inherent emotional value on their uterus that's separate from its biologi-cal function. Does it enhance your sense of femininity, or sexual responsiveness? Does it make you feel "whole"? Some of Dr. Chapin's patients actually find just the opposite when they sit down to think about it; they say that they have been bothered for years by sexual penetration that touches their cervix (the open-ing to the uterus) and will not be sorry to see it go. Or perhaps they've finished bearing chil-dren and think their uterus has done its job and is expendable. Other women see it quite differ-ently. How do you feel?

FOR MORE INFORMATION ON GENERAL GYNECOLOGICAL PROBLEMS:

AMERICAN COLLEGE OF OBSTETRICIANS AND GYNECOLOGISTS RESOURCE CENTER
409 12th St. NW
Washington, DC 20024-2188
202-638-5577

NATIONAL WOMEN'S HEALTH NETWORK
514 10th St. NW, Suite 400
Washington, DC 20004
202-347-1140

NATIONAL WOMEN'S HEALTH RESOURCE CENTER
2440 M St. NW, Suite 325
Washington, DC 20037
202-293-6045

URINARY INCONTINENCE:
HELP FOR INCONTINENT PEOPLE (HIP)
P.O. Box 544
Union, SC 29379
800-BLADDER

SIMON FOUNDATION FOR CONTINENCE
3621 Thayer St.
Evanston, IL 60201
800-23-SIMON

THE BLADDER HEALTH COUNCIL AMERICAN FOUNDATION FOR UROLOGIC DISEASE
300 West Pratt Street, Suite 401
Baltimore, MD 21201
800-242-2383

NATIONAL KIDNEY AND UROLOGIC
    DISEASES INFORMATION
    CLEARINGHOUSE
P.O. Box NKUDIC
9000 Rockville Pike
Bethesda, MD 20892
301-468-6345

INTERSTITIAL CYSTITIS:
INTERSTITIAL CYSTITIS ASSOCIATION
P.O. Box 1553
Madison Square Station
New York, NY 10159
800-HELP-ICA

ENDOMETRIOSIS:
ENDOMETRIOSIS ASSOCIATION
8585 North 76th Place
Milwaukee, WI 53223
800-992-ENDO

FIBROIDS:
AMERICAN COLLEGE OF OBSTETRICIANS
    AND GYNECOLOGISTS
See Hysterectomy

HYSTERECTOMY:
AMERICAN COLLEGE OF OBSTETRICIANS
    AND GYNECOLOGISTS RESOURCE
    CENTER
409 12th Street SW
Washington, DC 20024-2188
202-638-5577

HYSTERECTOMY EDUCATIONAL
    RESOURCES AND SERVICES
    (HERS FOUNDATION)
422 Bryn Mawr Ave.
Bala Cynwyd, PA 19004
610-667-7757

LUPUS:
THE LUPUS FOUNDATION OF AMERICA
1717 Massachusetts Ave. NW
Washington, DC 20026
800-558-0121

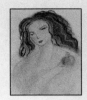

PART THREE

Menstrual Health and Cycles of Change

CHAPTER EIGHT

MENSTRUAL HEALTH

Each month
the blood sheets down
like good red rain.
I am the gardener.
Nothing grows without me.

—Erica Jong, "Gardener"

"She's got the curse." "She's on the rag." "It must be that time of the month." We've heard them all. Many women say they've had at least one slur directed at them—and often they're *not* recalling adolescence. Take the workplace as one example. Husband to wife in times of stress. Even harried *men* are accused of it mockingly—usually by other men.

Menstruation, a physiological sign of our femininity, has been the butt of jokes, the subject of irrational fears, the stuff of mystery and ritual, and—happily—even delight to emotionally healthy young girls who are comfortable with the notion of womanhood. My own mother was told that her period would kill the plants in her home. Men have been warned that menstrual blood is a threat to their sex organs. Orthodox Judaism holds it sacred to *avoid* sexual relations with one's spouse while she is menstruating, and women claim that this temporary abstinence prevents disease.

The myths, beliefs, and legends are countless. What is perhaps more striking than society's obsession with the act of menstruation is the remarkable process that takes place in our bodies to create it. For those of us who menstruate regularly, and who complain half-heartedly about the nuisance of it, we tend to take for granted the dramatic act that plays out in our bodies to bring menstruation about.

On average, at about age twelve, girls will menstruate for the first time. It can be scary—if you've never seen blood on your toilet paper or underwear before, you're apt to think something terrible is occurring. Some young women fear they have a fatal disease. If you're lucky, your mother, sister, aunt or some other knowing older woman is nearby for reassurance. That's if you're willing to speak up and report what has transpired. My maternal grandmother, who happened to be visiting when my big event occurred, beamed "welcome to the club." Clearly the culture of menstruation had changed somewhat in the 30-plus years since she had subscribed to the dead plant theory.

THE REPRODUCTIVE CYCLE

By their early teens, when menstruation has become the norm, most girls are looking for their periods and are relieved when it arrives. Earlier than that—and certainly much later—it can be upsetting. People generally don't like to be different, and young girls are no exception. But within a fairly broad age range, from about 10 to 16, menarche (the onset of menstruation) is normal. Before age 10 is generally considered *early* puberty; after age 16, late (often called "primary amenorrhea"—meaning primary lack of menstruation). We'll talk about some of the causes of this later in this chapter.

It's useful to understand the hormonal basis of menstruation for several reasons. First, the more you know about the normal workings of your body, the more you'll understand if any of those processes breaks down. Second, when it comes to treating menstrual problems and understanding menopause (the cessation of menstruation), you'll have a much better idea of what's happening in your body.

For starters, menstruation comes about by

an interaction between parts of your brain and parts of your reproductive anatomy. Here's a simple version of what's going on: Your hypothalamus, in your brain, gives a chemical signal to your pituitary gland to get the process rolling. Your pituitary in turn produces something called FSH—follicle simulating hormone—the signal to the follicles, the shells that contain your eggs, to start making the hormone estrogen. The estrogen "talks back" to the pituitary, letting it know to start producing another hormone, called LH (luteinizing hormone). With LH and estrogen at their peaks, the follicles do as they were told and release a ripe egg into the fallopian tubes, where it can be fertilized if sperm is present. The follicle, now "empty," is not done with its work. It becomes the corpus luteum, or yellow body, which makes the hormone progesterone. In turn, the progesterone helps thicken and prepare the lining of the uterus for a possible pregnancy.

If pregnancy does *not* occur, the progesterone level eventually drops off and the uterine lining breaks down and sheds. The result is menstruation—the start of the entire cycle once again. That "blood" you see is largely made up of uterine lining that wasn't needed to support a pregnancy. This is why menstrual blood is not liquidy like pure blood, but often slightly more clotted. Mucus also makes menstrual flow more clumpy.

CYCLE LENGTH

It's easy to see how any blip in the machinery—at the level of the brain, the chemical messengers or the reproductive organs—can throw a woman's cycle off track. It's amazing, in fact, that most women *do* have fairly regular cycles.

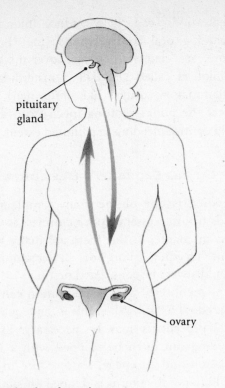

pituitary gland

ovary

Pituitary gland and ovaries

for just a couple of months—or even a couple of years—can have quite irregular cycles (missing occasional periods, for example) without arousing much concern. Of course, if they are sexually active and pregnancy is a possibility, every missed period deserves investigation—at least with an at-home pregnancy test.

In addition, cycles can change as you grow older. Some women find that after pregnancy, or for reasons they and their doctors never understand, their cycles that were immovable at 30 days suddenly become 26 days long—or vice versa. Some women find that their cycles shorten or lengthen with age, and that finally, in the premenopausal years, they can develop extremely erratic patterns (sometimes periods become less frequent, occurring one month and then not another; sometimes they seem to appear almost constantly). This irregularity can be extremely disconcerting, as it's unpredictable, can ruin clothing and cause embarrassment and discomfort. Talk to your doctor if your cycles become so erratic that they're hampering your normal activities. (For a more complete discussion of menopause and menopausal sensations, *see* chapter 10.)

Some women find that their cycles *never* become regular, making pregnancy prevention, ovulation charting and other related activities much more difficult.

DURATION AND HEAVINESS OF FLOW

Again, while there are averages, there's no such thing as "normal" flow length or heaviness. Healthy women menstruate for as few as two days and longer than seven, Dr. Debrovner says. On average, menstruation lasts for about five days, with bleeding heavier in the first 48 hours

For the average woman, the entire menstrual cycle just described takes about 28 days, but "normal" cycles can be much shorter or longer, from as few as 20 days to as long as 40-plus, according to most experts. A woman's first few periods are usually *not* on a scheduled pattern. According to Dr. Charles Debrovner of New York's Roosevelt Hospital, the key is regularity. If a woman has a 28-day cycle for several years and then switches suddenly to a 40-day cycle, she might want to investigate. If she has had a *regular* 40-day cycle for many years, she's probably perfectly healthy—and can count herself among the lucky ones who get fewer periods per year.

It can take a few years for your regular cycle to kick in. Adolescents who have had their periods and tapering thereafter. But there are perfectly healthy women with eight-day periods that are heavy from start to finish, as well as healthy women with very light two-day flows.

When should you worry about excessive menstrual flow? According to Dr. Jay Daskal of the Illinois Masonic Medical Center, you should *not* have to "double up" on protection. For instance, if you need a large tampon *and* a sanitary pad to protect you from just two hours' flow, for example, you may be bleeding excessively heavily. It's hard to say how many tampon or pad changes is normal, since some women change eight or ten times a day when their pads aren't yet saturated. As a general guideline, though, Dr. Daskal advises that if you are soaking ten tampons or pads each day (even after the first couple of days of flow), if the blood runs down your legs or is very thick and clotted, you might want to discuss it with your health care provider. Dr. Debrovner uses a general guideline of about 50% more blood flow than you usually have as a measure of newly excessive bleeding.

If you are losing excessive amounts of blood, you may be anemic (lacking red blood cells and iron in your blood); this can cause lethargy or other mood and energy problems. Your health care provider may do a simple blood test to see if you are anemic, and if you are, you may be put on iron supplements or encouraged to eat foods that are more rich in iron (*see* chapter 20 on nutrition for some examples).

Sometimes, extremely heavy flow is *not* a sign of problems at all, but just a variation on normal. In other cases, it can signal the presence of fibroid growths (for more on fibroids, *see* chapter 7), a hormonal imbalance, impending menopause or many other factors. Several medications can help reduce blood flow, including oral contraceptives (the "Pill"; for more, *see* chapter 11), and over-the-counter painkillers called NSAIDS (nonsteroidal anti-inflammatory drugs, like ibuprofen), which affect the body's clotting mechanism and can help control bleeding to a limited extent.

TREATING EXCESSIVE BLEEDING

Bleeding is one of the main complaints that leads to unnecessary hysterectomies, as we discuss in chapter 7. But there are many ways to limit bleeding short of hysterectomy that should always be considered first.

As mentioned above, medication can sometimes do the trick. When this is inadequate, surgical procedures may be necessary. Excessive bleeding can often be stopped with a D & C (dilation and curettage, a procedure in which the lining of the uterus is scraped off surgically) or with a high-tech procedure called laser ablation (or rollerball ablation) in which the lining of the uterus is burned away (the uterus is no longer functional after this procedure, but the organ is still intact). Neither of these procedures works for all women, but they are often effective. If heavy bleeding resumes, a second procedure can be tried.

WHEN SHOULD YOU WORRY ABOUT EXCESSIVELY LIGHT FLOW?

If your menstrual periods are normally light but quite regular, you probably have nothing to worry about. But if your periods suddenly become much lighter than usual, lasting only a couple of days with scant flow, talk to your doctor. While it could be absolutely nothing, you'll want to rule out rare problems that can result in scarring in your uterus (after an abortion or D & C, for example) or from Asherman's syndrome, in which adhesions in the uterus can cause the uterine walls to cling to one another, cutting off blood flow and preventing the shedding of the lining from portions of the uterus.

BLEEDING BETWEEN PERIODS

Minimal bleeding between periods may be normal for you, but if it isn't, or if your doctor doesn't know about it, it's worth investigating. The cause may be as benign as ovulation, or perhaps minor polyps or other cysts or benign growths. In rarer cases, it could signal a reproductive cancer, or an infection somewhere in the reproductive system that needs treatment. Sometimes hormonal imbalances can cause irregular bleeding, too. Pregnancy is another common cause of mid-cycle bleeding. Early in pregnancy, even perfectly healthy pregnancies, light bleeding or "spotting" or "staining" is quite common. Pregnancy-related problems, including miscarriage, also cause irregular bleeding.

USING TAMPONS AND PADS TO CONTAIN MENSTRUAL FLOW

There is no *right* choice for containing menstrual blood. The best choice is the option with which you feel most comfortable. Both tampons and pads are safe and effective, though women have their favorites and tend to swear by one or the other. Some women with heavy flow use both at once to avoid soiling clothing, but remember, if you're saturating both methods constantly throughout the day, your bleeding may be excessive.

There is no "rule," but there are guidelines for tampon use. You may have heard of a problem called toxic shock syndrome (TSS), which is caused when a certain family of bacteria that produces a toxin multiplies in the vagina and leads to a life-threatening syndrome of fever, vomiting, diarrhea, dizziness and ultimately shock. This condition, though quite rare, has been associated with leaving too-absorbent tampons (and other objects like certain barrier contraceptives) in the vagina for too long. The theory holds that the tampon absorbs and traps the bacteria, promoting its growth. How to translate "too long," however, is a bit of a problem. Most practitioners advise removing tampons after a couple of hours, even if you haven't yet saturated them. There are instructions regarding TSS inside leading tampon brand boxes. The message of caution is especially important late in your period, when you may be bleeding very little and could be tempted to leave a tampon in all day since there's little risk of staining. *Don't do it.* Use a smaller, thinner tampon for those light days so it will become moist enough to remove easily even if it isn't saturated with blood. With these simple precautions, tampons are extremely safe and many women find them more comfortable than sanitary pads, especially during exercise or when wearing close-fitting clothing.

OVULATION

We've been assuming that if you have a regular menstrual cycle, you're ovulating; that is, releasing an egg each cycle. In fact, that's not always the case, says Dr. Jill Rabin, chief of ambulatory and urogynecologic care at New York's Long Island Jewish Medical Center. It's possible to bleed (often irregularly) without ovulating. Some common obstacles to ovulation, she says, include obesity (which can lead to excessive estrogen production relative to other hormones) or extreme underweight (which can cause a *lack* of estrogen); thyroid problems (both high and low thyroid activity, but more often low thyroid, which can be associated with a newly deep voice, puffiness in the shins and eyes, slightly excessive weight, and erratic negative moods); autoimmune diseases, in which the body's own immune system turns on itself; and many others. To bring back ovulation, you must determine the precise cause of the problem and treat it directly: thyroid medication, weight gain or loss, and so on.

Ovulation normally occurs 14 days *before* the start of your next menstrual period; note that only if your cycle is about 27 days long does it occur at approximately mid-cycle. If your cycle is 33 days long, ovulation normally occurs at about day 20 in your cycle. For more on ovulation and treating ovulatory problems, *see* chapter 16, "Infertility: Causes and Treatments."

MENSTRUAL PAIN, WATER WEIGHT GAIN, AND OTHER PHYSICAL PROBLEMS WITH MENSTRUATION

Some women experience pain or cramping with their periods, often starting just before menstruation begins and reaching its peak in the first couple of days of bleeding. The pain is sometimes accompanied by other physical discomfort, such as nausea or appetite changes, fatigue and general malaise. In general, menstrual pain (as well as menstrual irregularity) seem to be worse at the early and later extremes of a woman's reproductive life span. For example, adolescents may have severe cramping once their periods kick in, and women in their late 30s who may be approaching the early changes of menopause often report newly severe menstrual pain. Some say that women who have never borne biological children may be at risk for more menstrual pain as they enter their 30s, but this is variable. (While menopause, the complete cessation of menstrual periods, occurs on average at age 51, the hormonal changes that lead to it begin much earlier for most women. It is possible to have hormone tests to chart your progress toward menopause. Increasing levels of the hormone FSH indicate a movement toward menopause, and can explain some menstrual irregularities.)

Most women have *some* discomfort with menstruation. Usually it comes in the form of abdominal pain or cramping, breast tenderness and, for some women, generalized achiness. Dr. Rabin urges women to look on the bright side of this pain; we're feeling it for a good reason, she explains. Our bodies are producing chemicals called prostaglandins that help stop menstrual bleeding before it becomes excessive. This spasm of vessels causes pain. If you have mild premenstrual pain, you'll usually be helped by over-the-counter painkillers, particularly the nonsteroidal anti-inflammatory drugs mentioned earlier. Some experts report that fewer women have been complaining of menstrual pain since use of over-the-counter NSAIDS became more routine. The best approach, according to Dr. Michelle Warren, head of reproductive endocrinology at St. Luke's-Roosevelt Hospital in New York, is to take one of these medications *before* your pain becomes severe. A good analogy, she says, is seasickness; once you've got it, there isn't much you can do to undo it. The same goes for menstrual pain; medications can't do too much to eliminate the pain you're already feeling. But when taken shortly before pain becomes severe, at the first twinge (most women come to know their systems well enough to recognize this threshold), medication can prevent the worst cramping for many women. Some practitioners advise taking a larger dose of NSAIDS at first, and then tapering to a smaller dose as pain abates. Discuss the proper dosing with your doctor.

Acetaminophen and aspirin are different stories. Many practitioners I spoke with report that acetaminophen (Tylenol) does little or nothing for menstrual pain. But they add that since it is a pretty benign medication, if it *seems* to help you, there's no reason to switch to another medication for pain. On the other hand, many practitioners advise *against* taking aspirin for menstrual pain, since it can increase both bleeding *and* the production of prostaglandins.

If your pain continues to be severe even while you're taking over-the-counter pain medicine, *do not* keep upping the dose to try to find relief. Discuss the situation with your doctor. While these drugs are nearly ubiquitous and one would like to think they're harmless, they can be dangerous in excessive amounts—causing harm to the lining of the stomach and other problems. Some NSAIDS are available in stronger doses by prescription; if your doctor prescribes them and monitors you appropriately, this is much safer than taking larger and larger doses of the over-the-counter forms on your own. For chronic discomfort, some doctors prescribe oral contraceptives—by "taking over" the menstrual cycle, these drugs sometimes break the pain cycle.

If your menstrual pain is extreme, you'll also want to be sure that nothing more serious is going on in your body. One example would be endometriosis, in which tissue similar to the lining of the uterus grows outside the uterus, causing spasms, adhesions and contractions (literally like having menstrual cramps in other parts of your body). Other pelvic problems, like fibroid tumors, can also worsen menstrual pain (as we discuss in chapter 7 on gynecological health). One bad period isn't enough to make doctors suspect serious problems. But if your pain persists for a couple of cycles, if it's worse than it was in the past and if it seems to get worse with time, you should be examined by a doctor—if only to rule out serious problems or find ways to treat your pain more effectively.

If more serious problems have been ruled out and your pain is thought to be related to menstruation alone, medication is not your only option. A wide range of non-drug therapies can help relieve your discomfort. Heat applied to the abdomen and warm-to-hot baths may help—although this is not an adequate solution, since you cannot take hot baths or apply heat pads at work, for example. Some women find that exercise helps relieve menstrual cramps, it's worth a try, if you can manage to get yourself up and working out. Other women find that regular exercise reduces the incidence of cramps in the first place, but this is variable. Dr. Warren reports that premenstrual problems (both physical and emotional) are relieved by reducing alcohol, excessive caffeine and sugar in the diet. (For a further discussion of menstrual discomfort "remedies," *see* chapter 9, "Premenstrual Syndrome.")

A smaller number of women have some pain at approximately mid-cycle, or the point at which the egg is released from the follicle, which may not in fact happen at the exact midpoint of the cycle (as discussed above). This usually brief pain comes in the form of a "twang" known as *mittelschmerz,* German for "middle pain." It's usually short-lived and relieved with over-the-counter pain medicine (acetaminophen or another mild nonsteroidal anti-inflammatory drug) at most.

As with cycle length, any *change* in the severity of your menstrual pain that persists for a couple of cycles is worth discussing with your practitioner. And, as we discuss repeatedly throughout this book, you'll only recognize change when you start to pay attention to how your body feels and looks in general. Being more attuned to your menstrual cycle and other body functions will help you and your doctor catch problems before they become severe.

How do you define too much pain? Most practitioners define it in terms of *function.* If your pain is getting in the way of your enjoyment of life's activities, your productivity at work or your relationships with others, that's too much pain for you—and you should discuss it with your doctor.

WATER RETENTION

Many women gain a few pounds of water weight before and during menstruation, and it can be uncomfortable for some. According to Dr. Michelle Warren, water weight gain usually sets in several days *before* menstruation and lasts for several days, so women may complain of a full week of bloating. Water gain of more than five pounds is unusual, she says, and may be caused by other problems, such as a large ovarian cyst that's retaining fluid. Water retention can sometimes be managed with behavior changes like restricted salt intake (watch out for items like pizza, chinese food, canned goods

and processed meats, e.g.), exercise and occasionally diuretics (under a doctor's supervision). While it may seem illogical, drinking lots of water is a good way to reduce water retention over time, since the more you urinate and sweat, the more you keep fluid moving through your body in a healthy way. Don't deprive yourself of needed fluids in an attempt to keep your water weight down—it's unhealthy for your bladder, kidneys and many other body systems.

PRIMARY AND SECONDARY AMENORRHEA

The first question your practitioner will ask if you're experiencing amenorrhea (lack of menstrual periods) is whether the problem is *primary* or *secondary*—that is, if you've never had a period before (primary), or if you used to have periods and then they stopped (secondary). We mentioned earlier that "primary" amenorrhea is usually defined by the lack of menstruation by age 16. There are a vast number of potential causes for primary lack of periods, and now that you understand how the normal menstrual cycle works, it will be easy for you to see that amenorrhea an be caused by problems anywhere along the brain-reproductive organ cycle. Just a few examples include trouble with the glands that send the chemical messages of menstruation, the ovaries or uterus that receives those messages and the hormones levels themselves. Another important potential cause of amenorrhea is excessive skinniness, often associated with the eating disorder anorexia nervosa, a condition in which a person starves herself of calories, and may exercise obsessively to the point of dangerous thinness and bone loss. The extreme lack of body fat connected with this problem, and the halt of estrogen production that ensues, can prevent menstruation from taking place. This is a serious and unfortunately common problem of young American women and must be considered when weight is dropping and periods disappear—or don't appear in the first place. (For much more on eating disorders, *see* chapter 23.)

Competitive athletes, because they have such high muscle mass and low body fat, can also be amenorrheic: consider the prepubescent appearance of 18-year-old gymnasts, or marathon runners. The power of body fat on hormone regulation should not be overlooked. Even small amounts of estrogen in the body created by body fat can help keep cycles normal. Naturally, any treatment for amenorrhea will be geared toward bringing on menstruation; that is the goal. Depending on the underlying cause of the amenorrhea, treatment can take many different forms—anything from weight gain to hormonal treatments to limiting athletic training.

Other more serious hormonal or structural problems in the reproductive system can also prevent menstruation. The best person to diagnose the cause of amenorrhea is a reproductive endocrinologist, who can run a number of sophisticated hormone and other tests to look for a cause. Many causes of amenorrhea are treatable.

When Your Periods Stop.

The first thing you'll want to rule out with secondary amenorrhea is pregnancy. No matter how old you are, if you are sexually active and have not yet reached menopause, this should be considered immediately. It is extremely important for all women to become familiar with their menstrual cycles, and to pay attention to the timing of their most recent periods, so that if pregnancy occurs, they're able to pinpoint the likely time of conception. Some practitioners tell of intelligent women who appear in their offices thinking they might be one month pregnant who are in fact closer to three months pregnant—simply because they've forgotten the dates of their last period. If you want to continue that pregnancy, you've lost important prenatal care; if you want to terminate the pregnancy, you may have brought yourself into a later and more dangerous time for pregnancy termination. *Pay attention to your body!*

Sometimes breast-feeding can hold off periods for several months if it's done absolutely exclusively (that is, no infant formula supplementation at all). Other causes of secondary amenorrhea include highly vigorous athletic training and eating disorders (as mentioned above); minimal weight gain of a few pounds or cutting back training intensity can often bring periods back. Ovarian cysts or tumors can interrupt menstruation; their removal will often restore normal menstruation. Thyroid problems may be the culprit; proper medication can return menstrual flow. Excessive male hormones, or the presence of a hormone called prolactin which can cause secretions of milk from the breasts even when breast-feeding is not taking place, can also interrupt normal periods.

Barbara Drinkwater, a research physiologist at Seattle's Pacific Medical Center, points out that while the lack of a period is not always a problem in and of itself (some women find it a relief!), the lack of hormones that bring on menstruation affects *other* body systems too, most notably the bones, which can become brittle and porous even in young active women.

So there are very good general health reasons to try to bring menstruation back as soon as possible, whatever the cause of its cessation. Oral contraceptives, which override the body's normal hormone production and create an artificial, regular cycle, may be the best temporary solution for some women.

Extreme emotional stress is another potential cause of missed periods. Again, remember the significant role of the brain and the chemicals it produces to bring on menstruation. A disruption in brain chemicals associated with stress, depression, extreme grief or some other powerful emotional upheaval can throw the delicate menstrual cycle off course. Time may cure the problem, but if the problems are severe and persistent, counseling or medication may be warranted (for more on mental health, *see* chapter 7).

Sometimes secondary amenorrhea is brought on by a problem that's easy to identify and just as easily reversed if bothersome. For example, some (but certainly not all) women taking progestin-only contraceptives (like Depo-Provera, the minipill and Norplant) lose their periods after some time on the medication. There are women who don't mind the absence of periods a bit, and others who find it quite disconcerting (enough so to switch methods).

OUT-OF-THE-ORDINARY MENSTRUAL PROBLEMS

At some point in your reproductive lifetime, or perhaps throughout all of the years you menstruate, menstrual problems can get out of control. Your physical problems may become extreme, getting in the way of your enjoyment and full participation in life. Your emotional changes may become volatile, extreme, unmanageable. When you feel that your menstrual cycle changes, both in body and spirit, have carried you past a point that you can handle with minor lifestyle adjustments and medical treatments, you may have premenstrual syndome or PMS.

Don't take your feelings lightly, or let others dismiss them as improbable or exaggerated. Seek the care you need and deserve. The next chapter discusses premenstrual syndrome, its causes, symptoms and management. There are a lot of women out there who feel the way you do—and an equally large number of treatments and approaches to handling PMS that have given life back to those women. Let yourself become healthy again.

FOR MORE INFORMATION ON PROBLEMS WITH MENSTRUATION SEE RESOURCES AT THE END OF THE CHAPTER ON PMS, PAGE 155

CHAPTER NINE

PREMENSTRUAL SYNDROME

Is it possible that there are lessons for women and men in PMS? Is the greater sensitivity experienced by women premenstrually something we all, as a society, need to learn about? Without wanting to glorify or romanticize their pain, I wonder what growth will come to women as they confront PMS. What would the world be like if men sometimes seemed to cry without reason? What would we then believe about vulnerability or sensitivity?

—Michelle Harrison, M.D., *Self-Help for Premenstrual Syndrome*

Since 1951, when the term "premenstrual tension" was coined, vast amounts of research and debate have surrounded this amorphous female "problem." It was given a fancy name, "late luteal phase dysphoric disorder," which was quickly discarded because it was too awkward. It seemed logical that the signs of PMS would be caused by a hormonal "imbalance" at a time when, as we saw in the previous chapter, both progesterone and estrogen levels are low. But so far, scientists have failed to prove that hormonal changes cause the symptoms many women experience. So skeptics crawled out from under worldwide rocks and said the problem doesn't exist at all—it's just in women's heads. Feminists jumped on both sides of the debate, some arguing that a strict definition of the problem would legitimize women's feelings and help bring needed research, others saying that a vision of menstruation as a disease process just catapults women back into the Dark Ages.

WHAT IS PMS?

In fact, arguing over whether PMS exists is of little use to most women. After all, while we don't know where it comes from or what exactly it *is*, we *do* know that many of us experience something uncomfortable around the time of menstruation, and that the degree of discomfort varies from mild to severe. Millions of women can tell you that, and they don't need a license or a title after their names to do so. The best definition of PMS is the one that fits *your* experience; premenstrual moodiness or achiness, physical or emotional discomfort—the only "real" definition is your own. The more useful question one can ask about PMS is what to *do* about it: How can we help people to feel better? And the answer is good news; there are quite a few solutions.

Whatever name you choose, premenstrual problems amount to a group of signs, symptoms or changes that occur to large numbers of women in the week or so preceding menstruation. These changes range from the physical (breast tenderness, abdominal discomfort, cramping) to the emotional (weepiness, irritability). Many women experience both kinds of problems. For some women, the symptoms linger into the first day or so of bleeding. And while the feelings are practically invisible for some women, they can be utterly debilitating for others. Most of us fall somewhere in between.

In this chapter, we'll look at some of the current definitions of PMS, and we'll consider the treatments that have proved most helpful to large numbers of women.

PMS: THE HARD FACTS

Studies and anecdotal reports show that about half of American women suffer some noticable discomfort in the week before they menstruate. And it is thought that about 5 percent of American women have "severe" premenstrual problems—that is, they're incapacitated by the problem. That adds up to an awful lot of women walking around in physical and emotional pain for at least a week each month, not to mention lost or impaired productivity, or the pain and suffering of loved ones.

WHO'S AT RISK FOR PMS?

Young women who have just started menstruating sometimes have premenstrual discomfort, and women who are heading toward menopause have their own set of changes to experience, including PMS. But the largest group of women who turn up in PMS clinics seems to be 30 to 40 year-olds, and often the mothers of two or more children. If your mother had PMS, you're more likely to have it, too. Furthermore, many women report that their premenstrual symptoms worsen with age, but as Jane Harrison-Hohner, director of the Menstrual Disorders program at the Oregon Health Science University points out, that could easily be a result of the increased pressures on many women as they grow older. Working outside the home while raising children and trying to keep a marriage healthy is highly stressful and is thought to contribute to PMS, as does any kind of outside life stress. This is *not* to say that emotional stress is responsible for PMS; it's just one reason why stress management is increasingly thought to be an important part of PMS treatment.

Other groups of women at high risk for PMS include those with underlying mental illnesses, such as chronic depression. If you're depressed, you're more likely to have premenstrual mood problems—and on the flip side, your underlying problems will often be exacerbated premenstrually. This is called "premenstrual magnification," and it's often treatable. Premenstrual magnification can affect physical as well as psychological health problems. For instance, asthma and herpes infections are known to flare premenstrually for some women.

PMS sometimes begins or worsens after some type of pelvic surgery, like tubal ligation (having the fallopian tubes "tied"), ovarian surgery or hysterectomy.

The bottom line, however, is that if you're female and you menstruate, you're at risk for PMS. You don't need any underlying additional problems to create PMS. That's one of the myths that we have to shake off if we're going to attack the problem rationally and effectively. If you've got it, you're *not* to blame. Dr. Jill Rabin of the Long Island Jewish Hospital in New York urges women to think about PMS as a normal process, not as a disease—and to keep in mind that it's often manageable.

PMS: WHAT YOU HAD TO SAY ABOUT IT

Judi, 44 years old

My family said even when I was in high school they could see when I was getting my period, but I didn't know it. It peaked about age 40–41. When I saw it interfering with my work, I knew it was something I had to deal with. I was very short, my coping skills were low. I work as a high school counselor, this is my 21st year. I'd get real chills, bad diarrhea, a cold sweat and horrible cramps. Combination vitamins really helped with the physical—I still take a B-complex vitamin, and a regular multivitamin and calcium. Five days before my period is always the worst. I'd feel out

of control, fearful of what I would say next. I'd get mad, fuming about little things that would never bother me the other 29 days of the month. It was like being outside of myself looking down. Somehow you feel justified being this angry at something that small. Such self-humiliation: I don't know—God forbid—what I'll do in that state, not physically, but what I might say to someone. Mad for no clear reason. Anything will tip me off. I would cry easily, feel very ugly, insecure and then on the second day of my period I again felt normal.

My biggest problem is being on overload, taking on too much, so now in the week before my period it's "say no to people." About four years ago I decided to see a PMS expert. Is this all in my head? I wanted validation that these behaviors were something to do with my hormones and menstruation. We looked at all the options—the first was to eliminate foods I craved, chocolate, caffeine, coffee, and eat lots of green vegetables instead. I felt fabulous. I was fearful of Xanax, we decided on a very small amount. I've discovered I need to take it *before* I get anxious or I won't realize that I'm escalating.

Ann, 33 years old

Lots of anger, just sort of out of control, not to the point of physical violence but feeling enough stress, and also extreme depression. The physical things weren't that bad, a little bloating and cramps. It comes on so fast, just an incredible depression and no energy, no motivation to do anything. It's been more apparent since I had my child, he's five and a half. It's almost an overnight change, I can tell when it's coming on.

Antidepressants didn't help. Being on the Pill seems to help. I gave up caffeine and according to my husband, and I agree with him, it made a big difference. Exercise helps a ton when I can do it, working on the equipment at the gym, jogging, and I'm starting to swim.

Jan, 46 years old
It was always there. I had a couple of triggers. I'm alcoholic, I had to deal with the PMS, not drink it away. I got a divorce, that was another trigger, the stress. I had more emotional problems than physical. I did have breast tenderness, and an inner rage. I would instantly trigger react, it was like I was looking in on myself, saying what *is* this? I thought I was going crazy, they were going to lock me up.

When there was finally a name for it (PMS) I could get treatment. We started with progesterone suppositories and diet. Cut the sugar out, cut the coffee down, increase the exercise. The clinic saved my life, if they didn't keep trying everything I think I might have committed suicide. With birth control pills for three weeks a month I would be symptom-free. The time off the pill was when I'd get the symptoms. I'm now symptom-free. Of all the things we tried, [the Pill] works best. There is help out there. Try and find a woman practitioner because they've been through things you're talking about. Be persistent. Keep searching for people to help you if people tell you it's all in your head.

ARE YOU SUFFERING FROM PREMENSTRUAL DYSPHORIC DISORDER (PDD)?

Recently, experts have categorized premenstrual problems into several distinct entities, such as premenstrual syndrome (PMS) the most loosely defined "popular" term, and premenstrual dysphoric disorder (PDD) a strictly defined problem listed in the diagnostic manual published by the American Psychiatric Association.

Jean Endicott, director of the Premenstrual Evaluation Unit at the Columbia Presbyterian Medical Center, a leading researcher on premenstrual changes, says that the PMS term used so widely by women and described in so-called "women's magazines" is actually a loosely defined group of mostly *mild* physical symptoms including breast pain and swelling, slight weight gain, headaches, fatigue and perhaps some minor irritability—most of which can be managed easily with over-the-counter preparations. Mention these symptoms to many women and they start nodding acknowledgment. To be considered PMS, the symptoms must occur regularly at the same phase of the menstrual cycle—that is, sometime in the two weeks before you menstruate, usually close to the time of menstruation. But there are some variations—for instance, some women feel crummy when they ovulate (that's at mid-cycle), then they feel better briefly and then crummy again just before their periods begin. Other women go up and down every day in the week or two before their periods. Some feel bad for the entire two weeks before their periods begin, and then feel terrific as soon as their periods start.

Far more serious, Endicott says, is PDD (premenstrual dysphoric disorder), a condition described in the The American Psychiatric Association's Diagnostic and Statistical Manual of Mental Disorders (DSM-4). To be diagnosed as having PDD, you must have at least five of the following eleven symptoms. They must occur in the last week before you menstruate, and subside when your period starts. Finally, these symptoms must markedly interfere with your usual activities, both social and work-related.

Check each symptom that applies, and if you check more than a few, consider seeking additional advice from your doctor and review the treatment section later in this chapter.

Do You See Yourself Here? Signs of Premenstrual Dysphoric Disorder (PDD)

In the week before your period, which of these feelings interferes with your daily life?

1. Markedly depressed, hopeless or self-deprecating?

2. Highly anxious, tense, keyed up or on edge?

3. Suddenly sad, tearful, more sensitive to rejection than usual?

4. Markedly or consistently angry, irritable or prone to personal conflicts?

5. Decreased interest in usual activities such as work, hobbies, friendships or school?

6. Finding it hard to concentrate?

7. Lethargic, easily fatigued, weak?

8. A significant change in appetite, a tendency to overeat or specific food cravings?

9. Needing to sleep more, or the inability to get to sleep?

10. A sense of being overwhelmed or out of control?

11. Physical discomfort, such as breast pain, breast swelling, headache, fatigue, bloating, joint or muscle pain?

It's important that your health care expert determine that these symptoms are not caused by any other problem, such as panic or depressive disorders.

As you can see, PDD can significantly disrupt a woman's life. Some experts feel that this distinguishes it from PMS, which is largely a syndrome of *mild* physical and emotional discomfort. But for the purpose of making this section accessible to more women, we'll use the most common term, PMS, to describe all negative premenstrual changes. You can decide for yourself if you fit the more severe or the more mild category.

Symptoms of PMS

Less strictly defined than PDD but certainly no less real, the list of PMS symptoms is longer than the Great Wall of China. I am amazed at how consistent women's reactions are when I read them the list—it just seems to hit home for a lot of women. "Classic" PMS is supposed to be a relatively minor problem, according to strict definitions . . . but we all know that what's classic often isn't what's universal. The following is just a sampling of the premenstrual problems, both physical and emotional, that turn up on just about every researcher's list—and remember, many of these symptoms continue into the first day or two of menstruation. You may experience one or many of these sensations, and they could be mild or severe. Perhaps they differ month to month. As we are individuals, so our feelings and interpretations of PMS often differ.

Physical Changes before Menstruation

- breast tenderness
- bloating, weight gain of several pounds

- abdominal cramping
- change in appetite; salty and sweet food cravings
- weakness, fatigue, lethargy
- change in sleep pattern; more sleep or insomnia
- nausea, vomiting
- acne
- headaches (including migraines)
- rapid heartbeat or pounding heart
- dizziness, clumsiness, shakiness, faintness
- joint and muscle pain
- bowel changes; diarrhea or constipation
- backache
- change in sex drive
- sweating
- other problems flare: herpes, yeast infections, hemorrhoids, allergies

Emotional or Psychological Changes before Menstruation

- anger, irritability (65% of Harrison-Hohner's patient population report that anger and irritability are their primary emotional symptoms before menstruation)
- anxiety, panic, paranoia, nervousness
- mood swings, outbursts
- intolerance, impatience
- pessimism
- tearfulness, depression, withdrawal
- poor concentration, forgetfulness
- hypersensitivity
- feeling "stressed out"
- vulnerability, insecurity

If you recognize many of these symptoms, and feel that they are getting in the way of your ability to lead a happy or productive life, or prompting you to hurt yourself or other people, you need to seek help for PMS.

Prevention and Treatment of PMS

Where to Find Help

The best place to get the help you need? Well that's debatable. In some areas, women's centers or specialized PMS clinics provide excellent resources to help you deal with your symptoms *globally*—that is, helping you to resolve your physical, emotional and family-related PMS problems. However, the term "PMS center" *can* be used merely as a marketing tool, a way of getting you in the door of a clinic to grab your business, since premenstrual problems are so common. The key in choosing care is to see someone who takes PMS seriously, thinks it is a *real* problem and not something you dreamed up in your head—be it your gynecologist, your family doctor, someone practicing at a teaching hospital, or someone who focuses her or his entire practice on PMS. As Endicott likes to say, "Vote with your feet and walk" if you are not treated with respect and understanding when you discuss your premenstrual problems. Read the rest of this chapter and you will be able to approach any health care provider with the information you need to demand the best possible care, without getting sucked into questionable or quack "cures."

Recently, several top PMS experts from around the country, including Jean Endicott, got together and reviewed much of the scientific literature on PMS treatment. They divided the different forms of treatment into five main categories, which I think is very useful for consumers, so I'm doing the same. Of course there is some overlap, but the five major types of treatment we'll look at are: lifestyle changes including diet and exercise, stress reduction through both traditional and alternative therapies, family therapy, non-prescription remedies like vitamins and minerals and medications.

Before we look at the many different treatments for PMS, keep a couple of things in mind.

First, many treatments for PMS are targeted at specific symptoms. So be sure that your health care provider has a good reason for suggesting a particular remedy, and that it matches *your* complaints. No use taking a great medication for breast swelling if your only problem is abdominal cramps. Many doctors won't bother to tell you what your particular drug does, so speak up and *ask*.

Second, it's a good idea to start with the simplest, least invasive, most "natural" treatments before moving on to the so-called "big guns." PMS is a condition in which lifestyle changes alone can cause a dramatic improvement in the way you feel. I must put a caveat here. Some PMS experts, including Dr. Joe Mortola of Beth Israel Hospital in Boston, question the scientific validity of so-called "lifestyle" cures to PMS. He wonders whether a strong placebo effect isn't involved, rather than a real effect of treatment. Probably, the truth is somewhere in a gray area: if you have clinically defined PMS, you likely will need more extensive treatment than lifestyle changes alone. If you have some premenstrual aches and pains, behavior changes alone may do the trick. So before you consider medication, which can have side effects, take a close look at the diet and lifestyle changes that may reduce or eliminate your discomfort.

Also, the earlier in life you start to treat PMS, the better off you'll be. That's not to say that it's too late to start if you're older, but since women have noticed that their PMS can worsen over the years, it's best to attack the problem as soon as possible, while you have more control over it.

Finally, keep in mind that PMS is *not* one static entity; it is constantly changing, and you might feel quite differently one month than you did the previous month. Listen to your body, and each month do what you think it will take to make you feel better now. If a treatment that worked for a few months starts to fail you, move on and try something different.

How can you best keep track of your symptoms, or be sure what's working and what isn't? *Chart them,* says PMS expert Dr. Michelle Harrison, author of *Self-Help For Premenstrual Syndrome.* Make a grid with the day of the month and how you felt that day, and study it to see when your symptoms peak and what, if anything, makes you feel better. Does napping help? Eating differently? Taking a painkiller? Exercising? The better you understand how your body changes and how it responds to your efforts to feel well, the better you will become at managing your premenstrual problems. And remember: for *most* women, the problems *are* manageable. So think positively and read on.

DIET CHANGES

As I mentioned earlier, for some women, lifestyle changes alone can make the difference between suffering premenstrually and feeling okay. A great deal of research has been done on what foods exacerbate premenstrual discomfort, and which ones alleviate it. There is certainly no expert agreement in this area—some PMS experts insist that all diet changes are hogwash, while others swear by them. The reason: these are very hard theories to test scientifically. Following are some of the leading theories. But keep this in mind: in order to make diet changes work for you, you *must* try to change what you eat *all month long*, not just in the days before your period. It takes the body some time to feel the impact of any kind of change, diet included. It can't hurt to try, since a diet that helps relieve PMS is also a generally healthful meal plan, so your entire body will be better off as a result of your efforts.

Eat Frequent, Small Meals.

Try not to let more than three hours go by without eating—and avoid eating large amounts at any one sitting.

Avoid Salty, Spicy and Caffeinated Foods.

It's thought that getting lots of salt and spice in your foods will contribute to the water retention or bloating which so many women complain about premenstrually. Bloating contributes to breast pain, another common complaint. Pastas, grains and vegetables that are served on the bland side are better choices than more zingy recipes. Caffeine, like salt, is thought to contribute to breast tenderness and breast cysts. However, quitting caffeine cold turkey can cause withdrawal symptoms, particularly headaches and sleep problems. You might try gradually weaning yourself from caffeinated beverages, rather than stopping them all at once. If you have three caffeinated sodas each day and a couple of cups of coffee, try cutting out one of the two beverage types first. Or reduce the number of each type of drink that you consume each day. Over several weeks, eliminate caffeine either completely or as much as possible.

Avoid Simple Sugars.

Before your period, you may crave so-called "simple" sweets like chocolate bars and cookies. Many women do. In fact, researchers have tried to understand if there is an important connection between the chemicals in chocolate and premenstrual problems. Experts say it's best to stay away from simple sweets because they cause rapid rises and falls of your body's blood sugar level and can make you feel groggy, irritable and weak soon after you eat them. Replace simple sweets with complex carbohydrate sweets—like fresh fruit.

Avoid Alcohol.

Many women report drinking excessive alcohol premenstrually, perhaps as a way of "treating" or numbing their unpleasant symptoms. In fact, Dr. Harrison points out that alcohol only makes things worse by keeping your blood sugar down and increasing your headaches, irritability, dizziness and anxiety.

Eat More Complex Carbohydrates and Less Protein.

Research has shown that eating more complex carbohydrate foods, like pastas, breads, grains, vegetables and fruits and fewer protein-rich foods like meats and fish, will relieve PMS symptoms. *However*—figure this one out for yourself—Dr. Rabin points out that some experts have noted the exact opposite to be true for some women!

EXERCISE AND PMS

A great tension reliever, sweat producer, endorphin releaser, self-esteem builder, oxygenator, blood flow promoter, and toxin eliminator, exercise is one of the best PMS "treatments" out there. Some women say that the better shape they're in, the fewer cramps they have and the more energy they feel before they menstruate. It's not a cure-all, but regular workouts that get your heart and lungs working and the sweat coming through your pores can make a big difference in how you feel premenstrually. Try vigorous walks, jogs, biking, playing sports, indoor exercise machines or the stairs in your office building. However you like to move your body, doing it can make a big difference in how you feel all month long, not just before and during your period.

STRESS MANAGEMENT AND PMS

One of our biggest challenges is to stop PMS from interfering in our lives—and that means both our personal lives and our career lives. Whether it's to keep our productivity from slipping at the office or to make our home lives more livable, managing premenstrual stress is a top priority for all women with PMS. Getting the best treatment, of course, is the right start, since it will hopefully lead to reduced feelings of irritability and stress before menstruation. But learning to work around your PMS is vital, too. Following is a list of tips:

- Exercise (see section above).
- Don't make major life decisions when "under the influence" of PMS. For instance, even if your boss is driving you crazy, don't quit your job. If your lover seems to be doing or saying everything wrong, don't leave him. Teach yourself to ride it out until you're not premenstrual. When you're feeling better yourself, *then* decide if you need a major change.
- If you can control your schedule, *don't* plan important commitments around the time of your period (an especially strong incentive for charting your menstrual cycle and symptoms). Dinner parties, family outings, staff meetings, spring cleaning— most can wait a week. If you absolutely must do a major project during your premenstrual time, which happens to all of us, try to clear your schedule of other unnecessary commitments so you can focus better and you won't feel overloaded. Nine in ten women with PMS say that it negatively affects their job performance. You can fight that statistic by working around your premenstrual changes.
- *Do* schedule high-performance tasks for the week *after* your period, when you are likely to feel your most energetic.
- Be *kind* to yourself before your period. Do the small things for yourself that make you feel better—a bath? a nap? more time exercising? a movie or a good book? Ana Rivera-Tovar, director of the PMS program at Western Psychiatric Institute and Clinic, says it's tough to get women to do things for themselves sometimes, because so many of us have been socialized to care for *others* instead. This is one time of the month when you have to break out of old habits.
- At some other time of the month, urge your loved ones to treat you more kindly and patiently when you're premenstrual. Discuss it calmly and not in an accusatory way. Ask for support. If they aren't capable of giving it, then ask them to make themselves a little more scarce and a little less demanding for a couple of days instead.

- Meditate, do yoga, try massage (if you can't afford a professional, a friend or lover can often do the trick. Reciprocate a week later!). Researchers have looked at the effect of many "alternative" therapies for PMS, from expressive arts and journal writing to acupressure, acupuncture and meditation, deep muscle relaxation and biofeedback. These relaxation techniques have been found to reduce PMS symptoms significantly in some women. Because so many medical doctors are skeptical about the role of alternative therapies in the treatment of PMS, Terry Oleson and colleagues at the California Graduate Institute recently published a formal scientific paper on the role of hand, ear and foot reflexology (cousins of acupressure) in relieving PMS symptoms. I witnessed a session of the technique, which, if nothing else, relaxed the patient tremendously. According to the study, though, the technique does more than just reduce stress. Published in the *Journal of the American College of Obstetricians and Gynecologists,* the study found reductions in physical and emotional PMS symptoms rivaling many drug therapies. Keep an open mind!
- Try formal psychotherapy, support groups, or some other form of psychological counseling. Delving deeper into your personal premenstrual feelings and challenges often helps you to deal with them better. Sometimes just hearing from other women with similar experiences can be helpful. Training in anger management techniques can be very useful for some women. You might have to shop around

for the kind of counseling that's best for you. Social workers, psychiatrists, psychologists, family therapists and a whole range of other mental health care providers can help you deal with PMS issues. The key is to find someone who takes your concerns seriously and has experience working specifically with PMS-related issues.

TREATING THE "PMS FAMILY"

After one PMS expert told me about treating the "PMS family," I though it was an interesting idea—but a bit eccentric. Soon I learned that, in fact, all over the country PMS treatment centers are taking a close look at the impact of one member's PMS on the family as a whole, and there's a trend to try to treat those who don't have the problem as well as those who do.

What does all that mean? Well, maybe you can relate to this: you wake up one morning with some of the signs of PMS. You're tired. You're achy. You're irritable, when nothing has even happened yet to be irritable about. You're ready to battle the world. Then your child or spouse or lover says something even slightly critical, or makes what seems like an enormous demand—but probably wouldn't seem like much on another day. You blow your top. Maybe you're nasty, loud, insulting or histrionic. Maybe you cry—but you have no idea why. A lot of women can relate to this scenario. Chances are, you feel remorseful fifteen minutes later. You feel guilty, and maybe even try to apologize. But it's not so easy for the other party to let go of what happened.

When it happens a few times every month, resentment builds. Your loved ones become guarded, as testy as you are during those times of the month. They don't forgive; in fact, they lash right back at you. The result? Your family becomes periodically dysfunctional.

Stephanie Bender of the Boulder, Colorado PMS Clinic sees treatment of the PMS family as one of the centerpieces of PMS treatment. You've got to ask for help from your family, express your feelings, say what you need, she urges, if you really want to see a change in the way your family operates around your PMS. What *they* don't know can hurt *you*. It's been observed that men absorb women's anxiety, irritability and even depression around the time of PMS. Some are frightened and frustrated by the problem; others are skeptical that it even exists. Furthermore, when they feel they can't be of any help, many men in PMS families develop a low sense of self-esteem.

Sometimes the family's understanding and expectations about you during your premenstrual time can make it easier for everyone to deal with the tension. A big part of it is education. Bender and other PMS experts from around the country are taking more and more time to help boyfriends, husbands, children and any significant others to learn about PMS, to become less judgmental and more adept at working both *with* and *around* the person with PMS when need be. Interestingly, other aspects of PMS treatment, like charting symptoms, can be used for the family's benefit; for instance, if you know when you're likely to feel your worst, you can warn those around you as well as preparing yourself.

Rivera-Tovar says that the bottom line in treating the PMS family is legitimizing the problem—making it *real* to others in the family—and building support and compassion. Loved ones can learn to make life a little easier

on the person with PMS—and they can also learn when it's simply best to steer clear of confrontations, waiting a day or two to raise controversial issues or make demands. Even a session or two with a trained PMS counselor can dispel myths, cut through a lot of resentment and make a *big* difference for a family dealing with PMS.

As I mentioned earlier, Endicott and several colleagues did us all a great service by taking a look at the results of many reputable studies done on the most commonly used PMS drugs and supplements, to see just how effective they really are. Here's what they said about the following treatments, many of which you'll probably read about or hear about from PMS caregivers.

NUTRITIONAL SUPPLEMENTS

Many women think that if you buy it in a health food store, it must be okay. This is not always the case—in fact, as you'll see below, sometimes the opposite is true.

Vitamin B_6.

A lot of studies have looked at the use of vitamin B_6 for treating PMS, so it's one of the first vitamins to appear in many pop magazine articles on the topic. Unfortunately, while some women report lowered depression and bloating when they take 200–500 mg a day, formal scientific studies find that it's no better than a placebo (sugar pill) at relieving PMS. Plus, in large doses, B_6 can cause severe side effects like dizziness, nightmares, headaches and painful tingling in the fingers and toes. Endicott says "don't waste your money," but if you do, stay under 300 mg per day.

Vitamin E.

This vitamin seems to make patients feel a little better overall but the improvements are not what scientists call "statistically significant"—that is, they aren't strong enough positive results to merit recommending the vitamin to women.

Calcium.

One study showed that calcium improves PMS symptoms, but it comes with side effects like constipation, flatulence and stomach upset. The fact is, women should be getting adequate calcium for bone health anyway (exact amounts are listed on page 404); there's no reason to start adding tremendous quantities of calcium to prevent PMS.

Evening Primrose Oil.

This combination of essential fatty acids is a another one of the popularized treatments for PMS; you'll probably find it mentioned in every book or article on the subject. The review found it ineffective against PMS symptoms in several studies.

Optivite.

This multivitamin, multimineral preparation got mixed results; one study said that it helps in high doses, other studies show it doesn't help at all. The best approach to vitamin supplement use, according to the experts I interviewed, is to make sure you're getting 100% of the required amounts of each important nutrient, but *not* to get caught up in the often costly and questionable practice of taking special (or mega) amounts of certain vitamins with unknown benefit. For a list of popular multivitamin supplements and their contents, see page 416.

MEDICATIONS FOR PMS

You must keep in mind that not a single drug is approved by the FDA for treating PMS. The drugs and other PMS remedies that you've heard about are usually approved for other health problems, and then prescribed by doctors to relieve PMS symptoms. As a result, there is wide disagreement about what works, what doesn't, and how much of a given improvement is a so-called "placebo effect"—that is, you feel better just because you're taking *something*. In their review of PMS treatments, Endicott *et al* tried to separate the wheat from the chaff and give at least some idea of which treatments are promising, and for which parts of PMS.

Diuretics.

These so-called "water pills" have been widely studied as treatments for PMS. Diuretics *do* help relieve the breast pain and swelling associated with PMS, and they help reduce general bloating by promoting water loss from the body. Rivera-Tovar notes that for some women with mild PMS, this minor physical relief is all they need—not surprisingly, their slight irritability subsides on its own when they are feeling better. Diuretics should be used with caution, however, since overdoing it can lead to dehydration, depleted potassium and other related problems. Some say they cause lethargy and a generally ill feeling. If you want to get a diuretic effect but prefer *not* to take a drug, you might try natural diuretics like drinking lots of water, eating foods like cucumber and watermelon that are loaded with water, or drinking herbal diuretics like raspberry leaf tea and chamomile tea or eating parsley and thyme.

Progesterone.

For many years, health care professionals have tried using progesterone products to relieve PMS. In fact, they aren't effective. Neither dydrogesterone nor progesterone (mostly given as a vaginal suppository) helps PMS. Progesterone can cause unpleasant side effects, too, such as moodiness, spotting and erratic menstrual cycles.

Antibiotics.

Are you surprised by this one? Some research has suggested that certain cases of PMS are caused by an infection of some kind—perhaps a bacterial infection. When treated with antibiotics to kill the potential infection, some women get better. We need more research in this area, but there is some promise at least for a subset of women afflicted with PMS.

Antianxiety Drugs.

Antianxiety drugs are sometimes given *during* PMS symptoms. They're mild tranquilizers, some of which have been found to help. Interestingly, one such drug, alprazolam, not only relieved some of the emotional symptoms of PMS but also the physical ones. It is important to take these drugs under careful supervision by a doctor in order to avoid withdrawal symptoms. One suggestion is to taper off the drug by the end of the menstrual cycle. Another antianxiety drug, called buspirone, caused sedation, constipation and dry mouth, but also helped relieve PMS.

Antidepressants.

One well-known antidepressant, fluoxetine (or Prozac), helps relieve a wide range of PMS symptoms in a large number of patients. It's thought to work by boosting a brain mood chemical called serotonin. Both this drug and its cousins, called serotinin re-uptake inhibitors, have dramatic impact not just on mood but on physical symptoms as well. Dr. Joe Mortola has found it effective in about 75% of patients with strictly defined PMS. Many of these patients had tried countless therapies before this one, without success.

But these drugs, which are in extremely wide use today, are *not* for everyone. They occasionally cause side effects like nausea, headache, dizziness, nervousness, insomnia, increased appetite and decreased sex drive in some patients. The side effects are quite variable; some patients have few or none at all. Even though they're thought to be safe, these drugs should not automatically be prescribed as a treatment for PMS before other nondrug remedies have been tried.

Another antidepressant, nortriptyline, helped eight of eleven women in one study. Lithium, commonly used for treating manic depression, was *not* found effective against PMS. The so-called tricyclic antidepressants, which have been around for many years, have been found to help some women who have premenstrual worsening of an already-existing depression. These drugs cause a long list of side effects, however, from dry mouth and stomach problems to urine retention, faintness and heart palpitations.

A type of mood-altering therapy called melatonin inhibition—that is, treatments that affect the hormone melatonin—also seems to help fight PMS symptoms. Melatonin is connected to our sense of time of day, light and darkness, and therefore is tied to energy and mood as well. Also, "light therapy," in which patients are put in front of banks of bright light to relieve depression, seems to help premenstrual depression. These treatments boost energy and vigor and reduce irritation. Sometimes a bit of this effect can be gained just by spending more time outside in daylight, but that's not always easy in certain parts of the country at certain times of the year (for instance, in the Northeast in the dead of winter when days are cold and short).

The following medications are used to suppress ovulation and have been tried as treatments for PMS. They hold back the release of an egg from the ovaries, preventing the body from going into the second half of the menstrual cycle, when PMS signs develop. This is an extreme approach to treating PMS, far more potent than most women will need. But if your condition is serious, and your doctor recommends one of these drugs, here are some brief descriptions:

Danazol.

This drug causes significant side effects similar to those associated with menopause (hot flashes and bone loss, for example), but relieves PMS symptoms in some cases. It is recommended only for the worst symptoms of PMS; most women will get by with far less potent medication.

Buserelin.

This drug is a so-called LHRH (Luteinizing hormone releasing hormone) agonist. It was found effective against bloating, poor mood and breast tenderness, which is quite good news, but it was *not* effective against irritability and fatigue. On the down side, it causes hot flashes, mood swings and lowered sex drive,

and potentially could cause bone loss over the long term.

SURGICAL REMOVAL OF THE OVARIES

An extreme measure to say the least, removal of the ovaries does help relieve PMS symptoms. But it certainly isn't the treatment of choice for relieving PMS—in fact, some would call its use for this purpose barbaric.

SO JUST HOW WELL DOES TREATMENT FOR PMS WORK?

While individual treatments seldom do the whole job, *comprehensive* treatment—for the body, for the mind and for the family—does often work. In one study at a comprehensive PMS treatment clinic, 95% of women were satisfied after a year of care. Eighty-eight percent said that their lives were better after treatment, which one could argue is the bottom line. Of course, "better" is in the eye of the beholder. Endicott finds that a lot of her patients do not expect to feel *great* before their periods begin. They just want to feel good, or better than they feel now. If your expectations are realistic, you are much more likely to be pleased with the result of your PMS treatment.

On the down side, there have been studies showing that when you scientifically measure improvement after PMS treatment, the results are disappointing. When given formal symptom rating scales, some women report that they aren't doing that much better after all—which is one reason you might run into health care providers who aren't sure it's worth trying to treat PMS. These are the folks who say, "It's just a natural process, don't try to treat it," or "It's all in your head." The best advice I can give you on this score is that you'll never know unless you try, and lots of women before you have found significant relief of their premenstrual symptoms. There's no reason you shouldn't be one of them if you apply yourself to getting better.

And keep in mind: information leads to empowerment. The more you learn about your particular symptoms and the options that are out there for treatment, the greater your chance of beating PMS. *Targeted* treatment is always best; the closer you come to having *your* PMS problems addressed, rather than some generic version of the syndrome, the more likely it is you'll get better. You must target all of your problems, from emotional distress to physical complaints to relationship issues, in order to be wholly well again.

FOR MORE INFORMATION ON PMS

NATIONAL PMS SOCIETY

P.O. Box 11467
Durham, NC 27703
919-489-6577

PREMENSTRUAL SYNDROME ACTION

P.O. Box 9326
Madison, WI 53715
608-274-6688

PREMENSTRUAL SYNDROME PROGRAM

40 Salem Street
Lynnfield, MA 01940

AMERICAN COLLEGE OF OBSTETRICIANS AND GYNECOLOGISTS RESOURCE CENTER

409 12th Street SW
Washington, DC 20024-2188
202-638-5577

NATIONAL WOMEN'S HEALTH NETWORK

514 10th Street NW, Suite 400
Washington, DC 20004
202-347-1140

NATIONAL WOMEN'S HEALTH RESOURCE CENTER

2440 M Street NW, Suite 325
Washington, DC 20037
202-293-6045

SEE ALSO THE MANY LISTINGS ON DEPRESSION AND ANXIETY ON PAGES 356–357

CHAPTER TEN

MENOPAUSAL HEALTH

It seems a pity to have a built-in rite of passage and to dodge it, evade it, and pretend nothing has changed. That is to dodge and evade one's womanhood, to pretend one's like a man. Men, once initiated, never get the second chance. They never change again. That's their loss, not ours. Why borrow poverty?

—Ursula K. LeGuin, *The Space Crone*

Menopause, with its countless physical and emotional manifestations, has pounced onto the pages and airwaves of the lay media after near-invisibility for decades. It just wasn't something women *talked* about in the old days beyond hushed whispers about "the change," "that time of life," and so on. Today, the topic of menopause is ubiquitous. As if there were something new about this near-universal female experience, and you aren't hip if you don't know the latest theory or trend or intervention for alleged menopausal problems. How much of what you read is true is subject to question—because there seems to be a study from *somewhere* in the world to support just about every treatment or intervention imaginable. Unfortunately, much of the data that's so widely quoted is already out-of-date, focusing on women from different times and different political, social and economic climates, and therefore drawing conclusions that don't necessarily apply to women of today. I have tried to focus on more recent data to keep the information as pertinent to *today's* women's lives as possible. As you read this chapter and collect new information from other sources, it is important to remember that: 1) every woman is different; 2) there is still so much to learn about this transitional phase of life; and 3) there is no such thing as a "typical" menopause. You would do best to cull from this material whatever is of most use to you and *your* personal menopausal experience.

What Menopause Is

In simplest terms, the menopause is the cessation of menstrual periods: the meno (monthly) pause. In fact, the entire menopausal experience is not a single event, but a gradual one that builds for several years before your periods stop (the perimenopause) and continues after your cycles have halted (postmenopause)—the rest of your life. The entire process (before, during and shortly after menopause) is sometimes called the climacteric. Health experts are pleased to announce that the postmenopausal years aren't the final few years of decline; in fact, most women will live at least a third of their lives *after* menopause. Since our older population is growing (between 1990 and 2025 the population over age 65 will increase 101%), postmenopausal women stand to represent even more powerful numbers in coming years.

On average, American women reach menopause at just over age 51. But there is great variability here; anywhere from the early 40s to the late 50s is still considered "normal." The process of course starts much earlier, usually in the 30s, when the ovaries begin to produce less estrogen and progesterone and we have fewer eggs available. Researchers believe that in the late 30s the rate of follicle loss speeds up and eventually doubles; if it did not double at this time, menopause would occur two decades later!

For a variety of reasons—including autoimmune diseases, problems with the ovaries, certain medications and other causes—some women will begin menopause as early as their 30s. This often comes as a complete surprise and can be terribly frustrating for women who delayed childbearing until later in what they hoped would be their reproductive years.

Because, as I mentioned, the menopause doesn't occur instantaneously but rather develops over time, there are objective measures of the hormone changes taking place in your body. Specifically, the hormone FSH (or follicle-stimulating hormone, responsible for telling the ovaries to produce an egg) starts to rise considerably as menopause approaches. You can think about this process as the FSH needing to shout louder and louder to get the ovaries to listen. Since there are fewer eggs available as a woman nears menopause, the body turns up the volume on FSH to try to get something going; eventually, it can't, and periods stop altogether.

Menopausal Sensations: Why Is a Natural Process Treated Like a Disease?

Menopause is a normal part of the life cycle; it's no more a disease than is menstruation. But because our bodies go through some major changes at this time of hormonal shifts, and because those changes are bothersome to a certain subset of women, many health practitioners have come to treat it and talk about it as an illness. And since menopause coincides with a time of life when other measures of health often start to decline, it's an easy scapegoat. Steven Austad, an associate professor of zoology at the University of Idaho, has tried to take a more refreshing approach to the study of menopause. He examined the evolution of menopause in women and in other female animals to see if it marks a *positive* adaptation to the physical tasks of later life. While he did not find this precise association, he does describe menopause as a beneficial adaptation that protects us from certain common diseases of later life. For example, since estrogen is associated with breast and other cancer risk, the drop in estrogen that occurs with menopause may be timed to protect us from cancer, he proposes. In this sense, it is a healthy event, not a disease.

We can't avoid the fact, however, that some of the changes associated with menopause can negatively affect our health. For instance, with estrogen loss, our bone loss accelerates and our risk of cardiovascular disease rises (as levels of dangerous blood fats increase). We may not feel these changes, but they are occurring in our bodies as our estrogen levels drop. Estrogen is a powerfully protective hormone that, in ways we don't fully understand, provides tremendous protection for the heart, vessels and bones over our reproductive lifetime. After menopause, that protection is largely lost. It is in this regard that many practitioners associate the menopause with illness, and recommend "treatment" that is actually more prevention than anything else. Dr. Janice Green Douglas, director of the division of hypertension and professor of medicine, physiology and biophysiology at the Case Western Reserve Hospital, warns her patients that many important risk factors converge at the time of menopause. Hypertension, high cholesterol, obesity and diabetes risk all climb at this time. It's a good opportunity to get a complete medical screening and, ideally, annual follow-up checks. We'll discuss some of those tests—and potential interventions (including and beyond hormone replacement)—later in this chapter.

Other changes that occur around the menopause are more obvious—they are feelings that we experience. Some call them "symp-toms," but again that traps us in the language of disease that really has no place here. Let's call them "menopausal sensations," in the tradition of Marilyn Rothert, acting dean in the college of nursing at Michigan State University. There is tremendous variability in the sensations women feel, as well as in the degree of those sensations. Our data in this area is skewed in certain ways, according to Sonja McKinlay, a well-known menopause researcher at the New England Research Institute. The problem, she says, is that too many studies of menopausal sensations have been done on clinic populations—that is, women who came to see doctors because of their discomfort! Naturally, when you focus on women with problems, you get the sense that most menopausal women have problems—and that, McKinlay says, is far from true. Another flaw in the available data is that it tends to focus on relatively affluent white women, to the exclusion of women of color and of different socioeconomic groups.

So while we know *less* about the menopausal experience of the average woman out in the community than most writers like to admit, we *do* know from McKinlay's and others' recent research that many women have at most *temporary* discomfort with menopause and still others have *no* trouble whatsoever. In general, it's thought that about 15% of white American women will have sensations bothersome enough to seek medical attention during menopause (I'll bet that number is smaller than you expected). For those who do have discomfort, though, the problems are quite real and sometimes severe. We'll discuss many of the most common sensations, and solutions, in this chapter.

MENOPAUSE: WHAT YOU HAD TO SAY ABOUT IT

Terri, 49 years old

I had a hysterectomy when I was 30 so I've been in menopause a long time. I've been on estrogen since I was 30. Originally for the first many years they had me on a pill, I don't remember the name, and what happened with me was the symptoms of menopause became absolutely overwhelming, and they kept increasing the amount of estrogen I was taking and my internist thought it was too high. They measured the amount of estrogen in my body and there was none! It wasn't getting into my system! I was frustrated because they kept giving me more and more medication and saying it's okay, but nothing was happening.

They switched me to the patch—I got welts wherever they put it. I was having the most violent hot flashes, at night you could wring me out, I had to change my nightgown nearly every night. The headaches were terrible. A lot of the time I was ornery, cranky, it was almost like PMS. Very painful drying out of the mucous membranes, vaginal dryness.

So they put me on estrogen shots. It's been working. I virtually don't get hot flashes anymore. It's just 100% better. I don't have a mood swings, I don't have the type of headaches and the flashes that were keeping me up at night, that's done. I just feel normal, I feel the way I'm supposed to feel. But one of my problems with estrogen injections is it starts to fade; it goes into my system in a rush in the beginning and then wears off. I've had some reservations about estrogen because of breast cancer. I get checked every six months, I have a mammogram every year, I check myself.

But for me the benefits outweigh the risks. I would hate to go off it. I'm not ready to take the chance now to go off and try vitamins or minerals. This works for me.

Helen, 64 years old

It was wonderful, no menstruation, no premenstrual tension. Very liberating, not one day did I feel crummy. My mother had a horrible menopause, so I expected that it was going to be quite awful. Instead it just kind of tapered off. I found that I didn't look much different, I was already dyeing my hair, I thought I looked pretty damned good! I had tons of energy, and I guess it was so unexpected after my mother's terrible time that I felt doubly lucky. I don't think he (my husband) even noticed.

Vaginal dryness was a problem, none of which my doctor discussed. He probably wasn't comfortable talking about it—and I wasn't comfortable talking about it either. Even doctors who really push estrogen said it's tough to tell you to take it, "if it ain't broke don't fix it." I probably was the best of all, my friends had terrible flashes—I didn't have a single hot flash! It's been incredible.

Lucy, 56 years old

I had hormone replacement therapy in a model program. It was a two-year program, a blind study. I started the protocol four months after I completely stopped menstruating. She tested me and my estrogen level was low enough. I have no family history that would contraindicate taking hormones.

I was having night sweats and flashes and lack of sleep, but nothing major. The night sweats disappeared (on the treatment) and I felt really good and when the study was over it turned out I was on a low dose of estrogen and progesterone, one pill, continuous and low dose. I was having mood swings, not incapacitating me. I realized I wasn't having any extreme swings of mood (once on the treatment). The vaginal dryness improved, not dramatically, so I used some topical stuff. They found I had maintained my bone—my bone looked good.

I didn't have problems, my friends had breakthrough bleeding and trouble regulating the balance of the estrogen and the progesterone. I have friends whose bust hurt, they put on weight and so on. I had breakthrough bleeding only once—it was really a very strong period four to five months into it and never ever again. I put on a little bit of weight, under five pounds, and my stomach was swollen, but I was exercising and doing a lot of walking—it definitely helped.

WHEN TO "TREAT" MENOPAUSE— HORMONES AND OTHERWISE

Most experts feel the best time to intervene and "treat" the sensations of menopause is as soon as they have begun to impair your quality of life. Naturally, different women will reach that point at varying levels of discomfort. Dr. Howard Judd of UCLA reports that some of his patients actually feel *guilty* for getting hormone treatment just for feeling "uncomfortable," and not for some more serious reason (threatened health), when there are treatment risks to be considered. Remember, you only get one life; living it as fully and as comfortably as possible is nothing to feel guilty about! Get the facts, and weigh those facts against one another: Don't beat yourself over the head for wanting to feel well. Also keep in mind that there is more than one way to "treat" the sensations of menopause. As we'll discuss in this chapter, lifestyle changes

and other nondrug approaches to feeling well can go a long way to restoring your sense of well-being at this time of hormonal change.

Also remember that there is another important way to manage menopausal sensations, and that is through *prevention* rather than treatment. The goal: to ward off or reverse some of the physiological changes that accompany the drop in estrogen and put us at risk for major diseases like heart disease and osteoporosis. We'll discuss some of these changes in a moment: increasing blood fats and blood pressure, accelerated bone loss, vaginal and urinary structures becoming atrophied and the consequent risk of incontinence or infections, and so on. Hormone therapy (estrogen replacement therapy, or estrogen plus progesterone) is sometimes used to mediate these problems, cutting the risk of heart disease by as much as 50%, reducing bone loss, and on down the line. Of course, it also carries a potential downside, including side effects for some women and a possible increased risk of breast cancer. Later in this chapter, we'll discuss the pros and cons of hormone therapy in greater detail, and we'll also go over the various forms in which you can take it.

MENOPAUSAL SENSATIONS

Here are some of the more common sensations reported, and a variety of solutions, both prescribed by doctors and anecdotally advised by women.

HOT FLASHES: SENSATIONS AND SOLUTIONS

You'll find data that anywhere from 28% to 94% of women have hot flashes in the years before, during and slightly after menopause. The most quoted figure is about 75%. This doesn't mean that ¾ of women will seek treatment for hot flashes, or that this number of women are even *bothered* by them; it just means that they occur. Margaret Lock, a medical anthropologist at McGill University, has studied the menopausal experience in different countries and has found, for example, that while hot flashes are quite common in the U.S. and other Western countries, they are quite *uncommon* in Japan. Lock also reports that women in Japan treat menopause with much less apprehension and disturbance than many American women do. Indonesian women also report fewer hot flashes than do Westerners. We'll discuss some possible reasons why later in this chapter.

Women often describe hot flashes as sudden bursts of heat that overcome their bodies, especially their upper bodies—the chest, neck and face. These areas may become quite red or blotchy as the heat builds, and finally after climbing to a peak, the sensation fades and is often replaced by a chilled feeling. The entire experience usually lasts for several minutes, but according to the National Institute on Aging, some hot flashes last 30 minutes! Flashes can occur several times an hour at their worst, or far less frequently. Unfortunately, they often occur at night, and can disturb sleep (which, as we'll discuss later, can set off a domino effect producing many other menopausal sensations).

Fredi Kronenberg, director of the Richard and Hinda Rosenthal Center of Alternative/Complementary Medicine, reports that there is great variety in how women experience hot flashes: some sweat profusely, some hardly sweat at all; some have significantly increased heart rates, while for others the increase is minimal.

McKinlay finds that hot flashes are most common in the years *before* menopause, peak at menopause and then rapidly taper off. She also finds that women who have more depression *before* menopause may be at increased risk for hot flashes around the time of menopause.

Hot flashes can occur anytime, but some women find that they are triggered by stressful events or stimulating foods (spicy or caffeinated items in particular.)

HERE ARE SOME SOLUTIONS FOR COPING WITH HOT FLASHES

Hormones.
As it does for many of the sensations of menopause, hormone replacement can greatly reduce the incidence of hot flashes. It appears that all three common preparations—combined estrogen/progestin therapy, estrogen alone or progestins alone (in small doses)—help to reduce hot flashes. Since progestins (synthetic progesterone) have powerful PMS-like side effects for some women, there is some hope that with the increasing availability of natural progesterone we'll have a more benign nonestrogen hormone therapy for hot flashes.

A 1994 study found that a so-called "progestational agent" called megestral acetate reduced hot flashes for women who could *not* take estrogen. Side effects were minor.

Other Prescription Drugs.
The antihypertension drug clonidine is used in low-dose patch form to treat hot flashes, with some (albeit limited) success. Dr. Bruce Kessel, head of menopause research at Beth Israel Hospital in Boston, notes that the side effects from clonidine can negate the hot flash

improvement for some women. These include drowsiness, dry mouth and fatigue.

Lifestyle Changes.

Certain behavior changes can make hot flashes less uncomfortable, but they probably won't decrease the number of hot flashes you'll experience. The National Institute on Aging recommends the following measures:

- sleep in as cool a room as possible
- use sheets and other bedding that breathe (some experts recommend all-cotton only)
- keep a glass of cold water nearby at all times and drink it as soon as a flash begins
- dress in layers so you can easily peel off clothing in the event of a hot flash, even in public

Avoid hot flash triggers, says Dr. Patricia Ganz, professor of medicine and public health at UCLA. These differ from woman to woman. For some, cutting back on caffeine or spicy foods may help; for others, avoiding stressful situations, when possible, will reduce the frequency or intensity of hot flashes. Joan Shaver of the University of Washington adds that sometimes moving from one room to another with a different temperature can trigger a flash. Try avoiding this type of "shock" to your system.

Vitamins.

Many women report using vitamin E with some success in preventing or reducing the severity of hot flashes. But the big problem here is that there is no guideline on how much of the vitamin is required—and how often it's needed—to make a difference. Not surprisingly, one woman may respond completely differently from another to a given dose of vitamin E—if she responds at all.

And there is little scientific data to back up the treatment. If you want to try taking vitamin E, it *is* generally a safe vitamin in reasonable doses, but it's not for everyone. Talk to your doctor about a safe range for *you*. Fredi Kronenberg says that the RDA for vitamin E does nothing to prevent hot flashes, so you'll have to go at least some degree higher for even potential results.

Dr. Veronica Ravnikar, director of Reproductive Endocrinology, Infertility and Menopause at the University of Massachusetts Medical Center at Worcester finds that many patients are taking magnesium to combat hot flashes. Again, there is little scientific data supporting that any of these vitamin remedies really work, and if so, how much to take.

Paced Respiration Training and Other Stress-Reduction Techniques.

There is an increasing body of evidence suggesting that slow, deep breathing and full-body relaxation can help reduce the severity of hot flashes. Stress reduction, in various forms, helps the body avoid overload and can be especially useful at night, when flashes are keeping you awake. Ideally, you should be trained to relax and breathe properly. One common technique involves lying down in a dark, quiet room and concentrating on relaxing each tiny part of your body until your entire body is loose. Start at your toes, then move up your feet, your calves, thighs and so on, letting your weight sink into the surface on which you're resting. You may fall asleep.

Take a Tip from Japanese Women.

Margaret Lock and others report that women in Japan have far fewer hot flashes than do Western women, and they're less bothered by those they do have. One prominent theory holds that the Japanese diet has a lot to do with this difference in menopausal sensations. The Japanese eat a great deal of soy-based foods (isoflavinoids) and lignans (such as sesame seeds, flax and grains like rye). The traditional Japanese diet contains about 40 grams of isoflavinoids per day—quite a lot! These foods have an estrogenic effect that *may* help prevent or lessen hot flashes. Interestingly, Dr. Kessel points out, the same populations that eat these estrogenic plant-based foods (known collectively as phytoestrogens) do *not* have high rates of breast cancer, which one might expect with extra estrogen activity in the body. So Kessel and other researchers hope that plants with an estrogenlike effect will prove to do some of the positive things that estrogen can do, without the negative side effects.

Herbs.

I hesitate to give information about herbal remedies for menopausal sensations because there is so little scientific data to support the use of these preparations. At the same time, it's impossible to ignore herbal therapies, because so many women are taking them *without* that data. Dr. Bruce Kessel is about to subject some of the more common menopausal herbal preparations (ginseng, black cohosh and don quai) to scientific study to determine formally if and how they work, if they behave like estrogens in the body, whether they are safe, and so on. There have been reports of vaginal bleeding with certain herb preparations, suggesting that they do have some sort of hormonal effect. According to new research by Kessel and colleagues, 15% of postmenopausal (mostly caucasian) women use herbal therapies to treat the sensations of menopause. A quarter use antioxidants. Other herbs commonly cited as menopausal "remedies" include motherwort tincture and licorice root. Unfortunately, there is neither quality nor quantity/dose control of herbs. They are not regulated like drugs; therefore, when you see a name on a label, you are *not* guaranteed that you'll find this ingredient inside the package. If you want to try herbs, then treat them like medication and find out how much you're taking and if you're actually taking the herb you expect.

It may cost you a pretty penny, but it's worth bringing an herbal preparation to the chemical laboratory of a nearby hospital to have the substance fully analyzed. I interviewed a chemist in Arizona who had found actual drugs like steroids and valium in supposedly pure herb preparations. He also discovered that some of the names and functions of the herbs, which were written in Chinese, were not listed correctly. This is not to say that certain well-controlled herbal preparations won't help relieve unpleasant menopausal sensations. But be a cautious consumer.

Lonnie Barbach, author of a book on menopause called *The Pause: Positive Approaches to Menopause,* acknowledges that there is a dearth of scientific information about herbal remedies for menopausal sensations. But she argues that it's only fair to recommend herbs as a reasonable option for some women, especially those who have problems with hormone replacement. So many women are *helped* by herbal and other "altrnative" therapies, Barbach states, that we can not ignore them. She feels that if women find reputable herbal advisers, they will avoid the dangers of herbal quackery. The trouble is, she says, finding a "reputable" herbal adviser is even harder than finding a reputable doctor—there are no sure ways to do it, and it's certainly not one-stop shopping. The best way to find someone is through word of mouth, Barbach says. But if you don't know anyone who has used herbalists or naturalists, her next piece of advice is to talk to a chiropractor that you know or someone you trust recommends, or seek the input of the owners of a health food store in your area.

Beyond herbal therapies, many women are using other unproven but anecdotally helpful unconventional treatments, such as massage, meditation, acupuncture and visualization. While there is no strong scientific data to support the use of these kinds of treatments, if you choose a harmless activity that makes you feel good, go ahead and enjoy it. It's always a good idea to clear the procedure or activity with your doctor, however.

Exercise.

Some women find that regular exercise reduces the frequency and intensity of hot flashes, although there isn't much in the way of data on what kinds of exercises are best, and how much to do. However, since weight-bearing aerobic exercise (walking is a good example) is an excellent way to combat some of the other physiological changes of menopause, like bone loss and heart disease risk, you can only help yourself by giving it a try. If your hot flashes subside too, you're ahead of the game.

Dr. Robert Wild, chief of the section of research on women's health at the Oklahoma Health Sciences Center, is concerned about the fact that health practitioners aren't customizing exercise "prescriptions" to their menopausal patients. Some midlife and older women, he finds, are sandwiched between obligations that make it hard to take time out to exercise. If

you're caring for an ailing loved one at home, for instance, it can be hard just to get out of the house. If you are a woman in this situation, consider getting an inexpensive stationary bike or other machine to ride at home in front of the TV. Or, if you have aching arthritic knees, swimming might be a much better option (at least to start out) than a more jarring exercise. If you are especially social, building exercise around social activities (joining a club or starting a neighborhood walking group, for example) is likely to keep you coming back for more. Workable individual guidelines are the only way to go if we truly want to change people's behavior, Dr. Wild insists. He sees it working with his own patients.

SLEEP PROBLEMS AND SOLUTIONS

Our sleep patterns change as we age, and at the time of menopause, some women experience notable shifts in their ability to get good quality sleep. Also at this time, there is often an increase in not just insomnia, but in a variety of other sleep problems as well. According to Dr. Quentin Regestein, director of the sleep clinic at Boston's Brigham and Women's Hospital, there is a surge in sleep problems for about a decade after age 50 in both women *and* men. For men, the increase is more gradual, he says, while women are hit harder and faster around the time of menopause. At this stage of life, women have five times the incidence of sleep problems that men have (25% versus 5%).

Menopausal sleep problems vary; some women report more fitful sleep, some have trouble falling asleep, others wake early. There is also more sleep apnea around the menopause. Sleep apnea is a condition in which we stop breathing for periods of time during sleep without knowing it. The condition can be benign, or quite serious, depending on the length of the breathing stoppages and their frequency. The hormone progesterone is a respiratory stimulant; when it declines, as it does with menopause, breathing can become more difficult. In fact, some *men* with sleep apnea are given progesterone treatment.

Certain sleep problems around the time of menopause are secondary to other menopausal sensations, particularly hot flashes. If you are awakened by a powerful flash, find yourself damp and then chilled, it can be quite difficult to get back to sleep. If this happens several times a night, extreme sleep deprivation can set in. Sleep deprivation, in turn, is associated with many other so-called menopausal problems, including irritability and depression. Dr. Regestein finds that a wide variety of self-esteem measures drop when people are sleep deprived, including self-confidence, thinking skills and composure. Some experts believe that getting regular high-quality sleep would erase many of the alleged menopausal problems we read so much about.

According to the National Institute on Aging, the quality of our sleep changes with age *regardless* of menopause. There are two kinds of sleep: REM sleep (rapid eye movement sleep) and non-REM sleep, which is much deeper. As we grow older, this deeper sleep decreases, giving a sense of less satisfying overall rest. (For more on sleep problems, *see* chapter 18.)

VAGINAL DRYNESS: SENSATIONS AND SOLUTIONS

After menopause, when the body has been deprived of estrogen for some period of time, the sensitive tissues of the vagina begin to grow thinner and more dry. The vagina actually becomes smaller and more narrow at this time, a process called atrophy. During our reproductive years, estrogen keeps the lining of the vagina plump and moist. Many women notice its absence after menopause, but not all are terribly bothered by it. For some, however, the dryness can be quite uncomfortable, and is associated with pain with urination and sexual intercourse, and an increased risk of vaginal and urinary tract infections. McKinlay reports that about one in six women find this menopausal sensation somewhat or very bothersome.

HERE ARE SOME SOLUTIONS FOR VAGINAL DRYNESS

Hormones.

Hormones in pill form or, in this case, in topical cream form can greatly improve vaginal dryness. If you want the benefits of estrogen but don't want too much of the hormone in your body, small amounts of cream applied to the vagina can be a good option. Remember, some estrogen from the cream is absorbed into your bloodstream, but much less than if you took pills or used the estrogen patch. Some researchers give tiny amounts of testosterone, the male hormone, to women with vaginal dryness and/or lack of sexual interest. It has proved helpful for some women but isn't backed by a great deal of research.

Water-Based Lubricants.

Water-based lubricants like astrogel and others can help tremendously in relieving vaginal dryness and in keeping the vagina moist throughout a full act of intercourse. Other types of lubricants, such as oil-based products, can be goopy, clog pores and don't tend to stay moist for as long as these water-based products. Dr. Richard Moss of Mt. Sinai Hospital in New York reports that about half of his patients with vaginal dryness are relieved by these artificial lubricants alone, with no need for medication. (*See also* list of water-based lubricants on pages 255–256.)

More Sex.

Both sexual intercourse and masturbation help increase vaginal lubrication. If sex is painful, try some of the other methods mentioned above—like lubricants or maybe hormone creams. It may take longer to get sexually excited, and for your vagina to get moist than it did during the years when you were menstruating. Don't rush sex. Gentle touching and other sensuous activities *before* intercourse will give your body more time to warm up. If your male partner is older and has experienced a typical slow-down in getting erections, he might appreciate a little time as well. Be sure to let your partner know when you are—or aren't—ready. If you have intercourse before your body is prepared for it you're more likely to irritate dry, fragile vaginal tissues, which will make you less inclined to have sex the next time—and that in turn will make it harder and harder to accomplish. Slow and steady wins the race.

Avoid Things That Further Dry the Vagina.

Perfumed soaps (any soap, really), certain douches, bubble baths and other scented bath products, and so-called feminine hygiene products can irritate and dry your sensitive vagina. Certain medications that dry the mucous membranes all over the body (such as those in your nasal passages or vagina) should be avoided—check with your doctor before using them.

DRY SKIN: SENSATIONS AND SOLUTIONS

Beyond vaginal dryness, some women experience generally dry skin at the time of menopause, as their estrogen levels drop. Marilyn Rothert of Michigan State recommends switching from hot baths or showers to cooler ones and from soap to gentle, dry-skin cleansing bars, moisturizing the skin and avoiding the sun. These methods usually solve dry skin problems in a short time. (*See* skin section beginning on page 59 for good general skin care.)

GASTROINTESTINAL SENSATIONS AND SOLUTIONS

Some women report constipation (and some diarrhea) in the perimenopausal years. Others report more generalized gastrointestinal upset at this time. Some portion of this problem may be secondary to other menopausal sensations and/or lack of sleep, in which case treating the underlying problem should help the stomach upset.

HERE ARE SOME SOLUTIONS FOR GASTROINTESTINAL UPSET

Laxatives.

With a proper diet, few women will need to take laxatives to relieve constipation; but for those who do, natural forms with the fewest additives (ideally, no chemical additives) are best. Those that are soluble-fiber based may have the added benefit of lowering your cholesterol, which has a tendency to climb after menopause. But you don't want to become dependent on laxative pills or powders; it's best to use them to get you on the right track, and then use dietary changes (*see* below) to keep yourself there.

Diet.

Marilyn Rothert finds that most women are relieved by diet changes alone, particularly by increasing dietary fiber with vegetables and fruit (both fresh and dried) and whole-grain breads, cereals and muffins that aren't laden with fat. Also extremely important is drinking several tall glasses of water per day, every day; six to eight 8-ounce glasses would be great. (If you're having trouble with urinary tract infections due to vaginal dryness, all this water will help that problem, too.)

Cross-Check Other Menopausal "Remedies."

Consider some of the lifestyle changes you've made since you entered the menopausal years and see if they might be causing stomach upset. For example, if you are taking extra calcium to protect your bones, your gut may be reacting to the form of calcium you're taking (some of which are quite constipating). Ask your doctor if it might make sense to switch types, perhaps to calcium citrate, which is a bit more easily digested than some other forms of calcium. Ask your doctor about the potential constipating or stool-softening effect of any other medications you may have started taking recently.

EMOTIONAL OR PSYCHOLOGICAL SENSATIONS AND SOLUTIONS

The idea that psychological changes occur as a result of menopause is quite controversial. When I raised the topic with Dr. Karen Hutchinson of the Yale University School of Medicine, she said that the idea of menopausal women having clinical psychological problems is nothing but a myth perpetuated by patients and doctors alike. It used to be taken as a simple

fact that menopausal women were more depressed, anxious, insecure and so on than premenopausal women. The older literature speaks a great deal about the "empty nest" phenomenon in which women, their children out of the home and their lives lonely, fall into a condition of despair. Today's information is quite different. Many menopausal women are active outside the home and are far from dependent on their children's activities and whereabouts. Postmenopausal women are in the workforce, out and about in the community, leading active, productive, personal and/or professional lives. There *are* certain mood changes associated with menopause, Dr. Hutchinson notes. The "blues," irritability and anger are common at this time. But we mustn't call these serious psychological problems, she insists. Rather, they are normal responses to a society that doesn't appreciate older women, as well as responses to physiologic changes like lack of sleep.

There is a definite subset of women who report "not feeling as psychologically well" as they did before the menopausal years, says Dr. Laura Bookman, director of the Menopause Wellness Center at Beth Israel Hospital in Boston. And while researcher Patricia Kaufert of the University of Manitoba does *not* find increased levels of depression associated with menopause itself, she *does* find that certain coincidental life events and physical sensations of menopause (*see* the list above) may predispose certain women to psychological distress.

THE "NEST RE-FILLING" SYNDROME AND OTHER LATER-LIFE BURDENS

Kaufert and McKinlay report that the empty nest syndrome, supposedly so common in the past, has for many women been replaced by something they call the "nest-refilling" syndrome. This occurs when adult children move back home with their parents due to economic or other social stresses, bringing with them significant problems and predisposing their menopausal mothers to depression. Whether these women would have suffered depression without the kids' return home is not clear. But it's increasingly rare to find menopausal women who are depressed just because of menopause.

For women entering menopause at a later age—and whose parents are older and becoming frail, ill or dependent—this can be an especially stressful time. We've read a lot lately about the "sandwich" generation caught between the needs and demands of young adult children and ailing older parents; if this "sandwiching" phenomenon coincides with the menopause, the emotional and physical toll can be quite difficult for some women. Again, it's not menopause itself that causes depression or emotional lability: It's the other demanding life events piled on top of this time of hormonal change that can push some women into depression. Nancy Woods, Director of the Center for Women's Health Research at the University of Washington, reports that most of the "blue mood" associated with menopause is a factor of other life problems, ranging from divorce or other relationship troubles to trying to meet the demands of too many roles ("parenting" both children *and* older parents, working, dealing with poverty and other stressors so common to women in this country).

HERE ARE SOME SOLUTIONS FOR LATER-LIFE BURDENS AND STRESSES

Depending on your budget, it might be helpful to try family counseling if the tension in your newly full home is getting in the way of healthy relationships. You may need to set some new rules now that your children are adults and back home: for example, as adults, they can take on adult responsibility in the home, helping with everything from shopping to meal preparation. Also, you must learn to respect each other's space as adults; it is your home, and you can set those rules, but keep in mind, for harmony's sake, that your adult children need privacy and respect as well (as long as they aren't stepping on your toes to get it). In many cases, they don't want to be back home any more than you want them to be there; be supportive of them, and they should be supportive of you in return.

If you are responsible for ailing older parents, avail yourself of whatever caretaking assistance you can afford or find for free. Many communities have volunteer support teams for elder care; even if it's a matter of someone coming to check in on your older parents a couple of times a week, or to transport them to a senior care facility when you just can't be there, it can help relieve you of some of the constant burden you're under. While you know what your responsibilities to others are, remember that you have some responsibility to *yourself* as well. Maintaining your sense of emotional balance and finding even brief periods of time for your own relaxation or pleasure is vital, not just for your mental health, but also to maintain your value and vitality in helping those around you.

While it may not be as common these days as in the past, certainly some women going through menopause do experience the proverbial "empty nest syndrome." If this is your case, your best bet is to get out of the nest yourself! Any activity that boosts your sense of worth and, ideally, helps others at the same time, will take your mind off of the past and fix it on the future. Work for pay or volunteer for the sheer satisfaction of it; learn something new; exercise; socialize; do whatever it takes to get you up in the morning and out of the house with a purpose. Or, if you like being at home but just miss the hustle and bustle that used to take place there when you were raising a family, bring your new friends/hobbies/companions back into the nest with you. Perhaps there's a project you can run from your own kitchen table: lots of people do it.

IRRITABILITY

There is a growing sense that increased irritability at the time of menopause—which a small subset of women report—is connected to one of two problems. First, hot flashes or vaginal dryness or other chronically uncomfortable physical sensations may bring on irritable moods. When we don't know what to do to lessen these sensations, it only gets more frustrating, and we become still more irritable. A second common catalyst to menopausal irritability is the woman's partner and/or other life companions. Dr. Vivien Burt, director of the Neuropsychiatric Institute/Women's Life Center at UCLA says that women who associate closely with people who value and respect older women do far better emotionally, at the time of menopause, than those whose loved ones are either panicked about aging *themselves,* or look down on older women.

OTHER SOURCES OF DEPRESSION

Dr. Burt reports a good deal of perimenopausal depression among women going through

menopause relatively early who have not yet had biological children, and feel a void in that area of their lives. With more and more career women postponing childbearing until their careers are on track, this is becoming an increasingly common problem. Even women who were pretty certain they did *not* want biological children can face menopause with great trepidation, Burt adds. It seems that the sudden reality that it might no longer be their *choice* can trigger fundamental depression. Add to those reality-based emotions some labile physical sensations in the perimenopausal years, and you end up with someone who feels chronically crummy, both mentally and physically. These women tend to be more sleep deprived, irritable and tearful, perhaps fitting what the media has put forth as the more stereotypical pattern of the menopausal woman.

SOME SOLUTIONS FOR IRRITABILITY AND DEPRESSION

There's no "right" time to seek professional counseling for chronic irritability or depression. Most mental health experts feel that when your negative mood is interfering with your ability to function properly during the day (to work, get along with others and enjoy family life) or night (you're having chronic sleep problems) it's time to seek help. Sometimes, talk therapy alone will bring you out of your funk. In other cases, medication can help. Don't ignore negative mood symptoms any more than you would ignore chronic physical pain; both are debilitating to your soul, and harmful to those around you as well. (For more details on mental health problems and solutions, *see* chapter 17.)

CHANGES IN MENTAL ACUITY

Some women report significant changes in their ability to process information—remember things, perform multiple tasks simultaneously, and so on—during the perimenopausal and menopausal years. Dr. John Arpels, founding member of the North American Menopause Society and a climacteric endocrinologist at the University of California at San Francisco, notes that many of his patients report such things as "premature senility," "the lights are dimming" and other similar complaints about mental functioning as they go through this time of hormonal change. They come to his office complaining of what he terms the "Post-it syndrome"—in which they have to put Post-its all over their homes just to remind themselves of everyday tasks. Dr. Arpels, who attributes these changes to the menopausal drop in estrogen levels, likens the problem to a camera in which the lens is working right, the picture is seen, but somehow the image isn't getting through to the film either because the connection is flawed or because there's no ink on the film. What he means is that the relative lack of the hormone estrogen, which is deeply involved in our thinking process through its impact on other brain chemicals and their swift connections, somehow short-circuits brain function in some menopausal women. Research by Barbara Sherwin of McGill University has revealed that estrogen replacement therapy helps maintain verbal memory *and* enhances women's ability to learn new material. (However, Sherwin stresses that she has yet to meet a menopausal woman for whom memory loss or loss of mental acuity is the *primary* sensation of menopause.)

Dr. Fred Naftolin, chairman of obstetrics and gynecology at the Yale Medical School and director of the Yale University Center for Research on Reproductive Biology, is studying the ways in which estrogen deprivation might affect brain function. There are no hard and fast answers at this time, but there are several theories. One is that estrogen is needed to insure proper information processing. Dr. Naftolin compares memory and thought processing to bank teller windows: they need to stay open long enough for you to deposit your money in the bank. If the windows shut down too early—that is, if your brain processing shuts or slows down—your "money" (incoming ideas) doesn't get deposited properly. As a result, they can't be recalled later on, and you *think* you have a memory problem.

Another theory of how estrogen affects brain function is through what Naftolin calls "connectivity"—that is, the links between brain cells that allow us to think clearly. When these essential connections are cut, we cannot think as clearly or as quickly, or perform as many different thought functions at once, as we used to do.

The result of these cut synapses, slowed processing and so on? Short-term memory and spacial reasoning may be affected in susceptible women, research suggests. What makes some women more susceptible to problems than others remains a mystery. Research by Dr. Dominique Toran-Allerand, a developmental neuroscientist at Columbia Presbyterian Medical Center in New York, shows that estrogen stimulates the dendrites—or cells that receive information—in lab animals. (Dr. Toran-Allerand notes that this does *not* prove that estrogen improves reception of knowledge in humans, however.) And in research by Bruce McEwen, head of the laboratory of neuroendocrinology at Rockefeller University in New

York, and others, estrogen has been shown to stimulate *new* synapses in the hippocampus or learning and memory center of the brain. Furthermore, McEwen notes: when you remove the ovaries of rats, thereby causing immediate menopause, certain brain synapses *disconnect*. Thus more and more pieces of the puzzle are falling into place, suggesting that estrogen's role in brain function is a vital one.

Dr. Wolf Utian, chairman of reproductive biology at Case Western Reserve University and director of the North American Menopause Society, argues that mental changes among menopausal women may not be the result of direct estrogen deprivation. Rather, he attributes the changes to various social problems, lack of sleep and irritability caused by hot flashes, and other physical discomforts associated with menopause (the so-called domino or snowball effect again). He notes that women who live in cultures where aging and menopause are valued and esteemed as signs of seniority (certain African tribes, for example) function wonderfully after the menopause, while women in youth-obsessed cultures like our own tend to have most of the so-called "mental acuity" problems we hear so much about.

Dr. Arpels argues that whatever the underlying connection between impaired brain function and the menopause, women who have symptoms should be given the *option* of estrogen replacement because "women deserve to be hitting on all cylinders, and with estrogen deprivation, they aren't." He compares the problem of estrogen deprivation to any other hormonal imbalance, such as thyroid deficiency or low insulin levels.

Some Solutions for Loss of Mental Acuity.
The old standbys like writing important things down on paper, getting adequate sleep and avoiding mind-clouding substances like alcohol and other sedatives will help boost clearheadedness for *anyone*. Some believe that physical exercise clears the mind, as do meditation and other relaxation techniques. Some experts feel that *mental* exercises like crossword puzzles and memory games help keep the mind sharp and clear. Cutting down on obligations when you're feeling vulnerable to overload is a nice thought, though not practical for some of us. Estrogen replacement has been shown to boost mental sharpness, but the same researchers who believe that the loss in brain function is due to hot flashes and sleep problems argue that estrogen replacement only helps by reducing or eliminating these cofactors.

SEXUAL PROBLEMS: LOSS OF LIBIDO

Earlier, we discussed the fact that when estrogen levels drop, some women experience vaginal dryness that creates pain with intercourse. This is a physiological problem. But there also seem to be, for some women, emotional issues surrounding sex that develop near the time of the menopause. Some women report a lack of sexual desire in these years, known as low libido. While physical discomfort is a sure deterrent to interest in sex, some women find that their lack of interest is unrelated to physical problems.

Ask yourself if the problem originates with you alone, or with your partner as well, advises Dr. Richard Moss of New York's Mt. Sinai Hospital. Sexual problems tend to be quite circular; if your partner is uninterested or unable to have sex, you'll get used to not doing it, and less interested in it yourself.

Some Solutions for Loss of Libido.

As mentioned earlier, testosterone, the male hormone, is sometimes used in conjunction with estrogen to boost sexual interest. It is not given in large enough doses to create a masculating effect.

If your lack of sexual interest is psychological in origin, and not physiological, hormones won't necessarily be the answer. Sex counseling can help you get to the root of your feelings. Are you interested in your partner? Are you depressed in general? Is your partner sexually responsive to you? Has the romance and passion you once shared drained in recent years, and is sex among the last things to go in your relationship? These are the kinds of questions a sex therapist will help you work through—ideally, along with your partner. Sometimes sexual fantasy games and other related tricks of the trade can help bring back that loving feeling. In general, sex therapists are seeing more lack-of-desire problems in women of all ages. Sometimes the demands of modern life tug our energies away from sex, and cutting down on obligations to make time for sex will renew your interest in it. (For more on sexual healing *see* chapter 14.)

Finally, some researchers have found that women who never enjoyed sex much *before* menopause *use* the menopause as an excuse to give it up altogether. If this is how you feel, you might want to take this time to evaluate why you never wanted sex in the first place. Have you ever been attracted to your partner? Do you feel comfortable about your own body? There's no reason to assume that it's "normal" for this latter third of your life to be sex-free. Lots of people have sex well into old age, and enjoy it. This is as good a time as any to take stock of your sexual life and sexual self-image and consider a wake-up call for this dormant part of your life.

SMOKING AND MENOPAUSE

If there is a single thing you can do to protect your health at the time of menopause, says Sonja McKinlay, it's to stop smoking. In almost every way, smoking and menopausal changes make for a poisonous mixture. Smoking not only brings on menopause earlier, but it exacerbates nearly *all* of the adverse physiological changes that accompany it. Smoking boosts the risk of heart disease and bone loss, two key menopausal risks. At *least* cut down—the less the better—but quitting is the real answer (*see* chapter 19 for smoking cessation tips and other facts about smoking and women).

A BRIEF WORD ABOUT NUTRITION DURING AND AFTER THE MENOPAUSE

As our bodies age, we have different nutritional needs. Older women have a lesser ability to synthesize vitamin D from sunlight, and may need to get more in the form of a daily supplement. We have less stomach acid as we grow older, so our absorption of nutrients like folic acid and vitamin B_{12} drops. Our bones need more calcium—up to about 1500 milligrams a day—which can be hard to get from foods alone. Perhaps a small calcium supplement would help you meet your goal. (For more on calcium in the diet, *see* chapter 20.)

There are also some nutrients we need *less* of after menopause, such as iron. Since we're no longer losing iron in blood through menstruation, our iron needs drop.

You might consider sitting down with your doctor or a trained nutritionist to evaluate the strengths and weaknesses of your diet at this important life juncture.

SURGICAL OR ARTIFICIAL MENOPAUSE

Menopause that is brought on suddenly by the removal of the ovaries or some other damage to the hormonal system tends to cause more dramatic sensations and problems than does natural menopause. Hot flashes, vaginal dryness, bone loss, a sharp climb in the "bad" cholesterol, earlier heart disease onset and a whole host of other problems are often exaggerated and quickened when menopause occurs suddenly. One reason for this may be that instead of gradually becoming accustomed to lower estrogen levels, which is what the body normally does in the perimenopausal years, the body is jolted into an estrogen-free state, and reacts more abruptly. Because of the greater potential for these sensations and the likelihood of climbing health risks, women—especially young women—who have a sudden menopause should be counseled about hormone replacement therapy.

Amazingly, not all women *know* that they're going into sudden menopause even *after* surgery. Dr. Janice Green Douglas warns that surgeons performing hysterectomies (removal of the uterus) sometimes don't bother to *tell* their patients if they removed the ovaries as well, or if the ovaries were damaged during surgery and therefore will not continue to function properly! Be sure to ask your doctor for his or her plan *before* surgery (with a full explanation if she

intends to remove your ovaries), as well as for the results *after* surgery. You have every right to know what's going on in your body so you can anticipate changes and protect yourself with appropriate treatments. (For more on hysterectomy, *see* chapter 7.)

MENOPAUSE: A GOOD TIME TO ASSESS YOUR MEDICAL VULNERABILITIES—AND YOUR STRENGTHS

This is an excellent time of life for a complete medical screening: it will help you determine if you're in need of lifestyle changes to improve your general health, and if hormone intervention is appropriate for you. Dr. Patricia Ganz of UCLA recommends having a bone scan to find out if you're *already* at risk of a fracture. The question is, which of the several bone scan tests to choose. There are several, and they vary in cost and in which bone(s) they measure. Dr. J. C. Gallagher, professor of medicine at Creighton University, urges women who think they're vulnerable to bone loss to pay the extra money (in the $200-plus range) for a DEXA scan, which measures the spine and femur. If you have greater than average bone density, he points out, you won't need to worry—nor will you need to repeat the test in the future, in most cases. If, on the other hand, you discover that you're beginning your postmenopausal life with weak or porous bones, many practitioners will urge you to take hormone replacement to ward off likely fractures and their serious subsequent health risks. Dr. Gallagher and other experts worry that postmenopausal calcium supplementation, while vital for women who get too little calcium in their diets, just won't provide enough protection for women whose bone is already quite weakened. The same goes for weight-bearing exercise; it's a great way to help prevent further loss, but once the damage has been done, drug treatment of some kind is more valuable protection against fracture. (*See* chapter 4, "Your Bone Health.")

OTHER MEDICAL TESTS AT THE TIME OF MENOPAUSE

A full range of blood tests can reveal how your lipids (blood fats) are holding up. Ask for a breakdown of your good cholesterol, bad cholesterol and your triglyceride level. Talk to your doctor about what the results mean, and if you should be modifying your diet or making other changes to protect yourself. Also, get your blood pressure tested, and be checked for diabetes. See if your weight is at a healthy level. Dr. Laura Bookman recommends this as a good time to review your family history of diseases; when it comes to the hormone replacement decision, particularly check your family history of breast cancer, heart disease and bone loss. Repeat these tests at an interval your doctor thinks is appropriate. If you are at high risk of major problems like heart disease, annual tests might be warranted.

HORMONE REPLACEMENT THERAPY: WHAT YOU NEED TO KNOW

To take or not to take hormone replacement: that is the question that plagues women and their health care providers perhaps more than any other health-related decision. And the choice is only made harder by the fact that just about everything you read about hormone replacement contradicts what you read before! What could be more frustrating than to see an article in your morning paper extolling the virtues of estrogen as protection against heart disease, the leading killer of women—only to see another article in the same paper the next week warning that estrogen causes breast cancer and should be avoided? The reason the lay literature seems so frought with confusion and controversy is that scientists are confused, too. They don't yet have all the important answers about hormone replacement, its risks *or* its benefits. Until recently, most of what we know about hormone therapy has come from so-called "observational" studies, which are far less rigorous (and the results less certain) than randomized controlled studies. Furthermore, most studies of hormone replacement have focused on healthy, affluent white women, which means we have little idea how hormone therapy affects women in poor health, women from lower socioeconomic groups and women of color. This is especially important because some major health risks associated with menopause, including heart disease, are far more prevalent in these latter groups of women—so hormone replacement might be of significant benefit to them. In 1994, a significant randomized, controlled study of hormone therapy (called the PEPI study) gave us some important new information about cmbined estrogen and progesterone treatment. Still, we need to know more, and continue to make our decisions about hormone therapy without enough solid, long-term data.

So what's a smart woman to do? The first intelligent step is to take a close look at what we *do* know about hormone replacement therapy (HRT), and an equally close look at what we *don't* know about it. Then you'll have to take that information and match it to your own particular risk factors for various diseases, to see if the evidence stacks up in favor of *your* taking it, or not. The answers aren't the same for every woman, and they certainly aren't easy to come by. This section should help you make up your mind by walking you through the important issues, but no one—and that includes your doctor—can make this difficult decision for you.

WHAT IS HORMONE REPLACEMENT?

As we discussed earlier in this chapter, when you approach menopause, the estrogen levels in your body begin to drop. In some women, the drop is more dramatic than in others. The results of this lack of estrogen are the many changes we've discussed in this chapter, including both problems you can *feel* (hot flashes, vaginal dryness, gastric upset, mood changes, sleep problems, etc.) and problems you *cannot feel* (an increase in your "bad" cholesterol level, a decrease in the strength of your bones, etc.). In short, your hormonal profile becomes more masculine, and with it, your risk of major diseases like heart disease come to mirror men's risk.

Hormone replacement means just what it sounds like: giving back hormones that your body is newly lacking to try to reverse the problems associated with estrogen deprivation. About 10–15% of American women over age 50 take estrogen, but about a third of those who are prescribed it never fill those prescriptions. Still others go on and off hormone therapy, trying to manage the changes of menopause and to limit the side effects or possible long-term risks of treatment. We know little about the health effects of this kind of self-treating, on-again, off-again therapy.

When estrogen is given alone, it's called ERT (estrogen replacement therapy). When *combination* hormone therapy is used (estrogen plus another female hormone, progesterone) it's called HRT (hormone replacement therapy). We'll talk about why you might choose ERT or HRT in a moment.

DEFINING YOUR GOALS FOR HORMONE THERAPY

The most important step in deciding whether or not to take hormones is determining what you want to achieve. It's a very bad idea to start hormone replacement (or any medication, for that matter) without specific goals in mind. Hormone replacement is given for two completely different reasons. It can be given to relieve feelings associated with menopause, such as hot flashes and vaginal dryness. This is a short-term goal: treatment usually lasts a few years, and the mission is to restore quality of life *now*. Interestingly, Dr. Howard Judd of the UCLA Medical School finds that many of his patients feel *guilty* about taking hormones "just to feel better." They tell him that they need a more "worthy" reason to take hormones. Don't get caught up in these kinds of feelings. The ability to feel good, to perform well and to enjoy life is a worthwhile goal in itself. Your much more important concern should be finding out if hormone replacement is a safe and effective option for you.

Hormone replacement can also be given to prevent disease down the road. This is a long-term goal, and may require taking hormones for decades—maybe for the rest of your life. With long-term preventive therapy, you won't have the immediate payoff you might experience if you were trying to combat current ill feelings. Experts still aren't certain what duration of treatment will provide long-term prevention of illness. The diseases in question are bone loss (osteoporosis) and heart disease; hormone replacement therapy can significantly reduce your risk of both of these problems. As we discuss in chapters 4 and 24, bone loss and heart disease affect a great number of women, robbing us of life years and productivity. Studies have shown that to get significant improvements in bone and heart health, you have to take hormones for many years—and it's possible that some of that benefit wears off when you stop taking hormones. As we'll discuss in a moment, the trouble is that when you take hormones over a long period of time, your risk of certain diseases climbs. That's why it's so important to establish a risk-benefit profile for yourself.

WEIGHING RISKS AND BENEFITS: A LOOK AT THE STATISTICS

If it were as easy as just taking hormones to prevent disease, with no downside, your decision would be simple. But of course, it's not that clear cut. Along with the upside come both the risks and side effects of treatment. We'll discuss them here. Most important, we'll take a look at some hard statistics (that is, as hard as any statistics are on this subject, which leaves quite a bit of room for improvement). Too often, the media's and even the health experts' evaluations of hormone therapy become treatises on hopes and fears, rather than on facts. Depending on whose opinion you're reading, these emotions can steer us away from the real

statistics that can help us determine if hormone therapy is right for *us.*

Let's start with the benefits of hormone replacement therapy. On the plus side, estrogen replacement alone (without progesterone) is believed to reduce the risk of both heart disease and bone loss. How big a difference does it make? That depends whose numbers you're looking at.

First, we'll look at bone health. The following data comes from a report by Dr. Deborah Grady and colleagues, published in the December 1992 issue of *Annals of Internal Medicine.* This study pooled the results of all available major studies on hormone replacement therapy to date. While we know that these studies had limitations, there is value in looking at *all* of them to try to tease out some important trends. The report says that a 50-year-old Caucasian woman has a 15% chance, on average, of suffering a hip fracture—and that estrogen replacement therapy cuts that risk to 12.7% You may have heard it phrased a different way: that estrogen replacement cuts the risk of a hip fracture by one fourth or 25%. Isn't it interesting to look at the *actual risk,* as opposed to the percent decrease? Naturally, if you have many risk factors for osteoporosis (see pages 43–44), the benefits of hormone replacement could be more impressive for you. Most experts say you need to start taking hormones within a couple of years of menopause in order to maximize the impact on your bone health, since about half of all bone loss occurs quickly (in the first seven years after menopause). However, one study *did* show a significant drop in the hip fracture rate among women over age 80 who were taking hormone replacement *plus* extra calcium and vitamin D. It remains controversial whether women who start hormone therapy many years after menopause will achieve significant bone benefits.

Now let's look at the numbers for heart disease from that same report. Estrogen replacement therapy cuts that same 50-year-old woman's risk of heart disease from 46.1% to 34.2%. Since the risk of heart disease is so great to begin with, this reduction is important and could save many lives. Some say the reduction in heart disease risk with estrogen therapy is even greater than these numbers indicate (perhaps as much as 50%!), but at this point there is no solid proof. But before you get too excited, consider this: if you add progesterone to the hormone therapy, which many do (for reasons to be discussed below), the heart disease benefits are blunted. By how much, no one knows for sure. All we do know is that some of the benefits that estrogen confers on heart health, such as reducing cholesterol, are *partially* negated by progesterone. The PEPI study mentioned earlier suggests that the negative impact of progesterone on heart disease risk is quite small, however and that when *natural* progesterone is used instead of a synthetic form, the cardiovascular benefits are almost as good as with estrogen alone.

Dr. Elizabeth Barrett-Connor, professor and chair of the department of family and preventive medicine at the University of California at San Diego (and an investigator on two major upcoming hormone studies), says that the protection from heart disease that one gets from estrogen is probably not as great as people are claiming. Why? Because the women who have been taking hormone replacement up to this point have been relatively healthy, from high socioeconomic groups, and Caucasian, and therefore are at lower risk of heart disease *to begin with* than many other women. This artificially skews the data in *favor* of hormone replacement, she notes. Given these problems with the available information, and the sheer *quantity* of information women have to sort through, Dr. Barrett-Connor laments the fact that women are trying to make their choice about hormone treatment based on 15-minute conversations with their doctors. It's easy to get caught up in big promises of long-term wellness, and to forget the fact that most of the data we have is spotty at best. It takes Dr. Barrett-Connor about one hour just to go through the big issues with women during an uninterrupted lecture; how can women sort it all out based on one office visit? Keep her concerns in mind when you talk to *your* doctor. If you don't feel you have all the pieces of the puzzle, ask for more information before beginning (or declining) treatment.

We've been talking about the benefits of hormone therapy. Now let's take a look at the down side. Estrogen alone *increases* your risk of endometrial cancer (cancer of the lining of the uterus). The average 50-year-old Caucasian woman has only a 2.6% chance of getting endometrial cancer; if she takes estrogen replacement alone, her risk jumps to 19.7%—a very significant increase. If you no longer have a uterus (you've had a hysterectomy) this is of no concern to you. If you *do* still have your uterus, however, experts recommend adding the hormone progesterone to your treatment regimen. When you take both estrogen and progesterone together (either continuously, or in a cyclic fashion we'll discuss later) you erase that increased risk of endometrial cancer. It's easy to understand why: progesterone promotes the shedding of the uterine lining, just as it used to shed with your menstrual period. So instead of building up and potentially becoming cancerous, the lining is sloughed off regularly. The trouble is that progesterone causes many unpleasant side effects for some women, as we'll discuss below. If you still have your uterus, can't tolerate progesterone, and want to take estrogen alone, you'll be advised to have an endometrial biopsy (a test of the lining of your uterus) every year, or whenever abnormal bleeding occurs.

Perhaps the most worrisome risk associated with hormone replacement is the risk of breast cancer. This is the issue that concerns women most, and may be the reason so many women who are prescribed hormone replacement never actually take it. According to the Grady paper, estrogen replacement increases the risk of breast cancer for that same 50-year-old woman from 10.2% to 13%. For all the press it generated, you may be surprised at how small this increase actually is. But since women fear breast cancer perhaps more than any other disease, even this small potential increase in risk frightens many of us away. There are a couple of things to keep in mind about the breast cancer and estrogen issue. First, it's thought that women who take estrogen for less than ten years may have *no* increased risk of breast cancer. The risk seems to go up for long-term users. (The trouble is, you may need to take estrogen for at least ten years to get heart health benefits, so there's a catch-22.) Second, it's possible that the kind of estrogen taken by most American women (a natural estrogen derived from the urine of mares) may be less likely to promote breast cancer than the kind of estrogen used by most European women (a more potent synthetic estrogen). To throw yet another issue into the mix, we simply don't know what the addition of progesterone to the hormone regimen does to breast cancer risk! Again, there are far more questions than answers.

What's the bottom line as far as statistics go? The Grady report only offers an estimate for estrogen replacement alone (ERT), since we have more data on ERT than on HRT. If you tally up the reduction in risk of heart disease and osteoporosis, and place it against the increased risk of endometrial cancer and breast cancer, you end up with an *increased* life expectancy for the average 50-year-old white woman of just under one year. In other words, the benefits outweigh the risks as far as life span is concerned. What that means to *you* is another story altogether.

If you have a very high risk of heart disease (let's say you have high cholesterol, high blood pressure, you're overweight, or have a strong family history of heart disease) and you're at low risk for breast cancer (much harder to predict, as we discuss in chapter 25), hormone replacement might add years to your life. If, on the other hand, you're at high risk for breast cancer, and very low risk for heart disease and bone loss, the scale for you might tip the other way—against taking hormones. This is all the more reason to have a complete health assessment at the time of menopause: if you find out how your heart and bone health are holding up, take a complete family history of disease, and have your breasts examined with mammography, you'll get a better idea of where you stand. As a *generalization*, Dr. Grady says that hormone therapy is probably best for women who have already had hysterectomies, and for women who already have heart disease or who have many risk factors for heart disease. Beyond these groups, she adds, you run into questions about long-term side effects and risk for basically healthy women—which raises important ethical questions.

MAKING THE DECISION YOUR OWN

Dr. Diane Meier, professor of geriatrics and medicine at Mt. Sinai Hospital in New York, is disturbed by the number of patients who come into her office saying they've been told by other doctors that they *must* take estrogen—that they should pop it like vitamin C. Dr. Meier considers the following problems strong indications for hormone therapy: debilitating sensations of menopause, below-normal bone density even before menopause, and heart disease. But beyond these clearer-cut cases, hormone replacement is *not* for everyone, she says. The bottom line is you have to wake up in the morning and feel you're doing the right thing! If you can't do that, regardless of your risk factors, you shouldn't be taking estrogen, Meier says. As much as you may want some authority figure to make this tough decision for you, it's one you *must* make on your own if you are ever to live with it comfortably.

Dr. Laura Bookman of the Beth Israel Hospital in Boston urges women who do choose to take hormones to attend lectures, group meetings and other information sessions on hormone therapy to learn as much as possible about what to expect from the treatment in both the short and long term. She observes that her patients who become highly informed are far more likely to be satisfied with hormone replacement therapy than those who don't. The fact is, no one wants surprises (especially uncomfortable ones) when it comes to their

health. The more you know (and the more your fears are replaced with information), the more empowered you will be—and the greater the chance that you will own your decision about hormone therapy.

HORMONE REPLACEMENT: YOUR OPTIONS

If you decide that hormone replacement is right for you, you'll have to decide when to start, what regimen to choose, and what form to take it in. Your choice of regimens includes estrogen alone daily, estrogen daily with progesterone only on certain days of the month (called "cycled" hormone therapy), or both estrogen and progesterone daily (called "continuous" hormone therapy). When progesterone is given continuously, it's given in a lower dose (a quarter to half as much) than when it's given cyclically—which means fewer side effects for some women.

Start out with an assessment of your overall health so that if changes do occur while you're taking hormones, your doctor will have something to compare them to (have a mammogram, full gynecological exam, blood fat screening, blood pressure and so on).

You'll be given a choice of types of estrogen to take. Most American women take Premarin, which is a natural estrogen called a conjugated equine estrogen. It is taken in pill form. There are other pill-form natural estrogens as well (which are less potent than the synthetic estrogens used in oral contraceptives). You can also take estrogen in the form of a patch worn on your body, a cream applied to your skin (placed on the dry, vaginal skin to moisten it) or by injection. When you take estrogen in pill form, it goes through your liver in the process of digestion. When estrogen passes through the liver it lowers your cholesterol level, which is a big part of how it protects you against heart disease. Estrogen taken by patch or cream does not pass through the liver. It goes straight into your bloodstream (in small quantities), and therefore doesn't have as significant an impact on cholesterol and fat levels. The patch protects against bone disease and many physical sensations of menopause, and the cream protects against vaginal dryness. Dr. Marjorie Luckey, director of the osteoporosis and metabolic bone disease program at New York's Mt. Sinai Hospital, says that if you *can* take the oral form of estrogen you *should*, since it provides more benefits than the patch or the cream. Women who can't take oral estrogen include those with an aversion to swallowing pills, those who get high blood pressure when taking estrogen replacement (a rare phenomenon), and possibly those with gallstones or liver disease, she says.

Estrogen gels, now available in Europe, will soon be available in the U.S.

The best time to start hormone replacement therapy is during the perimenopause, when your estrogen levels are dropping. This way you will avoid shocking your system with estrogen when very little is present. Experts recommend starting slowly with a low dose and building from there. (The same goes for *stopping* hormone therapy; going off it cold turkey can be hard on your system. Better to taper off gradually, according to a schedule mapped out by your doctor.) It's also valuable to start hormone replacement within a couple of years after menopause. Long after that, scientists just don't know how much benefit you'll reap. Dr. Veronica Ravnikar of the University of Massachusetts at Worcester, says that especially for *bone* protection, women

should start hormone replacement within two to five years after their last period. Much later and you may miss the window of most significant benefit.

No matter what hormone regimen you choose, be sure to alert your doctor *immediately* to any unexpected symptoms (bleeding outside of the time you've been told to expect it, or unusual breast changes, for example).

SIDE EFFECTS YOU MAY EXPERIENCE WITH HORMONE REPLACEMENT

Estrogen alone often causes breast pain and swelling, as well as fluid retention. Dr. Luckey finds that these side effects are more pronounced in women who start hormone replacement long after menopause; she likens it to an adolescent getting her first period—a jolt to the body. For this reason, she advises women several years past menopause to start out on a low dose of estrogen and build up gradually. And keep in mind, Dr. Luckey adds, that not all estrogens feel the same in your body. If one type doesn't agree with you, try another, and then another, until you find the right "fit." Progesterone (or more correctly, progestins, which are synthetic forms of progesterone) can cause PMS-like symptoms ranging from headaches to bloating to mood swings. Also, taking progestins means your uterine lining will shed once again, so you'll bleed—like having periods. The good news is that for women taking cyclic progesterone, bleeding normally stops after about 4–6 months.

Some find that continuous low-dose progestins cause fewer side effects than progestins given cyclically at a higher dose. Down the road, natural progesterone, rather than synthetics, may be used more widely for hormone replacement; it is thought that the natural form of the hormone will cause fewer side effects than the synthetics. Dr. Frederick Kuhn, director of preventive cardiology at Baltimore's St. Agnes Hospital, points to preliminary evidence that giving progestins just a few times a year instead of every month might reduce the side effects still further.

HORMONE THERAPY ISN'T FOR EVERYONE

The following women should avoid or be especially cautious about hormone therapy (there are some exceptions, at their doctors' discretion). Those with:

1. A personal history of breast cancer.[1]

2. Cancer of the lining of the uterus.

3. Liver disease.

4. Gallbladder disease.

5. Abnormal vaginal bleeding of unknown cause.

6. Clotting disorders.

Women with poorly controlled hypertension might also be advised not to take hormone

therapy. Talk to your doctor if you fit any of these categories.

We've listed the main physical contraindications to hormone therapy. But there are psychological or emotional ones as well. If after becoming informed about your risk-benefit profile you're still fundamentally uncomfortable with taking medication to prevent disease—or you just don't *like* the idea of taking hormones—don't let anyone push you into it.

HORMONE THERAPY: LIVING WITH A CATCH-22

Unfortunately, while the decision to take hormones may be relatively easy for women at extremely high risk for diseases on either side of the risk-benefit scale, the vast majority of us fall in a grey area. We aren't at *particularly* high risk of heart disease (although certainly we're at risk, since it's the number one killer of women). And we aren't at *particularly* high risk of breast cancer (but then again, three-fourths of breast cancers occur in women without major risk factors!) Our bones aren't strong as steel, but they aren't full of holes, either. It is for us—the vast majority of women—that this decision is so very difficult. We are forced to confront difficult questions, the most global of which is, *Are we willing to put ourselves at some known risk in order to avoid a potentially bigger unknown risk?* Perhaps the reason so many women walk around with prescriptions for hormones burning holes in their pockets is that it's ultimately easier *not to do* something than *to do* something; inaction is easier than action. But that's no way to make a major decision about your health. What we *don't* do can have just as strong implications for our health as what we *do*.

---

1. There was a time when a personal history of breast cancer was considered an absolute contraindication to taking estrogen. Now, even this long-held belief is being questioned. A 1994 review of the major literature on this subject failed to find significant evidence that hormone replacement was especially risky for breast cancer survivors. This remains quite controversial: at this point, you must discuss the issue with your health care providers (and consider also getting a second opinion from another medical center).

The trouble is, you can't let yourself off the hook by settling for something in the middle either, such as taking hormones for just a couple of years and hoping to prevent disease. Dr. Graham Colditz, coprincipal investigator on the Harvard Nurses' Health Study, a major study of women's health issues, feels the issue comes down to a painful catch-22. Since you need to take hormones for a long period of time to achieve heart and bone health benefits, he says, and long-term therapy has been associated with increased breast cancer risk, you can only achieve the benefits at the price of the risks. His advice to women in the gray area is *not* to take HRT, because there are so many ways to prevent heart disease through lifestyle changes, but so little you can do to prevent breast cancer. But plenty of other experts are quick to retort that you can catch breast cancer early, with mammography, while you may have a heart attack before any problem is diagnosed.

By now you can see that no matter how you analyze the issue, no matter how you break down the pluses and the minuses, the risks and the benefits, the answer will remain a tough one until the right kinds of studies are completed. All I can recommend is that you gather the information thoroughly and thoughtfully about both hormones in general and your own risks in particular, then look into your soul, and make the best decision you can for yourself.

OTHER MEDICATION FOR MENOPAUSAL RISKS

Cholesterol-lowering drugs might become necessary for some women at this time, as the "bad" cholesterol picks up steam. Hypertension medication may also be needed or, if you're borderline hypertensive (which many women are at this stage of life), lifestyle changes to cut blood pressure may be in order (*see* chapter 24 for specifics).

A special word to African-American women and other women of color: Many researchers feel that women in minority groups have been overlooked as far as managing menopause is concerned. Doctors aren't asking the right questions, and many minority women aren't seeking care at this time. Individual risk factors like excessive weight, high blood pressure and diabetes are more common in these groups, and when those factors converge and increase, the risk of fatal diseases (especially heart disease and stroke) jumps quickly. Dr. Janice Green Douglas urges African-American, Hispanic and Native American women to be screened for health risk factors at the time of menopause and every year thereafter. Furthermore, she adds, a myth has developed that African-American women do not have to worry about osteoporosis at menopause because their bones are generally more dense than Asian or Caucasian women's *before* menopause. Across the whole population, this may be true; but certainly many African-American women are at risk of bone loss that can lead to fractures, and should be closely followed by doctors to protect what bone they have and reduce the risk of further loss. Studies show that African-American women run a greater risk of death after hip fractures than do Caucasian women.

THE POSITIVE SIDE OF MENOPAUSE

As I mentioned at the beginning of this chapter, the menopausal experience is as varied as are women. While some have discomforts at this time, others have an almost completely positive experience. I was quite moved by a comment made by Mary Catherine Bateson, daughter of Margaret Mead, at a 1993 symposium on menopause called "Changing Views of the Change." Recalling her own movement into older age and experience with menopause, she smiled and said, "I reached a moment where I could grow my own silver jewelry." I looked at her, with her silver hair framing her experienced face, and wished we could all approach this stage of life as positively and as poetically as she had. Here are just a few physical and psychological reasons why we should.

BETTER SEX

Remember the problems with vaginal dryness and low libido we talked about earlier? Well for some women, menopause brings anything *but* sexual problems. On the contrary, some women report a sense of tremendous sexual freedom and openness around the time of menopause. Some reasons? First, for women who raised children, this may be the first time in years those kids are out of the house and mom is free to "do it" on the kitchen floor again! Privacy can do a lot for your sex life, and chances are, if you have kids, you haven't had much solitude in a long time. Second, menopause represents freedom from the fear of getting pregnant (be sure that you are well past your last period before you assume you are no longer ovulating; if you still have a period every several months, you may still be fertile—and should use contraception if you don't want to get pregnant). No longer needing to use messy, uncomfortable or otherwise bothersome contraception gives spontaneity to sex that may have been missing since you last tried to become pregnant!

Dr. Laura Bookman reports that many of her single menopausal patients (some newly single through divorce or widowhood) take up with new, younger and more vigorous sex partners than they've been with in years, and find that sex has never been better! The sheer variety can be exciting for some women who have had the same partner for years. (Of course, if you are having sex with new partners or multiple partners, use condoms to protect yourself from sexually transmitted diseases—even if you no longer need them for protection from pregnancy.) Others find new passion with lifelong lovers as they enter a new, independent phase of life as a couple once again.

A terrific sex life requires a vital sexual partner. If your male partner is experiencing trouble with erections or other sexual problems at a time when you are sexually charged, help him through this time with communication and support, as well as the name of an expert on sexual function (perhaps a urologist to start) who can try to correct any impediment to *his* sexual function. His sex problem is your sex problem, especially if you've never been more sexually awake, and he more asleep. Blaming is the worst thing you can do. Work the problems out together.

IMPROVED SELF-ESTEEM

With many of life's foibles and insecurities behind them, some women emerge at the time of menopause much stronger and more self-reliant than ever before in their lives. Sonja McKinlay's research turned up many women whose response to menopause was, "Is that all?"

Most of the women in her study felt fundamental relief at no longer getting their periods. Only two or three out of a hundred voiced any regret before *or* after menopause.

Many women recognize this as a time of life to pursue long-deferred goals or to reach the pinnacle of goals undertaken earlier in life. If you never got out and did things you hoped or dreamed of doing, this stage of life should be viewed as an open landscape of opportunity, a chance to reach out of your traditional worldview and become more vitally involved in the world around you. Take a job, go back to school, travel, volunteer in your community, take up a hobby, get fit. It can be a time of beginning, of change, not of decline.

Dr. Bruce Kessel predicts that as the baby boomer generation, with its social and political clout, reaches menopause, we might see a dramatic shift away from the negative, medicalized view of menopause toward a more positive definition of this as a time of strength and authority. Having menopausal women in Congress, at the top of major companies, and perhaps heading the White House in the near future, could change the image of menopause to one of gray-haired power and seniority. We can only guess if the negative sensations of menopause will abate along with this shift in attitude.

FOR MORE INFORMATION ON MENOPAUSE

OLDER WOMEN'S LEAGUE (OWL)

666 11th St. NW
Suite 700
Washington, DC 20001
202-783-6686

NORTH AMERICAN MENOPAUSE SOCIETY

c/o University Hospitals of Cleveland
Department of OBGYN
11100 Euclid Ave.
Cleveland, OH 44106
216-844-3344

NATIONAL OSTEOPOROSIS FOUNDATION

2100 M St. NW
Suite 602
Washington, DC 20037
202-223-2226

SEX INFORMATION AND EDUCATION COUNCIL OF THE U.S. (SIECUS)

130 W. 42nd Street
Suite 2500
New York, NY 10036
212-819-9770

MENOPAUSE WELLNESS CENTER BETH ISRAEL HOSPITAL

330 Brokline Ave.
Boston, MA 02215
617-735-3738

ALLIANCE FOR AGING RESEARCH

2021 K Street NW
Suite 305
Washington, DC 20006
202-293-2856

AMERICAN HEART ASSOCIATION

7320 Greenville Ave.
Dallas, TX 75231
214-373-6300

NATIONAL HEART, LUNG AND BLOOD
INSTITUTE

9000 Rockville Pike
Bethesda, MD 20892
301-496-4236

NATIONAL CANCER INSTITUTE
CANCER INFORMATION SERVICE

9000 Rockville Pike
Bethesda, MD 20892
800-4-CANCER

AMERICAN CANCER SOCIETY
NATIONAL HEADQUARTERS

1599 Clifton Rd. NE
Atlanta, GA 30329
800-ACS-2345

NATIONAL INSTITUTE ON AGING
INFORMATION CENTER

P.O. Box 8057
Gaithersburg, MD 20892-8057
800-222-2225
For information on exercise, nutrition and other
issues involving menopause and aging.

AMERICAN COLLEGE OF
OBSTETRICIANS AND
GYNECOLOGISTS

409 12th Street SW
Washington, DC 20024
202-638-5577

OFFICE OF ALTERNATIVE MEDICINE
NATIONAL INSTITUTES OF HEALTH

Executive Plaza
6120 Executive Blvd.
Rockville, MD 20892
301-402-2466

NATIONAL WOMEN'S HEALTH
NETWORK

514 10th Street NW, Suite 400
Washington, DC 20004
202-347-1140

AMERICAN ASSOCIATION OF RETIRED
PERSONS

601 E Street NW
Washington, DC 20049
202-434-2277

NATIONAL OSTEOPOROSIS
FOUNDATION

See Bone Health Chapter

ASSOCIATION OF SEX EDUCATORS,
COUNSELLORS, AND THERAPISTS

See Sexual Function Chapter

AMERICAN HEART ASSOCIATION

See Heart Health Chapter

PART FOUR

Sexual Health

CHAPTER ELEVEN

CONTRACEPTION

*We want far better reasons for having children than not
knowing how to prevent them.*

—Dora Russell, *Hypatia*

If you're a sexually active woman and you have taken responsibility for your own birth control method, at some point you've probably felt tremendous frustration at your limited choices as well as the drawbacks to many of those choices. Whether it's distaste for the drippiness after diaphragm use, the hormones of oral contraceptives, or the fact that your male partner doesn't like using condoms and complains every time you have intercourse, it seems there's almost always *something* undesirable you can point your finger at. If you're one of the rare lucky ones who's fully satisfied with your method of birth control, spread the word on what you're doing right!

The truth is, while we're complaining, the times we're living in now are the best *ever* in terms of contraceptive options. Not only are there more *safe* options than most women realize, but the fact that there are so many options *at all* represents important strides since even a generation ago. We have a long way to go, but we've come a long way, too.

In this chapter, we'll look at the pros and cons of each available form of contraception and how you can improve your odds of comfort and success with any given method. While no method is flawless, and the devices or procedures themselves can fail, many contraceptive failures occur because they are used improperly or inconsistently. Learning to use your method of contraception properly will greatly increase your odds of preventing pregnancy and, in some cases, sexually transmitted diseases as well.

For decades women have asked why the burden of contraception so often falls on *us*—why research hasn't led to a male birth control pill, for example.

At a recent lecture at the Harvard School of Public Health, speaker Rachel Snow assailed the U.S. government for its paltry spending on male contraceptives; of the more than 64 million dollars spent on contraceptive research and development between 1972 and 1991, only 12% of the money went toward male methods, she reported. One potential reason: there are still relatively few women in high-level scientific research positions. One would hope that as this situation changes, so will the output of female-friendly—as well as male-focused—contraceptive options.

Since reality dictates that we make due with what's available to us, let's focus on what we have available today. You may have to shop around, try two or three methods before you settle on one that's right for you and your partner. Some couples choose to use more than one method, or to switch among different contraceptive options. If you do this, be sure that you're always using at at least one effective method. A common cause of contraceptive "failures" is forgetting to use a new method after stopping a previous one. Don't rely on someone else to watch out for you: *protect yourself.*

CONSISTENCY MEANS GREATER EFFECTIVENESS

Whatever your selection, it's vital that you feel comfortable using it *every time you have sex.* Believe it or not, many of the statistics you've seen about contraceptive "failures" are not in fact due to a problem of the pill or the device, but rather to improper use or *not using* the method at all! This is why professor James Trussell of Princeton University, an author of *Contraceptive Technology,* says that the "best" form of contraception is the one you'll actually use correctly and consistently. According to the Alan Guttmacher Institute, 57% of all U.S. pregnancies are *unintended*—and half of those are caused by "contraceptive failure." And Dr. Phillip Stubblefield of Boston University reports that of the 1.5 million abortions performed in the U.S. each year, only half of the affected couples used contraception at all!

Experts divide contraceptive failure/efficacy rates into two categories: "perfect use" and "typical use." "Perfect use" requires using the method every single time you have sex, and using it and caring for it precisely as directed, without fail. "Typical use" includes the many human foibles that often get in the way of using a method properly, such as putting a condom on *after* inserting the penis into the vagina, skipping a birth control pill for one or two days, not checking to see that the strings of your IUD are where they should be, failing to add a dose of contraceptive jelly when using the diaphragm for repeat acts of intercourse, not showing up for a new injection of Depo-Provera until long after your scheduled date, and so on.

Take a look at the following chart from the 1994 edition of the text *Contraceptive Technology* (16th edition), which was assembled by leading experts in the field of sexual health and pregnancy prevention, and is based on the best available research. It shows the percentage of women experiencing an accidental pregnancy with both "perfect" and "typical" use of each available form of contraception *during the first year of use.* Keep in mind that as a rule, the longer you use any method of contraception, the better you get at using it. So your second, third, fourth and further years of use might offer better protection than this chart suggests.

Some women are startled by the significant differences between perfect and typical use for many contraceptive methods. The percentages for perfect and typical use of the same method can be so different that it seems as if you're comparing two completely different forms of contraception! In a sense, you are. Using a method wrong is sometimes as bad as not using it at all. Keep that in mind when you choose a method for yourself. Experts recommend that you think carefully about the kind of person you are, and perhaps what kind of person your partner(s) are, and figure out the likelihood of your using a given method optimally. If you're the type to forget your keys, lock yourself out of your apartment, miss appointments and arrive late for most meetings, you might just be the kind of person who will forget to take birth control pills. If you're very spontaneous and sexually passionate, and get carried away with the "moment," you may be less inclined to use a method of birth control that requires last-minute preparation, insertion or attention. If you often use mind or mood-altering substances before sex, like alcohol or drugs, you're far less likely to bother with a last-minute form of contraception, like condoms or female barrier methods, and may want something more reliable and user-independent, like an injectable contraceptive.

LIKING YOUR METHOD OF BIRTH CONTROL

As much as possible, it's important to *like* (at least relatively) your method of birth control. If

METHOD	TYPICAL USE	PERFECT USE
Chance	85%	85%
Spermicides (jellies, creams, gels, suppositories)	21%	6%
Periodic abstinence	20%	
Calendar		9%
Ovulation method		3%
Sympto-thermal		2%
Post-ovulation		1%
Withdrawal	19%	4%
Cervical cap		
if had previous children	36%	26%
if no previous children	18%	9%
Sponge		
if had previous children	36%	20%
if no previous children	18%	9%
Diaphragm	18%	6%
Condom		
Female (Reality)	21%	5%
Male	12%	3%
Pill	3%	
Progestin only ("minipill")		0.5%
Combined pill		0.1%
IUD		
Progesterone T	2.0%	1.5%
Copper T 380A	0.8%	0.6%
LNg 20	0.1%	0.1%
Depo-Provera (DMPA)	0.3%	0.3%
Norplant (6 capsules)	0.09%	0.09%
Female sterilization	0.4%	0.4%
Male sterilization	0.15%	0.10%

you like it, or at least don't dread it, you're more prone to look forward to and enjoy sex when you're using it. If you dread putting in your cervical cap, for example, you just might not bother having sex at all in order to avoid the hassle—or, worse yet (and more common) you'll have *un*protected sex "just this time." Many unwanted pregnancies and sexually transmitted diseases have resulted from "just this time" cases of unprotected intercourse.

CONSIDER WHAT YOUR GOALS ARE

There is more than one reason to use a given method of contraception. We use the terms "contraception" and "birth control" because these methods help prevent pregnancy. But these days, many women are using contraceptives to help prevent sexually transmitted diseases, as well as other health problems. The so-called "noncontraceptive benefits" of a given method of contraception can make it much more appealing for some women than another method with even greater protection against pregnancy. For example, the condom helps prevent transmission of sexually transmitted diseases. The Pill reduces your risk of certain cancers and cuts down on menstrual pain.

Unfortunately, experts report that noncontraceptive benefits have created a great deal of confusion among women. One classic misunderstanding holds that because the *condom* protects against sexually transmitted disease, so does *every* method of contraception! Of course this is not the case. You *must* take a look at the individual side benefits or risks to *your* method of contraception. Just as efficacy rates differ, so noncontraceptive benefits differ as well. Too

many women have come to believe that birth control and disease prevention go hand in hand—which is unfortunately far from the case. Dr. Michael Policar, former national medical director of Planned Parenthood of America, notes that many women believe that the vasectomy, or male sterilization, prevents the spread of STDs: this is *not true.*

Sometimes you'll have to use two methods of contraception to get the best antipregnancy benefits (say, from the Pill) and the best STD prevention benefits (from the condom, for example). Deborah Kowal, president of Contraceptive Technology Communications and an adjunct faculty member at the Emory School of Public Health, says people simply haven't caught on to the idea that you can use *two* methods of contraception at once. Nor have people realized that it's sensible to choose a method of contraception for the *short term* to meet your current needs, and then reevaluate those needs as time passes. As your needs change, Kowal says, your method of contraception should change with them. If you're in a long-term, mutually monogamous relationship, you may not need protection from sexually transmitted diseases. Be wary, however; experts say that many women who turn up in STD clinics were monogamous themselves, but learned the hard way that their partners *weren't.*

CONTRACEPTION: YOUR CHOICES— AND WHAT OTHERS HAVE CHOSEN

Every year the Ortho Pharmaceuticals Company, a leading maker of contraceptive materials, does a study of several thousand women to determine contraceptive preferences. The 25th anniversary study, released in 1993, finds that 45% of women in their childbearing years use a *reversible* method of birth control; that is, something they can stop using in order to become pregnant. (Even so-called sterilization, or "tying of the tubes," once an irreversible surgical procedure, is sometimes reversible with a delicate operation. Twenty-seven percent of women in their childbearing years use sterilization as a method of birth control.)

The 1993 Ortho study finds that the Pill is still women's leading choice—the choice of more than one-half of all women who use a reversible method. Nearly 17 million women take the Pill, for an average of five and a half years. The Pill is followed by the condom, at 17% of women; the diaphragm, vaginal suppositories and the sponge at 2% of women; and the IUD, douche, implants and jellies or creams at about 1%.

The most notable trends over the last ten years include an increase in condom use (doubled), and a decrease in the number of women using no contraception at all. Still, in this day of sexually transmitted diseases, it's disturbing that so *few* women choose condoms, and that so *many* women still use no protection whatsoever. According to Dr. Phillip Stubblefield, while in 1985 30% of women used no contraception at all, in 1991 that number had dropped to 19% (still one in five women!). It's a glass-half-empty, glass-half-full situation: improvement, but a very long way to go.

As for women's favorable opinions of the various contraceptive options, the Ortho study found the following results. Remember how important it is to have a favorable opinion of your method; you're more likely to keep using it, and use it right, if you like it.

PERCENTAGE OF WOMEN WHO HAVE A FAVORABLE OPINION OF THEIR METHOD OF BIRTH CONTROL

Pill	75%
Condom	63%
Vasectomy	62%
Tubal ligation	57%
Implants	33%
Diaphragm	29%
Sponge	24%
Foam	19%
Suppository	19%
IUD	18%
Cream/jelly	17%
Female condom	9%
Depo-Provera	9%
Cervical cap	8%

Cost.

Cost may come into play when you make your contraceptive choice. While there is great variability even in the cost of a given method (depending on where you live, how much your pharmacist bumps up the price, whether you have access to a public clinic, and so on), the following chart from *Contraceptive Technology* gives a good breakdown of the average annual cost of each major method—both the basic unit/device price and the annual costs.

YOUR CONTRACEPTIVE OPTIONS

Let's take a brief look at the various contraceptive options available to women and their partners today; their pros and cons, and their proper usage.

METHOD	UNIT COST	ANNUAL COST
Cervical cap	fitting and cap: $70–170	jelly: $85
Male condom	$.50	$50
Female condom	$2.50	$250
Diaphragm	fitting and diaphragm: $70–170	jelly: $85
Depo-Provera	injection plus hormone: $35 plus $140	
IUD	insertion and IUD: $160–170	Progestasert: $160 Cu T-380 A: $20 if used 8 years
Norplant	$350/kit plus $150–$250 insertion/removal	$130–$170 if retained 5 yrs.
Pill	$10–$20 per cycle	$130–$260
Spermicides	$.85/application	$85
Sponge	$4/pack of 3	$133

ORAL CONTRACEPTIVES: "THE PILL"

About 28% of women at risk of unintended pregnancy use the Pill.

When we talk about the Pill, which has been around for over 30 years, we're usually referring to the combination hormone pill containing both synthetic estrogen and a synthetic form of progesterone, called a progestin. There are several different pills on the market today, with different forms and concentrations of estrogen in them—*and* different forms and amounts of progestins. Older pills generally have more estrogen; newer ones are called "low-dose" pills because they have less estrogen. Most experts feel that women should avoid high-dose estrogen pills, for some reasons we'll discuss shortly; and in the last several years, the vast majority of women *have* made the switch to low-estrogen oral contraceptives. Try to use a pill with no more than 35 micrograms of estrogen, and a low progestin level. 98% of women can and should take low-estrogen pills. Dr. Policar, formerly of

Planned Parenthood of America, notes that a very small percentage of women *cannot* take low-dose pills because their failure rate will be higher than usual. One example: women taking antiseizure medication, because these medications can interfere with estrogen activity.

How the Pill Works.

In a sense, the Pill works by "tricking" the brain into thinking you're pregnant, thereby disrupting the flow of hormones that leads to ovulation. When you don't ovulate (release an egg), you can't conceive. Pills come in several different hormone combinations, to be used with different regimens. With some, you take the same amount of each hormone daily; with others, you vary the hormone intake throughout your cycle.

How Women Perceive the Pill.

The Pill is considered quite safe by medical experts. But many women won't accept that fact. In the past, there were many reports of problems with Pill safety, mainly in regard to cardiovascular complications (blood clotting, heart attack, etc.). Some women have remained fixed on this image of the Pill and won't try it as a result. In fact, cardiovascular risk was associated with *high-estrogen* pills—the newer, low-estrogen pills are thought to be quite safe. Furthermore, risks like blood clotting and other circulatory problems are far more common in Pill-users who smoke and are over the age of 35 than among all other groups of Pill-users. If you don't smoke, and use a low-dose pill, you should be quite safe; experts now believe that the risk of heart attack and strokes is no greater among nonsmoking low-dose Pill users than those who don't use the Pill at all.

Women with a strong family history or personal history of heart disease, clotting disorders, hypertension or diabetes are often counseled to avoid the Pill to remain on the safe side. That's because if you already have many risk factors for heart disease—high blood pressure, obesity, and so on—you don't want to add even another *possible* risk. If you're taking the Pill, just to be cautious, you should be alert to any potential signs of cardiovascular distress, such as leg pain or swelling, chest pain, sudden severe headache or coughing blood. But again, these problems are *quite rare.*

Women also fear that the Pill may increase the risk of certain cancers—particularly breast cancer. A major review study and other reports have failed to find a connection between overall Pill use and breast cancer risk. The only subset of women that raises some concern is those who started taking the Pill early (in their teens) and continued to take it for long periods of time (into their 30s or longer). There is possibly a small but significant increase in breast cancer

in this group, but keep in mind that this finding was based on high-dose estrogen pills. According to a study by the Centers for Disease Control and Prevention and the American College of OB-GYN, oral contraceptives add about 11 breast cancers per 100,000 younger women per year. Older women who have taken the Pill may actually have a *decreased* risk of breast cancer; the same report finds that the Pill may eliminate almost 18 cancers per 100,000 older women per year. When you bunch all ages of women together, the supposed increased risk in breast cancer risk is all but eliminated.

We know less about the low-dose pills than the high-dose ones, which have been around the longest. Experts believe that the lower-dose pills may be even safer than the higher-dose ones, which have been more heavily studied.

Other reports suggested suggest that Pill use might increase the rate of both benign liver tumors and an extremely rare kind of liver cancer; if it does, it does so extremely rarely. And Pill use *might* promote cervical cancer—but having a pap smear every single year will help you to detect any changes *before* they progress to cancer.

The Pill Versus Cancer.

When it comes to the Pill and cancer risk, what many women *don't* know could actually save their lives. All we ever hear about is the Pill and the risk of *getting* cancer. In fact, women taking oral contraceptives are *protected against* several forms of cancer, including ovarian and endometrial cancer (cancer of the lining of the uterus). This, according to experts across the country, is one of the best-kept secrets about Pill use. Some believe the word hasn't gotten out because Pill manufacturers hate to even discuss the word "cancer" in the same breath as oral contraceptives, for fear women will fixate on the breast cancer issue again. So they don't promote the issue at all. Overall, experts believe, taking the Pill will slightly reduce your chance of getting some type of cancer, rather than increase it.

Pros.

Public clinics can provide the Pill at reduced cost, you control it yourself, it provides excellent protection against pregnancy when taken consistently, and it allows sex to be spontaneous. It also protects you from several diseases (some are listed above—but there are other benefits, like reduced pain with menstruation, less pain with endometriosis, fewer ovarian cysts, and less pelvic inflammatory disease (PID). The Pill increases sexual interest for some women, perhaps because of the increased spontaneity of sexual activity. If you want to become pregnant, your fertility returns shortly after stopping the Pill (usually just a couple of months later).

Cons.

You have to remember to take the Pill every day. It can cause side effects like breast tenderness, swelling, water retention or slight weight gain for some women (more for others), and irregular or breakthrough vaginal bleeding. Some women experience nausea early in Pill use, others don't. Oral contraceptives may increase the risk of certain diseases, in certain women, as discussed above. Some research shows that every one of these risks is decreased when low-dose (that is, low-estrogen) pills are used, but the final word isn't in yet. Also keep in mind that the Pill provides no protection against sexually transmitted diseases, so if either you or your partner is not monogamous (or if your partner (s) already has a sexually transmitted infection) you're vulnerable.

The following women should not use the Pill, or should talk to their doctors about it carefully: Women with a personal or family history of heart disease, heart attack, clotting disorders, etc.; a personal or strong family history of breast or other reproductive cancers; a personal history of liver cancer or liver disease; smokers; those with diabetes, hypertension or gallbladder disease; those who are breast-feeding; those with abnormal vaginal or uterine bleeding; and those who are or must be immobile for long periods of time (since the Pill boosts clotting risk).

IUD (INTRAUTERINE DEVICE)

About 1–2% of women choose the IUD for contraception.

This is a significant drop from the 1970s when as many as one in ten women using contraception chose the IUD. The main reason for the switch: problems and controversy surrounding older forms of the IUD which are no longer in use (and the fact that the wrong women were often using the method, with some disastrous results). You've probably heard of the Dalcon Shield controversy of the mid-'70s, when IUDs became associated with severe uterine or pelvic infections. With disease and even death associated with IUDs 20 years ago, many women understandably dumped the device—and relatively few have returned. In fact, that reputation is largely outdated—at least for women with the safety profile listed below. In the old days, particularly the mid-'70s, the IUD was constructed differently. One particular device (the Dalcon Shield) had a string hanging from it that was made of a braided fabric that tended to act almost like a ladder for bacteria; sexually transmitted bacteria could literally "climb" from the vagina up into the uterus and fallopian tubes where they often caused serious, even permanent damage. Today's IUDs still have strings attached, but they're now made of a different material that does not promote the spread of infections.

IUDs are an excellent choice for women who are monogamous (have just one sex partner), whose partners are monogamous (don't assume that just because you aren't having sex with someone else, your partner also isn't), who currently have no bacterial sexually transmitted diseases, and who are therefore at relatively low risk for getting an STD. On the flip side, IUDs are not recommended for women who have multiple sex partners and are therefore at risk for sexually transmitted diseases. When IUDs are used by the right subset of women, they are extremely safe and effective.

How the IUD Works.
The IUD is thought to prevent pregnancy by preventing implantation of the fertilized egg on the wall of the uterus, but scientists are studying other mechanisms as well. The device, which sits in the uterus, is inserted through the cervix on an outpatient basis, during a normal-length office visit. The insertion can cause light cramping. There are two approved types of IUDs on the U.S. market. One type of IUD, made with 380mm copper and hence called the Copper T-380 A, is believed to deter the activity of sperm, says Dr. Policar—but scientists aren't completely sure of its other antipregnancy mechanisms. It may, Policar adds, be toxic to

the egg—or damage the sperm in some way that makes it unable to fertilize the egg. Another type of IUD, called the Progestasert, uses the hormone progesterone to inhibit implantation. The key to an IUD working properly is correst insertion in the first place— which depends on your doctor. Also, you must monitor the IUD regularly by checking for the string which hangs down inside your vagina. If the string is missing, or seems to be the wrong length, the IUD might be in the wrong place— lodged in the wrong part of your uterus, for example—or, you may have expelled it unknowingly (one of the risks of IUD use).

Pros.
The IUD provides very good protection against pregnancy. It's easy to use once it's in place— since you don't actually "use" it at all—it does the job on its own, letting sex remain spontaneous. One of the two types of IUD that are available, the Copper T-380 A, can be left in place safely for ten years! The other kind, Progestasert, must be changed once a year, which slightly increases the chance of infection. If you can use the copper type, experts recommend that you do so. Women who use the IUD like it a lot, notes Dr. Policar; in fact, they're more satisfied than users of any other contraceptive method. It's interesting, given that level of satisfaction, that so few women use it. Such is the legacy of well-publicized past problems.

Cons.
If you have sexually transmitted diseases or are exposed to them, or if you have multiple sex partners, the IUD can predispose you to pelvic inflammatory disease (PID). PID is a serious condition that can cause permanent sterility if

not treated fast—and since it is often silent, advanced disease can go undetected. PID occurs when infections travel from the vagina up into the reproductive anatomy, potentially destroying the fallopian tubes and other organs. Sometimes you'll have pelvic pain, fevers and other problems with PID; in a sense, you're lucky if this happens, because you'll get treatment. In other cases, PID is silent, wreaking havoc on your reproductive system—and sometimes causing irreparable damage. If the device becomes lodged in your uterus or elsewhere, you can have pain, bleeding, and other complications. But all of this is rare if the IUD is inserted right in the first place. Some women have increased menstrual cramping and/or bleeding when using the copper IUD; the Progestasert, on the other hand, can reduce bleeding. You may expel the device without knowing it, if you don't keep checking for the string; if you do, you're at risk of becoming pregnant and not knowing it.

Male Condoms

About 13% of all women at risk of pregnancy use condoms—but that number is much higher, at about 26%, for women aged 15–19. More women are thought to use the condom *occasionally,* or in combination with other methods, as a means of preventing sexually transmitted diseases.

Condom use increased during the 1980s, perhaps in response to the epidemics of several sexually transmitted diseases, including AIDS. But according to Jacqueline Darroch Forrest, vice president for research at the Alan Guttmacher Institute, that increase lagged in the 1990s—which causes great concern among STD experts. I cannot stress enough how valuable condoms are in preventing both pregnancy *and* sexually transmitted diseases—*when used properly.* It is unfortunate that even more sexually active teenagers aren't using condoms, since diseases that take root early can cause damage to the reproductive system that has lasting implications when women want to become pregnant later in life.

Even those who *do* use condoms often use them incorrectly, defeating the entire purpose of the device. *Proper* use requires putting the condom on *before* there is any contact between the genitals. Dr. William Masters of the Masters and Johnson Institute is concerned not only about genital-genital contact before the condom is on, but also hand-genital contact. He points out that since a woman often handles and stimulates her partner's penis before intercourse, she is exposing her fingers—and then potentially other parts of her body—to sexually transmitted organisms. So proper use means unrolling the condom *onto* the erect penis at the very beginning of sex play (or as soon as possible), leaving a small space at the end (between your pinched fingers) so the sperm has somewhere to go after your partner ejaculates. (You may want to bring your partner to an erection through his underwear, for example.) Proper use also means using a condom made with latex—*not* a lambskin condom—to protect yourself from sexually transmitted diseases. It means putting the condom on a *fully* erect penis, not one that's "almost there." And it means that if you are using some spermicidal jelly inside the tip of the condom, which is good, you don't use so much that the condom slips off the penis during intercourse.

All this is not to make sex seem antiseptic.

The point is to protect yourself. Once all of this becomes second nature, like brushing your teeth or riding a bike, you won't be focused on disease prevention at all—it will just be the natural way you use condoms. It's really no more difficult to use condoms properly than to use them incorrectly. It just takes more thought the first few times.

Common Mistakes with Condoms.

The most common mistakes made with condoms include letting the penis penetrate the body (the mouth, the vagina or the rectum) *before* putting the condom on—and then taking it out to put the condom on shortly before ejaculation. Not only is this unreliable (sometimes ejaculation isn't so well planned) but it's dangerous because whether you feel it or not, small amounts of fluid *do* leave the penis *before* ejaculation. In addition, if there are sores or other STD signs on the penis (often invisible), your skin will be exposed to them. Other common mistakes people make with condoms include pulling the penis out without holding the rim of the condom, so sperm leaks into the body; reusing a condom inside out (this is ridiculous); and using old, dried-out condoms that are prone to breakage or might have holes in them already.

There are a great many types and brands of condoms available on the market. You can choose among different colors, ribbed or unribbed, with or without spermicide, colored or clear, latex or natural "skin" condoms. If you want protection against sexually transmitted diseases, *choose latex only*. Natural skin condoms don't prevent the passage of some infectious organisms.

How Condoms Work.

Condoms work by trapping sperm and thereby preventing them from entering the vagina and the uterus. They help prevent sexually transmitted diseases by providing a barrier between the skin of the vagina and the skin of the penis and by keeping semen out of your body.

Pros.

Condoms provide good pregnancy prevention and STD protection if used properly (but can't protect you from exposure to sores or microscopic warts on the testicles or other uncovered parts). They're easy to obtain (except for those who are embarrassed to ask for them at a drugstore counter, which Penelope Hitchcock, chief of the Sexually Transmitted Diseases Branch at the National Institute of Allergy and Infections Diseases, says is a real problem). They're relatively inexpensive, and convenient to carry and to have on hand for unplanned sex. Some women find it quite nice to have the man take responsibility for birth control—a rarity, given the preponderance of female-controlled contraceptives. As soon as you want to get pregnant, stop using condoms; there's no delay in regaining your fertility.

Cons.

Some men feel lessened sexual sensation with condoms, and even refuse to use them as a result. Ask yourself if you want to have sex with someone who won't make this small sacrifice for you. (Interestingly, this reduction in sensation can have a benefit for men who suffer from premature ejaculation. Sometimes condoms slow the process down for them.) Condoms can interrupt the flow of sex, since they have to be put on before sexual contact. (Some experts recommend including condom placement as part of the sex act, to reduce this problem.) A small number of men (and women) are sensitive to latex condoms; others may be sensitive to the spermicides on the condoms. Some suggest that people who are allergic to latex use a lambskin condom with a latex condom on top of it (if the man is allergic), or the other way around if the woman is allergic. This provides protection *without* irritation.

Use the Right Kind of Lubricant with Condoms.

Never use oil-based lubricants with latex condoms; butter, mineral oil, petroleum jelly, baby oil, vegetable oil and so on will erode latex quickly. Instead, use a water-based lubricant such as the ones listed on pages 255–256. It's a good idea to use a lubricant with condoms to reduce the chance of breakage, especially for women whose vaginas don't lubricate a great deal (postmenopausal women experiencing vaginal dryness, for example).

SPERMICIDES (FOAMS, JELLIES, CREAMS, SUPPOSITORIES, FILM SHEETS)

Under 2% of women at risk of unintended pregnancy use spermicides alone as a form of birth control. But many more women use these agents *in combination with* other forms of contraception, such as the diaphragm, the cervical cap, condoms and so on.

Spermicides don't provide excellent protection on their own, although they're a lot better in "perfect" use than in "typical" use (as you can see when you look at the effectiveness table earlier in this chapter). If you follow directions carefully—

shaking the foam can vigorously before use, applying a new applicatorful for repeat intercourse if required, etc., you're more likely to get good results. When used with another form of contraception, spermicides make excellent backups for additional protection (in fact, the diaphragm and cervical cap should *only* be used with spermicide in order to be effective).

Keep in mind that while a small number of women—or their partners—are sensitive to or allergic to the spermicidal agent in a given product, sometimes switching to another brand or another form (cream to jelly, or foam to cream) can make you more comfortable. So before you give up on these agents, give more than one a try.

How Spermicides Work.

The main sperm-killing agent in these products (in this country) is nonoxynol-9. It not only kills sperm, but some sexually transmitted organisms as well. While spermicides can't *prevent* the spread of sexually transmitted diseases 100%, they can *reduce* the spread—particularly of bacterial STDs like gonorrhea and chlamydia, which pose serious problems for women's future fertility. There is some controversy over—and ongoing research into—the issue of spermicides and the spread of certain *viral* sexually transmitted diseases, including human papillomavirus (HPV—the virus that causes genital warts and sometimes cervical cancer) and human immunodeficiency virus (HIV—the virus that causes AIDS). There is some unconfirmed evidence that spermicides may irritate the skin of the vulva, vagina and cervix in such a way that it's easier for these viruses to gain entry into the female body. This is not certain—but it just serves to highlight the fact that if you are at potential risk of getting a viral STD from your partner (or if you're not sure about it), you should be using condoms along with spermicides (or better yet, abstain from sex until both you and your partner have been screened for all STDs including HIV—and until you are both monogamous).

Pros.

Spermicides are easy to use, and comfortable (they're soft and fluffy or smooth and cool, so they don't cause pain unless you're allergic to them). They add lubrication and can make intercourse smoother; as a result, they help prevent condom breakage. They're readily available without a prescription at most drugstores and supermarkets. They kill certain sexually transmitted organisms, and cut your risk of gonorrheal and chlamydial infections. You control their use, they're reasonably priced and they're thought to be extremely safe. If you want to become pregnant, just stop using them; there's no delay in regaining fertility.

Cons.

Spermicides can be messy, drippy and goopy after sex. They can cause irritation or full-blown allergic reactions in a small number of women (or their male partners). They provide inadequate protection from pregnancy when used without another method of birth control, such as the cervical cap, the diaphragm or the condom. They have to be inserted shortly before intercourse, which can interrupt the flow of sexual activity. If you are exposed to certain STDs, such as genital warts, spermicides can potentially irritate the skin of your vagina and make it easier for the virus to gain access—but this needs more research.

Experts warn that if you're using the film sheets or suppository forms of spermicides, it's important to wait several minutes before intercourse to allow the spermicide to disperse and give you adequate protection. It's also important to use another dose of the spermicide for repeat acts of intercourse; too often this is where women make mistakes and become pregnant.

STERILIZATION: FEMALE (TUBAL LIGATION) AND MALE (VASECTOMY)

About 25% of women and 10% of men at risk of unintended pregnancy use sterilization as their main method of birth control. The majority of these are women and men over the age of 35 who have already had biological children. About a million sterilization surgeries are done each year in the U.S.

In the right hands, sterilization surgery is quite safe, quicker than it used to be, and can be done under local rather than general anesthesia, making it even safer. Of course, finding "the right hands" is key. Choose a surgeon who does lots of these procedures, and one who has the most modern techniques—for example, the ability to do the procedure laparoscopically in women (with a tiny, rather than a major, incision), or using special microsurgical tools that are less likely to harm other pelvic organs.

One of the most important messages about sterilization is that while in *some* cases these procedures are reversible (but certainly not all) women and men should enter into them with the belief that the surgery is permanent. You can't count on reversing the procedure even if you've had the least invasive version done. Most people who have finished childbearing or who never want to have biological children are quite satisfied with sterilization and never look back. Others, for a variety of reasons including loss of prior children, remarriage and other major life changes, regret the decision. It is not one to be entered into lightly; most experts recommend a long thinking period in which you use a reversible method of birth control (condoms, injectables, the Pill, a diaphragm, and so on) until you're sure beyond the shadow of a doubt that you want surgery. Here are brief descriptions of the procedures available.

Tubal Ligation.

Sterilization for women can be accomplished several ways—either through clipping, putting rings on, or electrically burning the fallopian tubes. As with any surgical procedure, there is a risk of infection or of damage to other organs. As mentioned above, the more experienced your doctor, and the more precautions she/he takes, the lower those risks become. These days, with local anesthesia, women can leave the hospital quickly (after a few hours) and get back to normal life without much delay. You'll want to talk to your doctor about this option. After you're home, listen to your body for signs of problems—such as fever, cramping, bleeding or pain—all of which can signal infection or other postsurgical problems. Call your doctor immediately if you experience these symptoms.

If you are absolutely sure you want to have the procedure done, some experts recommend having it done at the same time as childbirth, or abortion, so you don't have to go back into the hospital or clinic for yet another surgical procedure.

Vasectomy.

Like tubal ligation, vasectomy procedures have become simpler, with smaller incisions and less time required. The vas deferens, a tube that carries sperm, can be either tied off or removed alto-gether, depending on the procedure used. While the procedure should be considered permanent, it's a lot easier to reverse a vasectomy done by clipping the tube than one in which all or part of it was removed. (For more on vasectomy and its reversibility, *see* chapter 16, "Infertility.")

Pros.

If the procedures are done properly, you can't find better protection against pregnancy. Also, sex becomes uninhibited, free, unencumbered by devices and/or hormones; you never have to think about birth control again. This often comes as a tremendous relief to couples who have been dissatisfied with birth control options, or who are extremely concerned about becoming pregnant.

Cons.

If you change your mind, regret can be strong—particularly if you discover that your procedure is not reversible. Even if you can reverse the operation, you'll have to spend a lot of money—and subject yourself to surgery at least once more—to return your fertility. *Don't count on reversibility.* The decision to be sterilized is a serious one that should be considered lifelong. If you're not sure, *wait.* Furthermore, don't confuse protection against pregnancy with protection against sexually transmitted diseases. If you are at risk of an STD, you still must protect yourself with condoms or other methods.

BARRIER METHODS FOR WOMEN: THE SPONGE, THE DIAPHRAGM, THE CERVICAL CAP AND THE FEMALE CONDOM

The barrier methods are so named because they form an actual barrier (the device) inside the vagina, in front of the cervix.

VAGINAL SPONGE (TODAY'S SPONGE)

About 1% of women at risk of unintended pregnancy use the sponge as their primary method of contraception.

The sponge *is* in fact a spongy object with spermicide inside it. You wet the device before using it, then insert it deep in your vagina where it acts as both a barrier and spermicide. You can see in the table earlier in this chapter that there's a big disparity between "perfect" and "typical" use success rates for the sponge; in actual use, the failure rate is quite high. There are several reasons for this, including the fact that women don't insert the sponge properly, the sponge dislodges and doesn't adequately cover the cervix, or women don't leave it in long enough (a full six hours) after sex. Dr. Policar says that women who have never had a full-term pregnancy have better success with the sponge than do women who have already borne children. This may be because once the vaginal muscles have been stretched, they don't hold the sponge snug in place quite as well. The effectiveness rate is much better (though still far from perfect) for women who have never had children.

Unlike other barrier methods for women, such as the diaphragm and the cervical cap, the sponge is disposable. It provides 24 hours' protection and then you throw it away.

Since the sponge contains spermicide (the same ingredient, nonoxynol-9, that's in most spermicidal foams and jellies) it can cause some of the same irritations (rare) *and* provides limited protection against certain sexually transmitted diseases.

An important caution about sponge use is that you should not leave the device in for more than 24 hours. While no one knows the exact time line for risk, it's thought that leaving it in too long will increase your chance of getting toxic shock syndrome (TSS), which you may have heard is connected to excessively long tampon use (discussed briefly in chapter 8). The point is, when you leave any absorbent object in the vagina for too long, you run the risk of trapping dangerous bacteria that can cause any number of infections, including TSS.

How the Sponge Works.
The sponge partially blocks the cervix, keeping sperm from gaining entry to the uterus; the spermicide in the sponge kills sperm.

Pros.
While some women find the diaphragm slightly uncomfortable to insert (because of the relatively rigid rim), the sponge is soft and malleable and therefore comfortable and easier to put in the vagina. It also has a loop that makes it easier to remove (some women have trouble getting hold of their diaphragm, on the other hand). The sponge is available over the counter, so you don't need to be fitted for it by a doctor (it only comes in one size) and you have the benefit of controlling your own birth control. It is competitively priced, compared to other forms of contraception.

Cons.
The sponge is relatively ineffective at preventing pregnancy, especially in "typical" use by women who have had biological children. It can cause burning and irritation or a full allergic reaction in a few women and men (as with spermicidal

jellies). Some men are bothered when they feel the sponge against their penis during intercourse. The sponge must be inserted several hours before intercourse, requiring planning, and can be drippy after intercourse (it must be left in place for at least 6 hours after intercourse, but for no more than 24 hours to reduce the risk of toxic shock syndrome). You must use it every time you have sex—which means you've got to be clearheaded and plan for sex several hours ahead or remember it in the heat of passion.

CERVICAL CAP AND DIAPHRAGM

We list these two together because they are closely related. As you can see in the table on page 191, their effectiveness rates are quite close in women who have never borne children—but the success for the cervical cap is lower in women who have already had biological children. Professor Trussell finds the effectiveness rates of both the cap and the diaphragm, even with "perfect use," quite discouraging. With some important differences we'll discuss below, the cervical cap can be thought of as a "two-day-diaphragm," says Dr. Policar.

About 5% of women of all ages who are at risk of unintended pregnancy choose the diaphragm as their main method of birth control.

This method along with the cervical cap is yet another example of where typical use is falling far short of perfect use. Women forget to add more contraceptive jelly for repeat acts of intercourse, they don't put the device in properly in the first place or they fail to have the device sized periodically by health care professionals. But there are other potential problems that women cannot control at all; for instance,

since these devices must be fit by a doctor or other health practitioner (they come in several sizes), a wrong initial fit can greatly impair effectiveness. Both methods are given by prescription.

Both the diaphragm and the cervical cap are rubber cups that are inserted into the vagina and placed over the cervix. The diaphragm is bigger and more shallow, so it doesn't hug the cervix tightly. The cap *should* hug the cervix when properly fitted. Spermicide is placed in the cup before insertion, so when the devices are in place, the foam or jelly is pressed against the cervix. Most practitioners advise women to put some jelly on the rim of these devices for further protection, but you don't want to make the device so slippery that it won't stay in place. Ask your health care provider to show you how much is appropriate *before you leave the office.*

There are several different types of diaphragms; they differ primarily by the type of rim (more and less flexible). Dr. Robert Sassoon of the New York Hospital/Cornell Medical Center reports that the less flexible (stiffer) diaphragms are easier to *remove*, because it's easier to get your finger under the ring. The flexible, so-called "spring" diaphragm is easier to insert, harder to remove, and more comfortable for some women, he says. However, few women feel the diaphragm at all once it's in place.

An advantage to the cap over the diaphragm is that it can be left in longer—up to 48 hours. The diaphragm must be removed after about 24 hours.

Unlike the cap and the sponge, the diaphragm does not provide continuous protection over long periods of time. Each act of intercourse requires the addition of more spermicide with an applicator—while the device is left in place. You can have multiple acts of intercourse without adding spermicide to the cervical cap.

Neither device should be left in the body for long periods of time (over 24 hours for the diaphragm, over 48 hours for the cap) because of the risk of toxic shock syndrome. The rationale is similar to that with the contraceptive sponge or tampons: the longer you leave a device in, the greater the chance of promoting dangerous bacterial growth.

How the Cervical Cap and the Diaphragm Work.

The diaphragm (which has been approved longer in this country) and the cervical cap form a barrier over the cervix, keeping sperm out; they are used with spermicidal foams/creams/jellies, which kill sperm and certain sexually transmitted organisms..

Cap Pros.

The cervical cap can be inserted up to 40 hours before intercourse, which is quite convenient compared to the 6 hours of continuous protection you get from the diaphragm (unless you add more spermicide *after* diaphgram insertion). You control the method. The cap, because it is small and hugs the cervix, is pretty unobtrusive; it doesn't change the feeling of intercourse and is easy to ignore. Because it's smaller than the diaphragm, some women find it easier to insert (others find the opposite, since they have to reach and become comfortable with their cervix, which can be awkward for some women). The cap provides limited protection from some sexually transmitted diseases; there are no systemic risks to the method; no hormones are involved.

Cap Cons.

Rarely, there is an allergic reaction to the device material or the spermicide. The cap can be a hassle to insert if you aren't comfortable with your vagina or body parts in general. It must be fitted and prescribed by a health practitioner, and can irritate the surface of the cervix.

A possible "con" for both the cap and the diaphragm is that some women report more urinary tract infections and more yeast and other organism problems when using these devices. Whether it's because of some trauma to the vaginal or urethral area on insertion, or because the spermicides affect the normal balance of organisms in the vagina, is subject to debate. The bottom line, however, is that some women can't use these devices because of chronic infections.

Diaphragm Pros.

With the diaphragm, you're in control of your contraceptive method. There are no systemic risks and no hormones. There is some protection against sexually transmitted diseases (with the caveat about spermicides and vaginal irritation discussed earlier). The diaphragm is easy to use once you have experience, and it's fairly unobtrusive (though not as small and snug as the cap).

Diaphragm Cons.

The diaphragm must be fitted by a health care practitioner, and cannot be left in for more than 24 hours. You must add spermicide for every new act of intercourse when using the diaphragm. It can be drippy and goopy after sex, can't be used with oil-based lubricants if made of latex, and insertion can be unwieldy for some women.

FEMALE CONDOM (CALLED REALITY)

After much hoopla, the female condom was approved in the U.S. in 1993. Hailed as a great advance in that women could control their own highly protective device against sexually transmitted diseases, the device has been somewhat disappointing. Many find it bulky, sloppy to use, and its effectiveness rate against pregnancy isn't as good as many hoped. The failure rate may be as high as 26 out of 100 users becoming pregnant after one year's use. But before we write off the female condom as ineffective at preventing pregnancy, Jaqueline Darroch Forrest of the Alan Guttmacher Institute notes that many of the pregnancies occurred when the method *wasn't used at all.* Certainly it's important that women failed to use the device, perhaps because it is unwieldy. But we shouldn't assume the worst about it yet, either.

Its STD protection rate may be more laudable than its pregnancy prevention, which suggests that the female condom might be a great choice as a second method along with other contraceptive methods. Dr. Policar urges women to consider the female condom a preliminary version of a potentially useful new device which needs a lot more fine-tuning before it should be relied on independently.

Made of polyurethane, which is stronger than the latex used in male condoms (in fact, some companies are developing new male condoms out of this material for its added strength) the female condom acts as a barrier not only for the cervix but for the entire vaginal wall and the vulva as well. With a ring on each end, the device is put inside the vagina and hangs all the way out, providing a tunnel of coverage and protection throughout the vagina. Like the male condom, it's designed for one-time use; but unlike the male latex condom, it *can* be used with oil-based lubricants since polyurethane doesn't break down with these products. It is inserted up to eight hours before intercourse, which is a distinct advantage over male condoms.

How the Female Condom Works.

The female condom works by trapping sperm and blocking it from entering the cervix and uterus. It prevents sexually transmitted diseases by preventing penis-vagina contact all the way down the vaginal canal.

Pros.

The female condom is another method of birth control that *you*, the woman, can control. It provides STD protection at a time when women are at extremely high risk of disease. It's painless, relatively inexpensive, risk free (no side or systemic effects) and can be put in eight hours before intercourse so it doesn't affect the flow of lovemaking. It's also disposable, and requires neither a prescription nor a fitting. This is the only contraceptive that protects the vulva, or outside of the vagina, from contact with potential sexually transmitted organisms—which is important because just covering the penis does not protect other parts of your genital skin (or your partner's) from coming into contact with bacteria or viruses.

Cons.

The female condom is bulky, and hard to use properly (which contributes to the high failure rate). It's also relatively ineffective against pregnancy, and some women find it uncomfortable because of the material that hangs out of the vagina (before intercourse).

PROGESTIN-ONLY METHODS OF BIRTH CONTROL: PROGESTIN-ONLY PILLS (MINIPILLS), NORPLANT, DEPO-PROVERA

These are hormonal methods of birth control. They differ from oral contraceptives (the Pill) in that they contain no estrogen—just synthetic progesterone, called progestins.

How They Work.

These methods work in several ways. First, they prevent ovulation by interfering with the body's normal hormonal pattern. Second, they change certain factors in the body, like the lining of the uterus and the cervical mucus, thereby blocking fertilization. Pills are taken by mouth, naturally; Norplant is inserted under the skin; and Depo-Provera is injected into the muscle.

Progestin-only Pills.

Often called "minipills," these progestin-only birth control pills have wide variability in their pregnancy prevention rates. The reason: when used properly and consistently—that is, taken right on time each day—they are extremely effective. When taken even slightly off schedule, however, their effectiveness drops considerably.

Norplant.

Approved at the end of 1990, the Norplant system consists of a set of six tiny silastic rubber sticks or capsules which contain progestin; these are placed under the skin of the upper arm and provide continuous protection from pregnancy for up to five years. The progestin used with this method is called levonorgestrel.

Dr. Anita Nelson of the Harbor-UCLA Medical Center reports great variability in women's feelings about Norplant. While some are delighted that their periods disappear (the progestin has this effect on some women) others are bothered by this change and constantly fear they're pregnant or sick. Some women will have irregular bleeding while using the device—those who are counseled and expect it usually don't mind, but those who are surprised by it often come back to have the device removed.

Depo-Provera (DMPA).

This is an injected form of progestin called depo-medroxyprogesterone acetate. It was approved in the U.S. only recently, in 1991, but should not be considered "new" in that it's been used in other countries and in millions of women for many years. Some concern about safety, which has largely been dispelled, kept it off the U.S. market for many years. The injections are given once every three months—just four times a year.

Dr. Nelson finds that certain subgroups of women are extremely pleased with injectable contraception. Teens who want long-term protection and privacy from their parents and are happy not to have to hide contraceptive devices at home, for example, particularly like this method. Nelson reports that her center is running out of its budget for this form of contraception—it's hard to keep up with the number of requests for it. In other parts of the country and in different practice settings, however, women are less likely to request injectable, long-term hormonal treatment. It's quite variable.

Pros.

Since many of the pros and cons of these progestin-only methods are similar, I'll group them here. Where there are exceptions, I'll note them. On the whole, these devices provide superb protection from pregnancy (with the exception of the minipills when not taken on a strict schedule). They're also safe for women who cannot take estrogen. Norplant and Depo-Provera provide long-term protection without your having to give a thought to birth control. This gives tremendous sexual freedom by removing the issue of contraception from each act of sex. With minipills and Norplant, quitting or removal of the device allow you to get pregnant with relative speed; with Depo-Provera, however, there may be a several month delay for the return of fertility. Menstrual cramps and bleeding are reduced with all progestin methods and endometriosis symptoms *may* be improved. With Norplant, there is a possible reduced risk of pelvic inflammatory disease (PID). Unlike with estrogen-containing birth control methods, most experts say it's safe to breast-feed when using these methods, although *some* steroid may get into the breast milk, which makes some practitioners leery. Dr. Robert Hatcher, director of family planning at Grady Memorial Hospital in Atlanta, says progestin-only methods like Norplant are quite safe primarily because they lack the complications associated with estrogen. Hatcher recalls a slide he saw in 1974 with the basic risks of Norplant on it: They are close to the same ones we know today, he notes—which he finds quite comforting.

Cons.

Progestins can cause many of the unpleasant feelings some women associate with premenstrual syndrome, like bloating, weight gain, breast tenderness, and moodiness; some women are bothered by irregular bleeding or spotting, or getting no period at all (others love this!). Minipills may increase the risk of ovarian cysts. With Norplant, some women develop irritations or infections where the device is inserted. You need an office visit for insertion (a minor outpatient procedure) and removal of Norplant, and it's expensive if you don't use it for the full five years prescribed (that is, if you have it removed early—although within a certain time frame you may be able to get some of your money back). With Depo-Provera, you have to remember to return for your shot every three months. Depo-Provera also can lead to some bone loss, which can be significant if you're already at risk of osteoporosis: However, bone seems to be restored when you discontinue use, says Dr. Stubblefield. You must remember to take your minipills every day at the same time—a problem for some women.

Keep in mind that while all of these methods provide excellent protection against pregnancy, they provide little or no protection against sexually transmitted diseases. These are not good *sole* methods for women with multiple sex partners or for those who are at high risk of getting sexually transmitted diseases for other reasons. Dr. Willard Cates Jr., former director of the division of training at the Centers for Disease Control and Prevention, is very concerned about the fact that these long-acting hormonal contraceptives give the *illusion* of total protection and freedom to have sex without fear of pregnancy. This sense of freedom can be very dangerous in light of the many sexually transmitted infections rampant in our society.

While we need more data on this subject, there is some evidence, according to Dr. Stubblefield, that Depo-Provera is associated with breast cancer—perhaps promoting the growth of already-existing cancers. The increased risk may not even be statistically significant, but it makes most practitioners feel that women with a personal or strong family history of breast cancer should avoid the method. In addition, some women with histories of certain heart problems including hypertension, migraine headaches and seizure disorders are advised not to use these methods. Talk to your doctor about it. Depo-Provera does not seem to affect the risk of ovarian or cervical cancer either way.

You may have heard news about problems with the *removal* of Norplant. In the right hands, removal of these small rods from the upper arm should be a minor, nearly painless 15-minute office procedure, says Dr. Robert Hatcher. But if your practitioner isn't properly trained, it can be much more complicated, take longer, hurt more, and result in infection or other problems. Worse yet, you *could* find yourself in an area where *no one* is trained to remove the device (if, let's say, you've moved away from where you had it inserted). As with any other procedure, you must make sure the person who is removing your Norplant device does this often and is trained to do so (don't be too shy to ask where and when they were trained, and if Norplant removals are a common part of their practice). Dr. Hatcher urges women only to have Norplant put *in* by a competent person who can also *remove* it. If you do have the device and move to a new region, remember to ask your new health care providers, including a gynecologist if possible, if they could remove the device if you changed your mind about it (or if the five years elapse). If the answer is no, do some legwork ahead of time so you know where to turn if you develop problems with the device, or if you decide you want to become pregnant.

FERTILITY AWARENESS

This global term is used for several methods of contraception—including the calendar method, basal body temperature monitoring, the sympto-thermal method, and so on—in which couples monitor the woman's ovulatory cycle and avoid intercourse at the most fertile times. About 2% of women at risk of unintended pregnancy use some form of fertility awareness as their main form of birth control. As you can see from the table on page 191, the success rates vary by the type of method used—all ovulation-monitoring methods are not equal. Here's a brief discussion of why.

There is a relatively small window in which you can become pregnant each month. The two key factors that must be in place include ovulation (your releasing an egg), and healthy sperm being present. Some women ovulate at mid-cycle, while others do not. Sperm lives in the body for up to three days on average (give or take a day); eggs live for about 24 hours. This should begin to give you an idea that there isn't just one day that you can pinpoint on which you might become pregnant. Sperm from several days ago can hang around and fertilize an egg released today; an egg released yesterday can be fertilized by sperm appearing tomorrow; and so on.

For this reason—the fact that cycles are variable and sperm and egg life unpredictable—counting days (the calendar method) is the least effective of all fertility awareness methods. The more methods you *add*, however, in determining your date of ovulation—and the more careful you are to avoid intercourse (or use alternative methods) during the several days *before*, *during* and *after* you may be ovulating—the greater your chance of preventing pregnancy.

There are several ways to be a better monitor of your ovulation pattern than just counting cycle days. You can examine your vaginal mucus (actually mucus that came from your cervix)—it tends to be more slippery and abundant around ovulation. You can study your so-called basal body temperature (called BBT), using either a special BBT thermometer (easier to read) or a regular thermometer. You'll learn that your temperature rises during and several days after ovulation. You can feel your cervix, if you're comfortable doing so: it tends to be softer at ovulation. And you can listen to your body for signs of ovulation, like pain (*mittelschmertz,* which means middle pain, occurs in some women at the time of ovulation). Some women have scant bleeding at ovulation, too. When you add all of these factors together—and it takes practice—your chance of correctly predicting ovulation is greatest. Next, you have to be willing either to abstain from intercourse in the days preceding and following ovulation, or you must use some other form of contraception at that time.

As we discuss in the section on infertility treatment, there are ovulation prediction kits (which test your urine) on the market now for about $25. They usually let you know when ovulation is *about* to occur. Most kits give you several days' worth of test materials so you can keep testing for a few days at approximately mid-cycle until ovulation occurs. Used alone, they might not give adequate protection (especially if your cycle is irregular), but used in conjunction with other fertility awareness techniques mentioned above, they can increase your chance of success.

Pros.

With fertility awareness techniques, there are no adverse health effects of the kind you might experience with hormones, jellies and other devices and products. You'll learn a great deal about your body and how it works if you use these techniques, increasing the chance that you'll get pregnant more easily when and if you decide you want to. *You* control this method, and if you want, your partner can participate. With fertility awareness, sex is unencumbered by devices and other messes. And most important for some women, these methods meet the requirements or values of certain religious and other beliefs.

Cons.

Fertility awareness methods of birth control provide no protection against sexually transmitted diseases. They have a relatively high failure rate compared to other forms of contraception, especially when fewer methods of detecting ovulation are used. If you won't use other forms of contraception, you'll have to abstain from sex for several days each cycle. It takes time and focus to get each cycle right.

WITHDRAWAL

Pulling out the penis before ejaculation is used as a primary method of birth control by about 2% of women at risk of unintended pregnancy. In typical use, it is not a reliable way to prevent pregnancy, since many men cannot control the time at which they ejaculate—and it doesn't protect against sexually transmitted disease, since some fluid is released from the penis even before ejaculation. With perfect use—that is, consistent use by a couple that has excellent control over ejaculation timing—it is much more effective. Withdrawal certainly has the benefit of being free of charge and free of the encumbrance of devices and hormones, but it shouldn't be high on your list of effective methods of birth control, especially in times of high sexually transmitted disease rates.

EMERGENCY POSTCOITAL METHODS OF BIRTH CONTROL

A number of hormonal methods of birth control, including oral contraceptives, progestin-only "minipills" and the still-unapproved RU-486 (the so-called "abortion pill"), among others, can sometimes be used after accidental unprotected intercourse (or rape) to prevent pregnancy. These methods usually require taking a larger than normal dose of hormones (perhaps two pills close together, for example) and therefore can cause unpleasant side effects like extreme nausea. If you absolutely cannot or do not want to become pregnant, however, they may be your only option. Talk to your doctor about the possibility of using a method of birth control you already have, or of contacting him or her at the time of a contraceptive emergency for fast help—ideally within half a day to one day of unprotected intercourse. Some experts say that emergency contraception could prevent nearly 1.7 million cases of unwanted pregnancy each year in the U.S.

ABSTINENCE

They say you should save the best for last, and if the best means the best efficacy, abstinence certainly belongs last on this list. Not having sex means no risk of pregnancy, and lower risk of sexually transmitted disease (There is still significant risk from other, non-intercourse sexual acts, and we can't rule out the "toilet seat" and "towel" theories completely, rare as they may be). Both anal and oral sex, in any combination, can result in the transfer of bacteria and virus-containing fluids from one person to another. Even hand-penis or hand-vagina contact poses risks of STDs. For protection against STDs you must use condoms or, for 100% protection, abstain from all sexual acts.

Abstinence isn't a popular topic these days—it's considered terribly unhip, if you go by the rules of peer pressure and popular culture. But remember that there's nothing hip about getting sick, nothing hip about getting pregnant when you don't intend to, nothing hip about becoming infertile because of a long-standing sexually transmitted disease, and nothing hip about being forced into doing things you aren't ready for or aren't interested in doing. Until you find a safe, disease-free, trustworthy and monogamous sexual partner, abstinence can be the healthiest thing you ever did for yourself.

CHAPTER TWELVE

ABORTION

It is the ability to choose which makes us human.

—Madeleine L'Engle, *Walking on Water: Reflections on Faith and Art*

The decision to have an abortion is highly personal, and yet has forever been politically, emotionally, morally, ethically and religiously charged. In the 1990s, with abortion clinic workers' lives at stake, clinics burned to the ground, and courts battling one of the most controversial issues of our time, abortion has been treated as anything but a health issue. Yet it is a women's health issue as well, regardless of your choice or values. This chapter does not address the myriad issues and conflicts that tear at the fabric of our diverse culture. Those issues are well beyond the scope of any single chapter—or to me, for that matter. Here, we will focus solely on the health and medical aspects of abortion—the techniques available at different stages of pregnancy, the risks involved and ways to reduce those risks. Too many women have lost their lives—and continue to lose their lives or quality of life—because of simple misinformation or inability to access essential health information about abortion. Your decision on whether to have or not have an abortion will no doubt be based on many factors. If you do choose to terminate a pregnancy, you owe it to yourself to do it in the safest way possible.

Today, more than half of all pregnancies in the U.S. are unintended. For teenagers, the cause of accidental pregnancy is often lack of contraception altogether, which points to a serious need for counseling at least at the time of the abortion to help avoid repeats. Unwanted pregnancies for women in their 20s and 30s are thought to be caused most often by contraceptive failures (which, by the way, includes the failure to use the contraceptive in the first place!). Half of those unintended pregnancies will be terminated by abortion, according to Dr. Richard Hausknecht of the Mt. Sinai School of

Medicine in New York. Pregnancy terminations reach 1.5 million each year in the U.S.

....

ABORTION: WHAT YOU HAD TO SAY ABOUT IT

Liz, 29 years old
The second time I had a lot of guilt. I felt really guilty. One time was understandable, a mistake and a fluke, the second time was carelessness. I thought God is going to punish me, I'll never have children, what goes around comes around. It increased my fears, my anxiety, and my guilt. I'm married now and happy, I would never have another one. I still keep thinking something's going to happen to [my son], or I won't get pregnant again. It's always in the back of my mind.

Lori, 29 years old
I was 24. I was very at ease with my decision. I knew I did not want to have it and I wasn't going to spend the rest of my life with [the father]. And I knew there were safe options, and I trusted my doctor. I did not have an emotional response. I wasn't cold about it, I was just resigned—it was an intellectual decision, maybe because I was raised with the idea that it was my choice. There was no pain, some grogginess. I didn't do it in a private office, I did it in a clinic, and the anonymity of it all was an advantage. I was surrounded by 13-, 14- and 15-year-old kids. I realized this was a method of birth control for some women. People were talking about this is their second or third one. I have friends who did have emotional reactions, not for religious reasons, but because they loved their partner and didn't know if it was the right thing to do to the product of that love. Some of my friends were devastated by the emotions. I did allow myself that if those feelings arose, I wouldn't brush them off. I'd deal with the grief. I was open to an emotional response, but didn't have one. A big part of it for me was having [the father] there, being supportive. He didn't question it. We knew it was the right thing. I never had a second thought about it. I was so young, and had so much ahead of me. I would have prevented all my goals from being reached. It was the right thing for both of us.

....

EARLY ABORTIONS: FROM CONCEPTION TO 14 WEEKS

In general, the earlier a pregnancy is terminated, the safer it is. The better we get to know our bodies, our menstrual patterns and so on, the better our chance of knowing we're pregnant early enough to have a simpler form of abortion. The earliest possible termination would be as soon as you test positive for pregnancy—or even, some would argue, when you suspect you're pregnant but don't know for sure—but *most* practitioners feel that you're better off waiting until about six weeks from conception (or eight weeks from the first day of your last period) to have an abortion. The best reasons to wait a couple of weeks: (1) you're more likely to miss the fetal tissue if you try too early; and (2) the cervix is harder to dilate (open) at the very beginning of pregnancy, and therefore your risk of lacerating the cervix is greater than if you wait a couple of weeks.

(NOTE: Before any abortion is performed, you should have a blood test not just to confirm your pregnancy but also to get your blood type and to see if you're Rh-positive or Rh-negative. If your blood is Rh-negative, you must be given a shot of Rhogam within about 96 hours of the pregnancy termination to insure that your body doesn't reject the *next* pregnancy you carry.)

The very earliest and least invasive form of abortion is called menstrual extraction, in which the lining of the uterus is removed without any form of anesthesia through a quick and simple office procedure. Some women prefer this method because it is done so early (that is, while you're strongly suspecting pregnancy but don't know for sure). This uncertainty is emotionally easier for some women.

In the early stage of pregnancy, from conception to 14 weeks, the most common abortion technique today is dilation and suction curretage—which means the practitioner will open your cervix and then use a suction device to "vacuum" the fetal tissue out of your uterus. This procedure is done under local anesthesia or something called hypnotic anesthesia, in which you're put to sleep but not as deeply as with general anesthesia. With local anesthesia, you should not feel any pain during the dilation of your cervix, but you may feel some cramping with curettage and during the suction removal of the fetal tissue. Under hypnotic anesthesia, there should be no pain at all. The entire procedure takes just a few minutes, but you will be asked to stay in the clinic, hospital or doctor's office for a couple of hours afterwards. Usually a mild painkiller will relieve the cramps that can last for several hours after the abortion.

After checking the tissue visually, if everything *looks* normal, your practitioner will send you home, but the tissue should *also* be sent to a pathologist who will determine more precisely that it is complete—that is, the whole placenta was removed (this can take a day or two). Very rarely, there will be a discrepancy between what the clinician saw and what the pathologist determines; if the abortion was not complete, or not done at all, you will be called back for a repeat procedure.

It is extremely important that your doctor confirm if the abortion was complete by studying the tissue collected *before you leave the clinic.* The reason this is so important is that (a) if the pregnancy was missed, you will need a repeat procedure, and (b) it is possible that the pregnancy is not in your uterus at all, but rather is ectopic (in your fallopian tubes or elsewhere outside your uterus). If this is the case, the normal method of abortion will not be effective and you will need immediate surgery on your tubes to protect you from a medical emergency. Ectopic pregnancy, which is more common in women with a history of pelvic infections, is not to be taken lightly and must be treated without delay. (Some abortion clinics will do a sonogram, a painless sound wave test, *before* performing the abortion, to be sure the pregnancy is in fact in the uterus. This is certainly preferable and helps avert some unsuccessful abortions, but not all centers have the ultrasound machine. It's a question you might want to ask beforehand. If needed, some high-tech, and potentially more expensive, offices will do a sonogram test *after* the abortion is complete, to be sure everything looks normal. This is probably the exception, not the rule.)

HOW YOU SHOULD EXPECT TO FEEL AFTER AN EARLY (FIRST TRIMESTER) ABORTION

If everything goes normally, as it usually does, you should expect to feel physically fine within hours, and be back to your regular activities almost immediately. The cramping should not be too severe after the procedure and probably won't last more than 1–2 hours or so—but some women find it quite uncomfortable at first. You will probably be advised not to insert anything in your vagina for a couple of weeks after the procedure to avoid infection—for instance, no sexual intercourse, no douching, no tampons and so on. Bathing and exercising and other normal activities are usually fine right away, but check with your doctor to be sure.

It is extremely important that you watch your body for any signs of trouble after an abortion, even if it's done early in the pregnancy and appears to go smoothly. If at any time in the several weeks following the abortion you develop a fever, nausea, cramping, bleeding, unpleasant-smelling discharge from your vagina or other signs that something may be awry, contact your health care provider immediately. While complications are quite rare in early abortions, they do occur. Sometimes, tissue will be left behind, and an infection can develop, or a pre-existing infection can be spread into your bloodstream. As mentioned earlier, this is a good reason to use a clinic where the extracted tissue is studied carefully after the abortion is complete. But no test is foolproof. You must guard your own health after you return home, and seek medical attention at the first sign of trouble.

SECOND TRIMESTER ABORTIONS: 14–24 WEEKS

There are two kinds of abortion procedures for the second trimester. In both cases, the procedure is riskier than early abortions and should be done by someone with experience and skill. Some centers, Planned Parenthood included,

will not do abortions after 18 weeks. Others will do these procedures up to 24 weeks, but only in a hospital or other appropriately equipped center, with properly trained practitioners for backup. Very few practitioners in the country are highly experienced in late abortions, in which the risk of injury is significant. Because the uterus is larger at this stage, its walls thin in some places and its blood vessels expand, the potential for injury is much greater than when the fetus can be removed by suction (as can be done up until about 14 weeks).

Second trimester abortions account for only 5% of all abortions done in this country. One of the reasons women have these relatively late procedures is major genetic complications in the fetus. But according to Dr. William Rashbaum, who serves on the affiliate medical committee for Planned Parenthood of New York City, there are other important reasons as well, such as not being able to face the fact that you are pregnant and therefore ignoring the problem too long, or not even realizing that you are pregnant in the first place. Whatever the reason for a so-called "late" abortion, the procedures are riskier and often the emotional aspects more significant at this stage. Support and counseling, which are important for *any* woman going through an abortion, become especially vital with later terminations.

PROCEDURES USED FOR THE SECOND TRIMESTER ABORTION

Dilation and Evacuation, Also Called the D & E or Laminaria Evacuation.
This procedure, which is done under local or general anesthesia, is divided into two parts. First, the practitioner will insert a thin rod

made of either sterilized seaweed (laminaria) or an extremely thin plastic strip into the cervix one or two days before the scheduled abortion. Over that time, the rod will absorb moisture and gradually dilate the cervix. This can cause cramping, which can be relieved by over-the-counter painkillers, but can be quite uncomfortable for women who have not had biological children. If the procedure is being done after 18 weeks and up to 24 weeks, the dilation process will happen over one or two days, with additional dilateria put into the cervix to open it further, after which the fetus will be removed using medical instruments. Dr. E. Hakim-Elahi, medical director for Planned Parenthood of New York City, urges women who are having this later procedure done to go to a hospital where bleeding and other complications can be managed on the spot. However, most 2nd trimester abortions are done in free-standing clinics. At the later stage, because the fetus is more developed, your practitioner will have to make sure that all fetal structures have been removed. Complications result more often than with early abortions.

Many practitioners feel that in the right hands, the D & E procedure is preferable to the amnio infusion procedure described next. The trouble is, it can be hard to find a practitioner trained in D & E in parts of the country—and practitioner skill is very important for this procedure. Sometimes, clinics that do early abortions can give references to skilled late-abortion practitioners in your area. You may have to travel to find someone reputable and experienced. Some resource groups listed in the information box at the end of this section can also help you locate practitioners near you.

Amino Infusion.

With this procedure, some type of noxious substance, such as saline solution, urea or prostaglandins is inserted into the amniotic cavity, causing labor to begin by the end of 24 hours. The solution is inserted by means of a needle placed through your abdomen (using local anesthesia) and into your uterus. Like natural labor, the contractions of your uterus will eventually expel the fetus, and, also as with natural labor, this process can be quite painful and time consuming. Patients need pain medication, and must be in the hospital for safety. This procedure, which many practitioners rate as worse for patients than the D & E described above, is usually done these days by practitioners who lack skill in D & E.

Depending on the kind of solution used to bring on labor, your symptoms will differ. Prostaglandins are more likely to make you feel sick (nausea, vomiting, diarrhea and fever); they are also more likely to cause bleeding and harm to the cervix. The drug pitocin is often used to speed things along, adding to the complications with this procedure. Saline solution has fewer complications, but takes longer to work and can be dangerous if the practitioner slips and gets some solution into your bloodstream (which is rare, but can be fatal). Certain medical problems, such as high blood pressure and kidney disease, make the infusion of saline solution impossible.

The recovery time for this procedure can be much longer than for the D & E. You may be asked to stay in the hospital for a day or two afterwards, compared to several hours with the D & E, and operative removal of the placenta is common, notes Dr. Rashbaum.

Hysterotomy.

The old-fashioned second trimester abortion, called hysterotomy, is outdated. During this procedure the uterus is emptied surgically as with a C-section. The risks of both complications (blood loss, perforations, injury to the bladder or ureter, and all other risks associated with major invasive surgery) and mortality are unacceptably high for most second trimester abortions. This procedure is almost never used today.

HOW YOU SHOULD EXPECT TO FEEL AFTER A SECOND TRIMESTER ABORTION

As mentioned earlier, your symptoms and length of recovery depends in part on what type of procedure you use for a second trimester abortion. If you have amnio infusion, you may need a several days to recover. The procedure is painful; it can take time both physically and emotionally to recover from that pain. D & E also can cause some pain and cramping, though the main portion of physical recovery—that is, the time it takes to feel physically better, for cramping to subside, etc.—tends to be a bit shorter (on the order of a half-day to a day) than with other procedures.

ABORTIONS AFTER 24 WEEKS

These are generally done only to protect the mother's life or health. As with earlier second trimester abortions, D & E is an option, as is amnio infusion. With amnio infusion, an injection is used to kill the fetus after 20 weeks. Only a few people in the country are properly trained to terminate pregnancies after 24 weeks.

RU-486

The coming to America of the so-called "abortion pill" RU-486 will, in the words of one abortion provider, forever change the landscape of abortion politics in this country. Only approved for closely guarded experimental use in the U.S. starting in the summer of 1994, RU-486 will almost completely privatize the earliest abortions (up to 12 weeks of pregnancy). The drug destroys the corpus luteum or "yellow body" which supports the early pregnancy by providing progesterone. In addition to RU-486, doctors often give patients prostaglandin drugs to make the uterus contract and expel the dead fetus. The experience with RU-486 as an abortion-inducer has been gathered in parts of Europe, where the drug is approved and widely used.

Further down the road, the anticancer drug methotrexate may also be used as an abortion agent.

RISKS OF ABORTION

The risks of abortion climb with increasing length of pregnancy. Mortality is extremely rare, at about 1 in 400,000 cases. The risk of dying in a first trimester abortion is many times lower than the risk of dying in natural childbirth in the U.S. Morbidity, or complications, are more common but also quite rare. About 1 in 20 cases will have a *minor* problem; these include mild infections that can be treated on the spot at the clinic, some blood in the uterus that can be easily removed, and so on. Less commonly, in about 1 in 200 cases, there will be major complications such as serious infection or bleeding or tissue left behind in the uterus. A major complication is perforation of the uterus, which occurs rarely in experienced practitioners' hands, but unfortunately, more often in less skilled hands.

Skill is a very important issue when it comes to abortions—especially as you get into a later stage of pregnancy. According to Dr. Hakim-Elahi, there have been no deaths after more than 250,000 pregnancy terminations in the history of Planned Parenthood, New York, which started doing the procedure in 1972. Of course, we all still read the horror stories in the paper about women who bleed to death after unskilled abortions; these problems exist around the country, but are almost always caused by inept practitioners, unsanitary or unsafe conditions, late abortion or centers with a total lack of backup for medical emergencies. We'll talk about some of the key questions you should ask in order to protect yourself later in this section.

RISKS OF REPEAT ABORTIONS

Studies show that having two abortions poses *no* additional risk to future pregnancies. There is not enough data on the risk of having three or more abortions using modern procedures. Most data showing added risk to future pregnancies is from foreign studies of multiple abortions using outdated techniques. We will have to wait for future studies to determine the impact of multiple state-of-the-art abortions.

AFTER THE ABORTION

Make sure, even if you're feeling well, that you return to see your practitioner about two weeks after your abortion. She or he will see if you are recovering properly, make sure the pregnancy is terminated and check for signs of infection. Get adequate rest, remembering that even if you feel physically fine, you also have been through a medical procedure and that can be *emotionally* exhausting, too. Pay attention to any instructions you were given about activities to avoid or symptoms to watch out for. Your period should return about a month to six weeks after the abortion; if it doesn't, call your health care provider.

QUESTIONS YOU SHOULD ASK OF AN ABORTION PROVIDER

Unfortunately, in certain parts of the country—especially if health care in general is scarce—you're going to get a "no" answer to many of these questions; or, if you get a "yes," it may not be the whole truth and nothing but the truth, as we'll discuss later. Certain things, like the need for emergency resuscitation equipment, are absolutely vital.

How experienced is the practitioner who is going to do the abortion? Has she/he done more than 100 of these procedures? (In most states it is not required that he/she be a board-certified OB-GYN in the U.S.—nor is there a formal cutoff number at which a practitioner should be considered "experienced." However, Dr. Richard Hausknecht of the Mt. Sinai School of Medicine, insists that the doctor's experience makes all the difference in the world. He has observed that the complication rate falls considerably after a practitioner has done more than 100 to 150 procedures. Since most doctors come out of medical school without any formal training in pregnancy termination, it's easy to end up in the hands of someone who's learning on *you.*

Is the clinic in which you're planning to have the abortion licensed? Ask to see a certificate. Some states require a license; in these states, it should be posted.

If the abortion is not being done in a hospital (most are *not*), does the person performing the abortion have the right to use a hospital for emergency backup?

Is the backup hospital nearby?

Is there good access for leaving the clinic in the event of a medical emergency?

Is there someone available at the abortion clinic or doctor's office who can take overnight or weekend calls for postabortion emergencies? Who is that person and what is her telephone number? Is there an emergency hotline?

Is there resuscitative equipment in the event of a respiratory emergency related to anesthesia or other problems?

Who is the anesthesiologist—and is that person board certified?

Who checks the fetal tissue after the abortion?

Is there someone available after the abortion procedure is complete to watch you and check your vital signs, and to give you instructions before you go home? Is a nurse available for these needs?

Is the tissue examined for evidence of a complete placenta after the abortion?

When will you next be examined after the abortion?

How does the clinic handle payment? If it accepts insurance, chances are it will be around to care for you if something should go wrong. If they take cash only and demand payment up front, be suspicious—the clinic's life span may be shorter than you expect.

Now that we've gone through the questions you might ask and have answered honestly in an ideal world, it's worth mentioning that there are some abortion experts who insist that *all* the questions in the world won't do you any good in certain situations where, for material gain, the abortion provider will give you false answers to any one of the above questions. As an example, Dr. William Rashbaum knows of a woman whose fetus was mutilated but not aborted in the office of an abortionist who did indeed have a "nurse." The so-called nurse was his wife, and she was never actually trained in nursing. This practitioner also had an answering service for late-night calls—but who knows what training the person answering really had. And so on. The truth of the matter is, you can ask all of the right questions, but because there is no formal certification or requirement for most abortion centers around the country, you put yourself at risk if you see a practitioner who hasn't been recommended by someone you know and trust—preferably your regular doctor. Dr. Rashbaum urges women to watch out for centers that heavily advertise special low rates, as well as those that are unlicensed. But again, some parts of the country have no licensed centers. This is a terribly unregulated area of medicine.

You'll also want to be sure to do some looking around at the clinic yourself. Does it look clean? Orderly? Your judgment or impressions count for a lot. If you feel there is something unsanitary or just plain wrong with the place, chances are your fears are valid. It may be worth traveling to a safer environment if there's nothing appropriate in your region.

YOUR EMOTIONS
AND THE ABORTION

Dr. Rashbaum calls abortion an "emotional minefield." The determining factor in how a woman feels, he says, has something to do with her reason for the abortion in the first place. Sometimes the decision itself of whether or not to terminate a pregnancy can be wrenching for women and for their partners. In other cases, the decision is easy, but the postabortion feelings more difficult. For later abortions necessitated by medical problems in the fetus, early membrane rupture or some other unexpected event, women often experience anger as part of grieving.

There is great variability in how women react to having abortions. In reputable centers, there are counselors—sometimes social workers—to help you determine that you have considered all of your options and are proceeding at your own will and without coercion. Keep your ears open; this discussion should not be laden with moral information or other suggestions on the part of the counselor. If it is, you may not be in an unbiased medical setting. Robin Herstand, director of social services for the Margaret Sanger Center of Planned Parenthood in New York City, warns women about the many centers advertising "reproductive services" and offering "counseling" on abortions, which show you horrifying films of abortions in an effort to persuade you *not* to have one. Herstand *also* warns against coercion from the other side; anyone urging you to *have* an abortion against your will should be avoided, too (and that includes both counselors *and* friends or relatives). Only accept counseling if you feel that you're being listened to, that your fears and concerns are being taken seriously and that you are not being pushed in either direction. Otherwise, get up and walk out, Herstand urges.

Some say that your emotional reaction to an abortion is closely related to how you felt going into it in the first place. If you were stable and unconflicted about the abortion beforehand, you're more apt to feel relief than distress afterward (although this isn't *always* the case). On the other hand, if you went into the abortion with deep uncertainty, or if you were pushed by a parent, spouse or other partner against your will, you may be vulnerable to postabortion emotional problems ranging from sadness to anger. One reason why deciding to have an abortion can be so traumatic, says Joan Mogul Garrity, a consultant and trainer of counselors in health care, is that for some women this is the first major independent choice they've made in their lives. This is especially difficult for adolescent women who are breaking away from the jurisdiction of their parents. This independence can be very frightening, Garrity says, and counseling can be quite helpful. One thing she advises women to keep in mind is that they should not expect to be *un*conflicted about the abortion, contrary to what many people will tell them. We're conflicted about just about every decision we make in our lives, Garrity says—including what to order for lunch. Why should we expect the decision of whether to have an abortion to be any different? If anything, it should be much harder. And anyone who presses you into thinking that you should automatically know the "right thing to do" just doesn't understand, she insists.

If you are feeling emotional pain after (or even before) an abortion, *seek professional counseling.* You not only have to deal with the emotional distress of the abortion itself, but with the other issues that put you in this position in the first place. (For example: Were you unable to resist the insistence of someone important in your life? Are you afraid either to have a child, or not to have one? Are you concerned that some aspect of your lifestyle, like excessive drinking or other substance abuse which contributed to the accidental pregnancy, will also make you an unfit parent?) All of these issues, and many more, must be addressed before you will feel emotionally strong again. Most important, counseling will help you not get into this difficult situation again. Robin Herstand finds that in most cases, as few as three sessions with a counselor can go a long way to resolving most doubts and fears. If you're in deeper trouble, with signs of depression (*see* chapter 17) or other significant emotional problems, you may need more long-term support.

If you have a religious background that doesn't approve of abortion, your decision to terminate your pregnancy and your feelings afterward may be quite painful. Sometimes your negative reaction will come immediately after the abortion; in other cases, these feelings will appear a month or more later, experts say. Religious women may fear punishment by God, and feel the need to be forgiven for their actions.

Usually, social workers and other mental health professionals who specialize in women's reproductive services are equipped to deal with these religious issues, because they come up so often. Contact a women's health center or Planned Parenthood chapter near you for a list of counselors' names. If you're feeling physically but not emotionally well after an abortion, you're not yet healed. Get the rest of the care you need.

FOR MORE INFORMATION ON ABORTION

PLANNED PARENTHOOD FEDERATION OF AMERICA, INC.
810 7th Ave.
New York, NY 10019
800-230-7526 (To find local PP Center)
212-541-7800 (National Headquarters)

NATIONAL ABORTION FEDERATION
1436 U Street, Suite 103
Washington, DC 20009
800-772-9100

CHAPTER THIRTEEN

SEXUALLY TRANSMITTED DISEASES

Just as you go to the dentist because you use your teeth, so you should go to be checked for STDs if you're using your genitals.

—Dr. Judith Wasserheit

The epidemic of sexually transmitted diseases (STDs) isn't likely to disappear anytime soon, for a very simple reason: people are having a lot of sex, with a lot of partners. Professor James Trussell of Princeton University finds that while 13% of women born in the mid 1940s had had sex by age 17, more than triple that number—40%—of those born in the mid-1970s had done so. Many women today have several sex partners before marriage. Sexually transmitted diseases are prevalent because of sheer exposure: the more sexual contact you have, the greater your chance of contracting an infection.

And women are at special risk. The first time I interviewed Dr. H. Hunter Handsfield, a top STD expert from Seattle, was at the First International Conference on AIDS in Washington, D.C. in 1987. His blunt, straightforward comments about sexually transmitted diseases and their impact on women have always stuck with me. "Sexually transmitted diseases are sexist," he pronounced. "They are among the most sexist diseases in existence." He went on to explain the many ways in which women are disproportionately harmed by STDs of all kinds. When he first started talking about these issues, he wasn't alone in his field, but he was a leader in terms of opening the public's eyes to the serious gynecological and psychological ramifications of sexually transmitted diseases among women. Today Dr. Handsfield says half of all Americans will contract an STD by age 30, with women bearing the brunt of the pain.

Why are women so hard hit? For many reasons. First, sexually transmitted diseases tend to "hide out" in the female body for long periods of time, without causing symptoms, evading detection by unaggressive doctors. Because they are often invisible, women don't notice them. The damage caused by STDs is accruing inside the female body, throughout the reproductive tract, away from sight. Yes, sometimes there are symptoms like pain, sores or discharge. But more often than not, there are no signs at all—or the signs so closely resemble common nuisances like yeast infections that women choose to ignore them. In fact, Penelope Hitchcock, chief of the STD branch at the National Institute of Allergy and Infectious Diseases, worries that many women who *do* have symptoms of burning, itching or discharge treat *themselves* with over-the-counter vaginal creams and yeast medicines. These make you feel better in the short term, but they don't cure STDs. They just further mask the problem.

STDs can have a devastating impact on women's reproductive systems, scarring the fallopian tubes and causing subsequent infertility or dangerous ectopic pregnancies (in which fertilization takes place in the tubes or elsewhere outside the uterus), miscarriage or fetal harm. This happens when the organisms that cause the sexually transmitted diseases climb up the reproductive tract from the vagina through the cervix and into the uterus and tubes causing problems sometimes referred to as PID or Pelvic Inflamatory disease. Many of these organisms, especially today, are quite aggressive and don't take long to make the journey upward. The American Social Health Association estimates that 300,000 women seek

treatment for infertility each year as a result of tubal damage from STDs.

Beyond harming the reproductive tract, some STDs have been associated with cancer of the cervix (more on this later) and damage to other major body organs.

It's time we started talking about STDs, opening up about how common and devastating they are, so we can protect women. Peggy Clarke, executive director of the American Social Health Association (ASHA), laments that the U.S. has more infections per capita than most other industrialized societies because we haven't been as willing to *talk* about the problem and *put money behind* the problem as they have. In Scandinavia, for example, where condom use is the highly publicized norm, STDs are less common. In Holland, where prostitution is legal and one might expect STDs to be rampant, their prevalence is actually quite low because of strict condom use. One of the most talked-about topics at the 1992 International AIDS Conference in Amsterdam was the fact that even among Dutch prostitutes, AIDS rates were extremely low, thanks in large part to condom use on the job. It's time the U.S. learned a lesson from our European friends.

Silence is a particular problem among young women, notes Penelope Hitchcock. She has learned that many teenage girls are afraid to ask potential sex partners if they've been exposed to STDs, because just *asking* implies they've already made a decision to have sex—which is considered inappropriate for the "girl" to do. Young women are at high risk of STD-related problems because they are physiologically vulnerable to STD damage: their cervical cells are more vulnerable, their immune systems are not as prepared to "take on" the organisms, and so on.

Teen girls seem to develop pelvic inflammatory disease faster than older women when exposed to STDs—all the more reason they should be screened regularly to protect them from permanent damage and infertility. Finally, teenagers often partake of risky, test-the-boundaries behavior, and sex is no exception. Because they seldom perceive themselves as vulnerable, they're likely to engage in risky sexual exploration.

Perhaps nothing is worse than the *psychological* toll STDs can take on their victims. Because our society is so tight-lipped about these illnesses, many who are diagnosed with an STD feel alone, frightened, singled out, humiliated. They may be afraid to have future sexual relationships, or they may be in chronic pain after certain treatments for the infection (more on this later). The lasting impact of sexually transmitted diseases on women has received far too little attention and, as a result, too many women have suffered too long, silently, feeling alone.

Cal Vanderplate, an expert on the emotional impact of sexually transmitted disease, says that patients initially react with disbelief and then anger when they're diagnosed with an STD. Quickly those emotions shift to feelings of depression, isolation, shame, and guilt. Many women report feeling "dirty," Vanderplate adds—and they develop fears of being "found out." Another common fear is telling partners: the average woman with herpes has told just two people about her infection. Vanderplate says it is *vital* for emotional recovery to tell someone you trust about your infection. But that takes a major leap, considering that many of his patients fantasize about *killing* the person who gave them an STD.

For whatever reason you've been avoiding facing the painful reality of STDs, it's time to wake up. These diseases have reached epidemic proportions in our country and threaten to cause permanent harm to women of all ages and backgrounds if we don't take action *now*.

WHAT IS A SEXUALLY TRANSMITTED DISEASE?

A sexually transmitted disease or STD (also called a venereal disease) is an infection that is passed from one person to another through sexual contact. Just as there are many different types of organisms that can cause diseases, so there are many different types of sex acts that can spread them. For instance, while many people focus on traditional penis-vagina intercourse as a means of passing STDs, these infections can *also* be spread by means of oral, anal and other forms of sex (man to woman, woman to man or between two people of the same sex).

Sexually transmitted diseases come in two main categories: those caused by bacteria (bacterial STDs) and those caused by viruses (viral STDs). Some common bacterial STDs include chlamydia and gonorrhea. Some common viral STDs include herpes, human papillomavirus and HIV, the virus that causes AIDS.

Bacterial STDs can often be treated and completely cured with the right antibiotic taken in the right dose for the correct amount of time. Let the bacteria sit around in your body for too long, though, and you are likely to develop lasting problems that cannot be reversed. Viral STDs cannot be cured at this time, but their effects can be controlled in a variety of ways (see more below). Viral STDs live in the cells of your body forever, sometimes causing symptoms, sometimes not. They usually do not have the same kind of impact on your reproductive tract as bacterial STDs, but they can cause problems during pregnancy and delivery, as we'll discuss.

THE HARD FACTS ABOUT SEXUALLY TRANSMITTED DISEASES

According to the National Institute of Allergy and Infectious Diseases (NIAID), 13 million people will be diagnosed with STDs this year at a cost of more than 5 billion dollars. That annual cost is expected to rise to 10 billion dollars by the year 2000, according to the National Institutes of Health. Two-thirds of those affected will be under the age of 25—including about three million teenagers. Somewhere between 10 and 40 percent of women with gonorrhea and/or chlamydia will get PID, or pelvic inflammatory disease, when the infection reaches higher into their reproductive tract. The biggest risk caused by PID: permanent infertility. According to ASHA, about 50,000 women are diagnosed as infertile each year due to chlamydia alone!

While women have always shared the nonfatal STD burden, we are increasingly sharing the AIDS burden as well; women make up the fastest-growing population of HIV-positive people. As a result, more infants are getting HIV from their mothers—at a rate of over two thousand cases per year. One in six Americans has genital herpes, one in three has the human papillomavirus that causes genital warts and can be associated with cancer of the cervix.

Here are some "hard facts" for the most common STDs:[1]

CHLAMYDIA

Four million new cases a year! Chlamydia, a bacterial STD caused by the organism *Chlamydia trachomatis,* is *the single most common* STD— and one of the most silent. According to ASHA, 75% of women have *no* symptoms of chlamydia. As a result, women often don't know they have it until it wreaks havoc on their reproductive systems.

According to Sevgi Aral, associate director for science in the division STD/HIV prevention at the Centers for Disease Control and Prevention, chlamydia is becoming increasingly asymptomatic. One of many possible explanations is that "silent" strains are becoming more and more resistent to treatment. That means you can live with the disease for many years and not know it: many women find out they have this infection when they try to become pregnant and discover that their fallopian tubes are destroyed. A relatively small percentage of people with chlamydia *do* have symptoms like discharge (both men and women), burning with urination and pelvic pain if the disease has spread. But most do not. The damage quietly being wreaked in your body is tucked away where it can't be seen or felt, in the upper reproductive tract.

Aral is concerned about the proper diagnosis

1. Note: There are other sexually transmitted infections that are not covered in this chapter. Some are more annoying or uncomfortable than they are serious health threats, such as pubic lice and scabies. Others you probably don't even think about as sexually transmitted diseases, such as several forms of hepatitis. If your regular doctor or gynecologist is equipped to screen you for any or all of these infections each time you have a new sexual partner (or when you are in a nonmonogamous sexual relationship), be sure to ask for screening; if you aren't comfortable talking to your personal doctor about sexually transmitted diseases, or if he/she isn't equipped to test you, consider visiting a full-service STD clinic for regular screening and care. Unfortunately, you may have to be persistent, since many of these clinics are overburdened and book up in advance.

of chlamydia. While culture tests are useful, high-tech polymerase chain reaction (PCR) tests are far more accurate, she says, and show that we may have been missing up to half of the chlamydia cases tested in the past. As PCR testing becomes cheaper and more widely available, testing speed and accuracy will increase.

Treating Chlamydia.

There's an important piece of information about chlamydia treatment: this infection can often be cured with a *single dose* of the antibiotic azithromycin. Other, less expensive antibiotics like tetracycline and doxycycline (and if you're pregnant, erythromycin) can also kill chlamydia, but you'll have to take them over the required several-day period to eradicate the bacteria. If you are in any way unreliable about taking medication regularly, or if you just want a "quick fix," try the one-dose therapy. (Your sex partner must be treated too, or you will end up passing the infection back and forth.) Then be sure to follow up with your doctor at whatever interval she suggests to make sure the disease has been destroyed and that you don't need one more dose.

Chlamydia and Pregnancy.

Dr. Judith Wasserheit, director of the division of STD/HIV prevention at the Centers for Disease Control and Prevention, calls chlamydia the "prime player" in infertility and ectopic pregnancy. But for those who manage to conceive and carry pregnancies to term with chlamydia, the results can be devastating. Over 100,000 babies are born each year with problems associated with chlamydia, according to the Alan Guttmacher Institute. Babies are at risk for a variety of chlamydia-related illnesses, including pneumonia and eye infections. This is why it's so very important to find out *before* becoming pregnant if you are clear of curable STDs. If not, you can be treated before you try to conceive. If you are diagnosed during pregnancy, you may be able to be treated in time to prevent some of the potential impact on your fetus, but you cannot use some of the more potent antichlamydia drugs during pregnancy. Usually erythromycin is given to infected pregnant women.

GONORRHEA

1.4 million new cases a year. Often silent (and like chlamydia, becoming more so), this bacterial infection can cause damage to the reproductive organs, resulting in infertility. When symptoms are present, they include burning with urination and, if the disease has spread, pelvic pain with possible fever and nausea. Gonorrhea can infect the genital tract as well as the eyes and throat. Like many STDs, it likes the warm moisture of mucous membranes. We've had some success in fighting this infection—the rate of gonorrhea infection dropped in the '70s and '80s—however, Dr. Wasserheit warns that there are several new, powerful strains of gonorrhea that resist treatment with conventional antibiotics. One of the reasons these strains develop is people don't take the prescribed amount of medication for the right amount of time when they are initially diagnosed. . . so a newer, stronger version of the infection lives on (it's like survival of the fittest: the strongest bugs live through the first couple of days of treatment; you stop taking your medication, and those strong bugs multiply).

Diagnosis is best made with a culture test. Other, quicker tests are available, but they're not as reliable.

When trying to protect yourself from disease, keep the following statistic in mind, says Dr. Edward Newton of the University of Texas Health Science Center in San Antonio: The chance of an uninfected woman getting gonorrhea or chlamydia from an infected man, with just a *single* episode of unprotected sex, is fifty percent! Men are luckier: their risk of getting it from an infected woman with one episode of unprotected sex is 5–15%. Just another look at the sexism of STDs.

GONORRHEA: WHAT YOU HAD TO SAY ABOUT IT

Elizabeth, 36 years old
My first contact with an STD, unfortunately, was when I was in high school, just after 12th grade. I contracted gonorrhea. We had been at a party and it was a one-time thing that we had intercourse, we were both drunk. That summer I heard my younger sister, who was friends with his younger sister, talking about a rumor that he had "something" and was being treated for it—a rumor that he was very sick and in the hospital. I didn't tell anyone, I took myself to the local clinic. I was very scared. There were several boys I knew there, and we were all very embarrassed to see each other. One boy took one look at me and said, "Oh, you slept with Jack." We agreed that we wouldn't tell that we'd seen each other there.

They took a culture and a Pap smear and I had to wait a whole month to find out my results, because I lived in the middle of nowhere and the tests had to be sent away. A month later I found I'd tested positive for gonorrhea and the way the doctor explained it, he said I'd just had a brush with it, just had it recently. I was scheduled to go

in for two penicillin shots. It was very scary. I did have information that I had just gotten in 11th grade health class, but the fear of the unknown . . . and I thought, "What if I hadn't gotten drunk?" Luckily the doctor was very friendly. My self esteem was in bad shape in the first place, I felt as if I was the dirt of the earth in the month I was waiting—and especially afterwards.

I felt so bad about it for a long time afterwards. For a little while I didn't have sex with anyone—for about a year and a half. There is a big difference between a man having an STD and a woman having one. It's something ingrained, we're the "bad" ones. *We* spread it to *them*. But I don't truly believe that. The sooner you can be responsible for your sexual health, the better. I've never heard from him to this day. I never saw him again.

Treating Gonorrhea.
Again, because it's a bacterial infection, gonorrhea can be cured with medication. Penicillin is the antibiotic of choice. However, it sometimes takes a combination of several antibiotics to kill the stubborn, resistant strains mentioned above. After you and your sex partner(s) are treated, go back to your health care provider after a specified amount of time and make sure the infection has cleared up. Since gonorrhea often turns up along with other sexually transmitted diseases, such as chlamydia, you'll want to talk to your doctor about the possibility of taking a drug with a broad enough disease-killing spectrum that it eliminates both infections at once. Remember, not all antibiotics kill the same bugs.

Gonorrhea and Pregnancy.
Gonorrhea can cause serious damage to a fetus. The baby's brain, lungs and blood can be

infected, as can its eyes and other vulnerable areas. Have a test for this and all sexually transmitted diseases before becoming pregnant, if you can time it that way. As with chlamydia, you can be treated during pregnancy, but not as aggressively as when you are not pregnant.

HERPES

Five hundred thousand new cases a year! Herpes, a viral STD, is astonishingly common: it's estimated that 30 million Americans have genital herpes. *Time* magazine gave it the cover in 1982 and branded it "Today's Scarlet Letter." Because it is caused by an incurable virus, it's likely to remain one of the diseases of the decades to come as well, unless we boost our prevention efforts. It's no wonder herpes is so common: the chance of an uninfected woman getting the virus from an infected man after a year of intercourse *with condoms* is 16%, says Dr. Newton. That's with good protection; without any protection, the chances soar.

When active, herpes shows up as blisters or sores on the genitals or mouth. It used to be said that herpes type 1 affected the mouth (cold sores), and that herpes type 2 affected the genitals, but there is actually a great deal of crossover, partly because of oral sex. The virus can cause a great deal of physical and emotional discomfort when it flares. Sores on the vagina, penis, anal area, buttocks and thighs can be quite painful.

Many people with the disease find that while the first outbreak is quite uncomfortable, it is often the worst. Subsequent outbreaks are less severe and less frequent, experts say—but this varies from patient to patient. (When herpes isn't causing symptoms, it's hiding in the gan-

glia or nerve cells at the base of the spine.) Triggers that bring the infection out to the level of the skin vary from person to person, but include emotional stress, lack of sleep and physical trauma. Sores usually appear near the place where they originally appeared, but you can spread your disease around by touching sores, then touching your eyes or mouth. Even non-mucous membranes on your fingers or elsewhere can develop sores if you're not careful about washing your hands after touching them.

What You Might Feel During a Herpes Outbreak.

Unlike the bacterial STDs discussed above, herpes, when active, can cause a great deal of discomfort. The only good thing about this is it lets you know you have a problem, so you can protect others from infection. However, some people carry the herpes virus and never know it; and during what's called "asymptomatic shedding" of the virus, can pass it on. According to Dr. H. Hunter Handsfield, director of the STD Control program at the Seattle–King County Department of Health, asymptomatic shedding may be much more common than we used to believe—which means the chance of infecting a sexual partner is greater than previously thought.

Herpes sores cause burning, stinging and itching. They can also cause pain or discomfort in areas around the sores, sometimes even before the sores appear—in the buttocks, legs or around the genitals. These pre-sore feelings are called prodromal symptoms; some women get them, some don't. You might have pain when urinating, pressure in your abdomen, fever, headaches, muscle aches that feel like the flu, vaginal discharge or swollen glands in the groin area. There is great variability in how much people are bothered by herpes. Some have severe physical (and emotional, as we'll discuss) symptoms; others hardly notice outbreaks. Those who have unhealthy immune systems, such as people with AIDS, often have more severe and long-lasting outbreaks of herpes, because their bodies cannot fight back quickly and effectively.

HERPES: WHAT YOU HAD TO SAY ABOUT IT

Susan, 43 years old
I was diagnosed ten years ago: just had my tenth anniversary. I had sores, and wanted to know what it was. I went to the doctor praying for anything else but that. That old line "herpes is forever". There was so little information out there, I assumed I'd always have sores and never have sex again. Then I got a little education.

I had a good suspicion who I got it from. I went back to him and said, "So how long have you had herpes?" He said he didn't think he had it, but then the sweat started pouring out of him.

At the time I was diagnosed even though I had an extremely strong support group—a lady I was living with, 2–3 other girlfriends knew by the end of the day, my mother knew the next day—I knew this would change my life. You go through, "I'm never having sex again." I felt dirty, that is a typical reaction when you have an STD. I know people who tell no one for four or five years. You gotta have someone to confide in, you have to talk about it. I had one day where I was crying my eyes out. The next day I was alright. You have setbacks. You go through emotions but I went through them fast forward because I had a lot of support.

Any time you have something that stays with you a long time, like diabetes, there is an adjustment period—when you take it forward with you to a new relationship. But the bottom line is everyone brings luggage with them, you just have an extra suitcase! Once you realize how common it is, you lose the fear, the isolation, and then you can get on with yourself. We're so two-faced about this, we sell perfume with naked bodies but when you have a friend with something "down there," you think—"WELL!. . . " This virus doesn't care who you are, or where you come from.

Diagnosing and Treating Herpes.
The best diagnosis is by viral culture, in which cells taken from an active infection are grown and studied in the laboratory. This test can give you not only a diagnosis of herpes, but a specific herpes type (1 or 2). A less useful test is a blood test that can show antibodies to herpes, which shows that at some point you were exposed to the virus—but doesn't show an active infection or tell what type of infection you have. If you get cold sores, for example, a herpes *antibody* test can come back positive; this does not mean you have genital herpes, however.

There is only one approved drug for herpes in the U.S. It's called acyclovir, and it can be taken two ways: orally, in pill form, or topically, as a cream applied to herpes sores. For those who have chronic severe herpes outbreaks, taking acyclovir pills regularly can help as a preventive measure, cutting the frequency and severity of attacks. However, some believe that when you take the drug this way, you're more likely to develop a resistance to it over time. If you get rare, not-too-severe herpes outbreaks, the cream form of the medication can help reduce pain and the duration of the outbreak, which is adequate relief for many people.

In addition to acyclovir, there is lots of anecdotal evidence about Chinese herbs and other vitamin therapy helping to reduce herpes symptoms. Because there is no solid scientific evidence that any of these potions helps, I advise you to proceed with caution: ask your doctor if the herbs you're thinking of taking can pose you harm—and make sure that the herbs listed on the container are actually the ones inside (you might have to send the herbs to a laboratory to do this)! There is no formal regulation of these remedies. If you have made certain that the treatment is safe, only then should you consider trying it for yourself.

What You Can Do For Yourself To Make Herpes Less Bothersome.

They say creativity is born of necessity, and since there is little to rely on medically for treating herpes, some health care professionals recommend simple "tricks" to reduce herpes pain or itching. First, wear all-cotton, loose-fitting undergarments and loose outer clothing when you are having an outbreak. After using the toilet, wipe yourself by blotting gently, not by rubbing or wiping the skin where the sores are. After showering, dry off as you normally would, but then take a blow drier, hold it far enough away from the affected skin that you don't burn yourself (about a foot away) and completely dry the area with the sores. This will speed their healing and increase your comfort before you put on underwear. Some believe that dusting sores with cornstarch helps. Dr. Newton recommends keeping your hands clean after handling sores, so as to reduce the chance of "secondary transmission"—spreading the virus to your eyes or elsewhere on your body. Soap and water will do the trick.

You can also avoid the common "triggers" to herpes outbreaks—like excessive stress in your life, fatigue, or irritation of the skin from things like sun exposure or sexual intercourse, or any other trigger that you've noticed affects *your* outbreaks. Some find that certain foods trigger attacks—but this is highly individualized. Oft-mentioned food triggers include chocolate, nuts and cola; possible herpes *deterrents* include yeast and high-lysine foods like liver, potatoes, milk and fish. If you haven't noticed any association between your outbreaks and these foods, don't start avoiding them or eating them just because you have herpes. Think about your own diet and behavior and whether there are any connections to your outbreaks. Start paying close attention to your body and you may discover other kinds of triggers you didn't recognize before, too.

Vitamin therapy is unproven: while some recommend either taking vitamins by mouth or applying them to sores, clinicians are skeptical about whether this actually works. Again, if what you're trying is safe (ask your doctor), you can experiment and see what makes *you* feel best.

Herpes and Pregnancy.

If you become infected with herpes during pregnancy, particularly in the first few months, you're at increased risk of miscarriage. Other problems for babies affected by herpes in utero include low birth weight and prematurity. Furthermore, if you have an active herpes infection at the time of delivery, you can have serious problems: if the baby is exposed to herpes sores, it runs a greater chance of serious permanent neurological and other damage. If active sores are *visible* at the time of delivery, your health care provider may recommend a cesarean delivery to protect the baby. Some practitioners recommend weekly herpes cultures in the weeks just preceding delivery, since you may be able to pass the virus to your baby even without visible sores. Others say that weekly culture testing isn't cost-effective, but this is a decision you can make with your doctor. Fetal infection is far more common if you have a *first* herpes episode during pregnancy than if you've had the infection for a long time before pregnancy. For this reason, if you are not infected with the virus, be sure to protect yourself from contracting it while you're pregnant. If your partner has it, use condoms and avoid intercourse when he has sores.

There is no reason to avoid becoming pregnant just because you have a history of herpes. You should not try to conceive during an outbreak, not because of the risk to the baby, but because you'll expose your partner to the sores (since presumably you'll be having unprotected intercourse). Don't worry about subsequent (as opposed to first-time) outbreaks during pregnancy. Then, simply watch (with your doctor's assistance) for the presence of sores at the time of delivery.

SYPHILIS

130,000 new cases a year. This age-old bacterial sexually transmitted infection was once considered nearly eradicated, but it has made a strong resurgence in the last decade, especially in certain communities (inner-city populations are hard-hit). In fact, in the 1980s, syphilis reached its highest level in 40 years! Approximately 130,000 new cases were diagnosed in 1990 alone. Many of these new cases were among lower-income, minority populations, but no one is immune to syphilis or to any STD, for that matter. While we think of it as a genital disease, syphilis can enter all kinds of skin through breaks or sores. Over time, if not treated, it evolves from a highly transmissible sore to a more systemic illness. It can be passed from mother to fetus during pregnancy, causing serious damage.

What You Might Notice.

Syphilis often starts out as a painless sore on the penis or in or around the vagina, then develops into a rash; it seems pretty benign on the whole. Men are four times more likely to get the sore than are women, says Dr. Newton. For this reason, women are at greater risk of moving on to a later stage of disease, he adds. Later, if not treated, syphilis can develop into *serious,* irreversible brain and heart problems. The later stages of syphilis are impossible to feel: after fevers and rashes abate, the infection can hide in the body for many years, until permanent damage is done to all major body systems.

Treatment and Diagnosis of Syphilis.

Blood tests are used for syphilis, and they are pretty reliable. The usual treatment is with penicillin, but other antibiotics can be used as well. Often the drug will be given in powerful doses by injection. Take advantage of the fact that this, like other bacterial STDs, is curable in its early stages. Get tested and treated fast, before permanent damage sets in.

Syphilis and Pregnancy.

If not treated early and effectively, syphilis is likely to be transmitted to a developing fetus, sometimes with devastating results—including death. Pregnant women can be treated, but the later in pregnancy you're treated, the greater the chance that damage cannot be averted. This is just one more in the long list of reasons for prenatal testing and treatment of all potentially harmful infections.

HPV: HUMAN PAPILLOMAVIRUS—THE VIRUS THAT CAUSES GENITAL WARTS

Five hundred thousand new cases per year. This viral infection is one of the most common STDs around, affecting an estimated 40 million Americans (and this is probably conservative). Some experts believe that almost everyone would turn up positive for this virus if we bothered to do the testing. There are about 60 different "types" of HPV, and according to the NIAID, about a third of them are sexually transmitted. These different types have been assigned numbers, and different numbers are known to cause different problems. For instance, certain types cause benign genital warts. Others—particularly types 16 and 18— are thought to be related to cancer of the cervix. Still others cause the minor warts we get on our hands and feet.

Peggy Clarke of the American Social Health Association notes that HPV has a devastating effect on romantic relationships, because it leaves open so many question marks—you can't say with *any* certainty when you were exposed (it could be weeks, months, or years ago) so blame and resentment can often be misdirected. Most people's reaction upon being diagnosed is to blame their current sex partner. Yes, that person *could* have given you the virus—but it's just as likely that your sex partner from last year was the culprit. (Also keep in mind that because HPV is often silent, especially in men, male sex partners usually don't know they're spreading it around.)

Dr. Karl Beutner of UCSF, who is on the HPV advisory board for the American Social Health Association, reports that he sees a college student with HPV every day—and often, they haven't even *heard* of the disease. While it is more common than herpes, Beutner says, many people don't know about it because scientists just started to learn about its prevalence when the AIDS epidemic grabbed headlines, stealing HPV's thunder. Some studies have found rates as high as 50% of college women infected with HPV.

HPV and Cancer of the Cervix.

Do *not* panic if you are diagnosed with HPV— don't assume that you will definitely get cancer of the cervix. Other cofactors like cigarette smoking or a poor overall immune system play important roles in causing cervical cancer. Having certain types of HPV puts you at increased risk of getting cancer of the cervix, so you should be on greater alert and have a doctor monitor the health of your cervix more closely. With regular gynecological exams, and the all-important Pap test every year at least, you will greatly increase the chance that you will catch any early, precancerous changes on the cervix when they are curable. Some feel that those diagnosed with HPV infection and abnormal changes on the cervix should have Pap smears every six months; after several years of normal tests, you may be advised to return to the once-a-year plan. (For more on the diagnosis and treatment of cancer of the cervix, see chapter 25.)

Dr. Beutner recommends screening of the

anal area for HPV as well, since this region is also sensitive to precancerous and cancerous changes. Penile cancer has been associated with HPV, too, but this is thought to be *extremely* rare.

HPV: WHAT YOU HAD TO SAY ABOUT IT

Sandra, 26 years old
I was diagnosed in 1991. I was in a steady relationship and so when I began to show symptoms, a little strange growth on my perineum, I didn't know what it could be. I had an abnormal Pap smear and my clinician said the growth was just the natural folds of my skin. They chalked it up to yeast and that was the end of it. I did have words with her later—I was angry—it's not the natural folds of my skin! Don't let anyone tell you anything about your body, you know it yourself!

The growth just continued to keep coming and proliferating, one after another they'd join one another. Two months later I made an appointment with a gynecologist who said, "You have genital warts!" I was lying on my back finding out I had genital warts, with tears running down my face into my ears, and she just gave me a pamphlet! It seemed like there wasn't any information coming from my doctor, I got pamphlets but no one said, "You need condoms, this is a virus you'll have the rest of your life, or if you need further information . . . "—nothing really! I knew nothing about it. I started trying to get a hold of anything I could find, I asked all the questions.

I felt so dirty and so gross, and (my boyfriend) made it no better. He totally freaked out, totally shut me out and I totally needed him at that time, I was grieving. He was very frustrated when we couldn't have sex during my treatments. He hurt

my self-esteem, he was really horrible. It was the beginning of my realizing how selfish he was, he didn't care about me. My genitalia wasn't in good working order and to him it was a bother! He never went to the doctor, I couldn't get him to go. The relationship lasted a year and a half longer, and finally at the end he went to the doctor and he had it, a little bitty nothing that had been there the entire time we were together. After what it did to my body, he got this little piddly thing!

I had cryosurgery, biopsies, colposcopy. I had to have all these endoscopic procedures, and they removed them. I had it two times last year and the little sons of bitches came back this year, so it's an ongoing battle. I had two on my cervix, in my vagina, inside the opening of my anus. I was covered. I couldn't go to the bathroom, I would bleed, it was like having a baby. I had a class 3 Pap smear, abnormal cells, precancerous cells.

Once I got rid of him I have not had an abnormal Pap since 1992. The more information I got the better I felt. My feelings about feeling dirty didn't last—I turned it to anger. I got really okay about it, I thought, "It's just a virus—we're animals, things live all over us, fungus, etc." The stress of not telling my parents was harder. For a year my parents ignored the hospital bills—I said, "You don't want to know," and they just said, "Do you need any money?" I just finally told my mother and she handled it pretty well. She's a Baptist lady, and for her to say "Jackass" is a lot—and that's what we call (my ex-boyfriend) now.

My father said, "Don't tell anyone." He was implying that it was something to be ashamed of. I told him I'm not ashamed of it. Now I have no secrets from my parents. I'm not much of a secret keeper anyway, I told everyone—I kept telling and telling and telling because I couldn't talk to my boyfriend about it. From my reading, it's estimated that a lot of people who have it don't know it and spread it around. I wear my infection on my sleeve. I don't tell someone I'm dating until I can trust them, but I tell them before they have any risk. Because of this I got interested in social health. I'm trying to go into nursing. I work for an STD hotline. As long as we all walk around acting ashamed of all this, there will be a stigma.

HPV and Pregnancy.

This is another of the STDs that can affect pregnancy. If warts are very large and not removed before delivery, the baby can come in contact with them and get warts on its outer skin, eyes or respiratory tract (this last can be serious). Generally, if HPV is controlled *before* pregnancy, the risk of transmission to the fetus is quite low—although some researchers argue that fetuses can get small amounts of HPV from the amniotic fluid in the uterus even when nothing is present on the mother. Again, this is *extremely* rare, and not all practitioners believe it. Treatment of large or widespread warts is sometimes recommended even *during* pregnancy to reduce the chance of transmission to the baby. As with all STDs, it's preferable to be diagnosed and treated before becoming pregnant, however.

Treating HPV.

There are several ways to eradicate the warts (visible or microscopic) caused by HPV. Usually on an outpatient basis in your doctor's office, you can have one of several techniques to eliminate infection on the cervix—including freezing with liquid nitrogen, "burning" with an electric current, conventional or laser surgery and—less commonly—injection with the drug interferon. There are also two topical medications that can be put on warts that appear on the vagina or vulva *(if you are not pregnant)* to shrink or reduce their number. The drugs are called podofilox, which you can apply on your own and rinse off after several hours, and trichloracetic acid (TCA) which is used by some practitioners. TCA can sting, but it acts fast; you usually feel better in a matter of minutes. Nothing completely rids you of the virus—just the outward signs of it. Most people who have HPV need repeat treatments over time to keep the warts under control—others are lucky and aren't bothered by the infection after one successful treatment.

Don't be surprised if you develop a recurrence of the warts (which you may be able to see, or your doctor may diagnose by means of a tool called a colposcope, a special kind of microscope). Often, the doctor will put vinegar on your cervix and around your vagina and anal area to "light up" hard-to-see warts. This should not be painful; you may feel just a bit of stinging on irritated skin. What *can* be uncomfortable is if your doctor takes a biopsy—that is, she might snip off a bit of skin that looks suspicious in order to have it checked out at a lab. If your doctor thinks it's likely that she will have to take a biopsy at your next visit, and since some people find this procedure painful, you might want to ask about taking a mild painkiller before you come in (say, an hour earlier). Your doctor can help you choose the right one—or might prescribe something.

If your warts, visible or invisible, turn out to cover a large area of skin (perhaps the cervix, vagina and anal area) your doctor might choose laser surgery in a hospital setting under general anesthesia. Laser surgery costs more than other treatments, but it's the best choice for extensive treatment. If this is your case, you might spend a few days in the hospital after treatment, and then have a several-week recovery period at home in which the uncomfortable skin that was treated with the laser gradually recovers. The lased skin will crust over, as if healing from a burn, and it will be quite sensitive. Extensive laser surgery can be quite useful in treating severe disease; however, it can also cause scarring of the genital skin and/or changes in the cells in that region, causing later discomfort (perhaps with sexual intercourse). These days, experts are trying to use as little laser as possible so as to eradicate the warts, but not destroy the normal surrounding tissue.

The biggest question about HPV treatment is, Should you treat asymptomatic (symptom-free) infection? When it's on the cervix, absolutely yes—since changes on the cervical cells can progress to cancer. But on the vulva, for example, if there is no pain, many experts are leaving well enough alone. Dr. Thomas Sedlacek, chairman of the department of gynecology at Graduate Hospital in Philadelphia, calls the treatment of asymptomatic, noncervical skin "the triumph of hope over reason." Since you can't eliminate HPV, having repeat, often traumatic or painful treatment for a virus you cannot feel doesn't make a lot of sense. Several years ago, practitioners were lasing and burning and freezing and giving medication to thousands of women who never even knew they had a problem. The invisible warts often returned, and treatment was repeated. Some doctors still treat asymptomatic infection: if yours does, make sure he/she gives you a good reason for it—and you might want to seek a second opinion before subjecting your genital skin to too much trauma.

A note about HPV transmission: Because this STD tends to be more widespread throughout the genital area than other STDs, it's hard to prevent spread to a sexual partner. Unfortunately, you can probably spread HPV even when warts are microscopic (one of many reasons the infection is so prevalent). Some estimate that two out of three sex partners of someone with HPV will contract the virus within a few months. Condoms can't protect the whole area, since they only cover the penis and the wart virus can be on the testicles or elsewhere, or on parts of the *woman's* genital anatomy that comes into contact with the testicles, etc. Spermicidal foams and jellies are of questionable value in protecting you from HPV as well, since some feel they irritate the delicate tissue of the vagina and can even make the condition worse. Talk to your doctor about this possibility, and how it fits into your overall plan for protecting yourself and others from all STDs. Oral transmission of HPV is also possible, though rare. Your best bet to reduce the chance of transmission is to make sure you are treated regularly to reduce visible warts. But with this STD, even more so than others, protection provides no guarantees.

TRICHOMONIASIS ("TRICH")

Three million new cases a year. Practitioners may suspect trichomoniasis after looking at your cervix: there is often a profuse discharge there. Trich is a common sexually transmitted infection caused by a parasite called *Trichomonas vaginalis.* You might not see the discharge yourself—sometimes it stays higher in your vagina—but in other cases you will see it, and it can be gray, greenish or yellowish. There is often a vaginal odor, some vaginal itch and occasionally abdominal pain. Trich is often mistaken for a simple yeast or bacterial vaginal infection. Your doctor should look at your discharge under a microscope to determine if your problems are caused by trich, and do a culture test to confirm it. Men may have a thin white discharge from the penis, or pain with urination.

Trich is easily treated with a single dose of a drug called metronidazole. Do not drink alcohol when taking this drug, as you may experience extreme nausea and vomiting. Male partners should also be treated, even if they are symptom-free, so you don't pass the infection back and forth.

HIV, THE VIRUS THAT CAUSES AIDS

HIV, or human immunodeficiency virus, causes the disease known as AIDS—acquired immunodeficiency syndrome. When you have HIV, you are said to be "HIV-positive." When you do not have it, you are "HIV-negative." We've come a long way since over a decade ago when we foolishly believed that AIDS was purely a disease of intravenous (IV) drug users and male homosexuals. AIDS is *everyone's* disease—if you have ever had sex, any kind of sex (oral, anal or genital), you are at risk. Worldwide, heterosexual transmission is the main route of passage for AIDS—and women are as hard hit as men.

In the U.S., women are increasingly at risk of getting HIV, with our rate of infection climbing faster than men's. Women now comprise 11% of U.S. AIDS cases, and in certain cities, the percentage is far higher. The World Health Organization predicts that by the year 2000, more than half of the new AIDS cases in the world will be among women. We are watching an epidemic in progress. And of course, a second epidemic is following closely on its heels: through women, children's infection rates are climbing, too, since about half of the infants of HIV-positive mothers will contract the virus. An important recent finding is that treating HIV-positive pregnant women with the drug AZT (azidothymidine) can reduce the chance that she will pass the virus to her baby. This is just one more reason it pays to find out your HIV status with an anonymous blood test.

According to Dr. Anthony Fauci, a leading AIDS expert and director of the National Institute of Allergy and Infectious Diseases, only 1.9% of HIV cases were transmitted heterosexually in 1985; in 1993, that percentage had jumped to 9%. That's a dramatic increase. At least twice as many women are infected heterosexually as men. HIV is much more "effectively" transmitted from the male body to the female body, Fauci notes, for reasons similar to those with other STDs: the vagina is warm and moist and provides lots of mucous membrane entry points; the cervix is often slightly abraded, making it easier for viruses to enter the bloodstream; and the vagina acts like a vault, holding semen for several hours, and transporting semen which may contain HIV up toward the cervix. In so many ways, women are physiologically vulnerable to STD infection, and the virus that causes AIDS is no exception.

The sooner women become aware that AIDS is our problem, too, the sooner we can begin to protect ourselves from this fatal disease.

How You Get HIV.
As important as outlining the ways you *do* get HIV or AIDS is listing the ways you *don't* get it. Let's dispel the myths about AIDS that have

unjustly made pariahs out of the many decent men and women who are suffering with this disease. AIDS is *not* spread by hugging, casual kissing, sharing cooking utensils, towels, bedding, toilet seats, or telephones. It is *not* spread by mosquitoes or by shaking hands. It is *not* spread by sleeping in the same room, or using the same shower. It is *not* spread by donating blood (a brand new, sterile needle is used for each donor). Most experts feel that "deep kissing," also called "French kissing," does *not* transmit HIV; however, the theoretical possibility cannot be ruled out that an open sore in the mouths of both kissers *could* provide a mode of blood-to-blood transmission. Again, this is *purely* theoretical. So you see, caring for, loving, being friends with and physically close to someone with AIDS does *not* pose a risk of transmission.

HIV *is* spread when infected body fluids carrying enough of the virus come into contact with uninfected body fluids. AIDS *is* spread through many kinds of sexual contact, such as penis-vagina intercourse, oral sex and anal sex (man to woman, woman to man, or between same-sex individuals). And AIDS *is* spread through sharing needles, which is common among intravenous drug abusers. In the past, AIDS was spread through blood transfusions— blood that was donated either before we knew about AIDS in the first place, or before we were able to test for it. Today, while no one can give a 100% guarantee that donated blood is AIDS-free, we can come extremely close to guaranteeing it.

AIDS has an important connection to other sexually transmitted diseases. When other STDs are present—especially those that cause open sores, but other types as well—HIV is more easily transmitted. The sores provide an open pathway, so to speak, that can let the AIDS virus in if you're exposed to it. You don't have to be able to *see* the sores to be more vulnerable. Irritated skin or just slightly abraded skin can also be welcoming to HIV. So having other infections or STDs and not using condoms puts you at significantly greater risk for contracting HIV.

You might think that with all we know about how AIDS is spread and how to protect ourselves, that people would be changing their risky behavior. But according to Dr. William Schaffner, chairman of the department of preventive medicine at the Vanderbilt University School of Medicine, 60% of college students are living just as they did before, thinking "chances are it won't affect me." Women must come to realize that they play a central role in the decision-making and responsibility burden of their relationships, Dr. Shaffner stresses. It's time women started carrying and insisting that their partners use condoms, and thinking hard about whether sex with unfamiliar partners is worth the risk. Remember, Dr. Shaffner adds, there's nothing you can tell about your partner's HIV status by *looking* at him, no matter who he is or what his background may be.

Generally, people become HIV-positive—that is, the virus shows up in their blood—several weeks to several months after they are infected. Some people get a flu-like illness around the time they're infected—others do not. After infection, you can live for many years—over a decade—seeming perfectly healthy, before the disease AIDS appears. You can see how easy it is for someone to spread HIV to sex partners if they don't know they have it, since they often look and feel perfectly healthy even though they're infected. Once full-blown AIDS sets in, most people live just a few years—and these are often deeply painful years.

Be compassionate, not ignorant. What you must keep in mind is that if you are not having sexual relations with someone who is HIV-positive, and you're not sharing needles, he/she poses no risk to you. In fact, it works the other way around. AIDS does not make you a disease-spreader: it makes you *vulnerable* to diseases, because your immune system is damaged. Minor infections that would never debilitate a healthy person can be life-threatening to people with AIDS. So if you are not infected with AIDS, and have the flu, and come into contact with someone with AIDS, you are putting *them* at risk. Keep this in mind the next time you find yourself afraid of someone with AIDS. Unless you are being exposed to their bodily fluids through sex or needles, your fears are irrational, and ostracizing a sick person serves no good purpose whatsoever.

Symptoms of HIV and AIDS in Women.
Some women will have chronic, low-grade problems while they are sick with HIV but not yet hit by full-blown AIDS. For women, these symptoms include chronic yeast infections and chronic flu-like symptoms. (Of course, these are quite common and can occur in HIV-negative women as well.) Dr. Deborah Cotton, an infectious disease specialist at the Massachusetts General Hospital, is concerned that many doctors and women themselves continue to ignore possible signs of HIV infection. If you have recurrent yeast infections despite treatment, she says, and no other explanation for them (such as diabetes or pregnancy), and you think you could have been exposed to HIV, you should be tested.

If you have had chronic gynecological problems—infections that return over and over again after treatment, terrible bouts with infections like herpes and yeast that cause others much less discomfort than they do you—and weight loss or other signs of poor health, talk to your doctor about having a test for HIV. You very well may *not* have HIV—but if you do, you'll be able to start life-prolonging treatment sooner.

For some, there are no early symptoms at all. As AIDS progresses, and the body's key immune cells start to deplete, more serious symptoms set in. When AIDS is in full effect, the symptoms are devastating, including everything from fevers, vision loss, pain, nausea, vomiting and wasting to cancer, pneumonia, seizures and ultimately death.

Women are often diagnosed with AIDS later than men are, and women also die faster than men with AIDS. Perhaps these two facts are linked: late diagnosis and treatment can make for a far worse prognosis. As we'll discuss later, AIDS treatment relies on delaying or suppressing symptoms, not eradicating them—so late diagnosis means falling behind at a crucial time. Much of the early research on AIDS drugs was conducted on men, which only adds to the relative dearth of information on women and AIDS.

Generally, HIV has hit populations of poor, minority women harder than middle-class caucasian women. Dr. Cotton says the disease is spreading fastest among young women of color in cities along the Atlantic seaboard, the rural south and major urban centers like L.A. and Chicago. According to the CDC, for every one caucasian woman diagnosed with HIV, 13.2 African-American women and 8.1 Hispanic women are diagnosed with it. For this reason, white, middle-class women have too long thought of themselves as immune to the problem. This is far from the case. While the middle-class white woman from Indiana is less likely to become infected than an African-American woman living in inner-city Newark, New Jersey, HIV is color-, education- and income-blind.

Dr. Fauci points out a worrisome potential parallel between women and gay men in the AIDS epidemic. Since gay men were initially hardest hit by the AIDS epidemic, that population started practicing much safer sex and, in some cities, infection rates started to level off. However, younger gay men who don't have as many friends and lovers infected with HIV have stopped protecting themselves as carefully—they don't perceive themselves to be at high risk, and their HIV rates have started to climb. Fauci predicts a similar problem among middle-class women who just don't believe they're an "at-risk" group: they don't practice safe sex, and their rates of HIV infection are increasing (albeit slowly). With time, this population stands to be at just as great a risk as any other. The moral of the story is if you're human, and you don't protect yourself, you *are* at risk.

Treating HIV Infection and AIDS.

There is no cure for AIDS, and no way to get rid of HIV. However, the disease can both be delayed and controlled to a certain extent with a variety of drugs. The first drug approved for treating AIDS was AZT (zidovudine or azidothymidine). Since then, several more have been approved, including DDI (didanosine) and DDC (dideoxycytidine). Just as cancer treatment often involves using several drugs in combination to get the best possible effect, so AIDS treatment has evolved to include multidrug treatment. Not only is the disease fought better this way, but drug resistance (when the drug stops working as well for you) is sometimes lessened when drugs are used in combination, or alternated.

One of the main goals of treating AIDS is to ward off the so-called opportunistic infections that make patients sicker, and often cause death. One of the most common of these diseases is Pneumocystis carinii pneumonia (PCP). Aerosolized pentamidine and other drugs can be used to prevent and treat this lethal infection. Many other drugs are used to treat the various fungal infections, wasting syndromes and other problems associated with both HIV infection and full-blown AIDS. With proper diet and treatment for the powerful physical and emotional trials of HIV infection, patients can be kept alive and well for several years. Drug therapy may help extend the disease-free period as well. What many people *don't* know, however, is that there are people out there living relatively healthy, productive lives *with* AIDS. I spent some time with one such individual while working on a story for CBS. He had full-blown AIDS for 6 years already, and was still working and socializing. Good medical care goes a long way to keeping AIDS patients alive. (Of course, it's also *very* expensive.) The longer they live, the better their chance of being here when a cure is found. Vaccine research for HIV is also marching forward, with the hope that early versions of vaccines might be helpful as treatments for people who are already infected.

So if you are diagnosed HIV-positive, do not give up hope. You only had to watch Magic Johnson coaching the Los Angeles Lakers or winning an Olympic gold medal if you needed an example of someone living life to the fullest with HIV. Immediately get counseling if you are found to carry the AIDS virus, since you are sure to experience a flood of difficult emotions. With time, though, as you absorb the news and get back up on your feet, you owe it to yourself and your loved ones not to give up before you've given a good fight. Access the excellent care that's now out there for people with HIV and AIDS.

EMOTIONAL ISSUES OF SEXUALLY TRANSMITTED DISEASES

Unfortunately, since our society attaches such a stigma to sexually transmitted infections, it can be emotionally traumatic to be diagnosed with one. To make matters worse, since many people discover an infection through infidelity (or at least suspect infidelity is involved), the emotional issues are even more charged.

Being diagnosed as having a noncurable, viral STD is sometimes hardest to handle, since people must deal with the idea that they will have this condition forever. Peggy Clarke of the American Social Health Association says that 80% of those diagnosed with herpes report feelings of depression; over half fear rejection by loved ones. Those with HPV report anger, depression and feelings of isolation. Dr. Richard Keeling, director of University Health Services at the University of Wisconsin in Madison, finds a strong connection between having an STD and low self-esteem. The relationship works two ways, he says: on the one hand, having an STD makes many women feel "tainted" or "damaged"; also having low self-esteem to begin with may predispose women to getting STDs, since it might prevent them from protecting themselves.

Dr. Keeling also notes that there are differences in the way men and women react to the diagnosis of an STD. Women are more likely to see themselves as less acceptable and somehow blameworthy or undesirable, while men are less self-deprecating on the whole. Keeling suggests that since our society paints male sexual activity as "prowess" and women's as "slutty," women bear the brunt of the negatives associated with sexuality. Thus a man with an STD may be perceived as "unlucky," while a woman with the same diagnosis is seen as culpable. We must fight these stereotypes in order to lessen women's emotional burden with STDs.

What's the best way to deal with emotional pain after you're diagnosed with an STD? First, get information: the more you know about the disease, the less it will frighten you. Next, if you can, share your worries with someone you can trust. Bottling the news up inside like a terrible secret is more painful over time, and besides, these diseases are so common, you're likely to discover you're not alone if you share the information. Seek counseling if you are feeling extremely depressed—and if you think it would help, find support groups and/or newsletters from groups like the American Social Health Association with supportive information about your disease (for more information, see the information section at the end of this chapter). Dr. Keeling urges women diagnosed with STDs to take good holistic care of themselves, eating well, resting and reducing stress in other areas of their lives. Not only might this decrease your chance of triggering a latent infection (like herpes), but it will make you better able to cope with the emotions you are feeling. And above all, remember that nothing about you—the inner you—has changed since you were diagnosed with an STD.

WHO'S AT RISK FOR STDS?

If you are sexually active—and that includes genital, anal, oral and other forms of sex—you are at risk for sexually transmitted diseases. It doesn't matter what you look like, what you wear, what kinds of friends and family you have: YOU ARE NOT IMMUNE!

The more sexual partners you have—or the more partners your partner has—the greater your risk. Sevgi Aral notes that many women who turn up in STD clinics were actually monogamous: their spouses or partners, however, were not. It's a painful way to learn about an infidelity. If you do not use condoms every single time you have sex, your risk of STDs climbs significantly. And condoms, while protective, give no guarantees.

There's a trend that's been noticed recently by STD researchers, and it's called "serial monogamy." With serial monogamy, people have only one sexual partner at a time, but they move from one partner to another after a limited period of time. People who are serially monogamous tend to think of themselves as "not promiscuous," and therefore not at high risk of STDs—after all, if you're just having sex with one person at a time, that doesn't seem so risky. Well, it is: each time you switch sex partners, you open yourself up to his or her collection of diseases (whoever came up with the line "Whenever you have sex with someone, you have sex with everyone they've ever had sex with, too" was right). Don't kid yourself. Whether you've had one sexual partner, one at a time, or ten different ones in a week—you're *all* at risk. Keep it simple: if you are sexually active, you're at risk for an STD, and you should be examined by a doctor regularly.

SYMPTOMS OF STDS: KNOWING WHEN TO WORRY

As I've mentioned, many STDs are silent—they create no symptoms at all. That's one reason you might want to pause before getting too angry at someone who "gives" you an STD—they may not have known they had it in the first place.

Occasionally, however—you might say for the lucky, since they'll be alerted to seek help—STDs do cause symptoms. These include abnormal discharge; blood or smell from the vagina or rectum (or the penis); burning during urination; itching in the vaginal or rectal area; pain during intercourse (or sometimes during the doctor's physical exam); generalized pain in the genitals, buttocks, legs, or abdomen; visible sores or warts on or near the genitals; swelling, pain or irritation of the genitals or rectum or surrounding area; swollen glands near the genitals or in the neck. If you have a male sex partner, he might notice any of the above symptoms plus a drip from the penis or pain in the testicles. Since men are more likely than women to have symptoms from STDs, be sure to communicate openly with your sex partners—and take a good look at his genitals when you get the chance. (The presence of a sore or other lesion should give you cause for concern but the absence of visible disease is no guarantee that your partner is STD free.) You may not be a specialist, but if you see sores or discharge or unusual irritation, speak up.

PREVENTING STD

The only way to prevent STDs is to abstain from all sexual contact and, in the case of AIDS, needle sharing. If you abstain, you are virtually guaranteed no STDs. There are of course certain exceptions—for instance, you might get pubic lice from using someone's unclean towel—but these instances are extremely rare. Often, cases that are blamed on toilet seats and hot tubs were really contracted elsewhere. This has been a big problem with diagnosing sexual abuse of children: when children are found to have STDs, towels are frequently blamed—incorrectly.

If you choose to remain sexually active, there are ways you can protect yourself—but there are no guarantees. To begin, Sevgi Aral recommends that every woman have an STD screening test two months after starting a sexual relationship with a new partner. Since many of us practice "serial monogamy"—that is, we have one sexual partner at a time, but several over a lifetime—we must recognize that we are at new risk with each new partner. Don't fall into the trap of thinking your partner is "not that kind of person." Sexually transmitted bacteria and viruses know nothing about your personality or morals; they like warm, moist skin and blood when they can get it.

First on the prevention list: condom use. The data varies, but experts agree that with *regular, correct* use of condoms *for all sexual acts,* oral, genital and anal, your risk of STDs drops dramatically. Aral worries that while more unmarried women are using condoms (the good news) they are *not* using them consistently (the bad news). Condoms are of significantly less value if you fail to use them every single time you have sex.

How to Use Condoms Properly.[2]
The fact is, since unwanted pregnancy rates are high in this country, and STD rates are soaring, we know that people aren't using condoms often enough—or if they're using them, they're not doing so consistently or correctly. For young people, the deterrent might be embarrassment, says Dr. Penny Hitchcock of the NIH. Condoms were shoplifted at such a high rate they were moved behind the counter in most stores; now, many young people are ashamed to ask for them. Another major deterrent to using condoms is that sex doesn't feel as good to the man when he's wearing one (we've all heard the "taking a shower with a raincoat on" line). While it can be very hard for some women to insist their partners use condoms, try to remind yourself each time you have sex what the consequences could be if you got an STD. Also ask yourself if you really want to have sex with someone who won't protect himself or you. In many cases, if really faced with the prospect of not having sex at all, men will use a condom. If you're threatened with the line, "I'll just find someone who won't make me use one"—again, ask yourself: Is this someone with whom I should be sharing my body?

You've probably heard of people who used condoms and still contracted STDs. There are several explanations. First, many people who use condoms use them *improperly.* Next, they *say* they use condoms, but they don't use them for each and every sexual act. Third, they don't use them with *all* of their sex partners. Finally, of course, condoms aren't perfect—even when used perfectly. They can tear, slip off or otherwise fail to give 100% protection. Abstinence is the *only* 100% guarantee. If you plan to be sexually active, know your risks, and take these precautions:

---

[2]Information on proper condom use is from the Department of Health and Human Services.

Unroll the condom onto the erect penis *before you have any sexual contact*. Many people are tempted to start sexual foreplay before putting on the condom—this increases the chance that you'll transmit a disease, and also puts you at risk of getting carried away with passion and not using the condom at all. Certainly don't let the penis enter your body without a condom if you are trying to protect yourself from disease.

Use latex condoms, not natural lambskin ones. Viruses and bacteria can't usually get through latex; they can get through natural skin condoms. Certainly natural condoms are better than using nothing at all, but they fall quite short of latex in terms of protection.

Be sure to leave some space (about a half inch) between the end of the condom and the end of the penis. This is where the semen will be caught. If the condom is too tight, there's nowhere for the semen to go, and the condom might burst.

Use a lubricant to help keep the condom from tearing. Always choose a water-based lubricant *not* an oil-based one like petroleum jelly. See a list of good water-based lubricants beginning on page 255.

Keep the condom on during the entire sexual act (whatever that act may be, vaginal-penile intercourse, oral sex, anal sex, etc.) and hold it by the rim as your partner "pulls out" so it doesn't slip off and spill semen into your body.

Never reuse condoms, and make sure to use ones that are still moist and strong (they should be stored in a cool, dry place and not for too long—wallets and glove compartments are *not* good long-term storage spaces for condoms). If the condom is dry or brittle or shriveled when you take it out, choose another one.

Add spermicidal jelly to your condom routine, putting a little bit (not so much that it slips) inside the tip of the condom before you unroll it onto your partner's penis, and/or inserting some into your vagina before sex. Spermicidal agents like nonoxynol-9 are thought to kill some viruses and may help protect against STDs. If your skin becomes irritated or abraded when you use these agents, however, avoid them, since by breaking your skin you may make yourself *more* vulnerable to infection.

Check for tears! A condom with a hole in it isn't much better than no condom at all.

FOR MORE INFORMATION ON STDs (INCLUDING HIV AND AIDS)

HERPES INFORMATION LINE
919-361-8488

NATIONAL STD HOTLINE
800-227-8922

NATIONAL AIDS INFORMATION CLEARINGHOUSE AT THE U.S. CENTERS FOR DISEASE CONTROL AND PREVENTION
P. O. Box 6003
Rockville, MD 20849-6003
800-458-5231
TTY: 800-243-7012

AIDS CLINICAL TRIALS INFORMATION
SERVICE (ACTIS)
800-TRIALS-A

CDC NATIONAL AIDS HOTLINE
800-342-AIDS (24 hours) or 800-AIDS-TTY,
or in Spanish, 800-344-SIDA

AWARE: ASSOCIATION FOR WOMEN'S
AIDS RESEARCH AND EDUCATION
San Francisco General Hospital
Building 90, Ward 95
955 Potrero
San Francisco, CA 94111
415-476-4091

AMERICAN FOUNDATION FOR AIDS
RESEARCH (AMFAR)
733 3rd Ave., 12th Floor
New York, NY 10017
212-682-7440

WARN: WOMEN AND AIDS RESOURCE
NETWORK
55 Johnson Street
General Building
Suite 303
New York, NY 10017

NATIONAL LESBIAN AND GAY HEALTH
FOUNDATION
1638 R St. NW, Suite 2
Washington, DC 20009
202-797-3708

AMERICAN SOCIAL HEALTH
ASSOCIATION
P. O. Box 13827
Research Triangle Park, NC 27709
National STD Hotline: 800-227-8922
Herpes Resource Center: 800-230-6039
Live Counselor: 919-361-8488

NATIONAL INSTITUTE OF ALLERGY
AND INFECTIOUS DISEASES
9000 Rockville Pike
Building 31, Room 7A50
Bethesda, MD 20892
301-496-5717

AMERICAN FOUNDATION FOR AIDS
RESEARCH
733 3rd Ave., 12th Floor
New York, NY 10017
212-682-7400

NATIONAL ASSOCIATION OF PEOPLE
WITH AIDS
1413 K Street NW, 7th Floor
Washington, DC 20005
202-898-0414

NATIONAL LESBIAN AND GAY HEALTH
ASSOCIATION
1407 S Street NW
Washington, DC 20009
202-797-3536

CHAPTER FOURTEEN

Problems with Sex

Sex is something I really don't understand too hot. You never know where the hell you are. I keep making up these sex rules for myself and then I break them right away.

—J. D. Salinger, *The Catcher in the Rye*

There is nothing more personal, more unique, or more private than one's sexual "personality." Sure, we talk with our friends about particularly funny, special or original sexual experiences. We tell about important sexual "firsts" as we grow older, daring places we've "done it," and so on. As working or parenting adults, we may joke about our sex lives as casualties of long hours, but we only joke. Overall, we tend to share only—or certainly *mostly*—the good news, not the bad. For the most part, women hold deep-rooted or persistent sexual problems as close to the vest as most any other intensely personal issue or problem. And partly because of that secrecy, these problems often fester, grow more serious and, worst of all, *persist*.

Part of the trouble is that it's hard to admit that one has a sexual problem when passionate, uninhibited sexuality is flaunted before us as a norm. You can't purchase an automobile or a bottle of perfume, can't watch TV or make it down the street without some reminder of the prevalence of raw, healthy sexuality. What would a billboard be without scantily clad women and men who can't seem to keep their hands off of each other, lustful becoming glances, outright references to sexual prowess. Because this society has defined sexiness, male promiscuity and a love of sex as a healthy norm, and those who have sexual problems or a lack of interest in sex as deviant or troubled, it's hard to acknowledge sexual problems—even to oneself. Well you might feel better after you take a look at some new, scientifically reputable data on Americans' sexual habits published by University of Chicago researchers in 1994. After interviewing 1,285 people aged 18–59,

Professor Edward Laumann and colleagues found a sexual landscape that was more sober than steamy. As we'll discuss in a moment, lack of desire and problems with orgasm are rampant. Only one in sixteen women had more than ten sexual partners; only one in a hundred women finds group sex appealing; 45% of current sex partners have known each other for at least a year, 85% for at least a month. Laumann also says there is a true battle of the sexes in sexuality; with dramatic differences in what "turns on" women and men. Many people with sexual problems convince themselves that their problems are temporary, or connect them with their partner and not themselves. Or perhaps they bring themselves to talk to health care professionals about a sexual problem, only to meet *their* embarrassed reactions in place of sound advice.

Another obstacle to getting good advice about trouble with sexual function is that it's hard to define a sexual "problem." After all, each of us is unique, and our mode of sexual expression is highly individualized. What's to say one person's "problem" isn't "normal" for someone else?

The best way to define a sexual problem for *you* is to answer the following questions: Do you enjoy sex? Did you ever enjoy sex? Do you or *have you ever* looked forward to sex? If you have an aversion to sex, is it because sex hurts you physically? Emotionally? Have you had disturbing experiences with sex in your past—such as forced sex with a stranger, or with someone you know? (Professor Laumann's study reveals that 22% of women were forced to do something sexual they did not want to do in the past 12 months—a disturbing statistic.) Has a past partner made you feel inadequate about sex, or made you take part in sexual acts that made you

uncomfortable or angry? Do you have sexually transmitted infections—or have you had them in the past—that make you physically or psychologically uncomfortable about sex? Have you ever had an orgasm—and do you ever have them now? There are a great many more issues related to, or blocking, "normal" sexual function—but these are a few of the leading ones.

Keep two key things in mind as you go through this chapter. First, there is no such thing as a "normal" sexual appetite. For some happy, loving couples, sex once every couple of weeks is just perfect. For others, breakfast wouldn't be complete if it weren't followed or preceded by sex. Some desire oral sex and have less interest in traditional sexual intercourse. Some love anal sex—others staunchly refuse to try it. None of these variations is more "normal" than the others. "Normal" or "healthy" for *you* means that you are comfortable with the idea and the practice of sex in some way, and that you are feeling sexually fulfilled by/with your sex partner(s). (These days, healthy sex also means *protection*—so if you have multiple partners, or your partners have multiple partners, do use condoms.) The second thing to keep in mind comes from sex therapist Judith Seifer. After years of successful sex counseling, Seifer finds that the only way to overcome sexual problems is to adopt the "this is the first day of the rest of your life" outlook. If you insist on remaining mired in the problems of the past, nagging your partner or yourself about sexual failures and complaining about lost years, you will never move forward successfully. The problems will be perpetuated, and you will not be satisfied. On the other hand, if you move ahead positively and commit yourself to sexual healing, you can recharge your sexual life at any age.

TYPES OF SEXUAL PROBLEMS COMMON AMONG WOMEN

LACK OF DESIRE

According to the University of Chicago report, nearly one in three women lacked interest in sex for at least two months in the past year. Nearly one in five reported that sex was not pleasurable, adds Professor Laumann, and among women who were forced to have some type of sex at some point, more than one in three lacked pleasure with sex.

There are naturally different degrees of "lack of desire." Sometimes, as we'll discuss below, we have a temporary lapse in our interest in sex. This is generally normal, short-lived, and caused by the outside interferences of a hectic modern life. At the other end of the spectrum, however, is total disinterest in sex: a feeling that you can't stand to be touched, or can never get aroused during sex. Perhaps your mind tells you you're not interested—or your vagina, which stays tight and dry, tells you the same thing. Early in a sexual relationship, you might brush this off as beginner's jitters or shyness with a new partner. But in longer-standing relationships—or if this happens to you in *all* sexual situations—there might be a more serious problem.

The most dire explanation for total lack of sexual desire—and one that has received a great deal of attention in the media and entertainment recently—is prior sexual abuse of some kind. In fact, while this horrible problem is quite real and deserving of long-term, formal therapy, it is *not* the cause of *most* cases of impaired desire. Some sex therapists are concerned that the sexual abuse "excuse" is being pushed too hard by experts, creating a "false memory syndrome" in which alleged victims

are led to "remember" events that never actually happened. If you, or a doctor or therapist believe that sexual abuse might be your problem, it is vital that you consult an expert or two in this area for counseling and treatment. With the right support, long-term therapy can help you regain your self-esteem and your ability to someday see the good in sex for the first time.

Other more common causes of decreased desire are much more mundane. Your relationship may simply have become stale due to busy schedules, a lack of appreciation for one another, or other life interruptions. Judith Seifer sees lots of women filling multiple life roles—employee, parent, wife, caretaker of older parents—who have come to see sex as just another thing they *have* to get done in a day. For these overtaxed women, sex becomes a chore, and with fatigue at the end of the day, often it's the chore that has to go. Worse yet, many women self-medicate with alcohol or other relaxants to make sex tolerable or interesting at the end of a long day, just to avoid saying "no" to their partners one more time.

The solution? Some experts say sex must be put at the top, not the bottom, of the priority list or it will become yet another casualty of too-busy modern lives. Doing the laundry, having dinner with friends, letting a cranky child fall asleep in your bed, making that one extra night-time business call might all have to be forfeited or postponed if you intend to keep your sexual relationship alive. While it might seem easy to put sex last, since you feel that your partner, more than anyone else, should be understanding, you may in fact be doing permanent damage to your relationship. Some say ignoring your own—and your partner's—sexual needs is a sure way to lead one or both of you into an affair. But worse than that, most experts feel, is the risk that your sexual relationship will get away from you permanently—that you will turn around one day in a few months when your schedule clears, and find that passion didn't wait around for you to make time for it.

Libbey Livingston, codirector of the Seattle Sexual Health Center, is seeing a lot of sexual problems among women with new babies—especially among those who waited until later in life to become parents. Some of these older moms have become accustomed to a romantic, just-the-two-of-us relationship in which sex is spontaneous, and energy and desire are high. With a new baby keeping them awake at night, the demands of parenting on their mind most of the time, sex moves to the back burner—and as the chicken and egg story goes, as desire drops, the less sex they have. Livingston counsels couples to feel okay about "grieving" over the loss of their freedom as a couple, and to learn to salvage romantic time together—albeit rare. Having a good caretaker helps a lot, she notes: couples who feel comfortable leaving their babies behind tend to revive their romance more easily, since their minds aren't tied to home at every second.

Sometimes, long-term repressed anger or resentment about things that have nothing to do with sex can impede sexual interest or maybe your heartfelt feelings about your partner are showing themselves physically: perhaps you are simply not attracted to this person, and you're trying to force it. Or it could be that your sexual styles are different, and even though you're attracted to one another, you can't seem to make your sex "fit"—so you grow less interested in trying. There are as many reasons for impaired sexual desire as there are people hav-

ing sex. The key is to find an expert on sexual function who can help you figure out *your* particular issue or problem, and get to work on solving it. I can't stress enough how much insight many of these counselors have when it comes to uncovering hidden sources of sexual tension. They've seen it all.

According to sex therapist and author Lonnie Barbach, one crucial step in determining the cause of lack of desire is learning if a woman is *ever,* or is *generally,* positive in her thinking about sex. If you had a fulfilling sexual relationship with someone in the past, and find yourself uninterested in sex *now,* it's possible that your situation may be solved with relative ease. For instance, hard as it may be to admit this to yourself, it's possible that you simply are not sexually attracted to your current partner. This can be very painful to admit, especially if the relationship is strong on other grounds—honesty, friendship, companionship. You will have to decide—and a sex therapist can help you—if it's enough for you to live with a "dear friend" or if you need a fulfilling sexual relationship at this time in your life.

If you *once* had a fulfilling sexual relationship with your partner, sex therapists can often help you rebuild sexual relationships "gone dry." A variety of sexual games, romantic scene-making, and bringing back playful or spontaneous sex can give a jump-start to failing sexual relationships. Working on bringing sexual fantasy back into your love life can take some creativity and thought, but it can liven the dullest relationships. Mutual masturbation can help revive or intensify a relationship in which orgasm has become too routine. There are a surprising number of ways to make sex more exciting and therefore pique your desire to come back for more. And the good news is that a loss of desire in an otherwise healthy relationship is often "curable" with *short-term* counseling: there's usually no need to delve into deep, long-term therapy to find answers. Lonnie Barbach urges self-help "tricks" like leaving sexy cards in your partner's underwear drawer or on the fridge, dressing up for dates and encouraging your partner to do the same, wearing your partner's favorite perfume and other such turn-ons that particularly appeal to the two of you.

Barbach also stresses that in her practice, it's the couples who *talk* to each other for at least 20 minutes a day who "make it"—and those who never connect with each other in areas *other* than sex who are doomed. Remember, she says, there is 30% less leisure time today than ten years ago—so make the most of it, or you're likely to regret it. If you're suffering from a lack of desire, ask yourself: When was the last time you really tried to turn your partner on—or vice versa? Maybe it's time to turn up the heat a little. With sex, as with anything else, you tend to get out what you put in. The worst thing you can do is to get caught in a 1-2-3 sexual routine that becomes automatic and mindless.

While some people are embarrassed to take their problems to a sex counselor, those who do go are amazed at the range of creative options out there that can make a sexual relationship strong—or stronger, even if it's pretty good already. Remember, there is nothing you can tell a sex counselor that she/he hasn't heard before. What you think is embarrassing conversation—and maybe your family doctor blushed at, too—is old hat to the sex therapist. I was amused when sex therapist Beatrice (Bean) Robinson of the Minnesota Medical Center Program on Human Sexuality said, quite mat-

ter-of-factly, "Sex is like tennis. Just let it flow, don't use your mind too much—but still you must focus." I could see that sex was, to her—and to others in her field—much like any other physical activity or skill (though perhaps a little more sacred). And as with other skills, sex therapists know that with practice and information, you can get better at it; that is, more excited about it, more interested in it, more creative about it, more giving and more orgasmic. Robinson also finds that couples who go for treatment of sexual dysfunction tend to have much stronger relationships than those who choose marital therapy. That's because, she finds, those who come for sex therapy often feel that their relationships are extremely strong and successful in areas *other than* sex. If there is a loving, firm underlying bond, and if there was *ever* a sexual relationship, therapy is likely to bring it back.

Still another cause of low sexual desire is low levels of the male hormone testosterone. Women have some testosterone in our bodies, too—and some clinicians find that giving extremely small doses to women with low sexual desire (especially postmenopausally) can increase sex drive.

Finally, a major cause of sexual apathy in women is depression. As we discuss in detail in chapter 17, depression is unusually common in women and one of the key signs is a lack of interest in sex, as well as apathy to other activities. Full-blown depression can mask your real feelings about other people and activities, blunting passions and interests that you once held dear. Sadly, the problem can become circular: You feel depressed or chronically tired and removed—you stay at work more hours or remove yourself from social situations—and you become more depressed and isolated. Before you let a sexual relationship die, look into some of the reasons you have become apathetic. Ask yourself if you experience joy in other aspects of life or if disinterest in sex is part of a broader pattern. Seek help from a qualified professional who is trained to treat depression (*see* the information section at the end of this chapter).

Sex therapist Shirley Zussman, editor of the "Sex Over 40" newsletter in New York City, makes an important observation about "normal" sexual desire. Rather than remaining at a constant "high," our interest in sex ebbs and flows like other interests, depending on what's happening in our lives. Normal, healthy sexual relationships have ups and downs just as all kinds of relationships do. The birth of a new child, an extremely pressured time at work for you or for your partner, having an in-law as a house guest in a small apartment—these and countless other interruptions can change the course of sexual relations for a time, she says. With healthy sexual function, a high interest in sex resumes in time. In other cases, when sexual activity becomes so rusty that you find you've lost interest in it altogether, it may be time to get help.

PROBLEMS WITH ORGASM

According to the University of Chicago study, more than one in five women were unable to experience orgasm for several months in the last year.

Trouble having an orgasm—or never having one in the first place—is another common sexual problem for women. Sometimes, again, the reason is simple and mechanical: for instance, if you can have an orgasm with manual stimulation (your own or your partner's hand), but you can't have one during intercourse, often the problem is *positional.* For most women, the clitoris must be stimulated in order to achieve orgasm, and depending on your own and your partner's body shapes, it's possible that the clitoris will get little or no stimulation during traditional intercourse. Bean Robinson hears this complaint frequently, and finds it relatively easy to treat. Sex therapists often recommend changing the position of sex: woman-on-top, for instance, provides much more clitoral stimulation and is often quite satisfying for men, as well. Or, if you're more comfortable with traditional sex, perhaps you'll have to learn to ask your partner for manual stimulation during or after intercourse in order to reach orgasm. These kinds of simple changes can make a big difference in your enjoyment of sex and your ability to have orgasms more often.

In other cases, the orgasm problem is more serious. For example, some women have never been able to achieve orgasm—or, while they can give themselves an orgasm, they cannot have one with a partner, regardless of the position or technique used. Sometimes this comes about as a fact of habit: if you have masturbated over the course of many years but have not had sexual partners, you might be "trained" to respond only to a particular type of touch. Or, if you're unfamiliar with the sexual workings of your body, and/or have had partners with the same degree of ignorance, you might not know how to have an orgasm in the first place. In other cases, the problem is psychologically based. The "treatment" for this problem requires retraining in the enjoyment of sex. It requires a great deal of patience from both you and your partner, can take time, and can be very frustrating. Sometimes just *trying* to have an orgasm can put a damper on the whole sexual experience, leaving both you and your partner feeling inadequate. This is a case where sexual counseling can be extremely valuable in protecting your relationship as you learn to grow together sexually. Sometimes a counselor or moderator can steer you away from the blaming and anger that often arise out of sexual differences and dissatisfaction.

Libbey Livingston cites yet another common cause of lack of orgasm: that is, the inability to *talk* about orgasm in the first place. She blames women—especially mothers—for not telling their daughters about orgasm and how to achieve it. She contrasts this silence to the relative openness (and perhaps machismo) of sexual discussions between fathers and sons. If more older women told younger women about how to achieve orgasm, we would come to expect it and perfect it, she insists. Keeping up the silence just means that more women will remain oblivious to the pleasure they *could* be experiencing.

According to Dr. William Masters, the well-known director of the Masters and Johnson Institute in St. Louis and author of the book *Heterosexuality,* many orgasm problems can be cured with self-help techniques. Here are a few of his recommendations:

1. Experiment with different sensations, touching your genitals with different objects and textures to see what arouses you the most. Some of his suggestions include fur, silk, velvet or water from a handheld shower nozzle.

2. Think sexual thoughts when trying to achieve orgasm. Let your mind wander into whatever sexual fantasy interests you.

3. Go through the motions of what you think an orgasm should be like—actually making the sounds and movements (for example, crying "yes-yes-yes-yes-yes!") that you associate with orgasm. Dr. Masters even recommends role-playing the aftereffects of an orgasm—what he calls the "warm afterglow."

4. Try using a vibrator, not just to achieve orgasm, but to learn what kinds of touch—how fast, how hard, how gentle—appeal to you.

Sometimes, nonsexual health problems can block your ability to achieve orgasm. Alcoholism and depression are two common examples. If you have a chronic health problem or trouble with substance abuse, getting the right treatment for that problem will sometimes eliminate the sexual difficulties as well.

Successful treatment of lack of orgasm takes, depending on the cause, somewhere between four and ten months on average, and first involves finding the source of the problem through talk therapy, and following up with sexual exercises and "games" to bring about orgasm.

Pain with Sex

When sex hurts, many women give up on it. How could it possibly be exciting or pleasurable when it causes pain? they ask themselves—and are soon resigned to being asexual people. Professor Laumann reports that 13% of women have had pain with sex for a significant period of time over the last 12 months. There are many causes for painful sex, and unfortunately, several of them are becoming more common these days. For instance, some sexually transmitted diseases—and the treatments used for them—can damage the delicate vaginal tissues and make sex quite painful. One example is laser surgery and other treatments commonly used to treat human papillomavirus. The procedure can damage the normal tissues of the vagina as well as those with signs of the virus. The result: less lubrication, and less flexibility of the vaginal tissues. Even if you feel excited about sex in your *mind,* your body can make it difficult for you.

Years ago, sexual theorists believed that most sexual problems were of psychological origin. Today, we know of countless medical problems and other physiological issues that can make sex painful or unpleasant. The more we learn about the physical body and sex, the more treatments become available to help women enjoy sex again—and the less often women are sent home with the hint that they've dreamed up their problem. Frequent causes of pain during sex that can be detected more easily with today's techniques include endometriosis, certain fibroid tumors, chronic yeast infections, and pelvic inflammatory disease (these are discussed further in chapter 7).

Sometimes, pain with sex disappears—or at least recedes—after treatment. What's troubling for many women, however, is that some of these problems can be hard to treat—or can recur even after successful initial treatment. It's important to coordinate the work of both the practitioner who's treating the physical problem and a sex counselor, for together they may be able to maximize your ability to engage in and enjoy sex sooner.

Another serious sexual problem for women, called vaginismus, causes severe pain during intercourse. The problem here is in the outer musculature of the vagina. With vaginismus, there can be tremendous tightness and pain with the insertion of any object into the vagina; a penis, finger, tampon or speculum at the doctor's office can be equally traumatic. Treatment can be successful if it is undertaken slowly and patiently and takes into consideration the cause(s) of the excruciating pain. Some common causes of vaginismus include a feeling of shame about intercourse or sexual relations, whether for religious or other reasons connected to one's upbringing; prior sexual abuse (here is a case where sexual abuse may be more prevalent as a cause of sexual dysfunction); or prior medical procedures that left scarring or other problems in the vagina.

Vaginismus is most successfully treated with both talk therapy and a gradual, slow process of stretching the vagina so it becomes accustomed to admitting various objects. You might start by inserting a tiny, thin, smooth object slowly and gently and letting it stay in your vagina for a brief period of time. Next, you'll move up to a larger object—perhaps the slimmest brand of tampon available. Next, you may move on to a finger. All the while, you and your partner work on massaging the perineal muscle (*see* chapter 3, "Your Reproductive Anatomy") so it becomes looser and more receptive. With time, many women with even severe vaginismus can succeed in having penile intercourse without pain. Eventually, a lack of pain can progress to actual *enjoyment* of sex—something about which these women know precious little. Effective treatment of vaginismus usually takes four to six months.

Counseling can be particularly important for the couple that has lived with chronic sexual pain over a long period of time. The reason: the sex partner of a woman who suffers pain during intercourse often becomes averse to sex him/herself. Over time, the partner becomes fearful of causing pain, and guilty about trying to have sex when it isn't pleasant for the other person. Or, it just starts to seem like too much work. Remember to keep your partner's feelings in mind as well as your own, and attend to them before your sexual relationship becomes permanently damaged.

Many people with sexual problems have more than one cause or type of sexual dysfunction. Robinson finds that about half to three-quarters of her patients have at least two of the above-mentioned common sexual problems—lack of desire, problems with intercourse and pain with sex.

SEXUAL "FIT"

The old-fashioned concept of "good chemistry" or a sexual "fit" is more than romantic fiction. Lonnie Barbach sees couples who love each other dearly, but whose sexual relations are always strained because their styles are so different. Perhaps one is a "puppy" and the other a "medieval dramatist"—Barbach's favorite examples. Each is turned off by the other's sexual style. She recommends to these couples a "my week, your week" game in which partners alternate taking control of the style of sex each week. For instance, when the "puppy" is in charge, sex is cuddly, sweet, gentle and giggly. When the medieval dramatist runs the week, sex is passionate, serious, sweep-you-off-your-feet dramatic (on the dinner table with the dishes pushed aside might be a good example).

The only rule, Barbach adds, is that neither partner can make the other perform a particular sex act with which he or she is uncomfortable. The environment, the setting, the mood, the clothing, are all part of the game, however. This technique has proved extremely popular among couples, particularly for the partner who felt her or his "style" of sexual play was getting short shrift.

Of course, at some point, a lack of sexual fit can terminate a relationship. Unless there is some basis for attraction to one another that distinguishes the relationship from a simple friendship, no counselor can create what isn't there to build on. Sometimes, a sex therapist can help salvage what's left of the good feeling between two people who care about one another but just can't make it work in bed. This can be an especially painful situation when *one* person feels unattracted, while the other still feels passion.

Extramarital Affairs.

Judith Seifer has seen an apparent big surge in the number of extramarital affairs in recent years. She attributes some of the new problems to women's appearance in the workplace: whereas in the past, men were much more likely to "trip over" sexual encounters outside the home (on business trips, in the office), now women are running into the same opportunities—and taking them.

Seifer and others insist that affairs often do *not* signal the end of a marriage. Surprisingly, while they can be devastating to deal with, they give couples a *goal* to work toward—and many couples grow stronger as a result of the healing process.

SEXUAL DIFFERENCES BETWEEN MEN AND WOMEN THAT CAN SEEM LIKE PROBLEMS

You must always bear in mind that there are some basic differences between the way men and women experience and appreciate sex—and that these differences need not get in the way of a healthy sex life. Sometimes just being aware of the differences can turn an apparent problem into a simple reality that you can live with.

For instance, after having an orgasm, men have a brief "refractory" period in which they physically cannot have another orgasm. How long that period lasts relates to several issues—the man's personal makeup, his age, his sexual experience, and other factors. Some teenage boys have a refractory period of under a minute. Some older men, on the contrary, can take a couple of days, and still be perfectly healthy. Women, on the other hand, do not have much of a refractory period; 15% of women are multiorgasmic—that is, capable of multiple, repeat orgasms (this is exceedingly rare in men). While for women after orgasm there might be a brief feeling of satisfaction and sense that there's no desire for more sex, women (of all ages) can become aroused again more quickly than men and may try to initiate sex before a male partner is ready. The result: women feel frustrated or rejected, and men feel inadequate. How about trying instead to encourage your partner to bring *you* to orgasm again *without* the need of an erect penis. In time, he may become aroused by stimulating you. If he doesn't, it shouldn't really matter—you can learn to enjoy other kinds of stimulation. It will make your partner happy to know he can satisfy you more completely—and in

different ways. Don't burden your partner with stories about the sexual prowess or endurance of past partners. Learn to accept your male-female differences, as well as your personal differences, and work them into a more fulfilling sexual relationship by becoming more flexible in your definition of sexual relations.

Another male-female sexual difference: orgasm during intercourse. Men almost always achieve orgasm during intercourse—and it's a good thing they do, for it helps the survival of the species. Women, as discussed above, often need additional stimulation of the clitoris in order to reach orgasm during intercourse. This can be learned through changing the position of sex, or by adding manual or oral stimulation before or after the man ejaculates. We must move past the very dated definition of intercourse as "over" after the man ejaculates. Your orgasm is just as important as his—so speak up and get the attention you deserve. You might just discover that your partner doesn't even realize that you aren't reaching climax during intercourse. *Communicate* calmly and warmly—don't criticize or complain, unless you feel you're becoming a broken record.

Particular sexual problems are somewhat age-dependent as well as gender-dependent. For instance, younger men are more likely to have problems with premature ejaculation than are older men. This may be a male problem, but women suffer the consequences as well! Be supportive, patient; and urge your partner to see a urologist and a sex therapist to discuss this common and often treatable condition. Men can learn to control, recognize and delay their climaxes in many cases, which gives you more time to enjoy sexual intercourse. Approach the problem as *both* of yours, not just *his,* and you're more likely to get results.

Older men are less likely to suffer from premature ejaculation, but *more* likely to have erection problems. Whether they suffer from total impotence or intermittent trouble getting or maintaining an erection, this is an area of abundant research and lots of success in treatment. We now know that most potency problems are physiological, not psychological in origin, and that medication (or getting off of certain medications!), surgery, "vacuum pumps" and implantable devices can all be used to improve potency. Don't take your partner's problem with erections as a personal insult, or immediately assume that he's having an affair or has lost interest in you: this is an ignorant and unproductive way to approach the problem. Instead, think of impotence as just another medical issue to be dealt with—like a sprained ankle, or heart palpitation—and seek medical attention from a qualified urologist and/or endocrinologist trained in sexual function.

Women too often fall into old stereotypes thinking healthy men must be chronically sex-starved, always anxious to hop in bed. But men have peaks and troughs of sexual interest just as women do, and they should be allowed some flexibility for it.

Dr. Barbach finds that a common sexual difference between men and women is the intensity of touch that they enjoy during sex. In general, she reports that men prefer a harder, stronger touch than women do (of course there are countless exceptions). A soft, feathery touch that can be quite sensuous to a woman can be totally unappealing to a man. On the flip side, a hard, more aggressive touch that might turn a man *on* will often turn a woman *off*. In general, women have a harder time making sexual demands than men do: we have to learn to say what we want, because no one's going to guess. There's nothing wrong with handling your sex partner somewhat firmly and asking him to handle you more gently.

A common *female* sex problem that *men* may fail to understand is lack of lubrication as we approach menopause. (For more on this, *see* chapter 10). As estrogen leaves our bodies, there are a wide variety of changes in our skin, our mood, our internal organs and so on. One area that's affected quite dramatically for some women is the vagina. The thin, highly sensitive tissues of the vagina become thinner still—and more dry—with the onset of menopause. Intercourse can become quite painful—so much so that some women avoid sex completely at this time. There's no need to do so. First, reassure your partner that you haven't lost interest because of any change in your feelings or attraction to him. Then, rectify the problem with one of several effective lubricants.

K-Y Jelly: A good choice that keeps up lubrication for several minutes, but not for as long as some other lubricants.

Replens: A slightly longer-lasting lubricant marketed specifically for vaginal lubrication. Many women like this product. It plumps and moisturizes the vaginal tissues.

Gynemoisturin: Similar pluses to Replens.

Astro-Glide: This excellent product may be harder to find in general stores, but can be ordered by mail, found in shops with sex supplies or ordered through a sex counselor. It is a superb, longer-lasting lubricant recommended by many sex therapists for its ability to keep the vagina moist for an extended period during sex, so you don't have to rush sex in order to avoid drying out before you're satisfied.

Aerogel and Slip: Two other longer-lasting lubricants in the Astro-Glide style.

Saliva: Sex counselors like to point out that one of the most cost-effective lubricants is in your mouth: lubricating your partner through oral sex or even putting saliva from your or your partner's hand onto your vagina can help. It's free, so it's certainly worth a try. But remember: sexually transmitted infections can be passed from the mouth to the genitals; if you or your partner have active herpes sores in your mouth, for example, you should temporarily avoid using saliva as a lubricant.

A note about Petroleum Jelly: While it *can* work as a lubricant, it's goopy, sticky, can clog pores and promote infection, and can wear out condoms quite quickly (if you haven't completed menopause and might still become pregnant—or if you're using condoms to protect against STDs—this could be an important issue for you). The same goes for butter and other fat-based lubricants.

SEXUALLY TRANSMITTED DISEASES AND SEXUAL FUNCTION

As briefly mentioned earlier, the symptoms of STDs and sometimes the procedures used to treat them can cause pain or discomfort during sex, and even make you averse to having sex at all. Certainly, the prudent thing to do (if you have more than one sex partner) is to learn to use condoms regularly to reduce the chance of transmitting the disease (and know, in the case of certain diseases like genital warts, that condoms do not provide perfect protection). Be open and honest with your sex partners to protect them and yourself. This can be extremely difficult, but it might be made easier at first by providing some reading material or even having a group chat with your doctor to ease your partner's fears—and your own. Because STDs are so incredibly common, most partners nowadays will have one of their own! (*See* chapter 13, "Sexually Transmitted Diseases," for prevalence rates, treatment, etc.)

But while we've been focusing on what you can do to protect your partners, a vital issue that doesn't get enough attention is what to do about the physical and emotional pain your STD is bringing to your sex life. There are no simple answers, which is one reason people don't like to talk about it. Dr. Seifer likens the damage caused by STDs to a "skinned knee for the vulva"—that is, the outer portion of the vagina. Lubricants (listed earlier) can help a great deal if your vagina is dried out from treatments. Keeping easily treated infections like yeast under control at all times will help relieve you of additional burning on top of already-sensitive skin. Warm baths before and/or after sex can relax you and soothe your skin, provided you don't use irritating soaps or bubble bath. Consider making the bath part of foreplay. Be sure to wait to have penetrating intercourse until you are fully aroused—the loosened vaginal muscles and lubrication will make sex more comfortable, and also will reduce the chance of developing tiny abrasions on the vaginal or anal skin, which can make STD symptoms more painful.

Finally, remember that so-called "ulcerative"

STDs—the ones that create open sores or fissures on the skin—make it easier for you to contract the virus that causes AIDS, since there's an easier entryway through your skin to your bloodstream. If you have broken vaginal skin, the best thing to do is avoid sex until the sore has healed. If you won't wait, absolutely use condoms and spermicides correctly (*see* chapter 13) and consistently. Don't be afraid to ask a man to use a condom: if he refuses, he may be a lot more stupid than you ever imagined—and if he sincerely believes that you won't have sex unless he wears one, chances are he'll put one on and enjoy the sex rather than holding hands or going home!

In closing, remember this: Don't wait for total abstinence before you seek help for sexual problems. Preventive medicine goes a long way in this arena, as in so many other types of health care. Some sex therapists think all couples should have a preventive sexual health "checkup" before settling into a permanent relationship. This may be extreme, but there is no reason why you should wait until your sexual life is painful or empty before seeking help. There's lots out there for the taking.

Sex as We Grow Older

In many ways, we come into our own sexually as we age. This seems to be true particularly for women, whose sexual drive increases over the years. Some of the reasons for our heightened interest in sex later in life: we're not worried about becoming pregnant, and many of us have grown past some of our hang-ups about enjoying sex, especially creative sex. Hopefully, we've come to accept our bodies for better or for worse, and we've long since stopped hiding under the sheets or behind towels. If we're in a long-term relationship, perhaps we've learned to make sex the best it can be for us as a couple. Maybe the kids are out of the house, and this is a good time to experiment with new kinds of sex, different rooms in the house—to revel in new freedom.

The loss of estrogen in the body after menopause can put a damper on sex if we don't do something about it, but many women have found their way around this time of vaginal dryness and irritation with hormone therapy or effective lubricants.

Another negative for sex in our older years might be a male partner's sexual problems. Impotence and other age-associated sex problems can impair a man's sexual function. Many cases of impotence are reversible, so there's no reason for you to give up on sex because your partner is having trouble. While he's being treated, try other kinds of sex that don't require an erect penis. You might just enjoy it!

If you are living alone, divorced or widowed, sex in later years can be a difficult issue for you. Our society has evolved in such a way that many "eligible" older bachelors are choosing younger women for sexual partners. Furthermore, it's hard to begin a new sexual relationship if you're suffering guilt after a long marriage, or have never had sex with anyone but your long-time partner. If you begin to date, and find yourself becoming interested in someone sexually, this might be a good time to sit down with a sex counselor to learn about getting-back-into-it techniques that might make you more comfortable. Just because you're older doesn't mean you have to jump past the hand-holding and kissing that preceded sex when you were younger. Getting back into intimacy slowly, one step at a time, can make it easier and will help you learn to be comfortable with a new partner. Many sex therapists recommend masturbation if you have gone through a long sex-free period (or if you want to avoid going through one!) to keep your sexual juices flowing. Some older women are averse to masturbating because of myths from childhood about the dangers or inappropriateness of self-pleasuring. A sex therapist can help you deal with these issues, as well. (*See* chapter 10 for more on later-life sex.)

When It's Too Late to Bother with Sex Therapy

Seifer puts it well when she says "if there's no glue left in the relationship," it's time to give up with sex counseling. Most couples know when the commitment to make things better is gone. If you *both* think it's not worth repairing, it's not likely that an outsider can be of much help. If you're not sure, if you're angry and frustrated and therefore unable to think positively about the relationship in any way, it may be worth a

couple of sessions with a therapist to see if there's a light at the end of the tunnel. But if it's clear—certain—to both of you that there's nothing worth working on, chances are it's time to move on, and move apart.

For More on Problems with Sex

The American Association of Marriage and Family Therapists
800-374-AMFT

The American Association of Sex Educators, Counselors and Therapists
435 N. Michigan Ave., Suite 1717
Chicago, IL 60611
312-644-0828

Sex Information and Education Council of the U.S.
130 West 42nd St., Suite 2500
New York, NY 10036
212-819-9770

PART FIVE

Childbirth

CHAPTER FIFTEEN

PREGNANCY AND DELIVERY

So I am often awake these days in the hours before the dawn, full of joy, full of fear. The first birds begin to sing at quarter to five, and when Sam moves around in my stomach, kicking, it feels like there are trout inside me, leaping, and I go in and out of the aloneness, in and out of that sacred place.

—Anne Lamott, *Operating Instructions*

You miss a period, maybe feel a little sick or sluggish over breakfast. The home test kit comes back positive. Your doctor calls with the news. However you discover you are pregnant, the news—or even the suspicion of it—can bring about a flood of emotions you could never anticipate. If you have been planning the pregnancy, and especially if you've been waiting for a long time for it to happen, this can be one of the most joyful occasions of your life. If you've had problems in previous pregnancies, you may be frightened. If you did not plan the pregnancy, your emotions can run from shock to despair. No matter how you approach the situation, one thing is clear: this is a life-changing event. How you handle it emotionally and physically will vary tremendously from woman to woman, but it's hard to find any woman whose outlook on life did not take a major jolt in one way or another upon learning she may bring another life into the world.

Even if you have wanted to be pregnant for a long time, the news can be startling. As a friend of mine likes to say, reality is what happens *after* you make your plans. It can take some time to absorb this kind of news, to incorporate it into your life's plans. Some think it takes the entire 40-week gestation, if not longer. If you are brimming over with a sense of good fortune, enjoy it. If not, don't assume you're abnormal. Talking to other mothers (including your own, if the relationship is good), to your doctor or midwife, friends and even counselors if you're very alarmed, can make a big difference in helping you let this momentous information sink in.

Some women will decide that this pregnancy is not right for them—it has come at the wrong time, with the wrong partner, at a time of medical risk, or many other factors. They may choose abortion (*see* chapter 12 for details), or putting their child up for adoption (*see* the information section at the end of chapter 16). Neither decision should be made lightly, and requires some of the deepest soul-searching a woman can do in her lifetime.

This chapter is for those who decide to go forward with their pregnancies, and want to do everything possible to bring about a healthy outcome. While there are certainly no guarantees in life, there are odds, and the odds show that with some effort on your part, you can significantly decrease the risk of problems in pregnancy. This is a wonderful opportunity to do things for your own basic health that you've been putting off for a long time. Your baby will benefit as much if not more than you will.

At the same time, because there are no guarantees, inevitable pregnancy problems should not bring guilt or self-blame. There is a lot that you and your partner can do, but there is an equal amount that you cannot control. If you take the kinds of precautions and show the kind of judgment recommended below, and things don't turn out as you planned, don't look inward and ask what you did or didn't do right. Nature takes its course in ways we can not deter.

BEFORE YOU BECOME PREGNANT

Let's take a step backwards for a moment. For those who are not yet pregnant, and want to conceive, there are a few important things to keep in mind.

First, you're a lucky bunch. It's better to *decide* to get pregnant before you actually conceive, since it gives you the opportunity to plan ahead for better health. The first thing you should do is visit a doctor for what's called a pre-conceptional visit. This is a chance to clear up any health problems that might interfere with your pregnancy. From a public health standpoint, this saves money: according to a 1985 report from the Institute of Medicine, a dollar spent on prenatal care would save $3.38 in the cost of treating low birthweight babies. From a personal standpoint, which is more important to *you*, prenatal care (and pre-conceptual care) will avoid many common pregnancy problems. The better your overall health *before* pregnancy, the greater the chance you'll have a healthy baby.

At your pre-conceptional visit, you should be tested for immunity to certain diseases: for instance, you'll probably be given a test for immunity to rubella (German measles). Even if you were vaccinated as a child, the immunity can wear off over time, and this disease can be disastrous in pregnancy. If you aren't immune, you will be vaccinated and probably told to wait a couple of months before trying to conceive, so that protective antibodies can build up in your blood and there's no theoretical risk of the vaccine itself causing problems for your fetus. You should also discuss your general health status, including your blood type, and whether your blood is Rh-negative or Rh-positive; whether you have diabetes or high blood pressure, and if so, how to get them under control before pregnancy; if your weight is in a healthy range; if your diet is well-balanced; if you have dangerous habits like smoking or alcohol abuse that should be eliminated before pregnancy; and so on. You should also be fully screened for sexually transmitted diseases and other infections of the genital/reproductive tract that might endanger a future fetus (*or* impair your fertility). Many bacterial sexually transmitted diseases can have a devastating impact on fetal health. The list of needed screening tests can be extensive.

It is known that certain nutrients are especially important in pregnancy for both your own and your baby's health. We'll discuss this in more detail below. But one major example that you should think about *before* conception is folic acid. Folic acid has been found to protect against a type of birth defect called an NTD (neural tube defect).

Another group of tests that should be done at your pre-conceptional visit include blood tests for heritable disorders common to your ethnic background. For example, Ashkenazi Jews should consider a test for Tay-Sachs disease, African-Americans for sickle-cell anemia, and Greeks and Italians for beta-thalassemia. These are genetic disorders known to run more commonly in particular groups. Most require *both* parents to be carriers for transmission to the fetus. If you are found to be a carrier, you'll want to have your partner screened, too. If you are not a carrier, there's no need to test your partner. Ask your doctor which of these tests is appropriate for you, and if both you and your partner should be tested.

These and many other tests and treatments can prepare your body for the major task of pregnancy. Going into the experience physically prepared will boost your chance of a healthy pregnancy outcome. As Dr. Mary Anna Friederich of the Maricopa Medical Center puts it, "Live the pregnancy life before you get pregnant" and you'll be okay. We'll talk more about the healthy "pregnancy life" later in this section.

TRYING TO CONCEIVE

In chapters 8 and 16 I go into more detail on the workings of the reproductive system and the factors that affect fertility. Here, we'll focus on the basics.

For you to become pregnant, your partner's (or donor) sperm must unite with your (or a donor's) egg. This sounds simple enough, but requires a good deal of information and precise timing. First, do you ovulate? That is, do you release an egg each month, and if so, do you release it on a fairly regular schedule? Next, does your partner produce sperm capable of swimming to your egg and fertilizing it? Third, are your hormones balanced properly, so that if conception occurs pregnancy will be sustained? For many of us, conception itself and continuing pregnancy are the answers to these questions. For others, infertility testing and treatment (*see* chapter 16) provide the answers.

When trying to conceive, you'll want to estimate your ovulation time. You basically have two options. You can go with averages at first: most women ovulate 14 days before their next menstrual period begins. This means counting backward from your next expected period, rather than forward from your last period, which many women incorrectly do. Let's say your menstrual cycle is 30 days long. Many women incorrectly estimate that the precise midpoint of their cycle is when they will ovulate: that is, day 15. In fact, on average, this will not be the day you ovulate. Day 16 is more likely—that is, 14 days before the start of your next period. As you'll learn, being a day off can make a big difference in your chance of conceiving each cycle.

The fact is, counting days is *not* the optimal way to predict ovulation—although it's the easiest and among the cheapest, and works for many couples. Other more precise methods, as discussed on page 210, include tracking your temperature and the quality of your cervical mucus. You may also want to invest $25 or so in a home ovulation kit which predicts ovulation shortly before it occurs, helping you plan the optimal time for intercourse. These tests are fairly reliable, and can be used over several days to increase the chance you'll catch the important hormonal changes.

However you compute ovulation, you'll want to time intercourse closely around it. Some recommend avoiding sex for several days before you try to conceive so your partner builds up a good sperm reserve. Most experts recommend that you try to have intercourse a day or two before suspected ovulation, then again on the day of suspected ovulation, and perhaps again a day or two later. Because the egg can only be fertilized for about 12 to 36 hours (probably on the shorter end of that spectrum), and sperm lives for just about three days (or a bit longer), you do have a little leeway, but you can see that being off by a full day can easily mean the difference between success and failure. For women who have spent the greater part of their reproductive years trying *not* to get pregnant, feeling as if it were almost inevitable without protection, it's an awakening to realize that it often takes a concerted effort to conceive.

It is believed that the traditional "missionary" position—man on top, woman on her back lying down—is most conducive to conception, because the vaginal canal tips back, helping sperm move toward the cervix and into the uterus with a little help from gravity. Some say you should lie on your back for a short while after intercourse to let the sperm make its journey unhindered. Of course, any position of penis-vagina intercourse can lead to pregnancy, and plenty of women who jump up to go jogging immediately after sex can find they're pregnant two weeks later, so there's no sense getting too clinical about this unless you're having trouble conceiving in the first place.

FINDING OUT IF YOU'RE PREGNANT

Each time you try to conceive, you'll have about a two-week wait to find out if it "worked." If you get a normal period, you can be pretty sure you're not pregnant. But some women do bleed during early pregnancy (the bleeding can be similar to your regular period, or sometimes lighter or spotty). And other signs of early pregnancy can also closely mimic those of menstruation; light cramping, for example, and fatigue. Don't assume you're not pregnant until a full normal period continues.

If your period is even a day or so late, you can use a home pregnancy test for a fairly reliable (99% accurate) answer. These tests, which cost about $15 apiece, measure the hormone HCG in your urine. HCG is the hormone made by a developing embryo—you don't have it when you're not pregnant, and you do have it when you are pregnant; pretty straightforward. If a home pregnancy test comes up positive, you can be fairly sure you are pregnant. If it's negative, however, you cannot be sure you *aren't* pregnant, because it takes some time for HCG to build up in the urine, and you probably conceived only a short time ago.

A more reliable test—nearly 100% accurate—is the *blood* test for HCG, which can be done in your doctor's office or clinic. Most practitioners will tell you to wait a week or so after your missed period before having the blood test, so HCG, if it's present, will be more easily detected. You'll be given a blood test for HCG even if your home urine test was positive, to confirm pregnancy and to see if your HCG levels are appropriate for your stage of pregnancy. This is very important. Early in pregnancy, HCG levels at least double every two days, keeping up this pattern for several weeks. If your HCG level is extremely low to start out with, you may just be in the earliest stage of pregnancy. If it's lower than your practitioner expects for your stage, however, she will probably retake the test in a couple of days to see if the number is doubling. If it is, things look good. If it isn't, this pregnancy *might* not be viable. When HCG is present but quite low and/or not doubling, doctors worry about tubal pregnancy (ectopic pregnancy that develops in a fallopian tube or elsewhere outside the uterus) or imminent miscarriage. These will be ruled out if suspected.

The final confirmation of pregnancy is called the "clinical" diagnosis, which your doctor may make in several ways—looking at your cervix, feeling your abdomen, or even looking at the small sac containing your growing fetus with a visual test called an ultrasound, in which sound waves are used to give an image of the uterus and its contents. Your doctor will also listen for the baby's heartbeat several weeks later to make sure things are developing properly.

If you test positive—and your "clinical" pregnancy is confirmed—you're on your way. You're already a few weeks into the 40-week journey to motherhood, since pregnancy dates are counted starting with the first day of your last menstrual period. This may seem strange, since on the day of conception you're considered two weeks pregnant already, and by the time you miss your period, you're about 4 weeks pregnant—but that's the way it's counted, so enjoy the concept that you're at least a tenth of the way there when your test comes back positive!

HOW YOU MIGHT FEEL

You might be nauseated and vomiting, and you might feel great: there is no way to predict these things. Dr. Palmer Evans of the Tucson Medical Center finds that about 80% of his patients have some nausea in the early months of pregnancy—but statistics vary. Some women are overwhelmingly fatigued, some have food aversions in which certain foods or smells make them feel sick. Some have cramps, constipation, weakness or dizziness. A large number of women have breast tenderness and/or swelling in early pregnancy—but again, not all do. A supportive bra can help. Some women have headaches during pregnancy—these are usually, not serious, unless combined with severe visual and other problems. And as pregnancy progresses, back pain is also common: try standing and sitting up straight, rather than slouching. Others feel absolutely terrific and don't change their habits a bit, if only stopping to wonder what all the fuss they've been hearing about pregnancy is all about. Interestingly, because so much has been made of the negative physical symptoms of pregnancy, some women who feel just fine think there must be a hidden problem! Many healthy pregnancies produce no unpleasant feelings at all.

Not only can you not predict how you're going to feel when you're pregnant, but you also can't predict if you'll feel the same way with every pregnancy. I've seen women who can barely pick themselves up off the floor in one pregnancy and do step aerobics classes throughout the next. Hope for the best, but if you feel lousy, *take it easy*. Dr. Richard Aubrey, director of obstetrics at the SUNY Health Sciences Center in Syracuse, urges us to bring back the days when pregnant women weren't expected to be superwomen, and when rest and self-care were acceptable and even recommended during pregnancy. This is the time to listen to your body, if ever there was one: if you're wiped out, sick, faint or queasy, take the pace of your life down a peg or two. For most women, these feelings fade or disappear completely by week 13—the end of the first trimester. So you won't have to move in slow motion forever.

PREGNANCY: WHAT YOU HAD TO SAY ABOUT IT

Tracy, 30 years old
I had heard so many stories of problems, I always just assumed it would take at least a few months to get pregnant, if we could conceive at all. So we started trying and didn't expect anything to happen immediately. When my period was late that first month, we were startled—sure enough, I was pregnant. The overwhelming excitement my husband and I felt was immediately dampened by the news that my pregnancy hormone levels weren't high enough, and miscarriage was likely. Even when they told me the chance of success was under one percent, we remained hopeful ("That's one out of a hundred," my husband said positively. "It has to work out for *somebody*."). As it turned out, the hormones didn't lie. I miscarried several weeks later.

We were devastated, frightened, worried about the next time, frustrated that we'd have to wait a couple of months to try again, to be sure my uterus was healed. We tried a few months later, and this time we conceived on the third month. I used a home pregnancy test when my period was only about five minutes late! My mother said I was nuts. But sure enough, the test came up positive. According to lab tests, the hormones immediately kicked in properly this time. I can hardly describe the elation we felt, the excitement about the future, the curiosity about what was growing inside my body, and the sense that we had already become a family of three even as this tiny being was no more than a few microscopic cells. I was lucky that morning sickness never arrived to quell these wonderful thoughts—but for about two months, exhaustion and breast tenderness certainly did.

Still, when I wasn't napping, we fantasized about hair and eye color, the baby's sex, talked about names and whom would it resemble. We prayed it would be healthy, our hearts in our throats at every prenatal visit. The first time we heard the baby's heartbeat, some curious blend of pride and relief washed over us both, and we cried at the fast, fluttering sound that echoed from somewhere deep inside of me. "Sounds like a boy," the doctor joked. But we couldn't get the idea out of our minds. "Do you think she was serious?" we asked each other as we skipped up the street, knowing she couldn't possibly have been, but enjoying wondering anyway. The next remarkable moment was the ultrasound test, when we saw our baby's tiny body for the first time. This imaginary creature had become a living being, and would seem even more alive in the coming months when it started to move inside of me. Some people complain that when you go the traditional "medical" route to delivery, it all becomes too clinical. Actually we liked having an M.D., and found security in the technology and expertise that came along with it.

Some evenings we would sit on the couch and just wait for the baby to move so we could see my belly swell and recede like an arched wave. We laughed, and rejoiced, and studied my growing abdomen day after day, week after week. "Is that you or the baby?," my husband would ask as my waistline expanded. The baby had this uncanny ability to sit absolutely still when my husband tried to feel it, and then to resume gold medal acrobatics as soon as he took his hand away. I realized then that there were aspects of this experience I would never be able to share with anyone. That feeling of fundamental attachment, the blending of another body into mine in the most literal *and* figurative sense, was at once thrilling and frightening. I knew that whatever I did over the next several months would have a lasting impact on this child, and that I had to begin parenting even before I knew who this little person was. I had already stopped drinking alcohol in case I conceived, but now I began eating not only for two, but for about six, just to be on the safe side! I made the mistake of becoming quite sedentary, partly because I was so tired in the first trimester, and partly because I was scared that something would go wrong with the baby if I hopped around too much—even though I knew intellectually that this wasn't true. The result of all that sitting was a

combination of irrational peace of mind and excessive weight gain by the end of nine months!

A new level of closeness set in between my husband and me, one that seemed to grow stronger as our child grew. Just about every topic of conversation was eclipsed by the new focus of our lives—this child we were barely beginning to comprehend as ours, connecting us to each other in a way marriage documents cannot.

Nine months went by faster than we expected, and I seemingly quadrupled in size. Summer arrived, and it was hard to move around outside in the heat. My face, legs and feet swelled, and I was always boiling hot. Two days before my due date, we went to sleep as usual—with me tossing from side to side in a vain search for comfort. At about 1 a.m. I felt a stomach pain that I attributed to bad food, and closed my eyes again. An hour later, the stomach pains were somewhat regular—about ten minutes apart. I started to bleed lightly. I'd always imagined this moment—saying "Honey, I think it's time"—so when I said those very words, it felt surreal, almost scripted. Within two hours my contractions were 4 minutes apart, but the pain wasn't too bad. We went to the hospital, thrilled, scared, charged with anticipation and the sudden realization that we had absolutely no idea what to do when the baby arrived and we had to bring it home. About 12 hours, some real pain, and an epidural later, Nicholas was born—skinny as a chicken, with lots of dark, wet, curly-seeming hair.

There will never be words for this moment, the joy, the relief, the astonishment, the feeling of being excessively alive that flooded me at that moment. They took him away much too soon for tests and to be cleaned up—I worried about his whereabouts in a way I expect to do for decades, with a little luck. When he was brought back to me after all the tests were complete, small and dark and serene and wrapped in white swaddling, my heart, my emotions swelled so large they pushed at the limits of my insides, up to my throat and down into my stomach. How can you ever convey what it means to create more of your history and family, more of someone you love and of yourself? I am certain there are no adequate words.

CHOOSING A PRACTITIONER TO CARE FOR YOU DURING PREGNANCY

Choosing the person who will guide you through pregnancy, answering your questions, tending to any health problems that may develop and making sure that both you and your baby are doing well is one of the most important "tasks" of pregnancy. For some women, the choice is simple and obvious: they stick with their regular health care provider, be she an obstetrician/gynecologist, a family practitioner or some other type of caregiver. In many ways this is a good choice, if you're pleased with the care you've been given, because the more the provider knows about your general health and history, the better she will be able to tend to your pregnancy needs. But some women have a particular kind of pregnancy care in mind, and feel that their regular health care provider isn't the person to give it.

You have several choices. You can go with a general practitioner or basic family doctor. You can go with a pregnancy specialist or obstetrician. You can go with a certified nurse-midwife (or C.N.M.), someone who is trained first as a nurse and then as a midwife. In some states, you can still choose a lay nurse-midwife, some-

one who delivers babies but has no formal training in the area (other states no longer permit them to practice legally).

It used to be that you would choose a particular style of care and be stuck with it throughout pregnancy. Today, pregnancy care has become more diversified. For instance, while medical doctors are often thought of as giving a quite clinical, "patient"-oriented approach to pregnancy and delivery, often using high-tech assistance in place of eyes and ears, many M.D.'s defy this stereotype and do in fact emphasize the human side of the pregnancy experience. On the flip side of the coin, while certified nurse-midwives are associated with a very natural, human approach to pregnancy and delivery, more and more they are working with M.D.'s to provide higher-tech medical assistance when necessary. In many ways the *team* approach to pregnancy care (doctors and midwives together) may offer the best of both worlds.

Of course, there are some basic differences in philosophy among the different providers. According to Theresa Marsico, president of the American College of Nurse-Midwives, she and her colleagues don't "deliver" babies—they assist women to give birth. Women do the birthing, she says, and nurse-midwives act as guides. Marsico emphasizes that the pregnant woman is in charge of the midwife-assisted birth, and that there is generally more flexibility in the birth process than with medical doctors. For instance, while many M.D.'s encourage women to lie on their backs for delivery (which is most convenient for the doctor performing an episiotomy or incision to facilitate delivery, and also a convenient way for the doctor to "catch" the baby) nurse-midwives encourage all kinds of birth positions, from squatting to lying on your side to even giving birth underwater! They also urge women to keep active during labor, walking, showering, taking baths, rocking back and forth. In a formal hospital or medical setting, these activities are sometimes prohibited or at least discouraged.

Marsico also points out that nurse-midwives are more involved with women *after* delivery than are medical doctors: nurse-midwives often give advice on feeding the baby, calming it when it cries, and so on. She calls midwifery "part art, part science": the artistic part means less reliance on high-tech care, and more on listening, seeing and feeling the progress of labor in order to best meet women's needs.

MIDWIFE DELIVERY: WHAT YOU HAD TO SAY ABOUT IT

Robin: 33 years old

The big difference between an ob and a nurse midwife was all the way from the beginning. It was a very calm, relaxing atmosphere, my questions were more than answered, someone was willing to talk and listen to me and I wasn't just another number, in and out, we've got 30 people behind you. Because of insurance problems, I was seeing a different ob with every visit.

I was in a clinic situation both times, so my situation may have been a little worse than someone with a private physician. Some real frustrating things happened to me. When I had my first baby I had an OB-GYN—they just looked at me and said "okay lie on the table and slap your legs like a frog," and it was my first baby and I was 21 years old. They had the attitude you're just another woman having a baby.

(The midwives) were very calm, very patient, very helpful to any concerns I had and any questions. They went above and beyond the call of duty for any ailments that can plague a pregnant woman. The other thing with certified nurse midwives, nothing is mandatory, "You're going to have an episiotomy, you're going to have an enema,"—it's much more individualized care. With a lot of ob's it's like, "this is what we do with all the patients and we're going to do it with you too," and the nurse midwives are totally different from that. Whatever you're comfortable with, these are your options. They'd make their recommendations. They're caregivers, they see you as an individual person.

We discussed different ways of delivery, squat or walk or be on your hands and knees, side delivery, if you want to be on your back that's okay too. They're skilled in giving women choices. I gained all kinds of insights with the birth of my 3rd child, it was just such a neat experience. The other thing about midwives is it's very rare for them to leave you, especially when you're in active labor. Now I'm going into the field. I guess I'm pro woman, there's just a big difference with how they deliver you, someone who's had a baby and knows what it's all about. They're just wonderful.

Another feature of nurse midwife-assisted deliveries is that, if you want them to be, they can become family events rather than couple-oriented events. Barbara Hughes, clinical director of the nurse-midwifery practice at Denver's University Hospital, had a memorable experience delivering a woman's tenth baby with the entire family present. The father was encouraged to keep his hands on the baby as it emerged, and all in all it was a family affair. While Hughes points out that fewer C.N.M.'s are able to assist home births these days (because insurance won't cover it in many cases), bringing the family to a birthing center can create some of that homespun feeling.

But clearly there's something more going on than just warm fuzzy care. Gwen Spears, director of nurse-midwifery education at Drew University in Los Angeles, points to studies showing that babies born with midwife assistance are larger, they're less often born preterm, have fewer cesareans, and the mothers are less anemic and tend to keep their prenatal care appointments better than with nonmidwife deliveries.

Clearly, there are excellent reasons to choose a medical doctor, too. First, they are trained to notice and intervene for many medical problems common in pregnancy like gestational diabetes and hypertension (both of which can be harmful to the fetus). They are also trained to use lifesaving technology as well as surgical delivery in an emergency situation where the mother and baby's lives may be threatened. They are trained to handle many of your health care needs, both those related and unrelated to pregnancy, so they can continue to provide medical care after delivery, prescribing medication if you need it, followup procedures if problems develop, and so on. Talk to your doctor about the extent of her ability to use high-tech care; the more specialized she is, the more medical options she will have.

If your pregnancy is high-risk in any way, specialized medical attention can mean the difference between state-of-the-art and inadequate care. For run-of-the-mill, low-risk cases, many different kinds of pregnancy care can be used. For this reason, many women seeking the best of both worlds choose combined care from nurses or nurse midwives *and* medical doctors. This is becoming more common around the country in hospitals, HMOs, birthing clinics and other settings.

THE RISK OF MISCARRIAGE AND BLEEDING IN PREGNANCY

Miscarriage is extremely common: about one in five pregnancies is lost to miscarriage or "spontaneous abortion." Its frequency makes it no easier to handle, and anyone who tells you "it was meant to be" is missing the point. Miscarriage hurts, emotionally and physically, and it takes some healing to get over it. Friends and family mean well when they tell you that "nature has its reasons," but chances are that information will do little to assuage your pain. The fact is, there aren't too many "right" things to say when someone loses a baby, other than "I'm here for you." Don't be angry if you feel others are diminishing the importance of your feelings—just try to let them know what you're going through, and remember that they're only saying what they think is appropriate or helpful.

Most miscarriages occur during the first trimester. Half of those that occur at this time are due to chance chromosomal problems, but others are caused by hormonal, structural and other problems. Up to 14 weeks of pregnancy, there is little or nothing your doctor can do to stop a miscarriage from happening, says Dr. Warren Crosby of the University of Oklahoma Health Science Center. Later in pregnancy, there is a lot they can do—which we'll discuss. It's vital that you pay attention to your body at this time, and alert your health care provider to the first signs of trouble.

MISCARRIAGE SIGNS

Many women bleed lightly or "spot" during pregnancy, especially in the first couple of months. Others bleed all the way through pregnancy, and give birth to healthy babies.

Sometimes bleeding is perfectly benign; in other cases, it signals trouble. Bleeding is more worrisome when it is accompanied by other symptoms like loss of breast tenderness or loss of other pregnancy signs, such as nausea or vomiting; cramping (although again, many women cramp during healthy pregnancies); and passage of clotted tissue in addition to blood.

Bleeding can be a sign not only of miscarriage but of pregnancy-related problems, such as ectopic pregnancy or a rare problem called molar pregnancy in which the embryo develops into an abnormal mass of cells instead of a fetus. Ectopic pregnancy, which is a serious and even life-threatening problem needing immediate treatment, often is marked by lack of periods and/or irregular bleeding, sharp one-sided abdominal pain, shoulder pain (if there is internal bleeding) and even fainting, sweating or dizziness, says Dr. Robert Sassoon, an OB-GYN at the New York Hospital/Cornell Medical Center. Women who have diseases affecting their fallopian tubes, like untreated sexually transmitted diseases, are at greater risk of ectopic pregnancy. If you've had a previous ectopic pregnancy, you're at greater risk of having another, so you should be especially vigilant in watching for untoward symptoms.

Sometimes bleeding occurs when you miscarry one fetus out of multiples: for instance, when one twin doesn't make it. Experts now believe that many women with painless spotting in pregnancy may be losing a twin without ever knowing it. Technology has given us information we never had before, sometimes for better, sometimes for worse. If you are told that your spotting indicates the loss of a twin or other multiple, it doesn't mean there's added risk to the other fetus(es), but you'll want to be

fully evaluated by your doctor to determine the status of the pregnancy as a whole. This can be a frightening experience. Tests like the utrasound will help confirm if the other fetuses look safe and protected in your uterus.

If you are bleeding during pregnancy, your doctor will want to rule out possible miscarriage with one or several tests. A blood test will often be done to see if the pregnancy hormones are developing normally. Ultrasound testing may be used to see if the sac in which your fetus is developing is normal, and if there is a fetal heartbeat—a very good sign. According to the American College of Obstetricians and Gynecologists, about half of women who bleed in early pregnancy miscarry and half do not, so don't give up hope if you have this sign.

If you do actually miscarry, you may experience strong cramps resembling a very bad menstrual period. Depending on how far along you are, you're likely to pass some fetal tissue along with blood. If you have the presence of mind to do so, collect some of that tissue for evaluation in a laboratory. You may get information that could be helpful in your next pregnancy. If your pregnancy is more developed, you might not pass all the fetal tissue without assistance. In this case, a procedure will be done to clean the uterus of its contents and help you move on to a full recovery.

If this is your second or third miscarriage, it's time for a complete evaluation by someone who specializes in or at least has lots of experience with miscarriage diagnosis. Your regular health care provider may be knowledgeable and kind, but specialization sometimes becomes necessary when unusual problems arise. You may be able to work with *both* your regular doctor and someone with extensive experience with pregnancy loss. You'll want a full workup to determine if you have hormonal imbalances or structural problems in your uterus or elsewhere that predispose you to pregnancy loss. Often, these problems can be corrected, either by taking supplemental hormones, or having surgery to repair a structural abnormality, *before* you try to conceive again.

Most women who miscarry go on to have healthy pregnancies in the future. Do not consider yourself a reproductive "failure" if you have one or more miscarriages. I once did a story on a brave woman in Boston who endured six miscarriages before having a healthy baby girl at the age of 42. She never gave up, and has a lovely child to show for it.

Miscarriage Later in Pregnancy

While most miscarriages occur early in pregnancy, some happen later. The later in pregnancy the miscarriage occurs, the more significant the physical impact on your body (hormones will take longer to fall back into place, your body will take longer to return to its pre-pregnancy shape, and so on). This can also make the emotional wounds take longer to heal—although it doesn't take a more developed pregnancy to make miscarriage emotionally painful.

Some causes of later pregnancy loss can and must be corrected before future pregnancies. For instance, a so-called "incompetent cervix," or a cervix that opens long before your baby is due, can lead to miscarriage. When the cervix or mouth of the uterus opens prematurely, the fetus can literally drop out of the womb. If you have an incompetent cervix, your doctor can sew it shut during your next pregnancy and open it only when it's time to deliver your baby. This is just one example of why it's so very

important to have a full workup and find a reason for pregnancy loss whenever possible.

Don't blame yourself for a miscarriage. It is seldom something you brought on through any behavior (or lack of behavior) of your own. Do, however, take reasonable precautions to keep the risk of miscarriage low. That means don't smoke or drink alcohol or do drugs during pregnancy, and keep your other health problems under as tight control as possible before and during pregnancy.

Other Causes of Bleeding in Pregnancy

Sometimes bleeding in pregnancy is coincidental, and has nothing to do with the health of the pregnancy itself. You may have an infection or other problem on your cervix or in your vagina, for instance. Many infections can be treated during pregnancy, while others will have to wait until after delivery. Bleeding can be a sign of premature *or* real labor, depending on the other symptoms that accompany it (*see* labor signs later in this chapter). It can also be a sign of various placental problems: Your doctor can determine this with ultrasound testing.

Caring for Yourself and Your Baby During Pregnancy

Substance Use and Abuse

I asked pregnancy experts from around the country what they thought were the most important things a woman could do *for herself* to make pregnancy healthier. At the top of everyone's list, before they could get another word out, was *eliminate substance abuse*. Stop smoking, drinking alcohol and using drugs (both illegal and prescribed), they pleaded, and a vast number of fetal problems will be eliminated. The American College of Obstetricians and Gynecologists reports that one in ten fetuses is exposed to illegal drugs, and a larger number are exposed to *legal* drugs that can be harmful. Smoking leads to a range of problems from low birthweight to fetal death, alcohol to a broad range of physical and mental defects in the fetus that can last a lifetime, other drug use to countless fetal abnormalities, fetal addiction and fetal death. If you do nothing else, they urge in unison, get off of these damaging substances or at the very least cut back as much as you possibly can (although even moderate use of these substances is associated with serious problems). Dr. Robert Sokol, professor of OB-GYN and dean of the medical school at the Wayne State University School of Medicine, says he has patients who worry about their diets and weight but think smoking during pregnancy is just fine. They're missing the point, he says. Substance use and abuse poses greater risk to a pregnancy than most other problems *combined*. Pregnancy is a great opportunity to get help for serious addictions that you did not have the strength to beat for yourself in the past; now you can do it for your baby's sake, and save yourself at the same time. (*See* chapter 19 for details and resources on quitting or finding help.)

GETTING HEALTH PROBLEMS UNDER CONTROL

Dr. Jennifer Niebyl, head of the department of OB-GYN at the University of Iowa College of Medicine, puts managing the mother's health problems at the top of the pregnancy health list. By getting diseases like diabetes and hypertension under tight, constant control, she says, you can greatly reduce the risk of many birth defects. Insulin can be used safely during pregnancy, as can many (but not all) blood pressure medications. Furthermore, she adds, it's vital to see your doctor regularly throughout pregnancy to be sure that if *new* health problems arise, you're able to catch and treat them immediately, before they affect the fetus. Two to three percent of women will develop gestational diabetes (diabetes during pregnancy), she notes, and a larger number will develop hypertension during pregnancy (preeclampsia) putting the fetus at risk of serious problems. Often, gestational diabetes can be controlled with diet, but sometimes, insulin is needed.

Regular doctor visits are especially important because health problems like the ones just mentioned often come without symptoms. You can feel great when your blood pressure or blood sugar levels are climbing—and it can be quite a while before other symptoms like swelling in the hands and face, sudden fluid weight gain, headaches, kidney problems and other trouble signs set in.

Some women are at greater risk for pregnancy-related health problems. "Older" mothers (over 35), younger ones (in their teens) and those who are quite overweight or who have chronic dietary problems may be at greater risk of trouble than others. But no one is immune to these problems, so everyone should be screened throughout pregnancy.

WEIGHT GAIN IN PREGNANCY

On average, a healthy woman who begins pregnancy at a normal weight for her height should gain between 25 and 35 pounds. This is an aver-age, and doesn't apply to every woman. Some exceptions include women who enter preg-nancy underweight: they should try to gain more, perhaps 40 pounds during pregnancy. Women who enter pregnancy already obese should gain less—perhaps as little as 15 or 20 pounds. Women who are carrying twins should gain more—40 or even more pounds can be just fine. Talk to your doctor about the right amount of weight gain for you, since averages aren't particularly useful. The key is that you *plan to gain* weight for the health of your baby. This is not a time to worry about your figure, to diet, or to think about getting into slim cloth-ing. If you find yourself obsessing about the changes in your body, talk to your doctor or a counselor about it. Remember, if you don't gain enough weight, your baby might be a lower than desirable weight at birth. Babies who weigh under 5.5 pounds have more problems than those who weigh more.

The American College of Obstetricians and Gynecologists charts the average weight gain as follows: 7 pounds in maternal fat, protein and other nutrient stores; 4 pounds in increased blood volume; 4 pounds in increased fluid volume; 2 pounds in breast weight; 2 pounds in uterine weight; 7.5 pounds in baby's weight; 2 pounds in amniotic fluid weight; 1.5 pounds in placental weight. It's easy to see how a pound or two extra here and there can make a big difference in your overall gain. For some women, fluid retention alone can add several pounds. Dr. Constance Bohon, chief of gynecology at the Columbia Hospital for Women in Washington, D.C., likes to see women gain one-third of their preg-nancy weight in the first two trimesters (at about ½ pound per week until 20 weeks) and then 1 pound per week for the next 20 weeks. She begins to worry when a patient gains nothing (or loses weight) in the first trimester. Some women, because they feel quite ill and find it hard to eat, will only gain a couple of pounds in the first trimester—and this is usu-ally fine. On the other end of the scale, Dr. Bohon worries when patients start gaining 3–4 pounds per week. This is seldom a problem for the baby she says (*sometimes* the baby will get too large), but it's more of a concern for the mother, who will have lots of excess weight to take off after delivery.

Regular exercise, which we'll discuss in a moment, is recommended as a means of keep-ing your body toned and helping prevent unnecessary weight gain beyond the healthy range. But again, the goal is health, not thin-ness. There's no reason to be proud of keeping your weight down during pregnancy. If any-thing, insufficient weight gain should worry you and your doctor. Don't listen to your next-door-neighbor who brags that she gained only 10 pounds during pregnancy: if things turned out fine for her, she was lucky, not smart. At the same time, you don't need to go crazy and start eating fattening foods that are of no use to you *or* the baby, like daily ice cream sundaes and potato chips. These high-fat, high-calorie, nutrient-poor foods will put fat on your bot-tom more than they'll help your baby.

Above all, learn to recognize the beauty of your expanding silhouette and think only about eating the healthy foods—and enough of them—that you and your baby need at this time. It helps if your partner is supportive in this, and doesn't cast a negative eye on your roundness. If you sense his disapproval, talk about it openly: explain to him the importance of adequate weight gain and, if you think it's necessary, ask him to talk to your doctor about the importance of your weight gain to the future health of your child.

NUTRITION IN PREGNANCY

The American diet tends to be loaded with calories and fat, and most major nutrients as well, which means that most fetuses get enough total calories. There are of course exceptions: women who live in poverty here, as anywhere else around the world, are at risk for imbalanced, inadequate diets and their babies may suffer. And as we discuss in chapter 20, even affluent women have several important nutritional deficiencies, among them calcium—something we need *more* of in pregnancy.

The key feature of a healthy pregnancy diet is that you want to replace unneeded foods with needed ones. Next, you want to get *more* of certain nutrients that are important for fetal growth and development.

Extra Calories.

You'll probably need fewer extra calories than you expect, because the baby is so small. The bigger change you'll have to make is moving from wasted, toxic calories in alcohol and junk foods, for example, to useful calories in foods like grains, dairy products and so on. During a singleton pregnancy (one baby) you'll want to add *about* 300 calories per day, on average, to your normal diet. Again, because this is an average, it isn't for everyone. Dr. Constance Bohon says she prefers to monitor her patients' weight than to count their calories, since some women become much more sedentary during pregnancy (and

thus need fewer than 300 extra calories per day) while others become quite active (and need more than 300 extra calories). Ideally, you should plot out your typical food intake for a few days and discuss it with your doctor or a nutritionist to see where you're getting wasted calories, and where you might boost intake for the health of your baby.

Certain groups of women need more than 300 extra calories per day when pregnant. Teenagers, because they are growing, too, need extra calories, and those who enter pregnancy underweight also need additional calories to ensure proper weight gain for both themselves and their babies.

Nutritional Guidelines.

Here is a list of the amounts of major food groups you'll need during pregnancy, compiled by the American College of Obstetricians and Gynecologists:

Protein: 60–90 grams, or 3–4 servings, of "high-quality" protein per day. A serving consists of 3 ounces of cooked meat, fish or poultry, ½ cup of cooked dry beans, peas or lentils, 2 tablespoons of peanut butter, or one egg. The leaner choices are best for your health—meat trimmed of fat, chicken without skin, etc.

Carbohydrates: At least half of your total calories per day. The best of these are the complex carbohydrates, the fiber-rich foods which women don't get enough of in general. Eat lots of grains, breads, cereals, pastas, vegetables and fruit, rather than the simple carbohydrates (candy). The ACOG recommends four or more servings of fruits and vegetables per day (a serving is a cup of raw vegetables, one medium piece of fruit, ½ cup of fruit juice, ½ cup cooked vegetables or fruit). They also recommend four or more whole-grain or enriched bread servings per day (a serving is a slice of whole grain bread, 1 ounce of ready-to-eat cereal, ½ cup cooked pasta, rice, oatmeal, etc.).

Dairy products: Four servings per day. A serving is an 8-ounce glass of milk, 1.3 cups of cottage cheese, 1 ounce hard cheese, 8 ounces yogurt, 1.5 cups ice cream. As with protein choices, it's best to select those with lower fat content, such as skim milk, nonfat yogurt, and so on.

Fat: Try to keep your fat intake to 30% or less of total calories. While you certainly need some fat for your body to function properly, you don't want to waste calories on fats that do little for your baby, at the expense of nutrient-rich foods both you and your baby can use. For advice on cutting fat in your diet, *see* chapter 20, "Nutrition."

NUTRIENTS YOU'LL NEED MORE OF IN PREGNANCY

Many practitioners recommend a so-called "prenatal vitamin" during pregnancy. While most women who follow a healthy pregnancy diet will get enough of these nutrients through diet alone, the multivitamin provides added protection against deficiencies, especially for those of us who live hectic lives and don't always have time to sit down for well-balanced meals. During the first trimester, if we're too sick to eat a lot of the time, a prenatal vitamin can pick up some, but not all, of the slack. But don't fall into the "more is better" trap. Pregnancy is *not* the time for megavitamins, or special supplements of particular vitamins or

minerals (other than the ones discussed below). Excessive amounts of fat-soluble vitamins like A, D and others can be dangerous during pregnancy, harming the heart and urinary systems of the fetus. Moderation is key at this time.

Calcium.

We don't get enough calcium when we aren't pregnant, so when we are pregnant and the RDA for calcium jumps from 800 to 1200 milligrams/day, we run the risk of a major deficit. This is a time to boost your intake of calcium-rich foods (for a long list of examples, see pages 405–406) and, many experts believe, it's a good time for a calcium supplement. The reason we need more calcium at this time is that we're trying to protect our own bone reserves as well as develop our babies' new skeletons and teeth buds.

Dr. Bohon notes that getting adequate calcium through diet is difficult for some women, especially in the first trimester, since many of us feel nauseated, gassy or constipated and calcium-rich foods can exacerbate these problems. Try spacing your calcium-rich foods throughout the day in order to spare your gut. Calcium *pills* can be more constipating for some women than calcium-rich *foods:* experiment for yourself. Sometimes the perfect balance is to get about 800 milligrams of calcium per day from foods and supplement with one pill—perhaps a 500 milligram tablet. If you can get it all with foods alone, even better.

Folic Acid.

As we discussed earlier, folic acid is vital during early pregnancy for protection against neural tube defects, a relatively common group of birth defects affecting the baby's brain and spinal cord. Some well-known NTDs include spina bifida and anencephaly (lack of fetal brain). Experts recommend .4 milligrams *starting before conception* or at least as soon as you suspect you *may* be pregnant in order to cut the risk of neural tube defects by at least 50%. Why *before* conception? Because the most significant impact of this nutrient in preventing NTDs occurs in the first few weeks of pregnancy, often before women even know they're pregnant. According to Dr. Richard Johnston, medical director of the March of Dimes Birth Defects Foundation, we can *conservatively* estimate that with proper folic acid intake, as many as a couple of thousand cases of NTDs each year will be eliminated. If you have had a previous child with a neural tube defect, you will be advised to take even more folic acid each day. Talk to your doctor about it immediately.

While folate, the natural form of folic acid, appears in many foods that are recommended during pregnancy (dark leafy greens, fruit juices, whole grain breads and others) it's quite hard to get an adequate amount from diet alone. This is an example of where supplement pills are the clear way to go for adequate protection.

Iron.
Because we menstruate and lose blood each month, most women enter pregnancy in a relatively anemic state—that is, low on iron. The fetus and uterus then take a large portion of the iron we eat, leaving us vulnerable to anemia during pregnancy. Dr. Warren Crosby, clinical professor of OB-GYN at the University of Oklahoma, notes that with the 25% to 50% increase in blood volume during pregnancy, we're "watering down" our blood iron stores even further, making anemia quite likely. For this reason, an iron supplement is usually rec-ommended during pregnancy. Because iron can be constipating, and pregnancy hormones already can have a constipating effect, ask your doctor to recommend an iron supplement with a built-in natural stool softener.

Do not eat your calcium-rich foods or take your calcium supplement at the same time that you take your iron supplement. Iron and calcium bind to one another, dramatically reducing the amount of either nutrient you'll absorb. Try to separate the two by about two hours.

HOW TO KEEP UP A HEALTHY PREGNANCY DIET WHEN YOU'RE FEELING SICK

Early (and very late) in pregnancy, eating can be quite uncomfortable for some women. During the first trimester, when you may be feeling nauseated or have severe food aversions, the last thing you may want to do is put food in your mouth. But you must do it for your baby. Experts recommend chewing more, eating more slowly, choosing bland and nongreasy foods that don't upset your stomach, and avoiding foods with powerful smells. Sometimes, eating many tiny meals throughout the day is easier than eating three big meals. This is true both at the beginning of pregnancy to reduce sickness, and at the end, when your uterus is large and pressing on your gastrointestinal system.

The most common recommendation for reducing "morning" sickness (which for some women lasts all day) is to eat crackers or dry toast even before getting out of bed in the morning, and to never let yourself get too hungry. Often, even though you may dread eating, you'll feel sicker on an empty stomach than on a partially full one.

You may find yourself constipated during pregnancy, thanks to a combination of pregnancy hormones (especially progesterone) affecting your gastrointestinal tract, and the baby's growing weight pressing on your intestines. For some relief, drink more water and eat more bulky fiber foods (like grains, fruits and vegetables). Also, don't be a couch potato: the more you move your body, the better you'll move your bowels.

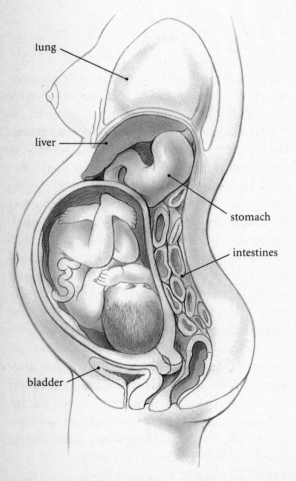

Internal view, full term pregnancy

lung

liver

stomach

intestines

bladder

EXERCISE DURING PREGNANCY

For a simple headline: Exercise is good—and recommended—during pregnancy. It's good for *you,* keeping your blood moving, your heart and lungs working, your muscles strong and your body free of some of the aches and pains that come with a sedentary lifestyle and growing belly. Plus, exercise still carries many of the healthy benefits it carried *before* you got pregnant: boosting your energy and mood (something you may be thankful for during pregnancy), keeping your weight in a healthy range, and keeping your metabolic rate high. Moderate exercise in pregnancy *may* also be good for your baby, increasing blood flow to the uterus. *Excessive* exercise, on the contrary, can be bad for both of you.

The basic rule is that with some exceptions and adjustments (listed below) you should be able to continue with your regular pre-pregnancy exercise routine. Dr. Raul Artal, a leading expert on exercise during pregnancy and primary author of the American College of Obstetricians and Gynecologists guidelines on the subject, warns pregnant women to avoid strenuous exercise for more than 30 minutes in an overly hot environment. If you're an avid exerciser, he urges you to get enough extra calories and fluids to make up for the added work your body is doing, particularly if you're working out in a hot, dry climate. Vigorous exercisers should clear their plans with their doctors, get more than the average extra 300 calories per day and drink water constantly throughout the day.

The main concerns about exercise during pregnancy are (1) overheating your body, (2) injuring joints and ligaments that become more lax in response to shifting pregnancy hormones, (3) falling or in some way subjecting your abdomen to impact, and (4) bringing your heart rate too high. This means that low-impact aerobic exercise is usually a great choice—brisk walking, swimming, cycling, and so on. Some feel that while running is safe for those who did a lot of it *before* pregnancy, the added weight and impact on your joints is not a great idea *during* pregnancy. If you are a serious runner, you might want to think about switching to lighter jogging or fast walking, or even changing sports during pregnancy. At least take the intensity of your run—the distance, speed, etc.—down a peg or two in consultation with your doctor. The concern isn't that you'll "shake your baby out," as many women fear. It's that you'll harm your own joints or, as Dr. Bohon warns, you'll stretch your uterine ligaments excessively, straining both your bladder and your uterus, and making you more prone to problems later in life. You'll also put extra stress on your knees and back, which are bearing an extra load at this time, and you could start feeling the effects of that strain as your pregnancy progresses.

Pregnancy is a good time to consider cross-training; that is, doing different activities on different days throughout the week. This is a good way to maintain overall body tone and strength, flexibility and balance (your balance will be shifting as your belly grows) and *not* overstress any particular muscle or joint system.

Most experts feel that light racquet sports like tennis are okay if you're used to doing them; doubles tennis is recommended over singles, however, fitting into the overall "take-it-down-a-notch" theory. Jarring stops on a hard court or slips on clay could be risky, especially as your balance shifts and your joints loosen.

When you're exercising during pregnancy, be sure to drink lots of fluids (even when you're not thirsty) and stay cool. You'll always want to be able to carry on a conversation, Dr. Bohon warns; if you're out of breath and can't speak, you're overdoing it. And while sweating is to be expected, you don't want to literally pour sweat or become drenched during exercise when you're pregnant.

If you were sedentary before you got pregnant, Dr. Artal suggests that you start exercising very slowly and find a relatively mellow activity that you enjoy, such as walking in the park or swimming at a local Y. He finds that pregnancy is often an excellent "healthy lifestyle window" in which women can pick up healthy behaviors, like regular moderate exercise, that may stick with them for life. The best guideline for sedentary women, he says, is to do what *feels good.* Your body is a good gauge of a healthy limit.

Many women want to know about the value of strength training during pregnancy—that is, lifting weights and other nonaerobic muscle-building exercises. Dr. Artal says that for women who lifted weights *before* pregnancy, this should be fine. He recommends sticking with lighter, 5–10 pound weights during pregnancy to avoid straining your newly lax muscles and ligaments. Don't *start* lifting weights during pregnancy if you never did it before, he advises—unless you're going to use the lightest weights (*up to* 5 pounds) with expert supervision to avoid injury.

An important caution about exercise during pregnancy is to *stay off your back* after about 20 weeks' gestation. When you lie on your back with a heavy uterus, you put pressure on the major blood vessels that divide and travel to your legs, which can deprive both you and your baby of needed blood flow. You may feel faint or even pass out if you stay in this position for a long period of time later in pregnancy. (This is why some women pass out in the dentist's reclining chair late in pregnancy.) You should also try to stay off your back during sexual intercourse and when sleeping at this stage: try to switch from your back to your side, using pillows for support if you tend to turn over during the night.

What are the benefits of exercise during pregnancy? No one can promise you an easier labor, but studies do show that fit women perceive the pain of labor to be slightly less severe than do unfit women. Also, women who exercise during pregnancy gain less weight than nonexercisers, while still having normal babies. They also tend to have fewer aches and pains throughout pregnancy, because their bodies are more toned to handle the physical stress.

Exercise Guidelines.

The American College of Obstetricians and Gynecologists recommends the following general guidelines for exercise during pregnancy. If you have any special risk factors during pregnancy, such as medical illnesses, vaginal bleeding or other signs that worry you or your doctor, talk to her about tailoring specific guidelines to your needs. These guidelines were published by ACOG in February 1994:

1. Regular exercise, at least three times a week, is preferable to intermittent activity.

2. Avoid exercise in the supine (lying on your back) position after the first trimester; avoid prolonged periods of motionless standing.

3. Stop exercising when fatigued and don't exercise to exhaustion; weight-bearing exercise can be continued but non-weight-bearing exercise will minimize the risk of injury.

ACOG also states that you should *not* exercise if you have premature rupture of the membranes, preterm labor, an incompetent cervix or other maternal health problems. Ask your doctor if there are any reasons why *you* shouldn't exercise during pregnancy.

There are some sports/activities *all* women should *avoid* during pregnancy. Generally, these are the sports in which you have a higher-than-average risk of falling or putting yourself at dangerous levels of air pressure. Some examples are scuba diving, water skiing, downhill skiing (although some experts I interviewed felt that expert skiers could proceed with caution if they avoid very high altitudes), sky diving, horseback riding and surfing. Use your good judgment; if there is a pretty good risk of injury with the sport, wait until after delivery to enjoy it.

SEX DURING PREGNANCY

Sex, another form of exercise, is usually perfectly safe during pregnancy. Some women—and their partners—have less interest in sex in the first trimester when they're feeling nervous about the pregnancy, or just tired and nauseated. If you feel fine, there's nothing wrong with keeping your sex life active throughout the entire pregnancy. Of course, be sure you aren't passing any sexually transmitted diseases or other infections between the two of you that could hurt the baby. If you had an initial loss of sexual interest, you may find that as your pregnancy progresses and you feel better, your interest in sex will increase—along with the girth of your belly. If you're creative and open to change, you'll discover many ways to have sex throughout your pregnancy. At times, when you are relatively large, it can take a bit of a sense of humor to make it work. Oral and anal sex are fine during pregnancy, too—again with the precaution that you aren't putting yourself at risk of disease transmission.

Dr. Warren Crosby notes that if you're bleeding or cramping at any stage of pregnancy, or if you're considered to be at high risk of miscarriage or early labor, you may be advised to abstain from penis-vagina intercourse and to choose other modes of sexual expression instead. This is because if you're on the verge of early labor, intercourse can trigger its onset (a combination of the prostaglandins in sperm and the force of the intercourse itself are thought to be the mechanisms). If you're not sure about the status of your pregnancy, or had prior bleeding that stopped, ask your doctor if sexual intercourse would be safe for you.

MEDICATION DURING PREGNANCY

We're usually quite cavalier about taking over-the-counter medications. It seems that if you don't need a prescription for them, they must be benign. That's not always true, and during pregnancy, it's often *false.* Even some of the most benign-seeming of all medications are not known to be safe during pregnancy. More often than not, you're going to hear the uncertain terms "*not known to be safe* in pregnancy" rather than definitive ones like "*known to be unsafe* in pregnancy" or reassuring ones like "*known to be safe* during pregnancy." The reason: drug makers don't test medications on pregnant women for fear of causing damage to a fetus. So it's only after the fact that we sometimes discover that a given drug caused problems in the offspring of women who took it—

and even then, it's often hard to prove cause and effect.

The moral of this story: err on the side of caution. Dr. Donald Coustan, chief of the department of OB-GYN at Women and Infants Hospital at Brown University, and the author of a book on medication during pregnancy, advises women to live by this general guideline: *Don't take anything you don't absolutely need.* This sounds logical, but many women don't follow it. We're so used to taking medication for minor aches and pains that we seldom wait to see what would happen if we took nothing at all. For example, Dr. Coustan advises, if your problem is self-limited—a bad cold, for example, that you know will be gone in a week or so whether or not you take medication—*don't medicate.* Later in this chapter I'll give some examples of nondrug remedies for some common minor health problems.

Lots of women ask about the safety of aspirin, acetaminophen (Tylenol) and ibuprofen (Advil and others) during pregnancy. These are among the most common over-the-counter medications, and ones women are used to taking for everything from minor aches and pains to fevers to menstrual cramps. Of the three, acetaminophen is thought to be the safest in pregnancy. This is the drug to take, in doses cleared by your doctor, if you have a fever or some other problem that you can't or won't handle without treatment. Aspirin, while it is actually *prescribed* in tiny doses to some women during pregnancy (those who are at high risk of hypertension), should *not* be used routinely by healthy women in pregnancy. Because it promotes bleeding, it carries certain pregnancy-related risks. Dr. Coustan advises patients to avoid ibuprofen and other nonsteroidal anti-inflammatory drugs (called NSAIDs) because we know less about their safety in pregnancy than we know about the other drug options just mentioned.

There are always exceptions, however. For instance, if you have severe, diagnosed arthritis and can barely get through the day without an NSAID because of chronic pain, then many doctors will say it's okay to take ibuprofen in controlled amounts during pregnancy. This is different from taking it for a little achiness after tennis. Each case should be individually monitored and guided by a physician.

Women often ask about the safety of cold and cough medications during pregnancy. In general, Dr. Coustan advises avoiding combination (that is, multi-ingredient) cough and cold preparations, since we know even less about drug interactions during pregnancy than we do about the effect of individual chemicals. There are certain drugs thought to be relatively safe in pregnancy—such as dextromethorphan for coughs (which you'll see in the letters "DM" after your brand name cough medicine), or sometimes Benadryl for congestion, says Dr. Bohon. But there are absolutely no guarantees about the safety of *any* drug during pregnancy. So anything you *can* avoid, you *should* avoid.

Another popular drug category is antibiotics. Some are thought to be safe in pregnancy, others less so. While erythromycin and penicillin seem safe, tetracycline does not (tetracycline taken during the second and third trimesters of pregnancy can discolor the fetus's teeth). We tend to be too casual about antibiotic use in general: often we fail to take the full recommended course of a given antibiotic regimen, or we go to the medicine cabinet and take whatever is left of an older antibiotic when we *think* we need it (for a sore throat, let's say). *Never*

take an antibiotic without a specific diagnosis and prescription (taking the wrong drugs at the wrong times promotes drug resistance and worse strains of infections). Pregnancy is a time to be especially vigilant about this. Unless your doctor okays it and prescribes it, don't take it.

Lifesaving Drugs.

Sometimes, when in a health crisis, you will have to make a decision balancing your life and health against potential risk to your baby. For example, if you have a life-threatening malignancy (cancer) and you need chemotherapeutic agents to increase your chance of survival, the risks these drugs pose to your baby may have to be put aside in favor of keeping you—and possibly your baby—alive. As with all medications, some are potentially more damaging to a fetus than others, so you will want to talk to your doctor about choosing a drug that will maximize your chance of recovery, but minimize the potential harm to your baby.

In other cases, such as heart disease, you may be able to switch from a drug that's not as well tolerated by the fetus (for example, ACE inhibitors) to one that is safer for the baby and still corrects your problem. Insulin for maternal diabetes is perfectly safe in pregnancy and recommended to keep mother's blood sugar in control and to protect the fetus from birth defects. On the other hand, oral diabetes medications are *not* recommended during pregnancy—they may cause the fetus's pancreas to produce too much insulin. For this reason, a woman whose diabetes was normally controlled with diet and oral medication may be switched to insulin for the duration of her pregnancy.

These days, even severe health problems do *not* have to prevent you from having a healthy baby. Dr. Patricia Cole of the Washington University School of Medicine in St. Louis notes that while some cardiologists refuse to care for pregnant women with heart disease, saying the situation is too risky, in fact *most* heart problems *can* be managed in pregnancy. Not only medications, but surgery (for mitral valve stenosis, e.g.) can often be done during pregnancy these days. The key is to find a practitioner experienced in your problem who will work closely with you throughout your pregnancy, monitoring both your own and your baby's response to your treatments. Since many of the symptoms of pregnancy (leg swelling, shortness of breath, fatigue and so on) resemble those of heart problems (as an example), Dr. Cole says it's all the more important to see someone trained in your particular problem who will recognize the nuances among symptoms and know when and if to treat you, and how those treatments might affect your baby.

Alternatives to Medication.

When the problem isn't serious, behavior changes alone are often enough "medication". The best medicine of all is often bed rest. When it comes to minor illnesses like colds, flus and other self-limited nuisances, rest can shorten the duration of your symptoms. Also, getting adequate fluids is very important in speeding your recovery. Enjoy lots of water, fresh juice, caffeine-free or herbal teas, hot water with milk and honey, light soups and other fluids as much as possible. Make sure to eat enough, even if you don't feel up to it—your fetus needs nourishment even if you don't feel hungry.

If you are congested, try using a vaporizer in your room, or even putting your face over some steaming water. It can provide at least temporary relief.

Overall, be patient and take it easy. If you give your body a break, it will recover faster. If you keep running yourself ragged, the illness may hang on longer and harder—or you may predispose yourself to catching yet another infection.

PRENATAL TESTING AND PREVENTION/ DETECTION OF BIRTH DEFECTS

All the testing in the world won't guarantee you a baby free of birth defects or abnormalities. The odds favor having a healthy child. But there are many problems we cannot predict or offset. About 150,000 birth defects occur per year in the U.S., and this doesn't count many problems we may think of as birth defects that are not classified as such (for example, fragile X syndrome or cerebral palsy, among many others). Each year, according to the March of Dimes, 1 in 115 live births has a heart or circulatory problem, 1 in 1600 has a neural tube defect, 1 in 900 has Down's syndrome, and 1 in 1000 has fetal alcohol syndrome. Some, but not all, can be prevented.

Dr. Richard Johnston, medical director for the March of Dimes Birth Defects Foundation and chief of the section of immunology at the Yale University School of Medicine, notes several areas where couples can make a dent in the rate of birth problems. First, he says, get rid of all infections before you become pregnant—or at least as soon as you discover you're pregnant. Chlamydia, syphilis and many other sexually transmitted diseases can harm various fetal body systems. The sooner you intervene, the lower the chance of problems. Next, test for infections like toxoplasmosis (a simple blood test says if you have immunity to this common problem). It's contracted by eating rare or raw meat, or from contact with cats (and their litter boxes). If you do not have immunity to toxoplasmosis, avoid these sources during pregnancy. Take folic acid to lower your risk of neural tube defects. Avoid alcohol to cut the risk of fetal alcohol syndrome (FAS). Stop smoking and taking drugs to reduce the chance of associated birth problems and fetal death. Avoid radiation and other workplace hazards like lead and other chemicals that might harm your baby. And remember, Dr. Johnston adds: this information goes for both mother *and* father. For too long we've ignored the impact of environmental and other toxins on sperm health and the subsequent effect that might have on fetal health. Even after conception, father's smoking and other habits can cause secondhand damage to the fetus, and can tempt mother into unhealthy behaviors she's trying to resist.

How can you screen for problems before your baby is born? You can start out, as we discussed at the beginning of this chapter, by testing yourself and your partner for common inherited illnesses that affect your ethnic group. Talk to your doctor or to a genetic counselor to determine the appropriate tests for you and your partner.

Once you are pregnant, there are variety of tests to predict fetal problems. These range from blood tests to measure pregnancy hormones, to more complicated blood tests measuring things like alpha fetoprotein, or AFP. The AFP test is an initial screening test for neural tube defects: if it comes back negative or normal, your chance of a baby with an NTD is quite low. If it's positive, you don't necessarily have a baby with a problem, but you will be advised to go on for further testing, such as an ultrasound test in which your doctor will take a look at the spine and brain structures of your developing fetus. You may also be offered (or you may request) a "triple test," or blood test for three factors—AFP, estriol and HCG. These three factors together have been found to predict as many as 70% of Down's syndrome cases. That's a remarkably effective test which puts you and your baby at no risk whatsoever (just a simple blood test). Not all centers are offering this combination blood test, but more are doing it all the time; it's worth asking about it, and finding out if a laboratory in your area will do it if your own doctor won't.

Ultrasound, or imaging with sound-waves, is offered for many different reasons. According to Dr. Fay Redwine, director of the perinatal center at St. Mary's Hospital in Richmond, Virginia, ultrasound testing at 20 weeks' gestation can give lots of useful information about the fetal heart, facial structures, hands, feet and many other body systems. It's also a good tool for dating pregnancies when women aren't sure when they conceived. A recent major study found that ultrasound testing is not cost effective (that is, it won't find enough problems to make it worth its price) in *low*-risk pregnancies. However, when the test is indicated, (and when it is done by experienced practitioners using good machinery, Dr. Redwine adds) it is an extremely valuable tool. Add a normal ultrasound result to a normal triple test (the blood test discussed above) and you've eliminated the risk of many—but not all—potential abnormalities.

The next step up from blood testing and ultrasound testing are the more invasive prenatal tests that check for chromosomal problems in the fetus—disorders like Down's syndrome and many other genetic abnormalities. You may elect (or be advised) to have high-tech, invasive testing for problems with your fetus if you fit one of several higher-risk categories. According to Dr. Sherman Elias, professor in the departments of OB-GYN and molecular and human genetics at the Baylor College of Medicine, genetic testing is indicated for the following groups: women who will be 35 or older at the time their babies are born; couples with a previous child with a genetic condition, such as hemophilia, cystic fibrosis, Down's syndrome or many others; and couples with a family or personal history of genetic conditions. Dr. Elias calls the family history the single most important prenatal test we have, so get all the information you can gather about your partner's and your own family history of genetic and other illnesses to help determine if invasive genetic testing is worth the risk.

Amniocentesis and CVS.

The two tests used for genetic prenatal diagnosis are aminocentesis and chorionic villus sampling, or CVS. Both of these tests carry a risk of fetal loss of ½%, or 1 in 200 cases. But talk to individual practitioners and you're likely to get different numbers. More often than not, you'll hear that amniocentesis is safer than CVS. Some centers have extremely low rates of complications in one or the other test because of their extensive experience with it. In general, it's a good idea to go to a center that does many of these procedures, since practitioner ability is thought to be related to risk. These tests should only be done when it's thought that the risks outweigh the benefits. For women over 35, the scales tip in favor of having the tests, since the chance of having a baby with a chromosomal abnormality is greater than the risks of the test. Some women opt not to have these tests even if the risks outweigh the benefits, however. It's up to you to decide to have the test or not.

According to Dr. Redwine, however, we're often comparing apples and oranges when we talk about the risk of having a baby with Down's syndrome versus the risk of losing a fetus to invasive prenatal testing. First, it depends on who you're talking to, she says. If you have tried to become pregnant for ten years, you're less likely to hear what doctors say about the benefits of testing, and more likely to focus on the unacceptable risk of losing this long-awaited fetus. If you become pregnant accidentally, you may be more concerned with the baby's health than with the idea of losing it. Everyone's concerns are different, and therefore risks have different meanings to different mothers. These are issues to discuss with a genetic counselor, who can give you an idea of the extent of the information you may get from these tests, and if anything can be done either to ameliorate the problem in utero (a rare possibility, depending on the medical problem) or to make delivery safer for a compromised fetus.

With amniocentesis, a needle is put through your abdomen and into the amniotic sac—ideally, with the guidance of ultrasound to avoid hitting the fetus. Some amniotic fluid is taken out and examined for chromosomal problems. With CVS, cells are taken from the placenta (not the amniotic fluid); these are obtained through the cervix or the abdomen. CVS can be done earlier than amniocentesis, at about 10–12 weeks' gestation. Amniocentesis is normally done at about 16 weeks, although with advances in technology, it can be done sooner in some cases, at certain centers. Earlier testing leaves the option of safer, earlier pregnancy termination for those who select it. (These days, with amnio results coming back quite quickly and the test being performed earlier, patients who choose pregnancy termination may still fit into a relatively safe time frame—almost equal to that following CVS.)

You may have heard that CVS has been associated with certain problems like limb injuries to the fetus (in up to 1 in 3000 cases), which frightens some parents and practitioners. Most experts say that when the test is done no earlier than ten weeks, the risk of limb injury is tiny, however. Dr. Joe Leigh Simpson, chair of the department of OB-GYN at the Baylor College of Medicine, says the evidence of this problem is not even statistically significant. The Centers for Disease Control and Prevention study which found that CVS increases the risk of fetal digit loss reported an increased risk of only .04%. And Dr. Simpson notes that two of the problem cases were done at eight and nine weeks' gestation, which is *not* advised for CVS. He therefore urges parents not to be dissuaded from trying CVS when it's in the hands of an experienced practitioner with good personal success rates and proper timing.

Dr. Redwine feels that CVS, since it's done earlier than amniocentesis, is a good choice for couples with an extremely high risk of chromosomal abnormalities due to one or both parents carrying an abnormal gene. The sooner these very high-risk couples get the information they need, the better. On the other hand, Dr. Redwine also acknowledges that at least at *her* center, amniocentesis is a less risky procedure overall than is CVS.

OTHER FETAL TESTS FOR LATER IN PREGNANCY: FETAL SURVEILLANCE STUDIES

There are many noninvasive tests to give you and your practitioner a sense of how well your baby is developing, and how it's doing in the uterine environment. These tests, which are generally done in the third trimester, range from the lowest-tech of all (having you count the number of times your baby kicks in a given day) to ultrasonography (getting sound wave-generated visual images of the fetus) to heart-rate monitoring both with and without stimulation of the fetus.

These days, many women ask for or are given an ultrasound test just to get the baby's first photograph. This practice may go by the wayside as health care costs are contained; a major study reported in the *New England Journal of Medicine* found that routine ultrasound testing for low-risk pregnancies did nothing to improve pregnancy outcome. But talk to some ultrasonography experts and they'll tell you of many important fetal abnormalities that can be discovered—or ruled out—by a well-performed sonogram. More and more, prenatal testing is going to be reserved for cases where it is deemed medically needed. If you have problem signs in pregnancy, general health problems, premature labor signs or late delivery (two weeks past your due date) you may get more high-tech testing than your neighbor got.

Some fetal surveillance tests that may be done along with ultrasound testing include the so-called "nonstress test," and, if the results of that test are abnormal, a more complicated biophysical profile which gives still more information about the fetus's overall condition.

THE PSYCHOLOGY OF PREGNANCY

We've been focusing on the physiological concerns of pregnancy, and the physical changes you may go through as your baby develops. According to Dr. Raphael S. Good, both a psychiatrist and an OB-GYN, the psychological changes of pregnancy are every bit as important and are too often overlooked.

Just as there are typical physical landmarks of pregnancy, like feeling the baby's first kick at around the 20th week of gestation, so there are important psychological landmarks as well. One of the most important is your growing sense that your fetus is part of you, rather than a purely separate entity depriving you of things you want to do (like drinking alcohol, or wearing a bikini). Women who don't perceive their fetuses as part of them are less likely to care for themselves and their babies properly, Dr. Good reports. They may not follow a healthy pregnancy diet, for example—and they may not even realize they're doing anything wrong, since the resentment is partly subconscious. Women who placed a high value on their figures as a measure of self-worth may be at higher risk of problems as their bodies change. If you don't feel your baby is part of you, or resent it for being there and depriving you of things you want in the short or long term, seek counseling before you do permanent damage to *both* of you. Start by talking to your doctor, but also ask for a referral to someone who does counseling with pregnant women. Birthing classes and/or new-mother groups are also a good way to find support and validation of your feelings. *Some* negative feelings about your pregnancy are perfectly normal, and often a good listener and some useful advice can go a long way to making you more comfortable with your situation, both now and as you look to the future.

Other important psychological stages of pregnancy include realizing that, while your baby is part of you, it is also a separate, unique person, and that it is forever connected to its biological father as well. This can be a very positive, automatic realization for many women. But if you have problems with (or no association with) the baby's father, this can be quite disconcerting. If you don't work out your feelings before the baby is born, you may impair your relationship with the child down the road because of these basic resentments.

Dr. Mary Anna Friederich advises pregnant women to resolve their feelings about their own parents—especially their own mothers in order to be happy and healthy parents. If your relationship with your mother was damaged, you may find yourself repeating mistakes from the past if you don't confront them before you become a parent yourself. Counseling can be very helpful with this process.

You also want to be sure that you and the baby's father have an equally positive outlook on this pregnancy. Some men become competitive with their offspring, vying with the baby for your attention. They may see your breasts as *their* domain, not the baby's, for example. These problems can become serious and interfere with your ability to grow as a family. Couples counseling is quite important here, and if you see problems setting in before your baby is born, get help before the baby arrives.

Dr. Richard Aubry, director of obstetrics at the SUNY Health Science Center at Syracuse, New York, is heading a project to help couples become effective parents *before* the baby arrives. He calls it "pre-birth parenting," and it involves becoming connected to and excited about the baby long before it arrives. Through massage, talking to the fetus, playing it music and many other activities, parents learn to become involved with their babies before they're tangibly in their lives. The goal is to improve parenting skills later on, especially in so-called high-risk families where there is a concern about later parenting problems. Preliminary data suggests that it's helping to improve parent-child relationships, but more study is needed. You have nothing to lose, however, by getting involved with your baby before it's born. If nothing else, it may build your excitement and help you through those long later months of pregnancy.

Psychological Stress and Pregnancy.

Many women, especially those who lead hectic lives with multiple roles, jobs and other obligations to fill, wonder if psychological stress is bad for pregnancy. We hear so much about physical stress—lifting too much weight, overheating our bodies excessively, and so on—but little about emotional stress. Unfortunately, we really don't know much about the impact of emotional stress on pregnancy. For instance, does emotional stress cut off blood flow to the uterus, as physical stress can do? Dr. Sokol points to animal studies showing that anxiety and worry lead to smaller offspring. He thinks this is reason enough to tell women to calm down during pregnancy and take life a little bit more slowly.

Dr. Aubry feels quite strongly about this issue. He worries a great deal about women who are expected or driven to perform "superwoman" roles during pregnancy, and who often suffer from more fatigue and physical discomforts during pregnancy than those who take time out to relax. Not only is it possible that emotional stress and excessive work and rushing about might have a direct, deleterious effect on the fetus, he says, but it also might predispose the mother to other harmful activities and habits. We know that stress often leads to cigarette use, poor diet and other unhealthy behaviors, so in this way alone it could be damaging to the fetus.

OLDER MOMS: PARENTING IN LATER YEARS

According to ACOG, by the year 2000 an estimated one in twelve babies will be born to women 35 and older. And while *on average* there are certain added risks to later childbearing (more miscarriages, more stillbirths, more low birthweights, more chromosomal problems, and more cesarean deliveries, to name a handful) there are also some distinct advantages to having a baby later in life. You may be psychologically better prepared for children when you're a bit older and wiser yourself; you may be more financially prepared for raising a child than you would have been ten years ago; and you may even be in better physical shape than you were in before (Dr. Raul Artal likes to call these women "chronologically advantaged," rather than "older".)

As we discuss in chapter 16, fertility rates drop as we grow older and near menopause. But if you *can* conceive, many studies show that older moms do quite well in pregnancy. If you're going to be 35 or older when your baby is born, you'll likely be advised to have more testing than younger women would be offered. It's up to you if you want to do it. You'll also be watched closely for some pregnancy-related health problems, such as hypertension, that are more common in "older" women. There's every reason to think, however, that if you follow the guidelines of healthy eating and other self-care that *all* pregnant women should follow, your chances are excellent of having a good pregnancy outcome.

Technology has brought about a new development in so-called "older" parenting, with the combination of donor egg programs and hormonal stimulation of postmenopausal women. Women over 50 and even 60 years of age who have already stopped ovulating have given birth to healthy babies with donor eggs and estrogen stimulation of their own bodies. Sound like a tabloid headline? It isn't. It turns out that in mid-life, when the ovaries are no longer functioning, the uterus is often still strong enough and healthy enough to carry a pregnancy. If the woman herself is strong and healthy, pregnancy may be perfectly viable. Later-life parenting has brought great joy to a variety of couples: those who never had children, remarried and wanted more, those made up of younger men with menopausal women and even older mothers who want to bring children into the world for their own infertile daughters. There are so many potential cases.

This phenomenon has ethicists up in arms, questioning the fairness of bringing children into the world whose parents will be close to 80 when they enter college. They question whether parents who are ready for an infant at age 60 will be ready for a teenager at age 75. And they also ask if it's fair to create a situation in which children may be orphaned by natural causes at an early age.

Those who support the concept of later-age parenting point to the advancing age of the American population, the fact that 80-year-olds can run marathons and climb mountains if they stay in shape, and the fact that every woman should be able to determine her own reproductive destiny.

One thing is for sure: this issue will become hotter as the technology becomes more widely available. As of now, it's still only being done in select centers around the world. If you are considering this procedure for yourself, be absolutely certain that your health is checked from head to toe and that you are aware of what you are getting into, both physically and psychologically, before you proceed.

WHEN YOU'RE IN LABOR

Is it time? You may feel you've been waiting so long it isn't possible. If you are feeling contractions of your uterus that last at least a half minute to a minute, occur in a regular timed pattern, and don't abate when you move around, you may be in labor. "False" labor tends to lessen with movement, and occurs in an irregular pattern. Other signs of labor include a rush of water or mucus from your vagina, some blood (called "bloody show"), and fairly constant pain. The fluid is released when the amniotic sac around the baby breaks and the amniotic fluid runs out; the mucus comes from something called the "mucus plug" that has been blocking your cervix all these months. True labor pains tend to originate in your back and move around to your abdomen; false labor pains are more often in the front only.

But let's get one thing straight: there are no hard and fast rules. If you're in pain, or feeling unusual, and the sensation lasts, call your doctor and talk about it. The last thing you want to do is wait too long and have your baby at home.

Get moving: your big day may be here!

Cesarean Delivery

You've probably heard that the cesarean delivery rate in the U.S. is quite high compared to some other countries, *and* that it's much higher than it used to be. The numbers are actually quite staggering: in the early '70s, about 5% of babies were delivered by cesarean section. Today, that number is about 24%, for a total of about 960,000 cesarean deliveries a year. Some experts believe that the difference is largely caused by unnecessary cesareans; as a result, many hospitals around the country are making a concerted effort to move away from cesarean births and back to vaginal delivery. Others defend the current cesarean delivery rate as a reflection of better surgical techniques, fetal monitoring technology, and other positive factors. However, even those who defend cesarean delivery rates for the most part admit that many surgical deliveries are done for the wrong reasons.

Why bother to lower the rate? First, cesarean delivery carries greater risk to the mother than does natural delivery. Make no mistake, the cesarean is *not* like having your tonsils out; it's major surgery, and carries risk of blood loss, injury to the bowel or bladder, blood clots, infection and other serious complications associated with major abdominal surgery. These problems are relatively rare, but must be taken into consideration. The recovery from a cesarean takes several weeks longer than with natural delivery, and you must spend a few extra days in the hospital after the procedure. The mother's risk of death with cesarean, though quite small, is four times greater than it is with vaginal delivery. So while cesareans are

quite safe in the right hands, we should not treat them as minor procedures. They should only be done when medically warranted.

The trouble begins when you start determining what "medically warranted" means. While there are some clear-cut cases, there is also a great deal of overlap between "appropriate" and "inappropriate" cesareans. Many "appropriate" cesarean deliveries can be criticized on "gray-area" grounds; the same goes for "inappropriate" ones. Dr. Robert Cefalo, director of the maternal-fetal division at the University of North Carolina School of Medicine, says there's a common saying among obstetricians: "I know *why* I did a cesarean, but I don't know if I *should* have done it." That's because in retrospect, if all went well, it's hard to say what *might* have happened if you had taken another course of action.

Cesarean Delivery: What You Had to Say About It

Isabelle, 29 years old
My pregnancy had gone so easily I assumed there would be no problem. My mother had no problems, my sister had no problems. I told my mother, "You had it so easy, so I probably will too." Well, later she told me, "Your other grandmother had a cesarean—your dad was born by cesarean."

My labor was progressing very slowly, but progressing and progressing. Seven centimeters. Eight centimeters. I guess at seven or eight centimeters I stayed there for 3 hours. They checked me every hour or two. Two to three hours—they said there was no change. My husband said he saw my face deflate when they said it. There were a few little scares, but the baby was fine. One in the morning. Two in the morning. The doctor came in after about 24 hours of labor and said, "You haven't dilated. This is when we think about doing a cesarean." He was gentle. I said, "I never expected this." He said he never expected it either. I was exhausted, and emotionally exhausted too. I said, "Fine, just get it out of my body."

At points (during the procedure) you feel nauseous, and I could feel him sewing me at one point. At times I felt sick. Immediately after I felt the lousiest I've felt in a long time. I didn't even see her when she was born, I remember thinking I'd almost rather be asleep. My husband held her up and he was saying, "She's beautiful, she's beautiful," but I didn't open my eyes. I don't know if it was physical or emotional, like this wasn't the time to see my baby for the first time.

Later I was lying in the room, my husband was holding my hand. I was feeling so awful, exhausted, I hurt, my stomach hurt, I was very thirsty and they said I could only suck on ice chips. I could barely talk. They moved me and said I could have a shot, a mild painkiller. I woke up five hours later completely different. Uncomfortable but recovered. I was really excited then—that's my baby! There she is. I was excited to see her and then I was like, "Now what?"

Four days later I could walk out, walking kind of funny. My back was sore, it hurt when I moved a certain direction. But I'm sure it hurts to walk after a vaginal delivery too! At two weeks I was pretty good. It was not as bad as it could've been. The operation itself was not fun. I'm not psyched for it to happen again.

Here are some cases in which a cesarean delivery is usually considered not only appropriate but necessary to protect the well-being of both mother and baby: (1) a problem called cephalopelvic disproportion—that is, the baby's head is too big to make it through the mother's pelvis; (2) fetal distress; (3) placenta previa (the placenta is below the baby or covers the cervix); (4) placenta abruptio (the placenta has separated from the wall of the uterus); and (5) *sometimes* breech position (the baby comes either feet or buttocks first). Others would add severe, life-threatening bacterial infections of the uterus and other medical emergencies to the list. But even some of these so-called "clear-cut" cases can be disputed, as we'll discuss in a moment.

Instead of trying to give hard and fast rules, let's look at some of the reasons cesareans are most commonly performed in this country— and how to maximize the chance that you'll get one only if you really need it.

COMMON REASONS FOR CESAREAN DELIVERY

The most common reason a cesarean is done, believe it or not, is usually unnecessary! It's the automatic repeat cesarean—an operation performed not because there's a problem, but just because the woman had one done the last time she delivered. About 300,000 cesareans are done each year just because of the old saying "once a cesarean, always a cesarean". Dr. John Larsen, acting chairman of OB-GYN at George Washington University Medical Center, feels that this is the area where we can make the biggest dent in excessive cesarean rates. Experts know that many women who had cesarean deliveries in the past do not need to have them repeated. They can become so-called "V-BAC" patients—which stands for vaginal birth after cesarean. Hospitals that are trying to lower their rates of cesareans are focusing heavily on these potential V-BAC patients, since they represent a substantial population that can avoid unnecessary surgery. According to the American College of Obstetricians and Gynecologists, six out of ten women trying to have a vaginal birth after a previous cesarean will succeed. And with statistics like these getting more attention, things *seem* to be improving: according to the National Hospital Discharge Survey, the number of vaginal births per 100 women with a prior cesarean rose significantly between 1982 and 1988, from 4.8 to 12.6.

Some women, of course, will *need* repeat cesareans: but the key is to get a good reason from your doctor. Just "because you had one the last time" is *not* a good reason. One factor your doctor will take into consideration is the kind of incision you had in your uterus the last time you had a cesarean. If the incision on your uterus was low and side-to-side (a so-called "transverse" incision), your chances are better of a vaginal delivery the next time around. If your incision was vertical and higher up (called a "classical" incision), a planned repeat cesarean may well be necessary, since heavy labor could be riskier and might rupture your old scar. You cannot see the incision I'm referring to (it's not necessarily the same as the scar you see on your outer skin, but rather is *inside,* on your uterus), so you should ask your obstetrician what kind of incision you were given last time around. It is especially important to get this information if you may be living in a different place or using a different practitioner for your next delivery.

The second most common reason for cesarean delivery is the labor's "failure to progress." This goes by other names, such as CPD (cephalopelvic disproportion, mentioned earlier). This category is often controversial, because determining whether the baby's head will fit or not can be quite subjective. According to Dr. Bruce Flamm, area research chairman for Kaiser Permanente in Riverside, California, it is *extremely* rare for a baby's head to be too big for the mother's pelvis. Unless the mother is a dwarf, or was deformed by polio in the past, or some other uncommon reason, most babies will make it through just fine with a little more patience on everyone's part. There are other less extreme cases, such as a narrow, five-foot-tall mother trying to give birth to an eleven-pound baby: True, this can be difficult, and a cesarean may be warranted. But for the average woman and the average baby, CPD is a weak excuse, Dr. Flamm says. Dr. Larsen adds that the biggest problem in these cases is "how long do you wait?" This is a highly personal question for the doctor (at this stage, it isn't much in the hands of the mother). Some will opt to wait it out and push for a vaginal birth; others will rush to cesarean delivery, and it's left to the armchair quarterbacks to determine if the play was the right one.

What are the options if a baby isn't making it through? For one thing, if the quality of the labor—the contractions—is not good, the mother can be given drugs to boost labor, or she may simply be encouraged to walk around for a while to get things moving. A lot depends on who's coaching the labor. A nurse-midwife, for example, may be a lot more patient about waiting for a baby to make it through naturally than someone whose penchant for the quick or high-tech solution is greater. You may be able to reduce unnecessary cesareans just by picking practitioners who value vaginal birth as much as you do—with, of course, your own and the baby's well-being in mind.

Another common reason for cesareans is "fetal distress." Once again, this is a highly controversial issue. Fetal distress is usually defined by fetal monitors, and often, cesareans are the immediate consequence of abnormal readings. Dr. Cefalo points out that fetal monitors were not developed or intended for this purpose in the first place and often, not surprisingly, fail to do a good job of it. Even when they indicate fetal distress, he says, they should be considered early warning detection systems that might point to giving the mother oxygen, turning her on her side, and other minor interventions short of cesarean delivery. In other cases, when distress is significant, cesareans may be appropriate. Fetal monitors read the baby's heart rate, and if that rate drops, they indicate some degree of fetal distress. Is the distress serious? Is the baby losing oxygen? Does the heart rate bounce back up, or is it staying down? A heartbeat that drops and stays down is *much* more worrisome than one that returns to normal. Fetal monitors are *not* the best diagnostic tools on earth: in fact, they give very *little* information about the baby's condition. However, the information they give must be acted on *fast*: this isn't a time for philosophical discussions. If your doctor feels it's time to get the baby out fast, who's going to dispute it on the spot? It is believed that lots of babies who are actually doing okay are delivered by cesarean because the doctor panics on seeing an abnormal fetal heart rate on the monitor. Certainly if the heart rate falls precipitously and doesn't recover, you know you've got problems, and a cesarean can save the baby's life. Other tests, like a scalp test for the baby's pH, can give additional information on the baby's level of distress. But many cases are in a gray area, and the doctor must make a quick decision. He or she smells trouble—or, if you're cynical, you can say that he or she smells malpractice suits—and figures why not take the baby out surgically and avoid any potential problems.

The harshest critics of unnecessary cesareans point to the doctor's financial incentive to do the procedure. The doctor makes more money doing cesareans, the procedure takes less time, and can be planned ahead—big advantages over vaginal birth from the doctor's viewpoint. No one can say whether this incentive accounts for a significant number of unnecessary cesarean deliveries, but it can't be ruled out as a factor in some cases.

Often, cesarean deliveries are performed when the baby is in an abnormal position (for instance, when the baby is breech—coming out feet or buttocks first). Vaginal delivery can be dangerous or impossible for practitioners who aren't adequately trained or experienced in breech deliveries. Dr. Flamm urges practitioners to try to *turn* breech babies a week before delivery, rather than counting on them to turn around themselves. At his hospital, simply by manipulating the mother's belly from the outside—with no invasive procedure whatsoever—practitioners can turn 50% of babies around, so they can be delivered headfirst. The procedure is slightly uncomfortable but certainly not painful for the mother. This is a good example of the difference you can make with low-tech medicine.

A fairly significant number of cesareans are performed because of health problems in the mother that are believed to make both pregnancy and delivery higher-risk. Some examples include maternal diabetes or hypertension, both of which pose serious risks to the baby

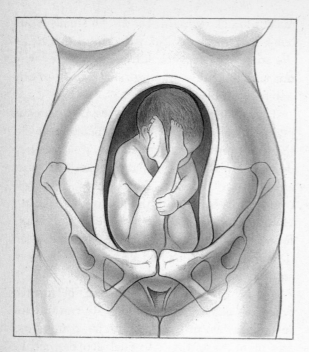

Full term pregnancy—breech position

when not tightly controlled.

Sometimes, multiple births (twins, triplets and so on) will be delivered by cesarean. This is *not* always necessary, but often is perfectly legitimate, especially when associated with other problems.

Maternal hemorrhage—which can occur with placenta previa, a condition in which the placenta covers the cervix—is considered a good reason to do a cesarean, since the lives of mother and baby would be at stake during vaginal delivery. The same can be said of placenta abruptia, in which much of the baby's lifeline is cut when the placenta separates from the uterine wall. These are cases where it makes sense to get the baby out ASAP, and cesarean delivery is the best way to accomplish that.

Questions You Should Ask of Your Practitioner. If you're concerned about having an unnecessary cesarean, do some investigating *before* you choose the hospital at which you're going to deliver. First, ask about the cesarean delivery rate at the hospital in question. The national average is 24%. Some hospitals have a high cesarean rate not because they're doing so many unnecessary ones, but because they tend to get a disproportionate number of high-risk births which *require* cesarean deliveries. Dr. Flamm warns, however, that this is an easy excuse for hospitals that may turn out in fact to have a perfectly average patient population. So do a little asking around: Does this hospital really have so many high-risk patients? Does it have a busy neonatal intensive care area, suggesting that it's staffed to handle high-risk pregnancies? And so on. In general, says Dr. Cefalo, teaching hospitals (where medical students and residents are trained) have lower cesarean rates by several percentage points than nonteaching hospitals.

Next, find out your practitioner's philosophy about cesareans. This does not have to be a confrontational conversation. Let him or her know that you would like to have a natural delivery if possible; that it is meaningful to you to have that experience. Find out if your practitioner works with a team that encourages vaginal birth; perhaps there is a midwife who can assist, for example. If your baby is in a breech position, do these practitioners make an effort to turn it around? How do they tend to interpret the fetal monitor—do they perform cesareans at the first sign of distress?

Remember, your practioners' primary goal (and yours), is to deliver a healthy baby. Ultimately, once you have chosen them, you have stated that you trust their judgment. If you end up with a cesarean despite everyone's best attempts to avoid one, and your baby is fine, you can't turn back the clock—focus on the fact that the most important end was reached, and begin to recover. Not all cesareans are bad: they often save lives. So avoid getting caught up in black-and-white philosophies on this issue, and after taking every step possible to avoid it, be thankful that technology was there and able to give you the best gift of all: your healthy baby.

AFTER DELIVERY: POSTPARTUM DEPRESSION

Every message we receive about a new baby's arrival—on covers of parenting magazines, in infant formula commercials and of course in our friends' photo albums—is *positive*. Smiling, teary-eyed mothers, beaming fathers, babies who never seem to make a fuss or have anything but blissful early life experiences. Sure, you know intellectually that this isn't reality. If you've had babies in the past, you know from experience that it isn't true. Still, when you're having a rough time during the postpartum period, it's easy to forget reality and come to believe that you're alone in your pain, your worries, and your depression. Everyone else can handle these emotions, you think—this is *supposed* to be a happy time. There must be something wrong with *you* if you're feeling miserable with your newborn by your side.

Well if there's something wrong with you, then there's something wrong with thousands of other new mothers, too. The fact is, some range of negative feelings, from the more minor so-called "baby blues" to the more serious postpartum depression (and the much rarer extreme of postpartum psychosis) are quite common. You don't hear too much about these negative feelings because they aren't considered "appropriate" in our society: you're expected to feel lucky and blessed with a new baby. People accept exhaustion, confusion, and worry from a new mother; depression, on the other hand, is still unacceptable to those who are ignorant about the syndrome. And just knowing that these feelings are frowned upon by friends and loved ones—especially those who have struggled or perhaps failed to have biological children—women clam up about their negative feelings, and grow increasingly ashamed of them.

It's time to break this taboo and talk about the facts. According to Ann L. Dunnewold, psychologist and president-elect of Postpartum Support International, the range of postpartum symptoms commonly goes from the "blues," with approximately ten days to two weeks of crying, anxiety, irritability, exhaustion and insomnia, to more severe depression that lasts longer (including the sensation that the "fog never clears"), with possible panic attacks mixed in. At the most severe end of the spectrum, postpartum psychosis, which is much more serious and far less common, involves confusion, hallucinations and other delusions that can be quite dangerous for mother and baby. The baby blues affect 50% to 80% of new mothers; postpartum depression, as many as 10% to 20% of women; and postpartum psychosis, about one per thousand women.

Marcia Biel, who serves on the board of Postpartum Support International, notes that with the baby blues, the "lighter" end of the spectrum, symptoms usually improve slightly each day until the new mother feels herself again in just a couple of weeks. Usually, just knowing that this is a common phenomenon, getting as much support as possible from your partner and/or other loved ones (both emotional *and* practical support), and attending the average new parent class or workshop will be enough to get you through the baby blues. If your symptoms have not improved after a couple of weeks, or if they're worsening, it's time to seek more structured help.

Postpartum depression often begins with sleep problems, changes in appetite (increased or decreased) and growing anger at oneself, one's partner or the baby, says Polly Kornblith, cofounder of the Massachusetts Depression After Delivery group. The problem is also often characterized by either an extreme *over*interest or *under*interest in the baby; that is, either the need to care for it and talk about it chronically and compulsively, or a total distancing of oneself from the baby. Other classic feelings of depression may also be part of the syndrome, including a sense of hopelessness, lack of interest in sex even after your body has healed from delivery, mood swings or a pure lack of feeling (numbness), and a sense of being isolated from the rest of the world. Many women begin to feel that they are inadequate mothers, that they aren't bonding successfully with their new children, and that something is fundamentally wrong with them. These feelings persist even when outside observers can see that their mothering is perfectly good. Ann Dunnewold recommends that women suffering from postpartum depression write down absolutely everything they've done over the past 24 hours: how many times they fed the baby, if they bathed it, changed its clothes, changed its diapers, etc. When women take a hard look at what they actually did in the course of one day, they're often startled to see how much they're accomplishing, she says. Writing it

down somehow makes it more real, and can have a tremendously reassuring effect on a woman who feels she's falling short in carrying out her obligations.

In addition to the feelings mentioned above, some women with postpartum depression have thoughts of harming themselves or the baby. If you have any or all of these feelings more than a couple of weeks after delivery, talk to your OB-GYN about them immediately, and ask for professional counseling by someone specifically trained to manage postpartum depression. Don't wait until your feelings are boiling over and you risk actively harming—or neglecting—yourself or your baby. You are still yourself underneath these terrible feelings, and the proper care will bring you back in very little time.

Postpartum depression doesn't always set in immediately after delivery. Sometimes it begins after you stop breast-feeding, or when you first begin menstruating again. It's thought that the new hormone shifts in your body are connected to the onset of these depressive feelings. You may be more susceptible to postpartum depression if you're socially isolated (living in a new community without friends nearby, for example) or if you've had postpartum depression in the past (in which case your chances are about 30% to 50% you'll have it again). Julia Dennis, a licensed clinical social worker in Memphis, Tennessee, gives the following additional risk factors for postpartum depression: prior mood problems of your own, or of family members; substance abuse; a troubled childhood; marital conflict; hormonal imbalances such as a thyroid disorder; a problematic pregnancy or delivery or a problem with the new baby; and many others. However, you can be seemingly risk-free and still suffer from postpartum depression;

and it's possible to have two smooth postpartum experiences and then to get PPD after your third child. *Don't blame yourself!*

If you are at risk of postpartum depression, but haven't delivered yet, consider getting some counseling *before* you deliver to set up a game plan that might lessen your chance of problems—or at least insure that you'll get the care you need should difficulties begin. Preplanning can go a long way toward alleviating the stresses that can tip you over into postpartum depression. Whether it's arranging for some additional paid help when you first bring the baby home, having the name of a counselor ready should you need professional support, changing your partner's or a friend's schedule so they're available to share the work—all of these preparations can be helpful. If you don't have the financial means to get help around the house, consider working out a plan with a friend or family member to take turns lifting each other's burdens so you can take some time out for yourself.

Treatment for postpartum depression should deal first with the immediate issues of concern: getting better sleep, eating properly, etc. Sometimes, medication helps; in other cases, some appropriate counseling is adequate. If you're breast-feeding, medication may not be an option—or you may be restricted to certain types. Marcia Biel urges women to enlist the help of people who have experience in dealing with new babies. Also, relinquish some control: let someone else do the laundry (or leave it undone for a couple of days); let someone else feed, burp or bathe the baby—and don't be ashamed to take some time out for yourself. Just talking about your feelings with someone you trust can he extremely helpful: stop hiding your feelings and assuming you're the only one who has ever felt this way. After you're feeling back on track a bit, you can start to face some of the underlying issues that may be getting in the way of your dealing with your new baby: self-esteem problems, dissatisfaction with your new lifestyle, and so on.

Some experts I interviewed were concerned that antianxiety medications are often given to women suffering from postpartum depression. Taking the wrong medication won't do a thing for your problems: be sure to get a firm diagnosis by someone experienced in this field before you accept any treatment. You OB-GYN should be able to refer you to a counselor familiar with postpartum problems.

It's important that both parents be counseled for postpartum depression. Educating the father so that he is nonjudgmental and supportive in the early months after delivery is vital, especially because there is so much misinformation about postpartum depression (some ignorant people may think of those who suffer from it as "going crazy"). Postpartum depression is a major marital stressor. But when partners learn how common this syndrome is, and that it can be successfully treated, the burden of blame and guilt can be lifted. Some fathers suffer postpartum depression, too, notes Biel. Group counseling with both parents present can be quite helpful.

As mentioned earlier, on the extreme end of the scale lies postpartum psychosis (PPP), a serious and dangerous disorder that requires immediate medical attention—medication and often temporary hospitalization. It sets in anywhere from three days to three weeks after delivery. Women experiencing PPP may hear voices, lose complete touch with reality and have harmful thoughts or take dangerous actions toward their babies. *This must not be confused with postpartum depression.*

BREAST-FEEDING

Throughout your pregnancy, your breasts have been gearing up for an important task: nursing your child. Chances are you've noticed some major changes in your breasts over the course of your pregnancy—they've grown larger, they may be tender to the touch, veins may be more noticeable on them, your nipple and areola may appear larger and different in color (usually darker) than ever before. There's a lot of work going on inside; the elaborate web of machinery that will produce food for your baby, if you choose to breast-feed, is rising to the occasion. Now you've got to decide: Is breast-feeding for you?

CAN YOU BREAST-FEED?

The overriding message from breast-feeding experts is that there are very few problems that are not solvable. Years ago, you'd hear a lot of women say, "I tried to breast-feed, but couldn't." The fact is, the vast majority of these women could have breast-fed if they knew how to work through common obstacles. But the American social climate was such (especially in the 1950s) that formula feeding was understood as the proper way to go; breast-feeding was seen as a peasant sort of activity that had pretty much seen its day. There was little support or encouragement for the "failing" breast-feeder—more likely there was a gentle nudge to give it up and buy plastic.

In the 1990s, it's safe to say we've come a long way, baby—pretty much full circle. Breast-feeding is back "in"—along with a host of support groups and a vast amount of literature on breast-feeding's health benefits, problem-solving tips, and so on. We still have a way to go, however: according to a Ross Laboratories survey, while one in two women in the U.S. starts breast-feeding in the hospital, only one in five is still doing it at six months. We'll talk about some of the obstacles that get in the way of breast-feeding stick-to-it-ive-ness.

If you want to breast-feed today—that is, if you're committed to it—chances are about 99 in 100 that you'll be successful. This is not to say that you should feel inadequate or guilty if you don't breast-feed. The choice is yours, and formula is a quite healthy alternative. Most experts would agree, however, that it's a second choice to successful breast-feeding. One important piece of advice, if you plan to breast-feed, is that you do so *immediately* upon your baby's delivery. Make sure your hospital staff does not give your baby a bottle or artificial nipple of any kind. If your baby even starts to get acquainted with pacifiers or bottles, the proper sucking motion for breast-feeding can be thrown off, and your task made harder. Also, the sooner you try to feed after delivery—and the more often after that—the better. You won't have actual mature milk right away—you'll have something called pre-milk, or colostrum. This is a remarkably nutrition-packed beverage, full of antibodies to protect your new baby. Colostrum has triple the protein of mature breast milk. Nature is telling us that immediate breast-feeding is a valuable thing. Within a few days, mature milk comes in and replaces it. If your milk has not come in after a week or so, talk to your doctor about a possible blockage or other treatable problem.

HEALTH BENEFITS OF BREAST-FEEDING

It seems nearly every day another potential health benefit of breast-feeding is identified. Just to give you a few big ones from the list, breast-feeding is thought to protect against gastrointestinal infections, respiratory infections, allergies, sudden infant death and ear infections, and even some later-life chronic diseases. Most experts advise breast-feeding for at least four months and ideally, longer—from six months to a year or more, to give your baby the most protection. There is some data, (albeit uncertain), suggesting that women who breast-feed are less likely to develop breast cancer than those who do not—but this is less firm than the information about the *baby's* benefits.

COMMON BREAST-FEEDING PROBLEMS—AND SOLUTIONS

According to Deborah McCarter, an international board-certified lactation consultant at Beth Israel Hospital in Boston, many of the very same set of breast-feeding problems crop up time and time again—and they can all be overcome with a little tinkering. Many women panic and give up before giving it their best shot. The reason? They're afraid of starving the baby. This is seldom a problem for well-nourished, healthy women. Here is McCarter's and other experts' list of common breast-feeding obstacles—and solutions:

Problem #1: Baby isn't getting enough milk.

The first question here, McCarter notes, is whether the baby is *really* not getting enough milk—or does the mother just *think*

this is so. The best way to measure this is to chart the baby's growth. Your pediatrician will help you do it using a proper scale. Also, is the baby emptying each breast in 10–15 minutes or so? This is another measure of success. If the baby truly isn't gaining properly, there may be a problem with inadequate milk supply, or with the baby's sucking ability. Here are a few solutions:

A) Feed more often. Don't wait for your baby to cry to feed her—put her on your breast more often. The more you nurse, the more milk you'll make. The system is designed to work this way—you don't have a limited milk supply. It's normal to nurse eight to twelve times in 24 hours with newborns. If your baby is sleepy and not eating often, wake her up and let her know it's feeding time. Ignore those who tell you to feed on a strict schedule, instead of on demand. All babies are different, and schedules imply that they can all fit a particular framework. If that were true, child rearing would be a lot easier!

B) Make sure the baby is positioned properly on your nipple. She should have her mouth wide open, her lips spread out, and her gums pretty much covering the areola as well as the nipple. The nipple should be centered in the baby's mouth, and the baby should be comfortably resting in the crook of your arm, tucked close against your breast or in the so-called "football" position, with her face looking up at you and her feet behind you to one side. The wrong position can make it harder for your baby to suck successfully.

C) Make absolutely sure that *you're* getting adequate nutrition and fluids by talking to a nutritionist. Remember, you need extra fluid, calcium and calories at this time. Don't wait until you're thirsty to drink—drink water, milk and other healthful beverages throughout the day.

Problem #2: Sore nipples.

This is very common early on. You may experience dry, cracked nipples, or just plain sore ones in the first couple of weeks of breast-feeding. If your nipples bleed, you will likely develop small scabs which crack and hurt when your baby sucks. In the early days of breast-feeding, many women would swear their newborns have teeth! This is one major reason many women "give up" soon after they get going.
The solutions:

A) *See* above for information on proper positioning. One of the main causes of sore nipples is the baby sucking on the breast improperly; when it's sucking directly on the nipple itself, and not the entire areola, you can experience great pain. If your baby gets an improper latch on your breast and you're in pain, slip your finger between her gums and your nipple, gently break the seal, and help her to get a better mouthful.

B) Feed your baby *before* she gets too hungry, so she doesn't latch on in a ravenous state. Signs to look for before crying include the baby gnawing on her hand or making a sucking motion with her mouth.

C) Massage your breasts before you put the baby on them. This will help "let down" some milk so your baby doesn't have to tug as hard to get it.

D) Let your nipples air-dry after feeding. If you're in a private place or comfortable around those in the room, leave them open to the air once in a while before replacing your bra or clothing. Sometimes, rubbing some milk into the nipples and then letting them dry is soothing—and better than using creams or lotions.

E) Be patient. Often, sore nipples get better within a few weeks even if you don't change what you're doing. It may seem like a lifetime, but if you can wait it out, you'll be surprised how much better you'll feel after your breasts get used to the new sensation. When the cracks heal, and you're feeling better throughout the rest of your body as delivery becomes a more distant memory, you may discover you actually *like* breast-feeding, and look forward to it as a relaxing part of your day.

F) Heat may help some women—ice may help others. Experiment with applying different temperatures to the breasts to soothe them. Standing under a hot shower sometimes does the trick.

G) Alternate breasts each time you feed. If your baby sucks from both breasts at each feeding, be sure to start on the opposite breast next time. Don't overwork one breast and leave one alone, *especially* if the baby tends to favor one breast. If one breast gives more milk and you start to ignore the other breast, the problem will get worse—the breast that produces less milk will produce less and less. Remember, the more you feed, the more milk you will produce.

H) Don't use products that make the problem worse. Avoid drying soaps and some bubble baths, for example.

Problem #3: Lack of support.

Often, even if a woman believes she wants to breast-feed, she gets negative feedback from others close to her—perhaps a husband who thinks breasts are "his" domain, a mother who used formula and thinks it's the best way to go, or friends who make her feel uncomfortable if she feeds in front of them.

The solution:

A) Call a breast-feeding support network like La Leche League International. They've heard it all—and have suggestions on how to deal with it all. Perhaps your partner, parent or close friend could benefit from some education on the benefits of breast-feeding, too.

Problem #4: Sucking problems.

Even with proper positioning and adequate milk supply, the baby can't get enough milk:
The solutions:

A) Occasionally (rarely) the baby will truly have a sucking problem that you can't do anything about. In this case, you have two options. If you want your baby to get breast milk, you can pump your breasts and then feed the baby your milk from a bottle. I know committed women who have kept this up for months, and are glad they did it. Or, you can switch to formula feeding from a bottle.

Some breast pumps are quite effective, and can be easier than you might expect: it takes about 10–15 minutes to empty each breast by electric pump. However, electric pumps (which you usually rent for a period of time) are costly. Pressing out your milk by hand is free of charge, and using manual pumps is relatively inexpensive, but both take longer than electric pumps. The nice compromise about feeding breast milk from a bottle is that your baby still gets the wonderful nutrition of breast milk, but others in the family can share in the feeding (and the late-night wake-ups!).

Problem #5: Inverted nipples.

If your nipples point inward rather than outward, you might just assume that you can't breast-feed—because there's nothing out there for your baby to latch onto. In fact, in the past, women with inverted nipples were told not to bother trying. This is a myth—with a simple solution:

A) Buy breast shells. These small plastic devices pull or suck the inverted nipple out so the baby can latch on and feed. Sometimes, after using the shells for a while and some good sucking on your baby's part, inverted nipples will come out more on their own. You can wear breast shells in your bra before delivery to "warm up" your nipples. Breast pumps also can help.

Problem #6: Infection: lactational mastitis.

If you have an infection, your breasts may be quite painful, swollen, red and might even develop pus. Many women give up breast-feeding as soon as they face this unpleasant, sometimes painful obstacle. Not only do they feel terrible, but they assume that it's bad for the baby to suck from an infected nipple. Actually, that's not the case.

The solution:

A) Soak your breasts in warm-to-hot water (don't burn yourself!), ask your doctor for antibiotics that will treat the infection but not harm your baby, and *keep* breast-feeding—the infection has no impact on your baby, and continuing to breast-feed, even through the temporary pain, will help clear the infection faster. You may need to have the pus drained: ask your doctor.

Problem #7: Blocked milk ducts.

If your breast(s) become hard, swollen and obviously aren't releasing milk despite your baby's sucking, you may have a blocked milk duct or clogged opening on the outside of your nipple (commonly called a milk blister).

The solution:

A) Massage the breast(s) and apply damp heat throughout the day (with warm wet rags or in the shower). Also let the baby continue sucking to work the milk out of your breast.

When You Cannot Breast-feed.

Some women truly cannot breast-feed, even if they do everything "right." Perhaps prior breast surgery damaged the ductal system that brings milk to the nipple (although these days the ducts can often be spared even with major breast surgery, such as surgical breast reductions). Maybe you have a medical problem, such as a thyroid problem, that severely impairs your milk supply. If you want to breast-feed but find that you just can't, talk to your obsetrician and to your general internist to make sure there's no medical problem that can be corrected. Sometimes, it's the baby who can't breast-feed, due to any number of problems with its sucking mechanism. (An option in this case, if you are producing milk, is to pump your breast milk and feed it to your baby in a bottle.) Whatever the reason you cannot breast-feed, *don't feel like a failure.* If you've given it your best shot and it isn't working out, the formula alternative is a good one—in fact, one that many baby boomers grew up on with great success.

Formula Feeding.

Commercial baby formula is very nutritious. It's not breast milk, but it's a very healthy alternative. There are a couple of major formulas on the market. Ask your pediatrician if he/she recommends one for your child. If it makes no difference (which is often the case), see which one your baby prefers and perhaps choose the less costly brand. Remember, your baby is a person, with personal tastes. If she doesn't seem to like one formula, try another. Or, if your baby has a problem with traditional formulas and your doctor okays it, try soy versions that are easier on the stomach.

FOR MORE INFORMATION ON PREGNANCY AND DELIVERY

U.S. DEPARTMENT OF HEALTH AND HUMAN SERVICES
NATIONAL MATERNAL AND CHILD HEALTH CLEARINGHOUSE
8201 Greensboro Drive, Suite 600
McLean, VA 22102
703-821-8955, ext.254

NATIONAL ASSOCIATION OF CHILD-BEARING CENTERS
3123 Gottschall Road
Perkiomenville, PA 18074
215-234-8068

ASPO/LAMAZE
800-368-4404

MARCH OF DIMES BIRTH DEFECTS FOUNDATION
1275 Mamaroneck Ave.
White Plains, NY 10605
914-428-7100

PARENTS CARE, INC.
101½ South Union St.
Alexandria, VA 22314
703-836-4678
(Support for parents of babies who are in the intensive care unit)

AMERICAN COLLEGE OF OBSTETRICIANS AND GYNECOLOGISTS RESOURCE CENTER
409 12th Street SW
Washington, DC 20024-2188
202-638-5577

AMERICAN COLLEGE OF NURSE-MIDWIVES
818 Connecticut Ave. NW, Suite 900
Washington, DC 20006
202-728-9860

POSTPARTUM DEPRESSION:
DEPRESSION AFTER DELIVERY
P.O. Box 1282
Morrisville, PA 19067
800-944-4PPD
215-295-3994

POSTPARTUM SUPPORT INTERNATIONAL
927 North Kellogg
Santa Barbara, CA 93111
805-967-7636

BREAST-FEEDING:
INTERNATIONAL LACTATION CONSULTANT ASSOCIATION
P.O. Box 4031
University of VA Station
Charlottesville, VA 22903

MEDELA, INC.
P.O. Box 660
McHenry, IL 60051
800-TELL-YOU

EGNELL/AMEDA, INC.
755 Industrial Dr.
Cary, IL 60013
800-323-8750

LA LECHE LEAGUE INTERNATIONAL
9616 Minneapolis Ave.
Franklin Park, IL 60131
800-525-3243
708-455-8317

CHAPTER SIXTEEN

INFERTILITY: CAUSES AND TREATMENTS

Infertility does not kill, nor is it a visible disorder. It is rarely discussed in public and its sufferers usually do not receive flowers or condolences. It is a private experience revealed only by one's childlessness and on occasion perhaps a few uncontrolled tears. No wonder so few people understand the impact of this devastating and growing problem.

—Linda P. Salzer, *Surviving Infertility*

Since childhood, many of us have been planners. We plan what we want to be when we grow up. If we want to go to college, we imagine where we'd like to be—and in high school, while we're still basically children, we are forced to plan that move. If we want careers, we imagine ourselves at the pinnacle of those careers, and plan our education or training to lead in the right direction. If we are interested in marriage, we plan—or at least envision—the proper time for that transition, too. We are *raised* to plan: Who can't remember being asked, before we're tall enough to reach the dinner table, "And what do *you* want to be when you grow up?"

As women, one of the most basic plans for many of us is to have children. And we usually think in terms of *biological* children. We might not know exactly *when* we want children, but in the backs of our minds, we have a picture of what would be ideal. Perhaps it's only after finding the perfect mate. Or after getting settled in a better position at work. Or after we can afford a home. Or after we've moved to an area more conducive to child rearing. Or when our friends or family members are having children. Or when we or our partner have more time to spare. The point is, most of us approach the issue of childbearing not as an *if* question, but as a *when* question. Even if we know, intellectually, that infertility does exist, most of us don't believe that it could happen to us. So we blissfully plan, or ignore the issue altogether, assuming that when the time comes, we will bear children.

Planning is a control issue: By looking forward to things, by pointing ourselves in a given direction, we have the underlying assumption that we can *make* these things happen if we work hard enough. And with luck and hard work, many of the things we plan *do* come to fruition. Others don't come to pass, and we live with the outcome. For about one in ten American couples of reproductive age, getting pregnant is that thing that doesn't come to pass—and according to women and experts across the country, the emotional consequences can be dire. In one study of infertile couples, 40% said that infertility was the most upsetting experience of their lives. Couples report emotional swings from anger and resentment to sadness and outright clinical depression when infertility persists. Some researchers find that the emotions are more deeply felt for women, who more closely link fertility to their sense of self-esteem, purpose and wholeness. But certainly men share the pain of infertility, and the stress on couples is tremendous.

The good news is this: while infertility is more common than most believe, successful treatment is common as well. The road to fertility can be long (depending on the cause), costly, and emotionally and physically stressful. The endpoint, however—bearing a healthy child—is very much in sight for most couples. The most important issue you will have to work out for yourself—and we will discuss it throughout this chapter—is how far you're willing to go to achieve the goal of pregnancy. Your chance of success can be hard to gauge, but we'll examine the various causes of infertility and some relative success rates for different problems. Keep in mind that you are not alone: 5.3 million Americans are dealing with the problem of infertility, and more is being learned about this problem every day. With the right information, patience and—unfortunately—a high financial cost as well, your chance of success is much better than you think.

INFERTILITY: WHAT YOU HAD TO SAY ABOUT IT

Kyle, 30 years old

It's not necessarily a system that works well at meeting your emotional needs. A lot of times the treatment interferes with work quite drastically, and trying to maintain a happy lifestyle. I was working 14-hour shifts and driving an hour each way for blood tests. Since '87 I've been going through this.

I'm 30 years old now. I was the victim of a very bad army doctor who did a procedure that was medically contraindicated. I have scarring in my uterus, and he lied about what he had done. He said he'd done a hysteroscopy—he didn't have the right equipment. My husband has a vasectomy which is too old to reverse, so I'm using donor sperm. It's a financial racket. I go through it month after month. I've tried in vitro fertilization. I became pregnant and had my third miscarriage. It was the most distressing thing that had happened, we had tried so hard, things went so well.

Having a baby boy (by adoption) helps, I don't think I could have done this without him. He came into the picture between the first and second surgery. He's the one very happy part of my life right now. With the infertility putting so much stress on the marriage, the marriage isn't good right now.

I've formed closer friendships with infertile women than anyone else in my life—you understand how desperately each woman wants to have a child of her own, how distressing it is each month you get your period. People are always going to baby showers, friends talk about babies. It felt like I was the only woman in public not feeding a baby.

Marriage is something you can accomplish by choice—pregnancy is not. At this point, we've almost exhausted our financial resources, we've exhausted our insurance. It's taken life away. I've put things on hold, vacations on hold. People say such flippant things, like "Relax, just take a vacation." In-laws put on so much pressure to have grandchildren. I think I would regret the rest of my life not being able to experience birth.

Lita, 36 years old
I was about 28 years old when I went to the first infertility doctor. I had been trying to conceive for a year and a half. I thought all I had to do was say I have an infertility problem and it would be taken care of. I got pregnant and miscarried, then I moved, and then I tried for five more years and had two more miscarriages. I was sure I wouldn't be able to have a kid. I was very depressed, totally sure I would never have a child biologically.

Having a child was out of the picture. It took 3 years to feel I could adopt, which turned me around a little bit—to think I could be a parent. The pain is worse for the woman. We are taught that is an important part of our roles in life, a critical, important part and men don't feel that as much. I don't think my husband ever felt the pain I felt.

I had lots of treatments, a GIFT cycle, two Pergonal cycles, and the doctor had me so messed up that there was no way I could conceive. He had me thinking I was in premature ovarian failure, that I would never ovulate again. I used a test kit at home because I thought I might never ovulate again. I ovulated on the twenty-first day—I hadn't taken anything then. I don't know what worked—I conceived!

The carrying was awful, I was sure I was going to have a miscarriage. It wasn't a happy pregnancy. Up to 2 weeks before I was due, I was afraid I'd have a miscarriage. My husband said, "If it happens now it won't be a miscarriage, it will be a stillbirth." The birth was the most exciting—it made all the pain and suffering worth it. It was like a miracle. It was truly as miraculous as it should be, the most exciting and miraculous event of my life. To watch a little person come out of your body is the most incredible thing.

I now have a girl and a boy, four and two-and-a-half. One month after I stopped breast-feeding the first one, I got pregnant with the second! I thought, "Better do it fast, it could be another five years and I could be in menopause."

My children came from nontreatment cycles, but some doctors say any pregnancy within six months of a treatment cycle is from the treatment. I've had plenty of infertile friends who had babies the same way. RESOLVE (the support group) saved my life, I wouldn't have been able to go through it without them. I wouldn't have had the stamina, that's what kept me going. The support system, the information. I still stay in touch with my support group, I'm having them over this Sunday. One woman is having her third child. We're the most fertile infertile group!

Debbi, 41 years old

When I got pregnant the first time my baby died for reasons we're just beginning to understand seven years later. When I got pregnant the second time I was very scared—it was two years later, and I miscarried at six weeks. I got pregnant a third time and miscarried four weeks later. It's a double-edged sword—you get pregnant, but you're so afraid. I had surgery to remove fibroids, then was on Perganol for two years and was unable to get pregnant after that right up to this day. We did Clomid for a couple of years, then surgery, then Perganol and we were at the point earlier this year where we were doing tests for in vitro.

I come from a really large family, lots of cousins, everybody has children. I've got nine nieces and nephews, and to me family is everything. That's what keeps me wanting to try each time. I get very scared each time I get more information. I just spent nine days in the hospital because I went through a test to see if I had any structural defects in the uterus. Unfortunately they did find a structural defect which no one knew was there, and unfortunately now I'm 41. I'm still sick, I had an abscess in my right fallopian tube, treatment let all this bacteria into my uterus.

I've sacrificed so much. I lost my position at work because of my fertility problem, I got demoted. They said, "Why can't you go to your doctor in the evening on your own time?" I had to do it in the morning, that's when they do the tests! I worked in the health care industry, a hospital, for 15 years. I'm a pharmacist. I've had my boss actually say to me, "When are you going to stop this nonsense?" This has been an almost unbearable stress, because I love my job. I've been out of work three weeks.

How much more of this do I want to do? The drugs make you crazy. "Perganol hell," we call it. Your feelings are out of control. We've been through hell these last few years. We're both uncomfortable with adoption. Four to five years ago it was an option, but now I'm at a point where it's so expensive, it's a very big commitment, and we've heard horror stories about adoption. Emotionally, I feel it's a closed door on adoption. Not for my husband. He's done so much for me these years, I feel I have to do something for him, so I'll think about it. My husband wants me to keep an open mind for the future.

I'm very lucky. Without my husband's support there's no way I could've gone on, it's part of who we are as a family. We got to a point where I wanted to do more, try in vitro, and he wanted to stop. It got to the point where we stopped communicating and we needed someone to step in—we saw a counselor. You need someone else. You feel like you're out there by yourself. It helps to know you're not. The counselor was able to put things in perspective. I wish we'd done it sooner. I'd tell another woman to be absolutely sure her husband is in it with her, because it really can be devastating to a couple. If there is any kind of counseling, get involved from the start. I'm finally leaning toward saying let's stop trying. For me to stop, it's like a big dark tunnel. I'm gonna need a lot of talking to the counselor, because to me, without children, it isn't a family. But we'll finally have some peace.

We've been through ups and downs, emotional upheaval. But I have to come to grips with something I didn't think I could live with.

WHAT EXACTLY IS INFERTILITY?

Infertility is defined as the failure to achieve pregnancy after one full year of unprotected (that is, no birth control) intercourse. The rate of infertility climbs with maternal age, but less so with paternal age. For example, the infertility rate in women aged 35–44 is double that for women aged 30–34, according to the American Fertility Society. The Society also reports that the rate of infertility is one in seven for couples ages 30–34, one in five at ages 35–39 and one in four at ages 40–44. There is a more upbeat way to look at it, however, notes Dr. Alvin Goldfarb of the Jefferson Medical College: and that is that about 95% of women who want to get pregnant and have regular unprotected intercourse will be pregnant by age 35.

Another term you'll hear in connection with infertility is "fecundity." That means the chance of becoming pregnant in any given month or menstrual cycle. For average, fertile, healthy people, the fecundity rate is about 20%—that is, there's about a one in five chance of becoming pregnant in a given cycle. These average, healthy, fecund people are in their early to mid-20s. Ninety-three percent of these average fertile people will be pregnant within one year of trying; 50% of them will be pregnant after just a little over 3 months. Age and many other factors reduce the fecundity rate. Logically, the smaller your chance of getting pregnant in any given cycle, the smaller your chance of getting pregnant in a year. For this reason, "older" women (in the reproductive sense)—usually those approaching or older than 40—will often be given a speedier fertility workup than will younger women.

Infertility isn't a diagnosis in itself: It is a symptom of some other problem(s). There are a wide variety of potential causes of infertility, and when you think about how conception takes place, it's easy to see why there are so many potential pitfalls. For conception to occur, a vast array of organ systems, hormonal signals and other physical factors must be in place in both the male and female partners. Sperm must be produced, and must be healthy, and must be able to travel out of the man's body and into the woman's. This alone requires a sophisticated set of hormonal and structural factors to be sound. Once in the woman's body, the sperm must be able to travel to meet the egg—which also had to be produced and transported via a sophisticated network of hormones, tubes and other structures. If there is a problem *anywhere* along the complicated systems of the male or female partner, infertility can occur. If more than one problem exists—as if often the case—fertility is further impaired. Frankly, once you understand what it takes to conceive, you're more amazed that so many pregnancies *do* occur than that so many *do not*.

TRENDS IN INFERTILITY PROBLEMS

There was a time when fertility problems were thought to be just *female* problems. Those days are long gone. In fact, those days were *always* long gone—male fertility factors have always been important—but some combination of sexism and resistance on the part of researchers to study and reveal male factor infertility held back the medical awakening which has added tremendously to treatment success (not to mention lifting the full burden of responsibility from women). As Dr. Kaylen Silverberg, a reproductive endocrinologist at the University of Texas, San Antonio puts it, "Infertility is a team sport." *Couples* sould be treated for infertility, not individuals—unless a person without a partner chooses to be treated with donor eggs or sperm. While estimates vary, it's thought that about 40% of infertility has some significant male factor, 40% has a significant female factor, and about 20% involves a combination of the two. In different parts of the country and in different regions within even the same cities, the causes of infertility differ. For instance, in inner-city populations, experts report that sexually transmitted diseases cause a relatively large proportion of fertility problems, while in suburban or rural areas, ovulatory dysfunction may be relatively more common (there are, of course, many exceptions on both sides, and the worst thing you can do is assume that you're invulnerable to one or another problem).

Dr. Victor Knutzen, medical director of the Northern Nevada Fertility Center and president of the Society for Assisted Reproductive Technology, is seeing a significant impact of sexually transmitted diseases (STDs) on fertility, especially in *younger* patients. Their reproductive organs have been damaged by silent infections like chlamydia and ureaplasma often because they failed to protect themselves with condoms. Dr. Michael Diamond of the Vanderbilt School of Medicine has noticed an increase in infertility caused by delayed childbearing: couples are waiting to have children until the "right time," only to find out that that time isn't under their control. In fact, Dr. Ronald Strickler, chief of the department of OB-GYN at the Jewish Hospital of St. Louis, finds older, two-career couples the toughest to treat of all, because they are so accustomed to controlling their tight schedules and meeting demands *on time* that when it comes to getting pregnant, they expect more of the same: conception on demand. Unfortunately, for many couples, it doesn't work out that way.

While most of this book has focused on women's health issues alone, in this chapter, we'll talk about the more common causes of infertility in both sexes. Treatment almost always requires both of you, and success certainly will affect both of you equally.

You will see how vital it is to find out the precise cause of infertility, since treatments are tailored specifically to different problems. In about one in ten cases, infertility will be called "unexplained." The other nine will be diagnosed by one of many tests on both the male and female partners, all of which we'll discuss below. Even those with "unexplained" infertility, however, can be treated successfully—though we may never find out what the source of the problem was.

Where to Begin with Treatment for Infertility

First you will have to decide what kind of practitioner to see to treat your fertility problem. Your regular doctor may have some experience treating infertility—and may be quite good at it—but it's hard for you to determine if this is the case. If you are attached to your doctor, it can be tempting to stick with him/her, especially at this emotionally trying time. But it's not always the best idea. There are people who specialize in the treatment of infertility. They are called reproductive endocrinologists, and they are board certified in the treatment of fertility problems. Some are subtrained in surgery for fertility problems. Another group of specialists—urologists—sometimes focus on treating male-factor infertility. Follow your best judgment; if you and your general doctor believe that you can get to the bottom of the problem without specialized help, go for it. If you are running out of time—that is, you are getting older—you may want to skip right to the specialists. Or, if it makes you feel more comfortable, perhaps you can find an expert who will incorporate your regular doctor into the treatment process.

No matter what, if it comes time for specialized treatments or high-tech fertility assistance, you would be wise to find someone with specialized training in your area of fertility management. For many types of fertility treatment, your first shot at treatment is your best shot. *See* the information box at the end of this chapter for some suggestions on where to find experts in various aspects of fertility care.

Giving Your Sexual History

When you sit down with your fertility doctor, you will be expected to give a fully detailed history of your sexual relationship. Be prepared to be candid and to remember specifics when possible, because this history can be key to understanding your infertility problem. Here are just a few examples. Let's say you and your partner do not have sex very often. Maybe you or he travel a great deal for your work, or your schedules make it hard to get together romantically. Perhaps one or both of you have had sexual problems—impotence, or lack of interest in sex. Maybe you don't have a good idea of *when* you need to have sex in order to get pregnant, so you've been trying in a haphazard way. All of these possibilities—and countless others—will come into play in determining how serious your fertility problem may be. For instance, if you have been having unprotected intercourse in the middle of your menstrual cycle (halfway

between periods) every month for a couple of years, you have probably given it an excellent shot. If, on the other hand, you have had sex at this most fertile time only a couple of times in a year, you may not have given natural conception much of a try at all. Your doctor will help you sort this all out.

In addition to your sexual history as a couple, you will be asked to discuss your sexual histories in general: any past sexually transmitted diseases, surgeries to the reproductive or urinary organs, and so on. Have you had miscarriages, abortions or other pregnancy-related issues in the past? Be sure that you are ready to be open with one another before you are open with the doctor. Holding back information can delay the diagnosis and solution to your problem. Also be prepared to discuss your lifestyle habits—including smoking, alcohol and other drug use. Again, if you and your partner are not forthcoming, your doctor's chance of helping you become pregnant is diminished.

Finding Causes and Treatments

Tests for the Woman

There are three basic fertility problems in women: (1) problems of ovulation (that is, trouble creating and releasing a mature egg, which can occur anywhere along the brain-reproductive organ pathway); (2) problems with physical structures (such as structural defects in the uterus, malfunctioning ovaries or blocked fallopian tubes); and (3) problems involving the health of the cervix, the mouth of the uterus, which may produce less than ideal mucus (and since mucus is needed to help usher the sperm into the uterus and on to the tubes, this factor can be quite important). There are a wide variety of tests for each potential problem, and a good fertility specialist will systematically examine each factor.

WHAT CAUSES OVULATION PROBLEMS?

There are enough answers to that question to fill this book. Ovulation problems can be caused by any number of irregularities stemming from the centers in the brain where hormone signals are created (the pituitary and the hypothalamus, in particular); the ovaries themselves, which can be "polycystic"[1] or otherwise malfunctioning; genetic abnormalities; excessive weight gain or loss; emotional stress; and many other potential causes. Most of these problems are treatable, either with hormone therapy, or with other medication or treatments to stimulate ovulation, weight gain or loss, and so on.

Ovulation Tests.

Like many of his patient-friendly colleagues, Dr. Russell Malinak of the Baylor College of Medicine in Houston likes to take a cost-effective route to detecting ovulation problems. He begins with the basal body temperature chart, in which the woman takes her temperature every morning for a full month (or a full menstrual cycle), writes it down and looks for a

"blip"—perhaps as much as a full degree, but usually less—at or near mid-cycle. This slight temperature rise indicates that ovulation probably took place: but it's not definitive (actually, no test for ovulation, other than conception, is truly definitive). There are special ovulation thermometers with a narrow range of temperatures that you can purchase for this test—but you can also use a regular thermometer if you read it carefully. Along with the basal body temperature chart, you can try the at-home ovulation kits (they are available in most drugstores and cost about $25 to $50). These simple tests check for the level of a hormone called luteinizing hormone (LH) in your urine, which would indicate that ovulation is about to occur. If the temperature chart *and* this test indicate ovulation at about the same time, you've got a pretty good clue that ovulation is happening.

There are other more costly and more definitive tests for ovulation, if you and your doctor still aren't comfortable with the test results. One is a blood test for progesterone several days before your period is due; another, which is slightly uncomfortable, is an endometrial biopsy, in which a sample of the lining of your uterus is taken and examined for signs that ovulation has occurred. Another higher-tech test—and the most costly of all—is the sonogram test, a painless exam in which sound waves are bounced off of your ovaries to give a picture of what's developing there. This test can reveal the development of follicles, which contain eggs, and can show with much better certainty if and when ovulation occurs (and from which ovary the egg emerged). If needed, your doctor will do several sonogram tests throughout your menstrual cycle to track the progress in your ovaries.

---

[1] Polycystic ovarian syndrome is a hormonal problem, often associated with obesity, facial hair growth, and acne, in which the ovaries malfunction and enlarge with many cysts, and ovulation is impossible without treatment.

If You Have an Ovulation Problem.

Ovulation problems are often treatable. If your only fertility problem is ovulatory, your chance of becoming pregnant after treatment is excellent. If you have a physical problem affecting a gland (say, a tumor on your pituitary) that problem will be treated. If you have any of a wide variety of hormonal problems leading to anovulation, you will be given one of several drugs that stimulate ovulation. The best known of these are clomiphene citrate (Clomid) and Pergonal. Clomid, which is taken in pill form, is less potent than Pergonal, but still carries certain risks and leads to twin pregnancies in about one in ten cases. Pergonal (also called hMG or human menopausal gonadotropin) is a powerful and costly drug that is taken by injection for up to two weeks in a row and leads to multiple gestation pregnancies in about one in five cases. If your problem is in the pituitary gland, with too much of the hormone prolactin being produced, you may be given the drug bromocriptine, which has a long list of unpleasant side effects including nausea, vomiting and headache. All of these drugs have side effects, ranging from breast and abdominal pain to headaches, dizziness and others.

Dr. Malinak stresses the importance of careful and constant monitoring while you're taking any of these drugs: the main risk is hyperstimulation of the ovaries, which sometimes occurs and can be dangerous. So be sure your doctor is keeping close track of your progress while you're taking these drugs. According to Dr. Deborah Manzi, director of reproductive endocrinology and infertility at the Creighton Women's Health Center of Creighton University Medical Center, the only way to adequately monitor ovulation stimulation is with both blood tests and repeat ultrasound tests. If it turns out that the ovaries have been overstimulated, Dr. Manzi notes, your practitioner can hold back further treatment and protect you from a medical crisis by NOT attempting fertilization during this cycle.

TESTING YOUR REPRODUCTIVE STRUCTURES

While the ovulation testing and treatment is going on, you will likely have your tubes, uterus and other physical structures studied for clues to your fertility problem. There are several tests with which this can be performed. One test is the hysterosalpingogram or HSG ("hystero" refers to the uterus, "salpingo" to the tubes, and "gram" to the X ray) in which your doctor will inject some contrast dye into your uterus and tubes and then x-ray the area to see if everything looks normal. The dye will pour into your fallopian tubes and show up on X ray only if the tubes are open: if they are blocked, they won't show up at all. The test is useful but not perfect, notes Dr. Silverberg, because sometimes the tubes will go into spasm as a result of the test itself, thereby appearing closed when there really is no problem.

Dr. Anne Colston Wentz, former president of the Society for Assisted Reproductive Technology, notes that for reasons we don't yet understand, some women will become pregnant *after* the HSG test—without any treatment at all. Whether it is, as she puts it, a simple "roto-rooter" effect in which the fluid pushes a small blockage out of the tubes, or some other mechanism by which the dye suppresses the immune system, something about this test facilitates pregnancy for a small group of women.

Another test that examines the uterus and the openings of your fallopian tubes is the hysteroscopy, in which a tiny scope is passed through your cervix and some gas is injected. Small abnormalities can be treated directly through the cervix with this test, which requires no incision at all. The test also can find larger abnormalities in the structure of the uterus, such as a septum or wall in the uterus that *can* (but doesn't always) impede fertility. (*See* illustration on page 36.)

The ultrasound or sound-wave test mentioned earlier can also be used to scan the uterus and ovaries for any obvious problems.

And finally, there is laparoscopy, a more invasive test for structural problems in various parts of the reproductive tract. This surgical technique, which has received a great deal of attention in the media in recent years, marks an advance beyond highly invasive abdominal surgery. Laparoscopy requires a *much* smaller incision in the abdomen than traditional surgery, and is generally safer and quicker in the right hands. The tiny incision is followed by the injection of fluid or some other substance into the tubes and other structures, and the insertion of a tiny scope with a light on the end that allows doctors to get a clear firsthand view of your pelvic organs. This test might reveal adhesions or scar tissue from previous problems that are blocking the tubes or other reproductive structures, or endometriosis (discussed further in chapter 7) which sometimes impedes fertility. Remember, however, that laparoscopy carries risks of its own—including perforation of the pelvic organs—so you'll want to find a practitioner with good experience using the technique. It's also a good idea to choose a doctor with experience in *treating* potential blockages, not just making diagnoses with the laparoscope, since treatment can be done at the same time as the diagnostic procedure. This is preferable to having a second doctor open you again to treat any lesions that were detected the first time around.

In addition to finding blocked tubes, the laparoscope can detect fibroid tumors, ovarian cysts and other structural blockages that might impede fertility. Most of these lesions can be removed and fertility sometimes restored surgically.

The American Fertility Society places the complication rate of laparoscopic surgery at about 3 in 1000 cases. Dr. Wentz, who admits that this recommendation does not make her popular these days, urges women to see specialists, not generalists, for laparoscopic surgery. While many general doctors are learning to do laparoscopy, and some are quite good at it, she feels that women boost their chance of success when they see someone who specializes in the laparoscopic diagnosis and treatment of pelvic problems—especially because the first attempt at this procedure usually has the best outcome.

Treating Blocked Tubes.

The fallopian tubes are highly delicate organs that can be disrupted by a number of problems. If they are severely damaged by past sexually transmitted diseases (gonorrhea and chlamydia are the biggies) or by some other type of pelvic infection, they often cannot be repaired. However, if they are only partially blocked or pinned down by small amount of cobweblike tissue or endometriosis, for example, treatment can be quite successful. The success of treatment depends in part on the location of the disease in the tube. Be sure to go over this with your doctor, because if the chance of success is small with your type of tubal problem, you may elect to skip tubal surgery altogether and move on to another form of assisted reproduction.

Dr. Miles Novy of the Oregon Health Sciences University specializes in treating tubal problems in women. He finds that if the problem is at the proximal end of the tube—the part closest to the uterus—surgery is often successful. If the damage is severe and at the distal end of the tube (that is, the part nearest the ovaries) surgery only works in only about one-fourth of patients. This is sometimes because the tiny, hairlike cells that line the tubes in this region (that are meant to usher the egg down toward incoming sperm) may be destroyed. Dr. Novy worries that some patients are given unnecessary surgery for severely damaged distal tubes—at the risk not only of surgical failure, but also of dangerous ectopic pregnancy (pregnancy outside the uterus, in this case lodged in the tubes). When the distal end of the tube is severely diseased, Dr. Novy puts the chance of ectopic pregnancy at about one in ten. He also stresses that while traditional surgery sometimes does the trick, microsurgery—which is performed with special, tiny instruments with the assistance of miscroscopic tools—can be even better in difficult cases. Microsurgery minimizes the amount of trauma to the surrounding reproductive tissues, cuts the chance of adhesions, and helps maintain a level of moisture in the tissues during surgery that promotes a better outcome in some cases.

The most successful tubal surgery, Dr. Novy adds, is that done for "peri-tubal" problems: adhesions or other disease *around* the tubes that may be pulling the tubes out of their normal position, for example. These problems are very amenable to repair, he notes.

Another type of procedure that can be done on tubes is reversal of tubal ligation or "tied tubes." If you had your tubes tied as a means of contraception and now have decided you want to become pregnant, surgery to rejoin the tubes can sometimes be done. Dr. George Henry of the Reproductive Genetics Center in Boulder, Colorado finds that when the tubes are healthy, tubal ligation repair is successful 80% of the time. Not everyone's numbers are that good: success greatly depends on the condition of the tubes and the extent of the previous surgery.

TESTING YOUR CERVICAL MUCUS

Sperm use your cervical mucus like a ladder when making the tough climb through your vagina and into your uterus and tubes. If the ladder isn't strong, or if it isn't properly structured, the sperm will get trapped or "fall down," never completing their journey. To find out if this is going on, you may be given a "postcoital test" around the time of ovulation. This test is an examination of your cervical mucus, with sperm in it, a couple of hours after intercourse. It's a good sign if the sperm are climbing through the mucus normally. If they are getting trapped in the mucus—or if they seem to be losing their ability to swim when they reach the mucus—there may be a problem. The test is painless (your doctor simply removes the mucus and sperm from your vagina), though some find it awkward or inconvenient to be examined so soon after intercourse.

Two potential problems with cervical mucus are (1.) that it isn't of the needed quality to usher the sperm upwards, or (2.) that there is an abnormal *immune* reaction taking place between the mucus and the sperm (that is, one of them is creating antibodies that "reject" the other, attacking it as if it were a foreign object). Sometimes, doctors will try drugs like mild steroids to try to suppress your own or your partner's immune systems. If the mucus problem is serious enough, you may be advised to bypass normal intercourse altogether and move on to some form of artificial insemination or assisted reproductive technology to put the sperm into more direct contact with the egg. We'll discuss this later in this chapter.

TIMING: GETTING THESE TESTS DONE, AND FAST

You may be thinking that it takes an awful lot of time, testing and treating to get to the bottom of a female fertility problem. If you're older and feel you don't have this much time, the process can look pretty daunting. The fact is, it *can* take a lot of time, but it doesn't *have* to. Dr. Wentz, noting that "time is the enemy of the infertile couple," says women should refuse to wait a year to get through all of the tests we just mentioned. Dr. Wentz, Dr. Silverberg and others around the country are advocating a much quicker, more aggressive approach to fertility treatment than is usually offered. They believe—and practice—that all of these tests and treatments can be completed in just three months (that is, three menstrual cycles). Other practitioners around the country are taking anywhere from one to three years to accomplish the same things! Dr. Maria Bustillo, head of assisted reproductive technology at the Mt. Sinai Hospital in New York, agrees. She is especially upset by cases of repeat tubal surgery with little chance of success, or endless ovulation drug therapy when it is known that pregnancy usually occurs within three months of treatment.

Dr. Wentz likes to use what she calls the "three times is enough of anything" rule in treating fertility. The fact is, she insists, if something doesn't work after three cycles (fertility drugs, for example) it is much less likely to work thereafter. Sometimes, you'll keep a treatment going, she says, but you should be adding/trying/doing something *new* as well, so as not to waste a patient's time with repeat failures. Repetitive, non-goal-oriented fertility treatment leaves some couples without pregnancy *and* without answers after several years in many doctors' offices.

Dr. Wentz points out a disturbing difference between fertility care and other medical care. With *other* medical care, she says, we expect a well-organized treatment plan. With fertility care, we seldom ask for—or get—anything this straightforward. We must start demanding a formal, laid-out plan of action in which we get diagnostic answers for every issue mentioned above, and a systematic treatment plan for each potential fertility problem. In the language of Monopoly™, she asserts, "Do not pass go, do not collect $200, go straight to a fertility specialist if you aren't conceiving and set up a goal-oriented plan of attack."

Dr. Malinek adds that for women nearing 40, or who have certain medical problems like diabetes, the general definition of "infertile after a *year* of unprotected intercourse" may be slightly shortened. He recommends at least starting fertility testing sooner in women with known medical problems that can interfere with fertility—perhaps after 6 months with no conception. On the flip side of the coin, he notes that for couples who are physically separated for large portions of each year (for work or other reasons), he might *delay* fertility treatment *beyond* the standard year, since they haven't officially tried conceiving for a full year.

Before we have every infertile woman running to her practitioner to complain about how long the workup is taking, however, there are several things to keep in mind. First, the faster you do the complete fertility workup—with tests on both the woman *and* the man—the more the process *costs,* and the more it *interferes* with your daily life. Some practitioners feel that if the woman is young, she should be spared cramming in these unnecessary costs, procedures and hassles. It costs more to go fast because you don't go through the low-cost, low-tech tests first, wait for results, then move to the next level, wait for results, and so on; instead, you plow ahead, regardless of cost, with all of the best tests at once. It takes more of your time because you have to commit yourself to many doctor visits and procedures in a short time frame, which can pull you and your partner away from work or other obligations for more time than you expect. But the fact is *you* should make this choice—not your doctor. If you are willing to spend more money, give more concentrated time and endure more hassle in order to reach your potential goal faster, it's your option, and no amount of dawdling should hold you back.

MALE INFERTILITY: CAUSES AND TREATMENT

Many of those I interviewed told stories of how the male partner had to be literally dragged into the doctor's office for fertility care, couldn't look doctors in the eye when talking about sperm function and otherwise denied any responsibility for the fertility problem. Even in the open 1990s many men resist acknowledging their part in fertility problems. Dr. Arnold Belker, a urologist who specializes in male infertility at the University of Louisville, says that many men are threatened by the idea that infertility could be their "fault"—while others simply don't want to be bothered by the workup. The denial is abating somewhat, at least in some cultures, now that there is so much clear information about the male role in fertility—and now that there are effective treatments for sperm and other problems. If you are trying to get your male partner to participate in treatment, rather than discussing it as a *male* problem versus a *female* problem, call it a *couple's* problem—and encourage your partner to join you in solving it as you would solve any joint issue.

FINDING AND TREATING SPERM PROBLEMS

There are several different kinds of sperm problems and they are treated differently. Testing begins with a fresh sperm sample: men may be asked to masturbate into a sterile container, sometimes at the clinic site, since sperm has a short out-of-body life span. If you live close to your fertility treatment site, you may be able to bring the sperm sample with you from home immediately after collecting it.

The sperm will be studied for several characteristics: first, the number of sperm in the semen sample; second, the motility of the sperm—how well they move and "swim"; third, the morphology of the sperm—that is, how they are shaped; and, fourth, if needed, the ability of the sperm to penetrate a test egg. These test eggs are either hamster eggs or parts of human eggs: the ability of sperm to penetrate either type is no guarantee that it can fertilize a human egg, or your egg, for that matter. But it gives some idea of the sperm's health.

The postcoital test, in which the sperm is examined within the woman's cervical mucus, is another test of sperm viability.

In addition to testing the sperm sample, the doctor should fully examine the man's physical reproductive structures, looking at and feeling the testes, and so on. This physical exam can turn up problems that the sperm test alone cannot detect. Blood tests may be done to check for hormonal imbalances.

Many factors can get in the way of normal sperm creation and function. Just as female ovulation is dependent on the right connections between hormones and reproductive organs, so male spermatogenesis (sperm making) is dependent on complicated, quite similar connections. Hormonal problems can affect the signals that trigger sperm production. Sexually transmitted diseases, fevers, infections, physical trauma to some part of the male reproductive tract, certain prescribed medications, past surgery, and use of illicit drugs, cigarettes or alcohol can all interfere with sperm production—to name just a few! Blockages of the tubes that carry sperm can interfere with even normal sperm's delivery. Even simple things that you'd never suspect, like wearing tight underwear that heats the testes, spending many hours in the hot seat of a truck or sitting in too-hot baths or hot tubs can impair sperm creation, which is very temperature-sensitive. Problems in the veins of the testes (one common example is varicocele, which is like a varicose vein in the testes) can also impede sperm production.

Still another cause of male infertility is retrograde ejaculation, in which the sperm, instead of exiting the body and traveling into the woman's womb, goes backward and travels into the man's bladder. This is harmless and your partner may not even know he has the problem. (Dr. Goldfarb notes that this problem can be resolved simply by retrieving the sperm from the urine, "washing it down" in a special way and giving it back to the woman with artificial insemination.) Of course, impotence can cause infertility as well: if the man cannot get an erection, have intercourse and ejaculate, conception cannot occur. There are now many treatments for both physiologically and psychologically-based impotence; these include drug treatment, surgical treatment, and psychological counseling. Urologists are generally the place to start.

Many of the other above-mentioned problems can also be treated. For instance, hormone treatment can sometimes stimulate sperm production. Interestingly, the same drugs that are used for women to boost ovulation are used in men to boost sperm production. Because sperm takes about 90 days to mature, you may have to be patient when waiting to see if treatment is taking effect. Treating varicocele, the testicular vein problem, is more controversial. Dr. Bustillo says that there is no clear evidence that treating varicoceles increases the chance of pregnancy. Many practitioners still do the procedure, but its efficacy has come into question.

TREATING BLOCKED SPERM DUCTS AND REVERSING VASECTOMY

Male sperm duct problems can often be corrected, too. We mentioned earlier that women can often have "tied tubes" rejoined in order to restore fertility. The same goes for men who have had surgical vasectomies and have now changed their minds. Dr. Belker, who does these procedures, says that repair is "almost never impossible," but that success rates depend strongly on how long it has been since the vasectomy was performed. The best success rates are at less than three years after the vasectomy, when there is a 98% rate of return of sperm to semen (the first measure of success) and a 75% pregnancy rate (the bottom-line measure of success). The rates get progressively worse as time goes on, with 3–8 years after surgery looking a little worse, and 9–14 years after surgery worse still. At 15-plus years after the vasectomy, the rate of return of sperm to semen is about 75%, and the pregnancy rate 30%. Dr. Belker urges patients to see the best practitioner right from the start, since repeat attempts to reverse vasectomy have lower success rates, even when sophisticated micro-surgery is used.

Surgery can also be done on other portions of the sperm ducts, such as a blocked epididymis (*see* illustration), the first part of the tube coming out of the testicle, or a problem with the ejaculatory ducts. When surgery fails, Belker adds, all is not lost: you still have the option of aspirating sperm from the testes with a needle, then using assisted reproductive technology (ART) to achieve pregnancy. This becomes quite costly, however, since the price of the aspiration (several thousand dollars) plus the ART (several thousand more) and sometimes micromanipulation of sperm to get it to enter the egg (a few more thousand) adds up quickly—with no guarantee of pregnancy.

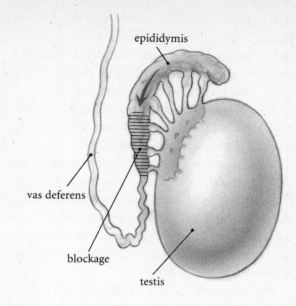

Location for male sterilization

Micromanipulation of Sperm.

As mentioned above, even when you can get some sperm, it sometimes fails to fertilize eggs. That's when micromanipulation comes into play. Using a series of new and highly technical procedures, doctors can place a microscopic sperm directly into a microscopic egg to achieve fertilization. Not all centers have the ability to do this, nor is it always necessary. But it's something you might want to ask about if you know that there are problems with your partner's sperm.

UNEXPLAINED INFERTILITY

You'd think from the laundry list of possible causes and treatments of infertility for both men and women that there isn't much left that the experts *don't* understand. Unfortunately, that's not the case. According to Dr. Malinak, about 5% to 20% of couples who go through a total fertility workup will be left without an explanation for their problem. These cases are called "unexplained" or "idiopathic" infertility. The situation is quite frustrating and painful for doctors and patients alike.

The positive side of it is that some of these couples will go on to conceive, either with "empiric therapy," (giving certain treatments even without a clear indication that they're needed) with the help of high technology, or with no treatment whatsoever. It might be comforting for some to know that even without treatment, 35% to 50% of couples with unexplained infertility will get pregnant in two years; and 60% to 70% will get pregnant after three years, according to the American Fertility Society. Dr. Ronald Strickler attributes these unexplainable "cures" to the "tincture of time." These couples are, after the fact, dubbed "subfertile," rather than "infertile." Others won't be as lucky, and will still fail to conceive after years of trying. This is rare: but it does happen.

Dr. Deborah Manzi warns that not everyone who is told they have "unexplained infertility" actually has it. She sees many patients who were told by other physicians that their fertility was a mystery, when in fact they were never given the full battery of fertility tests. This is why it is so important to be treated by a fertility specialist, she insists.

As we will discuss later in this section, infertility does *not* mean you cannot have children. Many options, including donor sperm, donor eggs and adoption have brought the joy of parenthood to the lives of thousands of couples around the world.

FERTILITY AS WE AGE

Several things happen to our fertility as we age. First, fertility drops gradually: there is a silent process in our bodies in which fewer healthy eggs are released with each menstrual cycle, the hormones in our bodies start to shift, and so on. This is the gradual process we talk about in chapter 10 on menopausal health. A couple of big dips in fertility occur after age 35, age 40 and age 45, on average. Many women can still conceive at these ages, but it becomes less likely per given cycle.

Two additional changes that affect our fertility as we get older are the miscarriage rate, which climbs with age, and the rate of chromosomal abnormalities, which also increases. Dr. Alvin Goldfarb criticizes the media for making 40-plus parenting seem so fashionable and easy, when in fact, it starts to get much tougher at this time. Women should be able to try to conceive whenever they want, he adds, but they should be informed of the risks of waiting until they're older.

Through research at his Reproductive Genetics Center, Dr. George Henry and colleagues have gained some insight into what goes wrong with eggs after a certain age. They have found decreased total energy in the eggs, particularly in their ability to divide, "sort" chromosomes and so on. While preliminary, these and other discoveries may lead to future treatments for aging eggs that will boost the chance of pregnancy for older women.

YOUR LIFESTYLE AND YOUR FERTILITY

If you have been diagnosed as infertile, you may be questioning what you did—or are still doing—to cause the problem. Usually the answer is *nothing;* it's not your fault, and you cannot control the situation. There are, however, a few exceptions. Smoking, drug use and alcohol intake *do* impair fertility. You may want to clean up these habits and see if it has any impact on your fertility. (*See* chapter 19 for resources that can help you break these addictions.) Short of severe nutritional deficiencies, diet isn't thought to be a major factor in fertility for either men or women. Certainly you and your partner want to eat enough, and eat well, when you're trying to conceive. Exercise, within reason (not to the degree where it makes you so skinny your ovulation stops) is great for your body and should not interfere with fertility. Some practitioners may tell you to reduce extremely jarring exercise while you're trying to conceive, but there are different opinions on this issue.

Sandra Allenson, nurse coordinator at the Northern Nevada Fertility Center, finds that many patients are burdened with the myth that stress causes infertility. While infertility does cause stress, it's rarely the other way around, she notes. Family members and friends who say "relax and you'll get pregnant" are showing their ignorance, but before you get angry, remember that they most often mean well and want the problem to go away as much as you do. (For more on stress and infertility, *see* page 327)

At a certain level, excessive emotional trauma can get in the way of fertility. Usually, we're not talking about day-to-day stressors, but those that have a powerful emotional impact, like grief after losing a loved one, or some other dramatic change in your life that sends your emotions reeling. The effect is sometimes seen in the form of lost ovulation; sometimes not. In these cases, trying to address the emotional issues head-on with therapy should be added to general fertility care.

ASSISTED REPRODUCTIVE TECHNOLOGY (ART)

ART jumped onto the headlines in 1978 when Louise Brown, the first "test tube baby," was born. Since that landmark occasion, the number of technologically assisted births has exploded: ART helped bring into the world over 33,000 babies between 1985 and 1992, replacing the pain of infertility with the joy of parenthood for many. While it has the power to change lives and pick up where nature slacked off, ART is not a cure-all: it doesn't work for everyone, isn't appropriate for everyone, costs a great deal of money—and is *not* covered by insurance in most states (there are exceptions).

The best known form of ART is in vitro fertilization, or IVF, which literally means "in glass fertilization" (done in a test tube). Your eggs, which are gathered through a sophisticated, tightly timed process, and your partner's sperm are joined in the laboratory, and then put back into your uterus after fertilization takes place. Usually, since several eggs are gathered, about three to four embryos (joined egg and sperm) are put into the uterus. Placing more than a few embryos can result in too high a risk of multiple gestations (triplets, quads, quints and so on)—which are riskier pregnancies. Placing fewer than that can lower your chance of getting pregnant at all. Leftover embryos that aren't used can be frozen at many centers and used at a later date.

Usually, a variety of sophisticated tests and procedures are done *before* IVF, such as micromanipulation of sperm, ovulation enhancement, and so on. The goal—and the reason it's so important to have an excellent laboratory working on your case—is to locate the healthiest sperm and the healthiest eggs in order to boost the chance that conception will occur and the pregnancy will be viable. Dr. George Henry claims, somewhat hyperbolically, that the "laboratory is everything" when it comes to successful IVF—but of course excellent care at every step of the process will boost the success rate. After "embryo transfer"—that is, placement of the joined egg and sperm into your uterus—you will be told to lie in place for a few hours at the center. A few weeks later, you will be told if you are pregnant. A negative result, especially if it's not the first try, can be devastating for couples: a positive one still requires patience, hope, and luck. If IVF fails, you will have to decide, with your partner, if you want to give the process another try. That means more money, more time and more vulnerability to disappointment. This is *not* an easy process, either emotionally or physically.

On average, the chance of becoming pregnant with IVF is 15% across the country. But success rates vary tremendously, for several reasons. First, maternal age, sperm function and other aspects of reproductive health can affect your chance of success. The older you are, for instance, or the more problems there are with the sperm, the lower the success rates. Certain cases are much easier to treat than others; for instance, if the sperm is healthy, you are ovulating and your only problem is that your tubes are blocked, the success rate with IVF can reach 40%. Some centers have poor success rates for reasons that have nothing to do with you or your partner—like sloppy lab work or poor timing of the tests that precede IVF. One way to

protect yourself from bad centers is to contact the Society for Assisted Reproductive Technology (SART), which tracks the records of many centers across the country and requires certain basic standards of members. *See* the information section at the end of this chapter for details.

You can also protect yourself from being misled about success rates by finding out exactly what a center is referring to when it measures so-called "success." For instance, *you* may be thinking in terms of the take-home-baby rate, while the *center* is quoting pregnancy rates. Since pregnancies don't always end in take-home babies, this rate can look better than the one you need to hear about. Furthermore, pregnancy is defined in different ways. Some centers will boast of a high pregnancy rate when in fact all they've achieved is a connection between the egg and sperm that doesn't persist past a few days. More important is the *clinical* pregnancy rate—that is, the existence of a fetus in the womb that can be seen with ultrasound.

A group called RESOLVE, which helps couples deal with a wide variety of infertility issues, as well as the American Fertility Society and other related experts, have created lists of questions to ask of ART centers you may be considering. Below are just a few of the questions from their lists that can help you locate programs that best meet your needs.

QUESTIONS TO ASK OF AN ART PROGRAM

1. When did you start your ART program?

2. How many cycles of ART have you completed for *my* fertility problem, and for *my* chosen procedure?

3. What is the training of your staff, including your medical director, nurse coordinator, embryologist, etc.?

4. What is your percentage of *live births* per egg retrieval since you started this center?

5. What is the success rate with *my* diagnosis, and *my* age group, in terms of clinical pregnancies *and* live births?

6. Do you provide emotional counseling for patients who want it?

7. What is your payment schedule—how much and at what stages do I have to pay; and how much of this, if any, is covered by insurance?

These and many other specific questions can help you get around the headlines and promises of a fertility center and get closer to the bottom line *for you.* Dr. Victor Knutzen complains that until recently, fertility centers have not been accountable to anyone. The lack of oversight has led to outright lies or misrepresentation of success rates. The Society for Assisted Reproductive Technology is starting to rectify this problem with the first audit of fertility centers—expected in 1995. In the meantime, Dr. Knutzen urges centers to report their results to outside accounting agencies as he and others have done for some time now.

OTHER KINDS OF ART

Beyond IVF, there are other high-tech procedures like Gamete Intrafallopian Transfer (GIFT), Zygote Intrafallopian Transfer (ZIFT), and others with different names that are slight variations on the same theme. With GIFT, instead of putting an already-fertilized egg into the uterus, doctors put the sperm and egg into the fallopian tube, where they can meet on their own. In the words of Kathryn Go, laboratory director of the in vitro fertilization and GIFT programs at Pennsylvania Hospital in Philadelphia, an advantage to GIFT is that "there is no laboratory any better than a healthy fallopian tube." She believes that one reason the pregnancy rate is better with GIFT than with IVF is that the egg and sperm naturally "like" to unite in the fallopian tube more than in a test tube. Other reasons for GIFT's higher pregnancy rate, she adds, have less to do with the procedure itself than with the types of patients often selected to have it in the first place: healthy tubes and normal sperm count, for example. Kathryn Go also notes that GIFT has a higher pregnancy rate for couples over age 40.

Some practitioners report that GIFT is being used *less* these days, for a variety of reasons, including the fact that unless pregnancy occurs, you don't know if fertilization ever took place. This leaves an important fertility mystery about the couple. GIFT is also falling out of favor with some clinicians because it requires laparoscopy, which is relatively invasive (IVF can be done through the cervix with no incision). If your tubes are healthy, and you are having a laparoscopy for *another* reason in your fertility workup, this is one opportunity to consider GIFT.

One advantage to GIFT is that it can save you money by averting the steep laboratory fees needed for IVF. However, some of that cost is replaced by the laparoscopy procedure, so don't be fooled: add it all up before you make your decision. GIFT has a slightly better success rate (both for pregnancy and live births) than

IVF—but some say this is because of more fertile candidates, and Dr. Bustillo suggests that because GIFT is often done at the same time as other treatments, other factors' contribution may boost the *appearance* of GIFT's success. Most experts agree, whether they generally support IVF or GIFT, that if there is a severe *male* factor problem (a sperm problem, that is) IVF is a better choice than GIFT, since with IVF you know beforehand if fertilization occurred—and if problems are detected, you can move on to high-tech procedures like micromanipulation of sperm and eggs.

When to Try ART

The decision of whether or when to use assisted reproductive technology is highly personal—and quite controversial among practitioners. As we've discussed, the cost in time, money, physical and emotional trauma can be high. If you have been told by a reputable center(s) that your chance of pregnancy with ART is quite small, and you are more interested just in being parents than in being *biological* parents, adoption may be a better choice for you. If you are driven by the need to reproduce biologically—or at least for ONE member of your couple to be the child's biological parent—ART may be worth the literal and figurative costs, no matter how small the chance of success. When it works, of course, it becomes priceless—in hindsight. While these high-tech procedures grab headlines, however, and are coming to be thought of almost as mainstream, of the millions of people who seek fertility treatment each year, only about 15–20,000 couples undergo high-tech procedures.

Dr. Mary Lake Polan, chairman of the departments of gynecology and obstetrics at the Stanford University School of Medicine, thinks that one of the most important things patients need to know about treatment for infertility—high-tech or not—is that they don't *have* to do it: they can *choose* to do it. She tells patients that infertility is not life-threatening, that you do not have to invest your time and money in treatments in order to *survive*. If you *want* to do so, it's your prerogative. Too many couples get caught up in the long process of treatment, swept along as if ending infertility at any cost were their sole option. Dr. Polan gives patients the option of being "liberated" from treatment, if that's what they really need. She often refers her patients to counselors who can help them decide if it's worth it to continue trying to conceive, or if they might prefer taking a different route to parenthood, such as adoption. Counseling is a good idea in any case, she adds, because of the enormous strain infertility can place on a couple. Deciding whether to quit—or keep going—can be one of the biggest stressors of all, especially when partners don't agree on how to proceed.

There are some clear-cut cases where ART is the only option, such as when the woman's tubes are completely destroyed by disease, and must be bypassed for pregnancy to occur. It was for this sort of problem that ART was first used. Since then, its use has been greatly expanded. Dr. Bustillo includes on the list of clear-cut cases those where the sperm is so weak or so few in number that other "natural" options won't succeed, or cases of "unexplained infertility" where no one knows exactly what to treat (and empiric therapy has failed). Some practitioners who are not skilled in ART will hang on to their patients too long, Bustillo says, or their patients will hang onto *them* for too long—because of strong emotional attachments or unrealistic hopes that something short of ART will work.

Some feel that ART should only be tried as a last resort after all other options have been exhausted. Both Dr. Strickler and Dr. Michael Diamond, director of reproductive endocrinology at Hutzel Hospital in Detroit, for example, insist that ART belongs where *all else has failed:* such as, when all previous tests have failed to find a cause of infertility, and "curative" treatments and/or empiric therapy have failed to bring on pregnancy in "unexplained" cases. Dr. Strickler is horrified to hear of cases—often moneymaking schemes—in which couples are referred to ART before even the most basic fertility tests have been done. To lure couples into emotionally draining, potentially health-threatening, invasive technologies before trying absolutely everything else is unacceptable, he insists.

Stricker has found great misconceptions among patients about ART (such as the belief that ART is 100% effective, 100% of the time). In order to put a dose of reality where less ethical practitioners have robbed it, Strickler and his colleagues now give two-hour educational sessions on ART each week. I suggest you inquire about similar lectures or information groups in your area, perhaps through infertility support groups. The more you know *before* you get involved in high-tech treatments, the more realistic your expectations will be, and the lower your chance of deep disappointment.

But the bottom line is this: no one can define the "appropriateness" of ART or any other procedure but *you.* Many of the experts I interviewed recalled patients who, for one reason or another, would not or could not wait for other options to bring on pregnancy. These were couples of all ages, backgrounds and fertility problems, some of whom probably would have conceived without ART. But since they had the strong desire, and the money to spend—or were willing to "do without," selling cars and other assets just for a chance at ART—they chose the high-tech route long before it was recommended by doctors. These kinds of choices, if you can afford them, are yours alone to make. Just be sure you're making them because you *want* to, not because you feel you *have* to. And proceed with a clear head, knowing that ART is not a solution for everyone, and that after all the effort, you can still come up empty-handed.

OPTIONS TO INFERTILITY TREATMENT

If you do not want to, cannot afford to, or have given up on fertility treatment, there are other ways to become a family. These methods are extremely satisfying, fulfilling and more than adequate for many families. If they are not desirable for you and your partner, that's your choice: but if parenthood is extremely important to you, you owe it to yourself to investigate the options.

DONOR EGGS/DONOR SPERM

If one member of a couple is thought to be fertile and the other not, donor sperm or eggs can be the answer. Naturally, only one parent would be biologically connected to the baby. But the other could be every bit as much a parent. Donor eggs and sperm can be given anonymously, sometimes through general fertility programs; they can also be given by friends or relatives. (*See* the information box at the end of this chapter for donor egg/sperm resources and places to go to discuss the physiological and emotional issues this process entails.) If you are part of a couple, the decision to use donor eggs or sperm is best made by *both* of you, since you will be partners in parenting. If you are a single woman considering insemination with donor sperm, the decision is yours alone, but is certainly best made after investigating the realities of single parenthood and how it would fit into your life. Specialized counselors, particularly those affiliated with fertility centers, should be equipped to address these myriad issues.

ADOPTION

You may decide, either after trying fertility treatment or even before, that adoption is the best way for you to become a parent. And remember, you are needed by these children as much as they are needed by you. There are countless children from around the world who could benefit from loving parents and stable homes. According to the American Fertility Society, 50,000 nonrelated adoptions take place a year in the U.S. Another 8000 children are adopted into American families from other countries.

Recently, the media has focused primarily on the down side of adoption, highlighting legal battles and tragic situations in which biological parents come back after years and try to regain custody of adopted children. These cases certainly do occur, but they are only one view of the adoption process. Many adoptions, the ones you don't hear about because they don't make juicy headlines, take place smoothly and develop into rich families with all of the usual joys and conflicts, no more and no less, than biological families.

There are several ways to adopt, but the two primary routes are through private adoption (with a private attorney), or through adoption agencies (public or privately run). You will have to investigate for yourself which process is best suited to your needs. In general, private adoptions are more costly, and may be quicker. Agency adoptions can take more time, but may provide you with more resources (both emotional and otherwise), and more legal protection of the adoption. Other variables include how much you want to know—or will be allowed to know—about the baby's birth parents; or how much they will learn about you. You will have to decide if you want to adopt an American baby, a foreign baby, a baby of your race or of another race. Perhaps you will want to adopt a child with physical or emotional problems; maybe perfect health is essential to you. You'll need to know if you want to adopt an infant, or an older child. These are not easy decisions, and not decisions to be made without outside advice (ideally, from adoption professionals *and* from other families that have adopted in different ways). Before deciding on ANY kind of adoption plan, do some reading, and contact some of the agencies listed at the end of this chapter. The more you learn about your options, including the rules in your state, the better the chance your adoption process will go smoothly and you will avoid problems down the road.

EMOTIONAL ISSUES SURROUNDING INFERTILITY

Infertility is an emotional hotbox for nearly everyone involved. Exceedingly rare is the couple that does not suffer some degree of emotional distress when confronted with the prospect of never conceiving a biological child. It hits at the root of how we perceive ourselves not only as human beings, but as female or as male. For some, it is seen as the most basic failure of all—the failure to re-create oneself for posterity. Aline Zoldbrod, a sex therapist in private practice in the greater Boston area, feels that medical language helps add to the negative self-image of infertile women with terms like "incompetent cervix," "habitual aborter," and "hostile cervical mucus." By depicting our body parts as bad or deformed, these terms confirm women's worst fears about their bodies as fundamentally defective.

Many women come to see their infertility as punishment for past "sins" or omissions. Still others believe that they alone have been singled out for suffering, and will never again be happy.

Yes, there are couples who deal with infertility issues much more positively, but they are rare. More often than not, infertile couples ride a roller coaster of hope followed by renewed pain with each menstrual cycle, the sign that conception has not occurred. It is absolutely vital that these couples seek help—and sometimes professional support—for the feelings they are experiencing. There may be some comfort in knowing that the pain is not only common, but often can be substantially relieved with proper care.

GRIEF

Much has been written about infertility as a symbol of loss, similar to the death of a loved one. Couples may first go through feelings of shock, then denial, then anger and eventually

resolution, this theory holds. Sidney Bundy, a marriage and family therapist who sees many infertile couples, notes that each new menstrual period renews the sense of failure and loss and can send patients into a spiral of pain once again. Every month, these couples grieve, she says. One of her goals in treatment is to get couples to take a look at their lives as a whole and to ask themselves, "What are we doing to have *fun*, and to be happy?" For many couples caught in this cycle of grieving, the fertility problem has become life itself; it permeates every aspect of their daily lives, from their timed sex schedule to their dealings with friends' and relatives' children. Ask yourself if you have stopped enjoying life, and each other—and fix the problem if you have. When you begin to focus on each other again, and on just plain having a date for dinner and a movie, let's say, at which you *cannot* talk about your infertility problem, you often find great relief, Bundy reports. Let go and live for the moment you are in, she counsels. A life focused on a *potential* future is empty. One that maximizes the joy between you as a pair, with or without children, *today* is important whether or not you ever conceive (or adopt). Sometimes just getting couples to talk about what attracted them to each other in the first place will shift the focus from the bad news they're facing to the good things they already share, experts say.

SEXUAL PROBLEMS

Having sex on schedule, feeling depressed about infertility, having sex measured or "scored" by doctors every month can do a lot to harm your sex life. Impotence, blaming and resentment can result. If your sex life is suffering as you go through infertility treatment, consider talking to a sex therapist or infertility counselor. Your problem is common, and there are solutions.

GUILT

Dr. Miriam Rosenthal, chief of behavioral OB-GYN at McDonald Women's Hospital, finds that one of the first emotions couples experience is guilt. "What did I do to deserve this?" is a common question couples ask. Was it having sex before marriage? The list of speculated causes is endless. Rosenthal finds that most couples will move past these feelings with time, but that a good number continue to have powerful feelings of both isolation and stress, as if they were singled out for this suffering. She recommends group therapy for couples having these feelings. In groups, couples discover that they are not alone in battling infertility. This in itself is extremely supportive, since some infertile couples are quite secretive about their problem, keeping it even from family members, and furthering their sense that they are in this crisis alone. Rosenthal recommends other methods of therapy, like stress reduction, not to "cure" the infertility problem, but to make patients—and couples—feel better.

(A note about group therapy: Dorothy Greenfeld, director of psychological services at Yale University's center for reproductive medicine, finds that the smaller the group, the better. She also reports that the best groups are made up of couples at a similar stage in the fertility treatment process. For instance, it's not a great idea for a young, newly infertile couple to share a group with a couple in their mid-40s that has been dealing with the problem for 15 years; it's too depressing and discouraging for the young couple, and not useful for the older couple. Furthermore, Greenfield recommends time-limited group therapy; instead of staying in groups for months on end, choose a program with a predetermined number of sessions. One reason: it's hard for some couples to see others in a group "succeed" while they are left behind, and this is a risk in groups that go on and on indefinitely.)

STRESS

Stress, except in extremely rare situations, does not cause infertility—infertility causes stress. Still, many loved ones are tempted to try to relieve the stress of infertile couples with uninformed but well-meaning advice, such as "relax, take a vacation, and you'll get pregnant." This is quite destructive and not based in fact. Several decades ago, the medical myth that infertile women were emotionally disturbed to begin with was quite pervasive, and to this day, some old-timers hang onto this view—despite the fact that it has been proved wrong by numerous studies. The rare exceptions to this rule, Dr. Rosenthal notes, are when clinical depression is present and ovulation stops; when psychological problems keep couples from having intercourse in the first place; or when mental anguish leads to disorders like anorexia nervosa, stopping ovulation and preventing conception.

In the vast majority of cases, infertility triggers emotional distress. Individual or group counseling can help you to deal with difficult feelings, with a marriage that has begun to suffer under chronic strain and discouragement, and with the decision of when to *give up* aggressive fertility treatment (which is highly emotionally demanding in itself).

INABILITY TO HANDLE SOCIAL EVENTS SURROUNDING OR INCLUDING CHILDREN

According to Dorothy Greenfeld, many infertile couples have trouble facing the holidays and other occasions at which children are the central focus. Baby showers, Christmas and so on can be anything but joyful when you feel, as Greenfeld puts it, "isolated in a fertile world." Infertile couples—particularly women who want the experience not just of having a child, but of being pregnant—tend to feel that everyone else in the world, from age 15 to 80, is getting pregnant while they fail. It's worst when a younger sister, for example, becomes pregnant. Anger, jealousy and resentment are common. Studies vary on whether it's best to face difficult social situations or to avoid them. Greenfeld and others tend to take the pressure off couples, telling them that if they can't enjoy the occasion, they should skip it. But there is data to suggest that an action-oriented approach to life, facing fears head-on, going to the baby showers and making yourself deal with them, can also help you work through painful feelings. You'll have to decide what you, as a couple, can manage, taking into consideration the companionship you may lose if you separate from friends and family versus the pain you may feel at facing what they already have, and you are still striving for. Find a counselor, Greenfeld urges, who lets you know that you aren't going crazy, that your feelings are normal, and that with work and time you will regain your positive view of life once more.

Consider the excellent advice given by Christopher Newton, a clinical psychologist at University Hospital in London, Ontario: he counsels couples to find and develop their own special holiday traditions and to celebrate them separately from the rest of their families. In this way, you can give special, personal meaning to the holidays that has nothing to do with children, and everything to do with you as a couple.

GENDER DIFFERENCES IN EMOTIONAL REACTIONS TO INFERTILITY

Women and men tend to react quite differently to infertility, and the differences in our reactions can put tremendous strain on marriages and partnerships. Women are often more open, more emotionally reactive, and more focused on fertility problems than are men—who are more likely to either bottle the problem up, or ignore it for long periods of time. One expert told me that in group counseling sessions, the women often say "I'm here because I have been unable to conceive for two years, and we aren't sure of the cause," while their male partners often say "I'm here because she wanted me to come." These are generalizations, but experts from all over the country point to them—as do scientific studies on the subject.

Christopher Newton finds that women are more emotionally expressive than men in dealing with fertility problems, showing a whole range of emotions including sadness, anxiety and frustration. Part of this, he says, may be that there's more added societal pressure on women to become pregnant than there is on men to impregnate. Men often cope with infertility, he says, by distancing themselves from the problem, controlling and regulating their emotions, turning inward. They may continue to behave as if nothing is wrong at all. This difference in coping styles puts great strain on marriages: women often interpret their partners' reactions as "not caring," while men think women are becoming "obsessed" with the fertility problem. Men, he finds, are more solution-oriented: if there is no immediate solution to the fertility problem, which there often isn't, men wonder "Why talk about it?"

One solution to these emotional differences, Newton finds, is to educate couples to understand each other's coping styles. Once each understands where the other is coming from, he says, you can build some sort of compromise in which couples meet each other halfway. Emotionally sharing conversations are often what women need; they aren't necessarily looking for immediate solutions, Newton reports. When men come to understand this, conversations can take on different meaning. Newton also recommends that couples have structured discussions about their fertility problem, setting aside a particular, limited time frame (maybe 30 minutes) to discuss the problem. After that, he urges couples to have fun together and leave the problem alone for a while. In this way, stereotypical male and female coping styles are both satisfied.

A final and important gender difference arises when couples must decide whether to give up on infertility treatment and move on with their lives. Men are much more likely than women to move past this decision smoothly, Newton says. Women may take much longer to grieve the loss and bring the entire ordeal to a conclusion. Counseling can be extremely useful at this painful decision-making crossroad, when mutual support is of the utmost importance.

WHEN TO SEEK HELP FOR THE EMOTIONAL ASPECTS OF INFERTILITY

When you and/or your partner feels a signifi-cant and growing sense of distance from the other, or when one or both of you is depressed to the point that you're having trouble eating or sleeping (or you're overeating or oversleeping), or when you're having trouble functioning normally at work or in your social life, or if your sex life has been significantly damaged, it's time to seek help. Don't wait until you're at the end of your rope: there's too much help out there. National groups like RESOLVE and others can help you find an appropriate counselor near you. Generally, couples counseling is more important than individual counseling for infertility. In some cases, however, if one partner is suffering particularly strong depression or guilt, concurrent individual therapy can be helpful.

FOR MORE INFORMATION ON INFERTILITY

RESOLVE INC.
NATIONAL HEADQUARTERS
1310 Broadway
Somerville, MA
617-623-1156
HELPLINE: 617-623-0744

AMERICAN SOCIETY FOR REPRODUCTIVE MEDICINE (FORMERLY THE AMERICAN FERTILITY SOCIETY)
1209 Montgomery Highway
Birmingham, Alabama 35216-2809
205-978-5000

SOCIETY FOR ASSISTED REPRODUCTIVE TECHNOLOGY (SART)
See above: American Society for Reproductive Medicine

SHARE
St. Joseph's Hospital
300 First Capital Drive
St. Charles, MO 63301
314-947-6164

ENDOMETRIOSIS ASSOCIATION
8585 North 76th Place
Milwaukee, WI 53223
800-992-ENDO

NATIONAL COMMITTEE ON ADOPTION
1930 17th St. NW
Washington, DC 20009
202-328-1200

NORTH AMERICAN COUNCIL ON
ADOPTABLE CHILDREN (NACAC)
970 Raymond Ave., Suite 106
St. Paul, MN 55114
612-644-3036

PART SIX

Energy and Mood

CHAPTER SEVENTEEN

MENTAL HEALTH

*Although the world is full of suffering, it is full
also of the overcoming of it.*

—Helen Keller, *Optimism*

Have you ever wondered if your weepy moods that last several days or weeks are something you should be seriously concerned about? Have you worried that your fears or anxiety about speaking in public, or confronting obstacles, are too extreme? Depression and anxiety are so common among women that it's hard to find *any* woman who hasn't experienced some degree of either problem. The key is to know what constitutes *too much* of these feelings, and when and where to get help.

Carol Landau, a psychiatrist and cofounder of Women's Health Associates at Rhode Island Hospital, calls depression the "common cold of women's health." She has no intention of trivializing the problem. On the contrary, she and her colleagues are trying to wake us up to the fact that depression is so common a problem, so prevalent and devastating to women of all ages, backgrounds and experience, that it has become nothing short of an epidemic. Both depression and anxiety disorders, two extremely common forms of mental illness, affect women disproportionately.

Before we begin to look at these serious problems and what to do about them, let's get one thing straight. It's time we started using the term "mental illness" appropriately. Depression, anxiety disorders and many other disorders of emotional health are mental illnesses. Mental illness is *not*, as it has come to be treated in this country, "craziness." That stereotype has done much to keep people with psychological illnesses in the closet, afraid to get help because they're terrified of being labelled "nuts." Just as a physical illness can be measured in tangibles—aches and pains caused by swollen

333

joints, broken bones, tumors and so on—so mental illness has tangible symptoms that manifest themselves as disturbances of your mind and mood. People who are depressed are suffering from mental illness, but they are certainly not "crazy." Especially today, as scientists learn more and more about the biological causes of mental illness (convincing the doubters that mental illnesses are "real"), we must drop the ignorant biases and stereotypes that prevent so many women from getting the care and support they need.

We'll focus in this section on both depression and anxiety, because these problems affect women far more than men, and because both can be treated with a great deal of success. But there are a vast array of different kinds of mental illness that also affect women more than men. For instance, eating disorders like anorexia and bulimia are forms of mental distress (with strong physiological components as well); these are discussed in chapter 23. Infertility can trigger strong emotional disturbances, as can childbirth. These issues are discussed in chapters 15 and 16. Other hormonally-related causes of depression, like PMS and possibly menopause (this is controversial), are discussed in chapters 9 and 10. Throughout this book, you will find references not only to the triggers that can disrupt our moods and thinking patterns, but also the ways in which mental illness can intersect with many so-called "physical" illnesses—illustrating the fact that we are complete beings, and our physical and emotional health are inextricably linked.

As you read this section, keep one important thing in mind: the *vast majority* of depression is treatable. As many as nine in ten women will find significant relief from their symptoms (with specialized depression treatments) in just 12 to 14 weeks! So what are you waiting for?

What Is Depression?

Clinical depression is a strictly defined illness that is believed to be caused by a network of both biomedical and social issues. While many people think depression means feeling sad or blue, it's actually much more complicated than that. We're too quick to use the expression "I'm so depressed" when we're just feeling down or frustrated. Yes, people with clinical depression might feel sad, but they don't *have* to feel sad in order to fit the definition of the disorder. Other common feelings of depression include a lack of interest in usual activities, a feeling of being slowed down or tired, and the sense that it's hard to keep going each day. See if you say "yes" to any of the following questions. They are drawn from the definition of depression in the DSM-4, or Diagnostic and Statistical Manual of Mental Disorders of the American Psychiatric Association.

HAVE YOU HAD ANY FIVE OF THE FOLLOWING NINE EXPERIENCES, FOR AT LEAST TWO WEEKS (INCLUDING EITHER #1 OR #2 AMONG THOSE FIVE)?

1. Are you depressed or irritable most of the day, most days?

2. Do you have a reduced interest or pleasure in most activities, most days?

3. Have you gained *or* lost a significant amount of weight or had a significant increase *or* decrease in your appetite?

4. Have you had trouble sleeping . . . *or* are you sleeping too much each day?

5. Do you feel either very agitated, *or* like you've slowed down?

6. Are you fatigued, or have you lost your energy?

7. Do you feel worthless, or do you feel inappropriate guilt—that is, do you think about an event or events constantly, blaming yourself, or feeling things are all your fault?

8. Do you have trouble concentrating or are you being indecisive?

9. Do you have recurrent thoughts about death (including your own death) or do you have suicidal thoughts or plans?

While each person is different and will experience depression differently, there are certain trends across age, for example, that have been noted by experts. For instance, notes, Dr. Nada Stotland of the University of Chicago, when it comes to appetite and sleep changes, younger women tend to eat more and sleep more when depressed, while older women tend to eat less and sleep less. There are certainly exceptions in both categories, but these patterns are most common.

Also keep in mind that while serious depression is a treatable disease, a certain degree of so-called "appropriate" depression is quite normal: for instance, after the death of a loved one, many of us experience symptoms of depression. Grieving is normal, if it is reasonably short-lived and doesn't take over our entire lives. Normal "situational" depression usually abates on its own after a short period of time. The length of time certainly differs from person to person, and from situation to situation. One clue that

grieving has become unhealthy is when you are unable to find joy in other life pleasures long after the painful event, or your unhappiness is preventing you from functioning properly at work, in relationships with loved ones, and so on. Don't wait until your feelings have hit rock bottom to seek help. Support groups as well as individual or family counseling help many people overcome problems that at first may seem insurmountable.

MINOR DEPRESSION

The criteria listed earlier apply to severe or major depression. Also quite common for women is something called "dysthymia," or minor depression. "Minor" by no means suggests that it isn't important, however: it's simply used as a comparison to more severe forms of depression.

If you say yes to the following questions, you may be suffering from minor depression:

1. Have you felt depressed more often than not, most of the day, for as long as the past two years?

2. In the last two years, have you ever been without the following symptoms for more than two months straight—a change in appetite or sleep habits, lowered energy, inability to concentrate, low self-esteem, hopelessness?

In general, if you find yourself unable to get enjoyment or interest out of your life, if you are withdrawing from society, refusing more and more often to see friends or to leave your home, if you feel hopeless or worthless and find that you can't perform routine tasks, it's time to get help.

According to Gwendolyn Keita, director of

the women's program of the public interest directorate of the American Psychological Association, there is a long list of physical complaints that often reflect underlying depression. Do you have chronic aches in the back, stomach or head that careful, attentive doctors cannot explain, or that standard medical treatment, rest and/or exercise don't relieve? Perhaps you are having physical manifestations of mental health problems. Too often, people dismiss this possibility as insulting, as if doctors are saying their physical pains aren't "real." While we don't want to fall back into the age-old problem (still all too common today!) when all of women's complaints were called "emotional," we should not eliminate the possibility that chronic, nonspecific, unexplainable aches and pains *could* be reflecting underlying emotional problems. Often, proper treatment of the mental disturbance will result in a "cure" of the physical symptoms, too, if you'll give it a chance. Too many people are hung up on the idea that it's embarrassing to have mental health problems, and this blocks us from getting the care we need.

DEPRESSION: WHAT YOU HAD TO SAY ABOUT IT

Renee, 31 years old
I had it all my life but could never put a name to it. Blue periods. As a child I would cry for no reason. My parents would get frustrated. My mother would say, "I hope you have a child like yourself." My real low ones—you get suicidal. I really felt suicidal. There is no hope. You never can finish anything. I had these big "I don't wanna's." Even though I know I'm intelligent, it would keep me from finishing anything. You feel desperate, and lonely.

I'm depressed because something's flowing wrong in my brain. I'd have these periods where I would just be paralyzed. I never had a boyfriend more than a month. There is no label on it, no way to describe it. You'd wanna go out in the sunshine, be normal. I never understood. It's a real disease. With medication I'm much more on an even keel. It was instant—the minute I started taking it there was a huge difference. I have a relationship for the first time in my life now.

With mental illness, depression, they consider you defective. Keep trying. It took me 30 years to find out what was going on.

Elizabeth, 36 years old
It's different for everyone. I had a lot of very bad days, just terrible, I couldn't concentrate, I'd cry for no reason at all. Tears would start. I couldn't talk. I couldn't think straight. I had stomachaches, and chest pain, and headaches. Things the doctor couldn't explain. I was thinking of ending my life. At that point I couldn't think straight, I wanted to give up. It's hard to explain. Your mind shuts down, you don't know where you're going, what you're doing. I could be talking with someone and all of a sudden I'd stop and I didn't know what I was saying. I would sleep maybe two hours a day, my mind would be racing constantly.

I went into the hospital because I had suicidal tendencies. I was fortunate I had a lot of people around me. My religious background, you just don't do things like that. I knew I'd have to save myself. I had a friend come over and spend the evening with me because I was so distraught. I had gone two–three weeks beforehand to national depression screening day. I'd read about it, signed things and went. What I saw was everything I had seen and I had felt. It just hit home. They gave me a listing of local organizations I could go to. One was a suicide prevention line. I called and the man I spoke to was so reassuring—someone could help me. Between that and having someone in the house, I went to the hospital and at the e.r. they took me right in right away.

I went through group therapy, this was very important because I could see other people suffering too—maybe not the same type, but I was able to confront my problems by talking it out with these people. I'm very stubborn, headstrong. I demand a lot from myself. Before therapy, I put my depression aside and just dealt with it.

I still have my bouts with depression. I now find because of my character I've been able to deal with issues that come up. I haven't been close to the depression I had before. Now it's due to stress, and the seasons changing. I find a way to deal with the stress. I tend to give myself the time where I didn't give myself the time before. I allow myself a moment, a day or two to recuperate. I have a very sympathetic family and that helps. I've adjusted pretty well. I've been out of the hospital two years now. I've kept in touch with people from the group who were in the hospital, too. If one feels down, we call each other. It's nice to know someone is out there who basically can understand what I'm going through.

THE HARD FACTS ABOUT DEPRESSION

There are 12 to 13 million depressed people in the U.S., and 7 to 8 million of them are women. One in 4 women will have an episode of significant depression in her lifetime. Remarkably, only 1 in 5 of them will receive needed treatment, partly because they do not know that help is available, and partly because we have stigmatized mental illness so powerfully that many women are afraid to seek help. According to psychologist Hanna Lerman of Los Angeles, depression rates in the U.S. have been climbing since the 1950s, with a greater increase among women (who started out with a higher base rate in the first place). As several experts are quick to point out, most of the leaders in mental health research are male—there is only a tiny handful of female heads of psychiatric departments, making it less likely that women's mental health is getting the attention it deserves.

Throughout the industrialized world, women's rates of depression outnumber men's, usually 2 to 1. A particular form of depression, called seasonal affective disorder or SAD, affects women four times as much as it affects men. This type of depression occurs during the dark, short days of winter—or in other situations where there is a lack of exposure to natural daylight. Many of the symptoms of depression set in at this time, and, quite logically, can often be relieved by spending time in front of banks of artificial bright lights that mimic sunlight.

Severe episodes of depression—again, the "major" depression described earlier—often last for about six to nine months and fade on their own, but without proper treatment many cases recur. For this reason, Ellen McGrath, chairperson of the American Psychological Association's national task force on women's depression, calls untreated major depression a "mental or emotional cancer," capable of lying dormant and then rearing its ugly head when you least expect it. It's a bad idea to let depression fester anyway, since no one has several months of life to toss away. Since treatment often takes effect quickly, it's a shame to let too much time go by without seeking help.

Experts have traced the rates of depression over the decades, and have found that while depression in general has become more prevalent over the past 40 years, the increase has been greater for women than for men. Some consider depression an illness of its own, while others call it a symptom of other, underlying issues and problems. Whatever you call it, it is treatable. The trouble is, too often it goes undiagnosed—so it *can't* be treated. Lack of proper treatment does not necessarily mean you failed to see a doctor. On the contrary, Carol Landau notes that two-thirds of people who commit suicide were seen by physicians in the month before they died! Are the wrong questions being asked, or are the right ones being omitted? Are women not acknowledging the depth of their pain to these health care professionals? We must discover what is blocking women from getting lifesaving *or* life-enhancing treatment for this epidemic of depression.

To make matters worse, even those women who *do* seek care for depression often find that their insurance doesn't cover that care. Mental illness coverage is notoriously poor, feeding the myth that somehow it isn't as valid or important or "real" as physical illnesses. Can you imagine an insurer that does not reimburse for the cost of treating pneumonia? Probably not. But somehow we accept the fact that treatment for mental illness gets short shrift when it comes to coverage. As often happens to women, particularly older women, sometimes the little coverage we do have disappears when we are widowed or divorced, and lose coverage from our spouses' insurance. In so many ways, from misdiagnosis to access to care in the first place, women with mental health concerns are neglected or ignored.

Who's at Risk for Depression?

Recently, the American Psychological Association convened a task force on women and depression to look at all of the scientific research and draw some conclusions about the prevalence, causes, and future research needs for this epidemic. Ellen McGrath headed the project, which resulted in a book that includes a strong agenda for renewed research and attention to depression among women. I interviewed McGrath and a number of other experts who took part in the project—as well as many other other experts on women's mental health. There was surprising agreement about the serious causes of depression in women, and lots of hope and ideas for resolving these pressing problems. Based on hundreds of studies, the experts determined that the causes listed below are the most important sources of depression among women.

Depression Cause: Abuse/Violence against Women

Abuse—physical, sexual and emotional—was at the top of the list of almost every mental health care expert I interviewed. Thirty to fifty percent of women suffer some type of abuse—half of it originating within their families. Police often don't take complaints seriously, and in many areas, shelters from abuse are unavailable. Gwendolyn Keita finds that some women fail to walk out on abusers not because they're afraid to leave, but because they have nowhere safe to go! In other cases, women stay because their children are threatened if they leave. To make matters worse, many women fail to recognize that they are being abused in the first place. While physical and sexual abuse are generally easier to define, emotional abuse can be more hazy. Are you often made to feel worthless, inadequate, or stupid? Are you made to feel like a servant, or powerless, under the control of someone else? Are you made to feel guilty, or put down, in the way you lead your life? Are you called names, like "bitch," so often that you've begun to think it's normal? Do you walk on eggshells, feel frightened of your abuser even in your own home? Do you feel "stuck" in your own life, afraid to make changes because of your abuser's reaction? Aline Zoldbrod, a Boston-area psychologist, believes that about a third of all depression among women is attributable to some form of abuse, and that women who aren't being physically beaten may not even recognize that they're being abused. Take some time to think about the way you are treated by your partner, boss or coworker—and think about how that makes you feel about yourself every day. Just as mental illness is no less important than physical illness, so emotional abuse is no less significant—or damaging—than physical abuse. The only difference is the bruises are on the inside.

Sexual abuse is another major problem and cause of depression among women. Dr. Jean Baker Miller, clinical professor of psychiatry at the Boston University School of Medicine and director of education at Wellesley's Stone Center for Developmental Services and Studies, points to the startling figure that 38% of women are sexually abused by the time they reach their late teens. Some would argue that this number is much too high, but regardless of where you place the final decimal point, most experts agree that the problem is serious and disturbingly prevalent. Depression and anxiety are common results of this abuse, and as we continue to uncover the extent of sexual abuse among women of all ages, says Baker Miller, we develop a greater understanding of many depression cases.

Advice.

If you are experiencing abuse of any kind and do not know where to go for help, start by talking to a mental health expert in your area. Stop keeping your terrible crisis a secret—reach out and open up. Start making stronger connections with people who support what you want to do in life, rather than those who tend to hold you back and mock or diminish your plans and dreams. Most important, seek professional counseling. If cost is a concern, look in the phone book for a community mental health center in your area. Your local health department may be able to steer you in the right direction. Often, payment for critical cases can be waived or put on a sliding scale to meet your needs. Or look for the number of a crisis hotline or center for abuse in your area. If you cannot get to an actual center, start with just a phone call and ask for the help you deserve. Often, it's hard to get away from the abuser for long enough to seek help. But trained crisis managers or therapists can accomplish quite a bit over the phone—at least giving you a start on your road to recovery. They will talk to you about issues ranging from finding a safe place to stay, alone or with children, and also about ways to protect yourself both emotionally and physically.

In cases of physical abuse, group therapy with the abuser present is *not* recommended, because often the abuser will later punish you for speaking up in front of others. However, women-only group therapy can be extremely helpful, as it proves to women that they are not alone and helps build a network of support. In cases of emotional abuse, couples therapy *can* be useful, but again, the problem of blaming and additional abuse in the privacy of home can still be a problem.

The laws in this country do not adequately protect women from abusers, and as a result, many women are too terrified to seek help for fear that their abuser will find out and accelerate the emotional or physical battering. The value of therapy, if you can find a way to get it cheaply and privately, is it will begin to help you discover options and solutions to your problem. You may be convinced that there are no options, but you are wrong. Too many other women have thought the same thing and stayed in abusive situations until it was too late to get help. You are not alone: millions of women are abused by family members, so-called "friends" and others every day. Professional group therapy and amateur support groups can help you realize there are other women like you out there, getting help for themselves and their families. Chances are that you have begun to think of yourself as a victim, and victims don't take charge of their problems; they are continually abused. Try to remember that no one is inherently a victim: you are only in that position as long as you allow yourself to be. Getting out from under an abusive relationship may be the hardest thing you ever did—or at this point, the hardest thing you can imagine doing—but you owe yourself what could come next: the rest of your free, empowered life.

DEPRESSION CAUSE: HAVING MANY CHILDREN; BEING AT HOME WITH THEM

High rates of depression have been found among full-time, at-home moms with many young children. Having more than two children under 5 is also associated with depression. Dr. Jean Baker Miller of Wellesley's Stone Center finds that the combination of a high-demand situation and the psychological isolation of being alone with young children all day can add up to severe depression. Women whose marriages are unstable or unfulfilling are, as you might expect, at even greater risk of depression. For instance, if you are unable to confide your feelings of depression to your spouse, you're at greater risk of serious problems. Many people are surprised to learn that depression is especially high among *younger* women who are at home with children. The traditional image of the depressed older woman, while certainly real in some cases, belies the fact that younger women are at very high risk of depression, too. Today, when women have so many more options than ever before, we must reject the *assumption* that younger women should be happy at home raising children. Some are, some aren't. The fact that so much depression exists in this population of women should tell us that something isn't right for many of us.

Dr. Marilyn Karmason, a psychiatrist at The New York Hospital/Cornell Medical Center, notes that the kind of community you live in often determines whether a given lifestyle will predispose you to depression. An at-home, full-time mother who lives in a community where most other women work *outside* the home may well suffer depression as a result of her unusual status. (On the flip side, Dr. Karmason notes, a high-powered investment banker who leaves her children at home with a nanny in a community where most mothers care for their children full-time may *also* experience depression.)

Advice.

Even small changes in your lifestyle can make a major difference in your outlook on life. If you're at home full-time with your children, making time for a single class each week so you can build toward a career when your children are out of the house, or taking on a volunteer project outside the home or even taking part-time work if you can arrange for child care, can build your sense of self-esteem and value in settings *other* than home. Self-esteem is a great antidote to depression. Connecting with others in your situation can also help; for instance, starting mother-baby playgroups and other support systems can help relieve your sense of burden. If you are already feeling too low to motivate yourself to make a change, start out with some counseling and move from there.

If you're working outside the home, maximize the enjoyable activities you do with your child in the evening or on weekends. Adding simple games, singing and other fun interactions will be more meaningful to you *and* your child than routine meals and bedtime. Also, talk with other working women about *their* "quality time" management. Communicating with others can relieve your sense of guilt and concern.

DEPRESSION CAUSE: A DEPENDENT, PASSIVE PERSONALITY STYLE

Some experts feel that women, who are more likely (on average) than men to have passive, dependent, negative personality styles, are more likely to become depressed. Do you tend to think that things are bad simply because the world is a hostile, unhappy place? Do you feel that you are miserable or unsuccessful because you are innately incompetent or untalented? Do you sense that your relationships with others are flawed because either you or they don't *deserve* closeness and happiness? Do you tend to let others walk all over you simply because you can't muster the energy to lead life differently? You may be trapped in the kind of negative thinking, outlook and personality that predisposes you to chronic, severe depression.

Susan Nolen-Hoeksema of Stanford University, author of *Sex Differences In Depression,* has found significant differences in the way women and men handle feelings of depression. While women are often more ruminative, she says, men are more active in response to depressive feelings. These are generalizations, of course, but she also reports that women are more prone to wallowing in our problems, blaming ourselves, while men are more apt to fight off "down" moods with sports, hobbies and other activities (unfortunately, sometimes they choose substance abuse over healthier coping activities). Nolen-Hoeksema says that women's bouts with depression are generally longer, and more frequent, partly because of our more negative, passive coping style. She urges women to take a cue from men on this score by trying to reject the passive, negative stereotype and taking action on our own behalf. Sometimes this can only follow treatment, particularly empowerment-based therapy discussed later in this chapter.

Advice.

A very effective, popular and often brief form of therapy called CBT, or cognitive behavioral therapy, might be the answer for you. This form of therapy or counseling, while it has a complicated name, actually is based on a very simple concept: that depression is often caused by faulty *thinking* patterns. The idea behind CBT is that we are depressed because of negative thinking styles, assuming that things are bad because *we* are worthless, or because the world is generally a negative place. With the help of CBT, you can learn to think more positively, more independently, and more aggressively—and by doing so, you can often melt away your depression.

Dr. Kelly Phillips points out that as our health care system moves gradually toward the HMO system, shorter-term mental health care might become increasingly common. Before we rush to criticize it, she says, we should recognize that brief therapy for certain types of depression or other emotional problems can be appropriate and effective.

While we don't often think about it this way, learning to be a more positive thinker is a *skill,* and like any other skill, with the right practice and instructor (or in the case of the therapist, the right guide), you can find your way out of a dark outlook on life. Sometimes, medication is used in combination with talk therapy.

DEPRESSION CAUSE: RELATIONSHIP PROBLEMS

Women, more than men, derive a great deal of self-esteem and optimism from healthy relationships—be they romantic, parent-child or friendship relationships. When relationships crumble, depression is often quick to follow for women. Women who are in unhappy marriages, for example, are 25 times more likely to be depressed than women in happy marriages. Men, by contrast, are less likely to become depressed as a result of a troubled marriage.

Relationship problems can trigger depression in several ways. For instance, in some cases, just the trouble in the relationship *itself* can cause depression. In other cases, while our own lives are going fine, we bear the burden of others' problems on our shoulders, worrying and becoming depressed *by association.* This is common in the case of mother-child relationships: our kids' problems often become our own. Certainly, these are generalizations; but researchers and clinicians in mental health fields have noted significant differences between men and women on this score. Having a child with a chronic illness, for instance, often drags a mother into depression. As traditional supporters, nurturers, and caregivers, both the health of others and our connection to them is vital to women's sense of well-being. When relationships suffer or crumble, so does our mental outlook.

Finally, the *absence* of important personal connections often causes depression among women. An example would be when close family members live far away—particularly at times of emotional distress. Women are vulnerable to depression when the nuclear family is dispersed, notes Karmason. The solution for this particular problem, Karmason suggests: form a "newclear" family of friends and associates. It takes time, Karmason adds, but school and religious associations, sports clubs and other social venues are good places to start. The approach has helped many of her patients, including older women who have been widowed or divorced, and find themselves needing to forge new social bonds.

Advice.

For relationship problems, a form of therapy called IPT or interpersonal therapy is designed to help people improve the ways in which they relate to others, helping us to stop making the same mistakes over and over, and to begin to forge healthy alliances with people that bring us joy and not depression. Some believe that IPT is especially useful for women, since it focuses on an area of great importance to women's mental health: namely, the success of relationships. In romantic relationships, couples therapy can be helpful in addition to individual therapy. But IPT is used to help resolve conflict in all types of relationships, teaching you invaluable skills of relating and interacting that will enhance all of your emotional bonds.

Depression Cause: Gender Bias

Bias in education is an important cause of depression, especially in younger women. Gender bias shows up in many forms, including girls getting called on less often than boys in class, girls getting praised not for the content of their work but for the neatness of their handwriting, and so on. Bias in the workplace is a major cause of depression in older women: it appears in the form of sexual harassment, unequal pay for equal work, condescension on the job, the glass ceiling and lack of control of one's time. Gender bias is everywhere and affects nearly every woman in our society at some time, in some way, on some level. Long-term discrimination of the sort we may even stop *noticing* over time is a tremendous contributor to depression among women. A chronic state of disempowerment and of second class citizenship in our world goes far in

making women doubt their own value, lower their expectations and dreams, and make the problem of discrimination and subservience a circular one.

I interviewed several teenage girls for a CBS story on educational gender bias in 1993. Most were well-spoken, outgoing and intelligent. Some were at the top of their class. They certainly did not seem the "types" to be oppressed by gender bias. I was astonished at the extent of their frustration and their resentment of the way in which they were treated not only by teachers but also by male classmates. The experience made them doubt their abilities, clam up in class, become too distracted to learn. These were talented and privileged girls, for the most part. If *they* were suffering from gender bias, one can only imagine the impact of these kinds of inequities on women of limited means and resources. We must realize that *all* women are vulnerable to gender bias, start to take notice of its subtle manifestations and support one another if we are ever to reach our potential.

Advice.

There are two forms of therapy that are often directed at women, and help solve the problems caused by chronic gender bias. One is called feminist therapy, and the other is assertiveness training. Feminist therapy, which assumes that women have become a subclass in need of elevation, can actually be attached to or incorporated into most other kinds of therapy. The basic concept is that a therapist, ideally a woman, enters an equal relationship with a patient/client on a first name basis. On this one-to-one, equal basis, the women work out issues and solutions to uniquely female concerns in our society. Assertiveness training, which is related to feminist therapy and is often behavioral in its approach, actually *trains* women to assert themselves in every realm of life, whether in their own homes with family members, in the workplace, or on the street when construction workers hoot and howl. Again, we're talking about building *skills*. Assertiveness can be learned, though years of submissiveness takes time to undo. Since depression is so closely linked to a lack of self-esteem and empowerment, a growing sense of strength and self-worth goes far to eliminate depressive feelings.

DEPRESSION CAUSE: DOING IT ALL— ROLE OVERLOAD

While at-home mothers are generally more likely to be depressed than working women, clearly there are variations on each theme. For instance, working women who have children at home and little help from spouses in the evening have very high rates of depression. The more roles you try to play without support, the greater your risk of depression. The superwoman image put forth by the media is a wonderful concept if only we had 48 hours in each day. But we don't, and when we try to do too much, our bodies *and* minds tell us we're pushing too hard. Margaret Chesney of the University of California–San Francisco points out that there *are* pluses to women having multiple roles: for example, more money, greater opportunities and the chance to find happiness in at least one domain (home and/or work). The downside, she says, includes increased stress hormones, high blood pressure and other measures of excessive stress on the mind and body. Depression often results.

Women are more likely than men to have two jobs, and we're also far more likely to be the at-home workers after a full day at the office. Professor and author Arlie Hochschild named it the "Second Shift," discovering that women are bearing most of the burden of home life even when both they and their partners work. Dr. Marilyn Karmason finds that when women lose the power struggle in two-career marriages, and are left to bear the brunt of childcare alone, depression often sets in. She calls this the "dark side of the new female power." Trying to be all things to all people—caring for children, jobs, aging parents, friends with problems—leaves us without support (and *time*) for ourselves. Exhaustion and depression—and often, the failure to do *any* of our many tasks well—are the frequent results. Some experts now believe that from fatigue and depression come reduced immunity, more physical illnesses and greater risk of other forms of depression such as that connected with PMS.

Advice.
It's easy to say *share the burden,* but that's hard or impossible for some women to do—especially if they get little support from their partners and/or have few financial resources to fall back on. One route you can take is to join forces with other women in your position. Perhaps you can take turns watching groups of children so at least you have *some* time for yourself, or a day or two each week in which you don't have to tear up the road getting home from work. Older children can be taught to chip in, especially in helping with younger ones. And by banding together with other women in your situation at work, you may be able to force the workplace to become more amenable to working mothers—perhaps by providing even

limited child care. What may seem impossible to accomplish as an individual can be far more attainable in large numbers.

DEPRESSION CAUSE: LOW-CONTROL JOBS

Women are more likely than men to be in jobs that offer little self-initiative, creativity or freedom. Too often, women are in strictly regulated jobs with limited break time, and we often report to more than one demanding boss. How many times have you been immersed in a deadline project when another superior dropped work on your desk and needed it ASAP? Do you feel like you have little chance for advancement in your current position, and that you are underpaid, undervalued, underacknowledged day after grueling day? Do others hold you back from advancement because they can't afford to let you move out of the dead-end position you're in? Add sexual harassment in the workplace to low-control, high-stress occupations and you have many depressed women in the workforce.

As we'll discuss more in chapter 24, "Heart Disease, Heart Health," low-control jobs create tremendous stress and can actually be harmful to your physical as well as mental health.

Advice.

If it won't cost you your job, start to speak up when at all possible, and set limits at reasonable times. The day a major project is due obviously isn't the best day to put your foot down. But for general day-to-day stresses and abuse of your time and ability, make your feelings known. For instance, let superior A know that you are working as fast as you can on superior B's project and that it will take until X o'clock to complete it. State that only *then* will you be able to begin the next task. If that poses a serious problem, suggest that the superiors work out a fair plan themselves—one that leaves you room to breathe and function effectively.

In your off hours, even if they are few and far between, try to get *some* type of training or education that will help you move forward in your career, or at least to move out of the position you're in now. Even a single class, one evening a week, can make a difference. Lots of people have gotten degrees or skills one tiny step at a time. Even if it will take you many years, you are gaining self-confidence the whole time and looking forward to something positive at the end of the road.

In general, whatever the cause of depression, taking action is a depression-beater. This can be a catch-22, since depression makes it quite hard to "get up and go." Motivating yourself may be the last thing on your mind, especially if you're having trouble just getting up in the morning or making it through the day. Take one small step at a time. Get together with others in your office who feel the same frustrations you feel, and try to work out solutions together. Often creative answers come out of group discussions. Could you cover for one another when the load gets too heavy on one of you? Might you be able to pool your talents and get more done in tandem than any one of you could have done alone? We spend so much time being competitive with one another that we often hold ourselves back, rather than building strength in numbers. Finally, never assume that there's nothing better out there. Keep your eyes and ears open for other opportunities (perhaps elsewhere in the company you work for), read the want ads religiously and pursue anything that looks exciting to you, even if it seems like a long shot. A potential employer might turn you down for now, but you never know—you could make a lasting contact, or get advice on a skill you might add to your repertoire that would make you a better candidate the next go-round.

As for sexual harassment, a major problem in its own right, experts advise that you document the problem. Tell at least one person you can trust what is happening to you: be calm, and be specific. Keep private written notes about what happened and when it occurred (it may be best to keep these notes at home). Speak up in the office and make a formal complaint to the appropriate superior. Dr. Margaret Jensvold, director of the Institute for Research on Women's Health in Washington, D.C., warns that some women will be told to see a psychiatrist after making a sexual harassment complaint. She urges women to refuse to see the therapist but to make a note that she was told to do so—with the date and the name of the person who made the suggestion. In dealing with a sexual harassment complaint, always be as professional, serious, and blunt as possible. Acting hysterical or out of control is likely to prejudice others against you. If you do not feel that your complaint is being taken seriously or that steps are being taken to rectify the problem, you may feel you have to take your complaint outside the office, retain an attorney, and file a suit. The more information you save and the more specifics you can give, the stronger your case is likely to be.

DEPRESSION CAUSE: SUBSTANCE ABUSE

You can find more detailed information on substance abuse (including alcohol, cigarettes and other drugs) in chapter 19, but because it is such an important source of depression among women, I mention it here. Depression and substance abuse are circular problems for women. On the one hand, depression can lead to so-called "self-medication" with alcohol, drugs or cigarettes. On the other hand, women who abuse drugs and alcohol are more prone to *becoming* depressed, which often drives them to further substance abuse. If you find yourself taking refuge in drugs or alcohol rather than dealing with your problems, it's time to get some help. Too often, women who abuse drugs and alcohol are ostracized by society because these habits are considered "unladylike," says Dr. Robert Millman of The New York Hospital/Cornell Medical Center.

Advice.

Both your depression and your substance abuse need treatment. The first thing you should do is enroll yourself in a program for detoxification. The AAP Task Force on Women and Depression found that a major obstacle to detox for women is the lack of child care facilities in most programs. Do you have someone—a parent, close friend or relative—who can help care for your children while you are receiving treatment? For entrenched alcoholism and drug abuse, inpatient treatment is often needed—that is, you'll need to stay in the hospital or treatment center for a period of time so doctors can monitor your safe withdrawal from your addiction. Therapy and sometimes medical treatment for your underlying depression and/or other problems begins in the detox program, but you're likely to need further therapy and care *after* you leave the center and resume life on your own. If you cannot afford these programs, call your local health department or one of the organizations listed at the end of this chapter for information on low- or no-cost treatment programs for which you may be eligible.

DEPRESSION CAUSE: POVERTY

There are over eight million women living in poverty in the United States: that means living on $5,778 or less per year. Seventy-five percent of the poor people in the U.S. are women and children. Women of color are particularly at risk. If you are in a financial crisis, you are at risk of serious depression. Dr. Margaret Jensvold notes that while women in general have worse access to health care than men, poor women are particularly disadvantaged when it comes to getting treatment for mental health problems. So the women who need care the most, get it the least. But your poverty should not deprive you of mental health care. While Medicaid provides little in the way of mental health care, you may be eligible for free, charitable programs through your local or community health department.

DEPRESSION CAUSE: GROWING OLDER

While the question of whether menopause contributes to depression is controversial, it is certainly a fact that the onset of old age in our society triggers depression for many women. Older women are more likely to live alone, see their friends and partners die, fall to a low-income level, have inadequate housing and medical care, poor health, increased sleep problems and other depression triggers than younger women. While certainly there are many older women who do *not* fall into these categories, the risks are there, and they are greater for older women than for younger ones.

DEPRESSION CAUSE: MEDICATIONS

The APA Task Force on depression notes that in addition to many social and biological causes of depression, certain medications that are taken either exclusively or primarily by women can promote depression as well. These include oral contraceptives and diet pills—both taken by millions of women. Certain chronic diseases are also known to contribute to depression, such as lupus (and other autoimmune diseases in which the body attacks itself), eating disorders like anorexia and bulimia, and thyroid disease.

DEPRESSION CAUSE: INFERTILITY

Read more about infertility, a common and serious cause of depression among women, in chapter 16.

OTHERS AT RISK

The APA Task Force on Women and Depression found several other groups to be at particularly high risk of depression: these included lesbians, adolescent girls with little parental support and ethnic minorities who have been exposed to racism and other problems associated with integration.

WHEN TO SEEK HELP—AND FROM WHOM

When depression is in any way impairing your ability to function properly—to do your job, relate to others, get up in the morning—it's time to seek help. Don't wait until you can hardly cope to seek help, urges Carol Landau. There are many different kinds of practitioners who can help you. Psychiatrists are medical doctors who can can offer both talk and drug therapy. Psychologists, licensed social workers and other kinds of mental health counselors can also provide excellent mental health care: see if they are open to consulting an M.D. should you need medication. Some feminist mental health practitioners think that female counselors are a must for female patients—others think this is a silly generalization. For certain kinds of highly sensitive, difficult-to-discuss problems like sexual abuse, you might feel more comfortable working with a woman therapist. But again, this is a personal decision—there are no hard and fast rules. You will be the final arbiter of which practitioner makes you feel comfortable, and who is doing a good job of making you feel well.

Talk to your health insurer about what kind of coverage is available for mental health care. It is likely to be minimal. Some insurers require that your practitioner have certain credentials; find this out before you choose a counselor.

Free or low-cost mental health care can be found in a number of settings, from university hospitals to colleges to community health centers to state health organizations. Charitable organizations also offer special programs for those who are unable to pay expensive mental health care fees.

Types of Treatment for Depression

Drug Treatment for Depression

Antidepressant medication saves lives. While some feel that these drugs are overprescribed, we cannot ignore their vital role in improving the lives of millions of people whose very existence is dampened by temporary or chronic depression.

Experts are quick to point out that many women "self-medicate" for depression with harmful drugs, cigarettes and alcohol. These substances can reinforce mental and physical health problems. The fact is, there are GOOD ways to medicate for depression. Sometimes, in addition to talk therapy for depression, antidepressant drugs play an important role. Hundreds of millions of dollars are spent on these medications each year in the U.S. Historically, there has been some concern about the overuse of antidepressants (as well as antianxiety medications) among women, who receive at least 70% of all antidepressant prescriptions. But when used correctly, they can be lifesaving and life-enhancing for many patients.

The keys to proper drug management of depression are (1) getting the right diagnosis in the first place, (2) careful monitoring and reevaluation by a physician on a regular basis while taking the drugs, and (3) compliance—taking the drug in the right dose, as prescribed. A large percentage of patients take antidepressant drugs incorrectly, reducing their effectiveness. One of the benefits of medication is that in just a few weeks, you may begin to feel better and stronger, and able to concentrate on talk therapy. Talk to your doctor about whether these medications might be right for you. Usually, if you are in a "major depression," (*see* symptoms on pages 334–335) medication will be recommended at least in the short term to help you get on your feet, literally and figuratively. Psychiatrists, because they are medical doctors, can prescribe these drugs, while psychologists

(Ph.D.'s) and other mental health professionals cannot. Often, non-M.D. health professionals will work with psychiatrists in order to make medication available to their patients. Discuss this possibility with your practitioner and see if this team approach to your care is possible.

Your regular family doctor—with an M.D.—can also prescribe antidepressant medication: in fact, the practice is quite common. Many psychiatrists (and other mental health experts) worry that nonspecialists are acting without the right background, information, diagnosis or follow-up. Landau worries about the fact that some nonpsychiatrists fail to make a proper diagnosis of depressed patients and give *antianxiety* drugs instead of antidepressants. Antianxiety drugs can behave like alcohol in the bodies of depressed patients, she says, adding an addiction on top of the depression! There is sometimes an anxiety component to depression, Landau adds, but certainly giving *only* antianxiety drugs to depressed patients is the wrong approach.

There are several categories of antidepressant drugs, ranging from the old-line tricyclic antidepressants, to the MAO inhibitors, to the newest so-called seratonin re-uptake inhibitors (like Prozac), which have received enormous amounts of media attention of late and are already among the most-prescribed medications.

The older drugs tend to have many more side effects, ranging from dry mouth, constipation and decreased sex drive to still more debilitating feelings—but they have their place in modern treatment and can be very effective in battling certain kinds of depression. MAO inhibitors can actually cause dangerous, violent side effects if taken at the same time as certain foods like cheese or wine, but again, they are appropriate for certain subgroups of patients. The newer antidepressant drugs have fewer side effects than the older ones (though they do have side effects like nausea, headache and others for some patients). They're also more effective than older drugs, for some patients and some problems—but they tend to be much more costly than older drugs, too.

You may have heard about the tremendous controversy over the drug Prozac a couple of years ago, when studies suggested that the drug itself might predispose patients to commit suicide. Every mental health expert I interviewed felt that the results of those studies were seriously misinterpreted—and that the increased suicide rate in some patients taking Prozac was attributable to the fact that this is a severely depressed, high-risk population to begin with. Drugs in this class are in fact considered relatively safe and effective, and are providing tremendous relief to many thousands of people. Some worry that their use is becoming so common it's almost faddish.

Talk to your doctor about the pros and cons of each type of antidepressant medication, and whether drug treatment is appropriate for you in the first place. Be sure to discuss all possible side effects, because these drugs differ tremendously in their effects: if you find one type intolerable, another might be right for you.

Nondrug/Self-help Therapy for Depression

While a true clinical depression requires formal treatment (talk therapy and/or medication), there are a variety of lifestyle and behavior changes that can help you heal. For less severe cases of depression—"the blues"—these self-help measures alone can make the difference between feeling good and feeling crummy.

Exercise.

Regular, vigorous aerobic exercise goes a long way to boost energy, mood and self-esteem. It is a much healthier approach to "self-medication" than overeating or drinking. Not only will your *physical* health get better as your body becomes more fit, but your *emotional* outlook will improve almost immediately after you begin a regular exercise program (as the so-called "feel-good" chemicals, endorphins, are released during exercise). Down the line, as you start to look and feel better, your self-esteem will climb. So just when you feel you want nothing more than to lounge in bed, force yourself to get up and start walking outside. Once around the block and you may feel you're ready for more. (For more on starting an exercise program, *see* chapter 21.)

Bright Light.

As mentioned earlier, a certain kind of depression, called SAD (seasonal affective disorder), occurs during dark winter months when we are deprived of sunlight week after week. Depression, weight gain and carbohydrate cravings are common among women with this disorder. While formal treatment for SAD involves sitting under bright banks of special lights for specified periods of time, just spending more time outdoors during the brief periods of daylight can make a big difference. Even if it's cold outside, bundle up, pack your sandwich and take your lunch break outside, walking around the block a few times.

Take Some Kind of Action, However Small.

Ellen McGrath calls *action* the antidote to depression. When you use your negative feelings in some small way, you can help transpose them from negatives into positive energy. Appropriate, strong, negative feelings are healthy: don't fight them or hold them inward. Some positive actions McGrath recommends include writing your negative feelings down on paper, drawing pictures of people who anger you and tearing them up (this is especially helpful if you have been abused by the person you are shredding), and creating what she calls a "family of choice"—that is, forging deeper bonds with people whom you respect and who respect and support you, and letting them function in a sense as family members. With time, and sometimes with treatment, writing feelings down and shredding paper should grow into more direct confrontations and solutions for your problems.

Landau notes that strong bonds with others—even with one important confidante—can sometimes be similar to therapy. But she warns that reciprocity is important: do not drag your confidante down, or vice versa—empathy, support and positive reinforcement are what you're looking for.

A WORD ABOUT ELECTROSHOCK THERAPY

For the treatment of certain, severe cases of depression, electroshock therapy is making a comeback in the psychiatric community. While many of us think about the procedure as barbaric, and associate it with oppressive mental hospitals of the past, in fact electroshock therapy has been improved and updated and can be both appropriate and helpful for a small, select group of patients.

Summary

If there is a bottom line about dealing with depression, it is this: in almost every form, from every cause, it can be treated successfully in most patients. Every day you go without seeking help is a day in which you *could* be moving forward with a better, happier life. Ellen McGrath notes that only one in five women suffering from a depressive or anxiety disorder is getting adequate treatment. You wouldn't leave your broken leg out of a cast. Don't leave your broken emotions in the same state of neglect.

Anxiety Disorders

There are several kinds of anxiety disorders, including panic disorder, generalized anxiety disorder, social phobia, individual types of phobias (called "simple phobias"), obsessive compulsive disorder and post-traumatic stress disorder. While all of these anxiety disorders are important, I'll focus on the two kinds of anxiety disorders that affect women disproportionately: panic disorder, and generalized anxiety disorder.

What is Panic Disorder?

Everyone suffers from anxiety at some point: before a test, before giving a speech, before confronting another person. Anxiety in these situations is perfectly normal and can be healthy: it gets our bodies revved up for the task at hand. Sometimes, though, anxiety stops being useful and normal and begins to impair our ability to function normally. At the greatest extreme, anxiety shows itself as panic attacks. Nearly one in ten Americans has had a single panic attack at some time. This does *not* constitute a panic disorder. About four million Americans have full-blown panic disorders—nearly two and-three-quarters million of them are women.

Because women are more than twice as likely as men to suffer from panic attacks, anxiety disorders are often thought of as women's health problems. Of those who enter clinics for treatment of panic disorders, 70% are women. According to Dr. William Apfeldorf, former director of the anxiety division at New York Hospital/Cornell Medical Center, panic disorder is a critical women's health problem primarily because it is often overlooked, even by health professionals, and can cause major, long-term impairment in women's ability to lead productive lives.

The disorder affects *young* women more than older ones, often starting in the late teens and early twenties but not being diagnosed for another ten years at least. The average age at which women appear in Dr. Apfeldorf's clinic is 40—for many women that's two decades after their first symptom! It is thought that this long delay may be shrinking somewhat since panic disorder has received so much more media attention. Often women will recognize their symptoms in a lay article, and realize after so many years that (a) they aren't going crazy and (b) there are others in the same shoes—and finally, they go for help. By this time, the disorder is often far more advanced than it ever had to be.

According to Dr. Robert Pohl, director of the panic disorder program at the Wayne State University School of Medicine, one reason women have traditionally been at higher risk for panic disorder is we've been less likely to work outside the home. While there certainly are exceptions, people who have to get out of the house every day are less likely to suffer from panic disorder, he says. With more women in the workforce, we just might see an impact on the incidence of panic and other anxiety disorders.

Just as we throw around the term depression when we're feeling down, so we're quick to say "I panicked" when describing a frightening situation. When you look at the list of panic attack symptoms below, however, you'll see that they bear little resemblance to the short bursts of anxiety or worry we so often label as "panic."

Psychiatrists define a true panic attack as consisting of at least four of the following thirteen symptoms. The symptoms usually occur suddenly—in about ten minutes, you'll go from no unusual feelings at all to at least four full-blown panic symptoms. The definition of a panic disorder also requires that at some point, panic attacks occur spontaneously—that is, they are not triggered by an obvious stressor.

WHAT A PANIC ATTACK FEELS LIKE

- heart palpitations
- shortness of breath
- choking feeling
- chest pain or discomfort
- hot flashes or chills
- sweating
- dizziness or lightheadedness
- nausea/vomiting
- numbness or tingling
- feeling like you're having a heart attack
- feeling like you're going to lose control

Paula Levine, a psychologist in private practice in Coral Gables, Florida, notes that while panic attacks only last a few minutes, they feel as if they are lasting for hours.

ANXIETY DISORDER: WHAT YOU HAD TO SAY ABOUT IT

Judy, 38 years old

I believe I had symptoms in my grade-school years because I had school phobias. I had different periods where it kind of hits its peak and comes back. I was going to the emergency room almost every week, I was 22, 23, or 24 at the time. I wouldn't go out of my house. I'd go twenty-some days without solid food because I was afraid I'd choke. I was eating instant breakfast drinks. I said I was having a heart attack. I was dying and had a son and my mother would say this is just another one of my attacks. But she'd go along and take me to the emergency room.

I went to so many doctors and psychiatrists and psychologists and internists and neurologists and nobody knew anything back then. I had no control over it, it would come at any time. I left grocery bags at the store. I was driving on a freeway, it was pouring rain and I told my friend I had to get out of the car, I thought I would die. I was pouring sweat, my heart was pounding, I got back to my house, my mind was outside my body. My skin would crawl, nobody would understand, that's what got me the most—people would say it's all in your head.

I'd start out with drinks and that got me depressed and suicidal. I couldn't even picture living. They were medicating me with Valium, and it didn't do anything and I started abusing that. A good three years I couldn't work, I basically couldn't function. Then I did hook up with a doctor who put me on an antidepressant, I know now it wasn't the right one but I felt a difference. I could go places, but I still had to be able to escape—but at least I was trying.

I got a new job and those feelings started coming back. I had to quit my job. When I started to eat I'd choke. I read everything I could on panic disorder and anxiety but didn't believe anything would help me. I answered an ad looking for people to participate in a study. I couldn't participate because I had already taken medication but that's how I found Dr. X. He believed it was biochemical and by then I had tried too much behavior therapy to know I had no control over this, no matter how much breathing I did. I'm on Prozac now. I feel I'm the person I was meant to be. If I hadn't found Dr. X I might be dead. I couldn't live like that. If it takes 20 doctors, it takes 20 doctors. Don't give up. I'm a whole different person, I haven't had a full blown panic attack in three years. I feel I just began living three years ago.

Peggy, 46 years old
It was diagnosed as panic disorder with agoraphobia. The first symptoms were at about age 35. It was pretty terrible, it probably took about ten years to be diagnosed. That's the major frustration. I had extreme dizziness, shortness of breath, feeling like I couldn't breathe, feeling like I was going to die, like right then would be the end of my life. Sometimes a couple of times a week, I couldn't go to work. Finally I checked myself into a psychiatric ward. I would shake, tremble in my hands and legs. Then the panic attacks would be almost continuous, 50 a day. They checked for thyroid disease and I was even diagnosed and treated for it. They told me I was depressed. I was treated for diabetes. One doctor put me on diabetic medication for five years. I wasted a lot of time. I thought I was going crazy. I couldn't drive my car by myself, I didn't like to stay alone at home, I was afraid I was going to die. It was like living hell.

I told the psychiatrist my symptoms and he said I might have panic disorder. It was the first I'd heard the words. I was put on an antidepressant and an anxiety drug, he told me to read this book on anxiety disease. It took much longer than I would've liked, it took three weeks to a month to see changes. Within two months I went back to work and I haven't missed a day since. I think I'm pretty much coasting or recovered at this point. I've tried to get off medication, but there must be some biochemical part of it because I can't. I worked extensively with cognitive and behavioral changes, exercise. Positive thinking is really important. Saying affirmations, setting goals, imaging myself doing all the things I couldn't do, staying alone, traveling out of town. I'm so good now.

You can find light at the end of the tunnel. It's so wonderful, nobody should have to suffer that long. The medical community doesn't know enough about this disorder. Try anything that works, don't knock the medication and don't knock the behavioral changes. Approach it from every angle. Get a good psychiatrist, get a support group, read all the books around. I have another friend who has not left the house alone in ten years. Some people just don't find the right answer. But I've met hundreds of people who've done really well.

HOW PANIC DISORDERS GET WORSE WITH TIME

Since panic attacks can occur without any external stressor, women with the disorder often develop something called "anticipatory anxiety," which is just what it sounds like: the fear of becoming anxious or of having a panic attack. Since it's impossible to predict when an attack may occur, those with panic disorders start to avoid public places—generally stores, crowds and public transportation—where they are afraid an attack might take place. Over time, the feared locations grow in number, until sufferers can become completely housebound. This part of panic disorder, which is known as "agoraphobia," is quite common. Dr. Thomas Uhde, professor and chairman of the department of psychiatry at Wayne State University, notes that while men tend to abuse alcohol and drugs more often when confronted with anxiety problems, women tend toward these so-called "avoidance behaviors"—like agoraphobia.

Treating Panic Disorders

Sadly, Dr. Uhde adds, many health practitioners who do not specialize in mental health are unaware of the symptoms of panic and other anxiety disorders, and of the social ostracism that can stem from them. As a result, patients often doctor-hop, going from one specialist to another to try to decipher the individual symptoms that are part of their particular brand of panic attack. If they suffer from heart palpitations or shortness of breath, they often will see cardiologists. For vomiting, they might see a gastroenterologist. Often, the specialist will rule out serious physical illness in *her* area of expertise, but won't offer information or treatment about possible anxiety disorders. According to Dr. Pohl, some women are overexamined when they present with panic disorder symptoms. They're given thousand-dollar tests, every kind of high-tech scan available. When all the tests are negative, Dr. Pohl says, women are often sent home with the proverbial "It's all in your head" diagnosis.

To make matters more confusing, there *are*

some physical health problems that cause similar symptoms to panic disorder. These include hyperthyroidism, and a rare tumor that causes an adrenaline rush, high blood pressure and headaches.

Sometimes, treatment is delayed because women believe they're going crazy and won't admit the problem even to their doctors, reports Dr. Uhde. Others live with anxiety disorders for decades, never even telling their spouses about the problem. Dr. Apfeldorf describes one patient, a mother of a six-year-old, who out of sheer terror was unable to go to the grocery store to get food for the child. After treatment, her ability to function as a parent and as a person were restored.

When recognized and treated properly, panic disorder can be eliminated. Experts estimate that about 80% of cases can be successfully treated with medication, nondrug talk therapy or a combination of the two. About one in four patients needs combination treatment to find relief, but most others do fine with one or the other form of treatment. At this point, there's no solid evidence that combination drug and talk therapy is better than either one alone, says Dr. Pohl.

Surprisingly, drug therapy for panic disorders centers around *antidepressant* medication (both the older-line drugs, and the newer ones, as listed in the depression section above). Certain antianxiety drugs, including the potentially highly addictive benzodiazepines (like Xanax), are also useful for some patients; other, newer forms (like BuSpar) have fewer side effects and are less addictive. Some experts feel that the risk of addiction to certain antianxiety drugs usually is related to taking the drug for the wrong reason, in the wrong dose. When they are prescribed for the right problem, and taken in the right dose, these drugs are useful and can be safe. Careful monitoring by a doctor is always important when taking these or any other long-term medication.

Drug therapy for panic disorders does not *always* need to continue for years at a stretch, though some patients will stay on medication for a lifetime. For some patients, short-term drug treatment is all it takes to release them from the bonds of a panic disorder. With time, they can be tapered off the drugs and do fine without them. *Don't* just quit taking the medication when you feel better, however. Taper off slowly, gradually, in order to avoid problems with withdrawal. Also keep in mind that there is a high relapse rate when medication is discontinued. Some say that cognitive behavioral therapy, a form of talk therapy discussed earlier in this chapter, can lessen the relapse rate. But this has not been proved.

Cognitive behavioral therapy or CBT is quite helpful in treating panic disorder. Alone, CBT can benefit 80% of panic disorder patients who try it. There are generally two components to treatment, including both an educational portion (teaching patients that panic symptoms like chest pain are *not* necessarily signs of heart disease) and also retraining patients to have calm, rational thoughts in place of the irrational ones that often accompany panic attacks. Relaxation exercises are also taught; they can be used when an attack occurs.

Generalized Anxiety Disorder: GAD

GAD is a completely different form of anxiety disorder that also affects about twice as many women as men. It is characterized by extreme, excessive, irrational chronic worry that impairs one's ability to get through the day and perform normal tasks. The strict definition requires that patients have two different areas of irrational worry over a six-month period. It is seen more often in later-middle-aged women.

Yes, we all have times when we're excessively worried, and usually it's normal. But when you find yourself chronically obsessing over fears about every issue that affects your life—such as your health, your finances, how the mayor is doing in your town, problems at your job—you may have a problem. Patients with GAD have trouble concentrating, often startle easily and have shakiness and palpitations. They seem a little like frightened animals, jumpy and unable to function properly.

According to Dr. Apfeldorf, "GAD waits forever to be seen." While ultimately, patients *usually* will see doctors for panic attacks, GAD often goes untreated for even longer, because it's hard to pinpoint the line that defines "excessive" worrying. This delay is a tragedy for many GAD sufferers, since treatment (including several types of antianxiety medication and cognitive behavioral therapy) often works quite well. Doctors discuss with GAD patients the *realistic* chances that their worst fears will come to pass—and with time, they learn that there is little on which to base their anxiety in the first place.

Paula Levine says GAD patients forget what it feels like *not* to be anxious. They may wake in the morning with feelings most of us associate with performance anxiety: in a pool of sweat, with tremulous hands and legs, and a feeling of doom even about the anxiety itself! The syndrome can be exhausting and debilitating.

SUMMARY

Anxiety disorders, like depression, are quite common in women, too often overlooked by health professionals and too often kept in the closet by women who suffer from them. Treatment works: don't wait to start it, and certainly, don't go for month after month on a treatment that doesn't work, urges Dr. Uhde. Be sure from the start that the practitioner you chose is not wedded to just one type of anxiety disorder treatment. If one treatment fails, try something different for your panic disorder, just as you would go on to try a different drug for your hypertension. You *can* take your life back—many women have.

Note: In this chapter, we discussed depression and anxiety disorders separately. In fact, in more than half of all cases, there is some blend of the two. The key is to determine which problem dominates, and to tailor treatment to that problem first. In addition, there are certain drugs that are known to work best in "combination" depression-anxiety cases. Ask your doctor if any of these might be helpful in *your* case.

FOR MORE INFORMATION ON MENTAL HEALTH

NATIONAL INSTITUTE OF MENTAL HEALTH

Free Information Service on Panic Disorder
500 Fishers Lane
Rockville, MD 20857
800-64-PANIC

ANXIETY DISORDERS ASSOCIATION OF AMERICA

6000 Executive Blvd., Suite 513
Rockville, MD 20852-4004
301-231-9350

NATIONAL DEPRESSIVE AND MANIC DEPRESSIVE ASSOCIATION

730 North Franklin
Chicago, IL 60610
800-82-NDMDA

DEPRESSION AWARENESS, RECOGNITION AND TREATMENT

D/ART Program
National Institute of Mental Health
5600 Fishers Lane, Room 15C-05
Rockville, MD 20857
301-443-4513
301-443-8431 (TTD)

NATIONAL MENTAL HEalth ASSOCIATION

Information Center
1021 Prince Street
Alexandria, VA 22314
800-969-6642
703-684-7722

NATIONAL ALLIANCE FOR THE MENTALLY ILL

200 North Glebe Rd., Suite 1015
Arlington, VA 22203-3754
800-950-NAMI
703-524-7760

NATIONAL FOUNDATION FOR
 DEPRESSIVE ILLNESS
2 Pennsylvania Plaza
New York, NY 10121
800-248-4344

AMERICAN PSYCHOLOGICAL
 ASSOCIATION
750 1st Street NW
Washington, DC 20002
202-336-5500

AMERICAN PSYCHIATRIC ASSOCIATION
1400 K Street NW
Washington, DC 20005
202-682-6000

NATIONAL ANXIETY FOUNDATION
3135 Custer Drive
Lexington, KY 40517
800-755-1576

PHOBICS ANONYMOUS
P.O. Box 1180
Palm Springs, CA 92263
619-322-COPE

CHAPTER EIGHTEEN

SLEEP AND FATIGUE

O lightly, lightly tread!
A holy thing is sleep.

—Felicia Dorothea Hemans, "The Sleeper"

Without sleep, we cannot survive. Without *adequate* sleep, we cannot function properly. Without adequate sleep over prolonged periods of time, everything that we are—our personalities, our interests, our ability to relate to others and perform tasks—collapses. Too numb to react, nerves too raw to withstand even minor demands, the chronically underslept watch helplessly while every aspect of their lives gradually becomes dysfunctional. Amazing, and frightening, isn't it, that millions of Americans are living this way?

It's not surprising, given the prevalance of sleep disorders, that we can't seem to get enough information about them. It's a sleep-deprived nation's national obsession! The Puritan ethic of "hard work for a good reward" has translated itself, in the 1990s, to "hard work to stay afloat." I'm constantly reminded in my role as a television producer that sleep disorders top the list of promotable issues for broadcast: whenever it comes times for "sweeps" series on television—the time when ratings have to be highest and therefore topics universally appealing—sleep problems rival only sexual dysfunction and bad backs for a place on the airwaves.

Literally millions of Americans suffer from clinically defined sleep disorders. Combine them with the crowd who are just plain chronically exhausted from stress and work overload, and you end up with a mammoth audience. You know what they say: people love to hear about themselves.

Women are at particularly high risk of certain kinds of sleep disorders, especially at vulnerable life junctures (times of hormonal shift, such as the menopause, for example). The most common of all is insomnia: at all ages, women are at greater risk of insomnia than are men. According to Dr. Quentin Regestein, director of the sleep clinic at Brigham and Women's Hospital in Boston, women make up two-thirds of all insomnia patients who seek treatment. Other common sleep problems, such as sleep apnea, have historically been considered male problems. However, new research shows that many women suffer from this problem, too—and with age, the gender gap may even erase. Women with sleep apnea may be missed because practitioners think of this as a male problem and don't always ask the right questions of women. We'll discuss insomnia and sleep apnea later in this section.

Most of the chronically tired among us do not have certifiable sleep disorders. In fact, many of us would feel just fine if we slept a little more each night, consistently. We are *sleep deprived*. It's not good enough to sleep into the afternoon on Sunday only to fall short most nights of the week. You can't trick your body into feeling rested, no matter how you try—but I'll discuss some ways of becoming more rested without having to quit your job, or ruin your family or social life. Napping is certainly one option: Dr. Regestein notes that in Greece, people who take an afternoon siesta have lower heart disease rates—and are a lot more cheerful than those who don't take naps. We'll discuss naps, when they are appropriate and how to use them, later in this chapter.

For those who do have real sleep disorders, symptoms can be a lot worse than just fatigue. Sleep disorders are associated with serious physical and mental health problems that won't abate until the sleep problem itself is resolved.

Treatment for sleep disorders can involve both behavioral therapies (lifestyle changes) and medical therapies (drugs or surgery). Too often these disorders are dismissed as trivial or not valid by friends and health practitioners ("Just get a little more rest and you'll be fine"). But with the advent of sophisticated sleep laboratories, in which various types and quality of sleep can be carefully tracked, sleep disorders have become increasingly legitimized and sleep science a fascinating area of study. The result: better, targeted treatments for specific sleep problems.

In this chapter, we'll discuss several common sleep and fatigue disorders that affect women (we don't have room for all of them!) and how they can be treated, both with self-help and medical treatment. We will also discuss the difference between feeling chronically fatigued and having actual chronic fatigue syndrome: a distinction that many overworked, underslept people fail to make. As you'll soon see, while you may be chronically exhausted, chances are you do *not* have CFS. This is a far more complicated syndrome than we were all led to believe by sound-bite-driven news reports.

SLEEP PROBLEM: WHAT YOU HAD TO SAY ABOUT IT

Tonya, 24 years old
I'm tired all the time, I have no energy, when I wake in the morning I feel like I didn't sleep a wink even after twelve hours. I fell asleep at the wheel and jumped a curb and that brought me to a sleep expert.

It's very frustrating. I'm getting married and I'm trying to plan my wedding, we'll have company and you could pay me a million dollars, but I can't stay awake! I fall asleep when my fiance is talking to me. I happen to be one of those people who needs nine hours of sleep, they said. I get six hours. My alarm goes off at 6:20, it takes one hour to get to work, one hour to get home, I go straight to the gym, then I go home and eat. If I got nine hours sleep my life would be eat, work out and sleep—I need to spend some time with my fiance!

I have to go back to the sleep lab, but they don't even want to talk to me until I get nine hours sleep every night for a couple of weeks. It's too hard for me. When I get my life together, get married, I'll get more sleep.

Barbara, 48 years old
Sleep Apnea: I was snoring, I wasn't sleeping through the night, never. Toward afternoon I would drag, I'd have to take a nap. I never felt really rested. It's been a long time I've been having this problem, I'd say about 25 years. The snoring was very disruptive, my husband is a lawyer, it was at the point where if he had court, we couldn't sleep together. I literally stopped breathing for short periods of time.

They suggested CPAP (an airway device during sleep). You look like a space cadet, it's not the most attractive thing to wear. I just started using it the last month and a half. I notice more energy, I don't have to nap. I notice a difference, my daughter's noticed a difference. I can go through the day and not be as draggy. It's hard to get used to, but I'm finding it easier now to fall asleep with it.

I'm overweight and they said if I'd lose weight I wouldn't have to use the machine all my life. I would need to lose about 75 pounds. Every once in a while I go upstairs and put this contraption on and think gee I wish I didn't have to wear this thing, but you do what you have to do. If I had diabetes I'd take insulin, right? I mean what are my choices?

Carol, 59 years old
I'd get a creepy crawly burning stinging I've-got-to-move-my-legs-or-I'm-gonna-die feeling. My legs start moving like a puppet is pulling the strings, I can't concentrate on anything else. At night when I'd get in bed I'd swish my legs like scissors across the sheets and I couldn't get to sleep and I'd get up and walk around. I absolutely went for years without really sleeping and at 5 a.m. I'd finally fall asleep. Crazy—people think you're crazy, you walk around like a zombie.

I was diagnosed as a manic depressive, for eight years I was told I had M.S., that I was in denial. They do not hear you, they do not listen to you, they just make up their mind and write it down.

I did more or less everything but I did it half-heartedly, I wasn't enjoying anything, when my husband would say something about being happy I wouldn't know what happy meant, I didn't feel joy or pleasure or anything. Sex was impossible, I don't think I had enough sex to have children, I adopted children.

Dr. X diagnosed me and she has me under control better than any of the people I speak with; she has me on a heavy group of medications, I keep a sleep log and there's a lot of information on it. I am very regimented about my medication. It's like being alive again. Not sleeping is without a doubt the most dreadful thing a person can be deprived of. It's helped my desire for my sex life, but the actual physical act still isn't easy. But I'm like a new person as far as my self-esteem, my personality, my outlook on life.

WHAT IS A SLEEP DISORDER?

There are several kinds of sleep disorders, some involving chronic lack of sleep (insomnia), some involving excessive sleep (hypersomnia), and some involving physical problems during sleep (such as sleep apnea). Other common disorders of sleep include sleep walking and so-called "night terrors," which are related to panic attacks in sleep. Generally, if under normal circumstances you have trouble getting calm, regular sleep over a significant period of time (not simply caused by an erratic overburdened lifestyle, or disruption of your normal routine), you may have some kind of sleep disorder. Other classic signs of sleep disorders are chronic daytime drowsiness and the inability to stay awake even for important tasks. Your problem might be as minor as the need to try a different mattress or change the air quality in your bedroom; it might be as serious as a physical or biological problem in your body that needs to be corrected before you can sleep soundly; it might indicate the use or abuse of the wrong substances before bedtime; or it might not in fact be a sleep disorder per se, but rather a symptom of a different, underlying problem (depression, for example).

The first thing you need to do, with your doctor, is to figure out just what your sleep problem is—what triggers it, what makes it worse or better, how long you've had the problem. Only then you can move on to determine the right course of treatment. Anyone who visits a doctor for sleep problems should be given a complete physical and psychological workup in addition to a discussion about the sleep problem.

THE HARD FACTS ABOUT SLEEP DISORDERS

Forty million Americans suffer from disordered sleep. Five to ten million Americans have sleep apnea, a breathing problem in sleep that threatens heart and lung health. Only a small fraction seek help. People with insomnia are more likely to have automobile accidents, to function poorly at work, and to have trouble thinking clearly than people who sleep normally. Millions of people who may not in fact have definable sleep problems still feel chronically sleepy, weak, unrested, unable to function or think effectively. An extremely small percentage of those who suffer from chronic tiredness and sleep problems suffer from a complex syndrome called CFS—chronic fatigue syndrome—which we will discuss later in this chapter.

SLEEP APNEA: WHO'S AT RISK, AND WHAT ARE THE SYMPTOMS?

If you're overweight, have high blood pressure, a tendency to snore (enough that your bed partner or roommates are often kept awake), feel tired or have chronic headaches in the morning, or need naps during the day, you may have sleep apnea. Observant bed partners may notice that you seem to catch your breath during sleep—or seem to stop breathing altogether for several seconds. If you have 5 breathing stoppages per hour, you have relatively mild sleep apnea; if you have 20 or more episodes per hour, your case is significant. The breathing stoppages of sleep apnea are usually followed by a loud, gasping sound, which can be quite disrupting to bystanders, and later quite embarrassing to those who suffer from the disorder. People with sleep apnea report being forced to sleep outside tents on camping trips, being reprimanded by people in adjacent hotel rooms, scorned on public transportation and shunned by their own bed partners.

Formal testing in a sleep laboratory can determine if you do in fact have sleep apnea. Dr. Susan Redline, codirector of the sleep disorders center at the Cleveland Veterans Administration Hospital, has found that sleep apnea is more common in women than previously thought. We used to say that women accounted for only one in ten cases of apnea. In fact, the ratio is closer to three to one (men to women) for younger people, and close to one to one after the age of 55. Among several reasons, experts say, is a decrease in the hormone progesterone after menopause. Progesterone is a respiratory stimulant—less of it means poorer breathing function.

Dr. Redline believes that women have held back discussing apnea symptoms with their doctors because it's an "unladylike" problem—women don't want to be associated with snoring and snorting. As a result, the number of women with sleep apnea has been greatly underestimated. Dr. Rochelle Goldberg, clinical director of the sleep center at the Medical College of Pennsylvania, believes that women with this problem also may underreport their symptoms because they consider sleep apnea to be a *male* problem. Dr. Goldberg also notes that male bed partners are less apt to notice women's snoring, perhaps because they snore themselves.

There are several kinds of sleep apnea, and depending on the type you have, treatment will differ. For instance, you may have a problem in which your brain "forgets" to tell your body to breathe (called central sleep apnea); this accounts for about 10% of sleep apnea cases in sleep clinics. Much more common is obstructive sleep apnea, in which the upper airway is either floppy or small, making it hard for air to get through. Some people have a combination of the two forms of the disorder. Finally, sometimes obesity alone causes the problem, and alcohol and/or other sedatives before bedtime can make sleep apnea worse.

TREATING SLEEP APNEA: LIFESTYLE CHANGES

Why bother treating a sleep disorder that seems to be merely socially unpleasant? Because sleep apnea can be dangerous, not just noisy. Long-term health problems associated with sleep apnea include pulmonary hypertension, heart rhythm disturbances and even heart failure, according to Dr. W. Shain Schley, chairman of the ear, nose and throat department at The New York Hospital. And motor vehicle accidents can result from the severe wake-time sleepiness associated with this disorder. So it's important to get sleep apnea under control before it becomes serious.

You may be surprised to learn that weight loss alone can eliminate sleep apnea for many patients. Obesity is clearly the major risk factor for this problem—getting rid of the fat often means getting rid of the sleep disorder. Naturally, losing weight takes time—and since sleep apnea can be unpleasant and even dangerous (if your breathing stoppages are long), you may want medical intervention while you try to peel off the weight. Also, make sure that the environment you sleep in is conducive to clear breathing: you'll want a well-ventilated, clean bedroom at a comfortable temperature. Avoid any kind of bedtime sedatives; for example, don't consume alcohol within 3–4 hours of bedtime. You'll also want to make sure your head and even your back are properly supported during sleep: raising your upper body, on pillows or other devices, can improve air flow and make it easier for you to breathe clearly.

Treating Sleep Apnea: Medicine and Surgery

There are very effective mechanical and surgical treatments for sleep apnea, and less effective drug treatments. One of the most effective treatments is to use a mechanical device called a nasal continuous positive airway pressure appliance (NCPAP). It is worn over the mouth and nose at night to facilitate breathing. The device actually works quite well, if you can tolerate wearing it. Dr. Schley says it's effective for 90% of patients. Some people find the device uncomfortable and don't want to use it, while others do quite well with it. Other appliances sometimes suggested by oral health experts reposition the mouth and tongue to facilitate breathing, if it turns out that there is a problem in this area. As you can see, it's vital to find out the cause of your sleep apnea before choosing a treatment, since if your problem is at the level of the respiratory muscles, for example, a mouth appliance isn't going to do you much good. If your palate or tongue are misplaced, these dental appliances can help.

There are several surgical techniques to treat sleep apnea, some more invasive than others. For those who have a so-called deviated septum in their nose (a common problem that does *not* always predispose one to sleep apnea), it can be corrected, and sometimes patients find relief. Other nasal or airway obstructions can also be relieved surgically, with removal of tissue from the back of the nose and throat. It's vital to have an experienced surgeon, since excessive removal can cause permanent problems with swallowing or other activities. Some of these procedures are being done with lasers now, says Dr. Rochelle Goldberg, which reduces the surgical risk. But on the downside, the laser procedures are fairly new so you might have a hard time finding someone experienced who can perform them.

Sometimes, removing polyps or large adenoids (tissue at the back of the nose and throat) can help relieve sleep apnea, Dr. Schley notes. And in the past, the upper airway was bypassed completely with a tracheostomy (a surgical hole in the windpipe) to eliminate sleep apnea. It did the trick, but this kind of extreme procedure is rarely used for sleep apnea these days.

Drugs are sometimes used to treat sleep apnea, although for the most part they have been disappointing, reports Dr. Goldberg. One of the goals of drug therapy is to improve so-called upper airway tone, which is a problem in sleep apnea. One drug that has shown some promise in *milder* cases of sleep apnea is a tricyclic antidepressant called protriptyline. Unfortunately, like many of the drugs in its class, it has some unpleasant side effects like dry mouth and constipation. The female hormone progesterone is also used with some success to treat sleep apnea, as are a group of drugs that acidify the blood (such as diamox), says Dr. Regestein.

Chronic Fatigue: The Symptom, Not the Syndrome

If you're chronically fatigued, join the club. It's a very '90s phenomenon, particularly for women, which some believe is caused by overburdening: too many roles to play in the home and on the job, too little time for sleep, poor diet, lack of exercise, and high rates of both depression and anxiety. Electronic gadgets from faxes to modems have egged on the lengthening average work week, making it possible to "produce" around the clock, blurring the line between office and home. Patricia Prinz, director of the sleep and aging research program at the University of Washington in Seattle, has noted a tremendous drop in vitality among women who have too many responsibilities for others and no time to work out their own needs and pains. The sad fact is when we are exhausted, we perform poorly, it takes longer to get things done, and the problem is compounded.

Mary A. Carskadon, director of chronobiology at E. P. Bradley Hospital and professor of psychiatry and human behavior at the Brown University School of Medicine, discovered that the impact of poor sleep habits on flawed performance starts early. Looking at adolescents, she found that girls get up earlier than boys before school in the morning, and overall get less sleep than boys on weekdays. She also found that kids who sleep less at night are more prone to oversleep in the morning, and to drop off to sleep during the daytime. If we start these habits as teenagers, imagine how entrenched they become by adulthood. They can require a great deal of undoing.

We make 10–15 million visits to the doctor's office for chronic fatigue each year, and while *some* (relatively few) cases are explained by a physical problem (a hormone imbalance for example) the *vast* majority are explained by a chronic sleep deficit: week after week, month after month, even year after year, getting less sleep than you need to feel and function well. Because there is no magic number of hours we need to sleep each night (eight has become a standard, more because it's an average than because it holds any special meaning), you should try an extra hour or two a night steadily for several weeks before you decide you have a dire medical problem. Until you have slept your added hour consistently (weekdays and weekends, the same number of hours) for several weeks at a stretch, you cannot rule out sleep deprivation. In addition to adding sleep time, see what happens to your energy level when you add just 30 minutes of some kind of exercise to your day—*early* in the day is best. That might mean walking to work, or taking a quick jog or using a machine like a stair-climber—something with which you can control the time, since you're clearly short on time in the first place. Now you may be thinking that adding one to two hours of sleep, plus a half hour of exercise to your day is impossible. For most people, if you become efficient about how you spend your time, it really isn't. Maybe instead of taking a lunch hour or half-hour in the middle of the day, you could take your walk with a friend or colleague, sandwich in hand. Consolidating your time this way will release hours you didn't think existed.

Also, follow the *sleep hygiene* rules listed in the "Insomnia" section below. Good sleep hygiene is key to restoring normal sleep *and* wake patterns.

Finally, if you cannot find an extra hour's sleep at night or in the morning, maybe you can steal a half hour for a refreshing nap during the day. The key to successful napping is that you do it every single day at the same time. Otherwise, like poor nighttime sleep, you'll throw off your delicately set schedule.

Insomnia

A major cause of chronic tiredness is poor quality sleep—or a complete lack of sleep even when you are lying in bed. If you have insomnia, you probably know it. The disorder affects women at a higher rate than men, can be powerfully stressful, and has 30 to 40 potential causes, by one expert's estimate. Some of the best known causes of insomnia are depression and anxiety. Sometimes, simply poor "sleep hygiene" can lead to insomnia. We'll discuss this in more detail shortly.

Thomas Roth, chief of the division of sleep disorders and research at the Henry Ford Hospital in Detroit, notes the irony that while women suffer more from insomnia, research on this disorder has focused largely on men, since drug treatments are thought to be risky for potentially pregnant women and since hormones can fluctuate with menstruation, interfering with study results. As a result, the treatments we use for insomnia—both the drugs and the dose—might not be optimal for women. Unfortunately, it's all we have to go on. As we've seen, this is an all too common problem in women's health care, as women for decades have been left out of important treatment trials.

Because insomnia is often a sign of *other* problems, it should be thought of as a *symptom,* not a disorder in and of itself. The solution, therefore, is to treat the underlying problem or eliminate the behavioral triggers, and the insomnia will abate. Some behavioral triggers for insomnia include exercising shortly before bedtime, drinking that "nightcap" before you go to sleep and eating dinner too close to bedtime. (*See* more on behavioral triggers to insomnia under "Sleep Hygiene," below.)

Depression and anxiety disorders (discussed in chapter 17) are extremely common problems among women, and can trigger insomnia. Usually, when these illnesses are treated properly (through both drug and talk therapy) normal sleep is restored. Too often, though, mental illnesses are overlooked as causes of sleep problems—partly because patients tend to see non-mental-health experts first and they in turn may ignore questions related to emotional health. It could be incumbent upon *you* to raise the possibility that your emotions are playing into your sleep problem.

Poorly managed physical pain also interferes with sleep. Older women, for example, who run a high risk of several forms of arthritis, can have sleep problems due to chronic pain. Often relieving the physical pain, even partially, will restore better sleep. Talk to your regular physician about trying new or different forms of painkillers: there have been advances in pain and inflammation management. Physical therapy can also help relieve chronic pain of many sorts, giving you a better chance at painless sleep.

Sleep Hygiene

Many sleep experts I've interviewed say that *nothing* is more effective against insomnia than good *sleep hygiene.* The goal: consistency, regularity and purity in your sleep habits. As Dr. Regestein puts it, "Regularity is the stuff of which physiological control is made." Few of us practice it faithfully, and it's not a big problem if we don't have a sleep disorder. But if you have insomnia, poor sleep hygiene can push you over the edge, making the problem worse—and persistent. What is sleep hygiene all about? It means making the place where you sleep *sacred* for the purpose of sleeping only. Some examples follow.

Do not eat, study, work or worry in bed—if you must worry at some point each day, then schedule it for the afternoon so you get it out of your hair. This might sound peculiar, but give it a try before you rule it out. Not eating in bed means *never* eating in bed: no snacks. Not studying in bed means *never* studying in bed: don't read even the last page of an assignment. And so on. These must be hard and fast rules.

Sleep in the same place as consistently as possible: train your body to think of the bed, or couch, or wherever you prefer to sleep as the only sleeping place.

Don't watch TV in your bedroom. If you have one television and like to watch it, move it into another room and watch there. If you refuse to break the TV-before-bedtime practice, then watch only the most calming entertainment before going to sleep.

Be as physically active during the day as possible: for some, that means getting formal exercise; for others, it just means getting out of the house and walking around, seeing friends or grocery shopping. Then take the action down a bit as bedtime nears.

Set regularly scheduled sleep and wake times, and try *never* to stray from them, even on weekends. 7-day-a-week consistent wake times are most important of all, because they set your internal clock.

Avoid caffeinated beverages.

Avoid alcohol in the evening, especially before bedtime. The "nightcap" is a terrible sleep disrupter, since dropping alcohol levels in the middle of the night will often wake you up.

Don't smoke. Nicotine is a powerful stimulant, and stays in your body for many hours. Even an afternoon cigarette can cause sleep problems at night.

Make your room as sleep-friendly as possible: dark, quiet, clean, well-ventilated and at the temperature you like; wear bedclothes you find cozy; use the right kind of pillow.

Avoid nasal decongestants, especially late in the day.

Take a warm or, even better, hot bath before bed.

Simmer down before bedtime: watching adventure movies, reading thrillers or watching violent news is not conducive to calm sleep: do something that calms *you* (this will of course differ from person to person).

Treatment for Insomnia: Medication

There is often a fine line between proper use and abuse of sleeping pills. When taken in the appropriate doses and at the right times, sleeping pills play an important role in managing sleep disorders (especially when the problem is short-term: for instance, triggered by jet lag or other interruptions of your schedule). But it's very easy to use sleeping pills *incorrectly*, especially when you aren't getting the results you hoped for. There's a temptation to take more pills, or to take them more often, when you are desperate for sleep. The result can be addiction, overdose or excessive side effects. To use Dr. Regestein's analogy, Prometheus got fire, and found that it can be used for good or for evil. The same can be said of sleeping pills.

In general, sleeping pills are best relegated to use in temporary sleep problems—such as insomnia that occurs just a few days a year. Even for this limited use, sleeping pills are major sellers: about 2.5% of Americans use sleeping pills on this occasional basis (fewer than 30 times per year).

You may have heard the controversy over the relatively new sleeping pill called Halcion, or triazolam. Headlines blared that this short-acting sleeping drug could cause dangerous, violent mood disturbances. Its use was banned in England. In fact, most sleep experts here in the U.S. think that Halcion is safe when used properly, and can play an important role in sleep management. The key, always, is that your sleep problem must be diagnosed properly and your use of these drugs must be carefully monitored. Furthermore, you must strictly adhere to taking the drug *as prescribed*. This is true not only for this particular sleeping pill but for all of them, both short and long-acting.

What kind of sleeping pill should you take? That depends on the kind of sleep problem you have. First of all, you'll want to discuss with your doctor the difference between short-acting and long-acting sleeping pills. Pills that have a shorter action have what's called a "short half life," meaning they are cleared from your body faster than drugs with a "long half life." Some feel that older people should avoid longer-acting sleeping pills because they can be too heav-ily sedating for aging bodies. But longer-acting sleeping pills have an important role in the treatment of sleep problems, too—particularly when certain other diseases are present.

After choosing the length of action for your sleeping pill, go over the different side effect profiles for several drugs in the category you're considering. The side effects vary, and if you have problems with one type of sleeping pill, you can try another in the same category. Do *not* mix different kinds of sleeping pills—or any medications, for that matter, without your doctor's consent.

The fact is, there is a great deal scientists still don't know about the newer sleep medications appearing on the market. For this reason, vigilance on both your own and your doctor's part is quite important. Watch for side effects, see if the drug is accomplishing what you hoped it would, and so on. Don't keep taking it if you aren't satisfied with the result.

There are also many over-the-counter sleep preparations. While again in the *short term* these can sometimes be useful, there is a great potential for abuse of these drugs (since you're less likely to be under a doctor's supervision). Taking them incorrectly can create a sleep deprivation/oversleep cycle in which you constantly rebound and need more and more medication to get adequate rest. This is a potential problem with *any* sleep medication, in fact—both prescribed and over-the-counter. Be extremely careful about the use of these preparations, and always mention to your doctor that you're considering taking them. Over-the-counter sleep preparations can make you groggy in the morning, and can cause dry mouth and eyes, experts warn.

Finally, for those who use alcohol as a sleep "medication"—an extremely common practice—you're on the wrong track. While alcohol may encourage you to fall asleep faster initially, you're likely to wake up once or repeatedly during the night and to have trouble falling back asleep as your blood alcohol level drops. Alcohol should *not* be used as a sleep inducer.

OTHER THAN FEELING BETTER, WHAT'S SO IMPORTANT ABOUT GETTING ENOUGH SLEEP?

If feeling better, having more energy, doing better at tasks, lowering your risk of injury and just being more pleasant to be around aren't enough for you, then consider the fascinating work of James Krueger, professor of physiology at the University of Tennessee in Memphis. He has found that sleep loss actually *hurts* the immune system by cutting down the action of disease-fighting cells. On the flip side, he notes that animal studies show that adequate rest boosts recovery from infections. So maybe when your doctor said, "Get some rest and plenty of fluids," she was hitting on something important. Before we know it, we'll be returning to "an apple a day."

HEADACHES

Lack of sleep, stress and other lifestyle triggers we'll discuss in a moment, all contribute to one of American women's greatest chronic enemies: the headache. Headaches are trivialized in our society ("not tonight, honey . . . ") but they are serious health problems, demolishing both quality of life and productivity. Until recently, many headache experts categorized headaches as migraines, tension headaches, sinus headaches and so on. Today, leading experts believe that all headaches are *some* form of migraine— that is, a type of headache caused by swelling of blood vessels in the brain and around the head. In fact, while it was once alleged that tension headaches were caused by tense muscles around the head, studies of the electrical activity in this area has shown that this is not really happening. Dr. David Buchholz, director of the neurological consultation center at the Johns Hopkins Medical Institutions, explains that you tend to feel headache pain where the blood vessels are swollen: for so-called "tension headaches," the vessels are swollen in the back of the head, for so-called "sinus headaches," the vessels are swollen in the sinus areas. Whatever you call them, and however you group them, women suffer from headaches twice as often as men, he notes— particularly during the menstruating years.

Why are women so vulnerable to headaches? Perhaps because of the role of hormone shifts in the body. In general, it is thought that headaches are related to the hormone estrogen, since many women develop headaches when taking estrogen-containing oral contraceptives or estrogen replacement therapy, and since headaches often subside after menopause. Many women suffer for years without realizing that birth control pills or hormone replacement are the cause of their headaches. But headache patterns aren't always that straightforward: For example, Dr. Buchholz notes, many women find that their headaches are worst in the days *before* they begin menstruating, when estrogen and progesterone levels are falling. Perhaps it is the *change* in hormone levels that contributes to headaches, experts say. Or it's possible that different *types* of estrogen (and/or other hormones) are more or less likely to promote headaches. There is still much to be learned in this area.

What Classic Migraine Headaches—and Milder Versions—Feel Like

You're having a good old-fashioned migraine headache if you feel throbbing pain primarily on one side of your head, often over the eye, and if this pain is accompanied by dizziness, nausea, vomiting and sensitivity to light. In the most severe cases, patients have trouble talking, see flashing lights and/or feel numbness and tingling, and suffer loss of memory for minutes or hours after the headache. This kind of headache usually lasts from a few hours to a few days. Less severe forms may involve two-sided head pain, and may last longer (for days or weeks) but have none of the accompanying stomach or vision problems.

Headache Triggers.

Lack of sleep (and sometimes excessive sleep) and stress are at the top of the list of headache triggers. But foods and medications are other common culprits. Keep in mind that it's easy to overlook headache triggers because they don't always take effect immediately. It's possible to eat a food trigger and not get the headache for 24 hours. So think about your eating pattern over the past day or two before your headache set in.

Some Common Foods/Ingredients That Trigger Headaches

- Caffeinated foods and beverages
- Foods containing nitrites or nitrates, such as processed lunch meats
- MSG (which sometimes hides under names like "hydrolyzed vegetable, soy or plant protein" or even "natural flavorings," Dr. Buchholz warns)
- Alcohol (particularly red wine and champagne)
- Foods containing tyramine, such as aged cheese, yogurt, sour cream, nuts and peanut butter
- Citrus fruits and juices (which contain phenols)

Some Common Medications That Trigger Headaches

- Certain antihypertensive drugs, such as beta blockers and calcium channel blockers
- Some tricyclic antidepressants (others can *help* with migranes—ask your doctor)
- Oral contraceptives
- Some drugs used to *fight* headaches, such as Anacin or Excedrin (both of which contain caffeine). (Does it sound strange that a drug used to prevent headaches would do just the opposite? Dr. Buchholz reports that because these drugs constrict blood vessels, they create a rebound effect in which the vessels expand once again, possibly worse than before! Some sinus and decongestant medications fall into this deceptive category as well.)

Preventing and Treating Headaches

Some women will find relief with lifestyle changes alone. For them, getting adequate rest and eliminating food triggers is all it takes to eliminate even chronic, severe headaches. The way to find out if foods are triggering your headaches is to eliminate *all* of the common headache triggers and then start adding them to your diet one at a time to see which one causes a problem.

Unfortunately, lifestyle changes alone aren't enough to prevent headaches for some women. For them, preventive medication might be necessary. And certainly, in the event of a severe headache, the drug sumatriptan (given by injection) can give acute relief quickly, before a headache gets out of control.

Chronic Fatigue Syndrome (CFS): When the Symptom of Chronic Fatigue Is Part of a Complex Syndrome

In the late 1980s it became almost fashionable to say someone had "chronic fatigue syndrome." So many people are chronically fatigued, we just assumed they fit the bill of this highly publicized "yuppie" disease (especially since media reports centered on the symptom of exhaustion over and above the many other complicated signs of this disorder). In fact, CFS is so much more complex than just chronic fatigue, and involves such a vast array of symptoms unrelated to sleep, that people usually know they *don't* have it as soon as they read the definition. Called everything from chronic mononucleosis to the "yuppie flu" to chronic Epstein-Barr virus, this condition is still largely a mystery to scientists.

The syndrome affects about two million Americans—striking women twice as often as men—and while it affects people of all ages and backgrounds, young adult Caucasian women turn up most often in clinics (hence the "yuppie" dub). Whether this is because these women are more likely to access health care in general or because they do in fact get this disease more often than others is still subject to debate. In either case, Patricia Prinz says that 88% of cases affect women in their middle adult years. CFS can be particularly troubling to women of reproductive age, since the symptoms tend to worsen premenstrually.

Defining CFS

While the diagnosis of CFS is one of exclusion as much as inclusion, the Centers for Disease Control and Prevention has devised a useful working model for the disorder that appeared in the March 1988 issue of *Annals of Internal Medicine*. The goal was not only to create a usable definition for clinicians and researchers, but also to distinguish this disorder from other similar problems (such as fibromyalgia, for instance, which includes a long list of muscle aches and other nonspecific symptoms; as many as $\frac{1}{2}$ of those who fit the criteria for this disease also fit those for CFS: close, but no cigar). Dr. Stephen Straus, chief of the laboratory of clinical investigation at the National Institute of Allergy and Infectious Diseases, notes that in the 19th century, a disease similar to CFS was attributed to women because they were considered "inherently weaker" than men. A related theme appeared in the early 1900s with the idea that women were more "neurotic" and hence sicklier than men. So CFS-like illnesses are not that new after all.

Happily, while we haven't quite made it out of the Dark Ages in terms of women's reputations and health care, we do have a more objective working definition of CFS based on physical findings, not bias and speculation.

Summary of CFS Definition by Centers for Disease Control and Prevention (with some changes to lay language)

Two "major" criteria *both* must be met:

New onset of persistent or relapsing, debilitating fatigue or easy fatigability in a person with no previous history of similar symptoms, that does not resolve with bed rest, and that is severe enough to produce or impair average daily activity below 50% of the patient's previous activity level, for a period of at least six months.

Other clinical conditions that may produce similar symptoms must be excluded by thorough evaluation, based on history, physical examination, and appropriate lab findings. These conditions include [here I summarize] malignancy, autoimmune disease, any infections, psychiatric disease, drug abuse, chronic lung, heart, intestinal, liver, kidney or blood disease.

Out of 11 "minor" criteria, you must have at least *six* symptoms, if you meet two or three *physical* findings; or *eight* symptoms if you have *no* physical findings: and these must have begun at or after the onset of fatigue and must have lasted or recurred for at least six months (not necessarily at the same time):

- mild fever: oral temperature between 99.6 and 101.5 degrees Farenheit if measured by patient—or chills
- sore throat
- painful lymph nodes in the front or back of the neck or underarm
- muscle discomfort or myalgia
- prolonged (24 hours or greater) generalized fatigue after levels of exercise that would have been easily tolerated in the patient's previous state
- pain in the joints that moves from place to place without joint swelling or redness
- neuropsychologic complaints (one or more of the following: sensitivity to light, brief blind spots, forgetfulness, excessive irritability, confusion, difficulty thinking, inability to concentrate, depression)
- sleep disturbance (excessive sleep or inability to sleep)
- the main symptoms developed over a few hours to a few days

Out of three physical criteria, you need at least two; and they must be documented by a physician on at least two occasions, at least one month apart:

- low-grade fever (oral temperature between 99.6 and 101.5 degrees Farenheit or rectal temperature between 100 and 101.8 degrees Farenheit)
- inflamation of the throat with no visible deposits
- palpable or tender neck or underarm lymph nodes

Dr. Anthony Komaroff of the Brigham and Women's Hospital gives a breakdown of the frequency of some of the more common CFS symptoms:

SYMPTOM:	% OF CFS PATIENTS WITH SYMPTOM
night sweats	50%
can't leave home	19%
chronic low-grade fever	36%
sudden onset of syndrome w/flu-like illness	85%
hurting muscles	89%
painful joints	75%

Is your head spinning yet? As you can see, CFS is a far cry from the overworked/underslept syndrome. Because people with CFS are so very ill—some completely bedridden and debilitated—they find it quite frustrating to see this disease trivialized and simplified in the lay literature for so long. Sufferers say the disorder comes on like a Mack truck, as a sapping, cloaking exhaustion, a devastating flu that just won't go away. Sadly, health care workers cannot make promises or even point to a light at the end of the tunnel, since the course of CFS is so unpredictable and people's reactions to treatment differ widely.

For many CFS patients, these symptoms wax and wane over months and even years. And while the following symptoms didn't make the CDC list, the Massachusetts CFIDS association (an advocacy group for people with CFS) finds the following symptoms also quite common: shortness of breath, sensitivity to heat and cold, intolerance of alcohol, irritable bowel syndrome, diarrhea, abdominal pain, dry mouth and eyes, hearing problems, rashes, hair loss and muscle twitching.

CFS and Psychiatric Disorders.

Several years ago, some research came out connecting CFS with psychiatric illnesses like depression. Scientists drew so many parallels between the disorders that many came to assume that CFS was a mental illness and therefore, because of the stigma we attach to them, somehow not *real*. This was a tremendous setback to the cause of getting people to recognize CFS as a true "disease." In fact, it has recently been shown that while people with CFS *do* have more depression and anxiety than people without CFS, most of that mental anguish developed *after* CFS kicked in—not before. Alison Mawle of the Centers for Disease Control and Prevention is a CFS researcher investigating hundreds of potential causes or triggers of the illness. While she knows as well as anyone that there are more questions than answers about this disorder, one thing she now says with certainty is that CFS is *not* "just in your head."

CFS Causes

If you can think of it—and even if you can't—it's probably being tested as a possible cause of CFS. Everything from viruses (certain herpesviruses, for example) to heavy metals (arsenic, lead, etc.) to hormonal abnormalities to immune dysfunction have been suggested as potential culprits. Some believe that a combination of multiple triggers might be at fault, with one trigger setting off another—creating fireworks in the immune system. For instance, some think that old viruses in the body reactivate, setting off an immune response that itself might run amok in the body. Other proposed triggers are quite different, ranging from personal grief and stress to automobile accidents.

Because we have no definite leads on the *cause* of CFS, we are terribly limited in our ability to *treat* it. As you will see below, the goal of treatment at this point is not to eradicate the disease, but rather to control the individual symptoms that make life so difficult for CFS patients.

Treating CFS

Providing comfort and assuaging fears may be the most important feature of CFS treatment.

Many with CFS have gone through a mind-boggling array of tests and procedures to rule out other frightening, sometimes fatal illnesses. They have feared they had AIDS, cancer and other progressive or degenerative diseases. They imagine not waking up the next morning, or never regaining their former happiness and vigor. For these reasons, warm, gentle, constant support is necessary from both health care providers and loved ones. Patients should be reminded over and over that their condition is more likely to improve than not, and that it is *unlikely* to get significantly worse than it already is: one-half of those with CFS will recover fully and many others will improve substantially after six months to two years. That may seem like a long time—but it's a lot shorter than an eternity.

After providing comfort, the next goal is to relieve symptoms. *There is no cure for* CFS. But there are a number of treatments that can make patients feel better—which goes a long way to boosting outlook and mood. The three key features of CFS which can be ameliorated are pain, lack of sleep, and depression. In some cases, nonaddictive, low-dose antidepressant medications can help with all three symptoms. Dr. Straus of NIAID notes that some patients do well on combination antidepressants—but this requires specialized treatment from an expert who does lots of work with both antidepressant drugs *and* CFS. The dose should always be *low* for CFS patients, as they often cannot tolerate higher doses of psychological medications.

Dr. Dedra Buchwald, a specialist in chronic fatigue at the University of Washington in Seattle, finds that nonsteroidal anti-inflammatory drugs (NSAIDs) can be extremely helpful in reducing muscle aches and pain. These come in over-the-counter forms (ibuprofen, for example) and also in prescription strength. Talk to your doctor about starting a carefully monitored regimen of nonsteroidals. Do not treat these drugs as candy just because they're widely available. They do carry risks of their own and when taken over the long term, should be monitored like any other medication.

Even though CFS saps its victims of the energy it takes just to get through the day, let alone exercise, Dr. Straus insists that regular moderate exercise is an important part of CFS treatment. If possible, just daily walks on one's own or light workouts with a rehabilitation specialist can build strength and endurance and boost mood. Many CFS patients feel especially debilitated immediately after exercise, so these outings should be as untaxing as possible.

It's easy to say "get adequate rest" when you're treating other ailments, but when you're talking about CFS, that recommendation can be quite frustrating for patients. While they are deeply tired, often they cannot sleep. A sleep disorder center may be able to help them find techniques or "tricks" for learning to sleep longer and better. The more high-quality rest, the stronger the body, and the better the chance of becoming well. (*See* "Sleep Hygiene" advice, page 366.)

While there is no strong data proving that a given diet makes CFS patients better, there is anecdotal evidence that the more complete and balanced your diet (and the fewer stimulants and depressants you take, like caffeine and alcohol), the better you will feel. Do *not*, however, get sucked in by quack promises of miracle diets—or any other miracle cure, for that matter. If someone offers you a magic bullet to cure your CFS, you can be pretty sure they've got a scam that will cost you money—and perhaps even compromise your health further. Because this is a disorder with so many open-ended questions, there's room for the many charlatans out there who claim to have the answer to your prayers, warns Alison Mawle. Resist the temptation.

Some other treatments you may have heard about include immune system boosters like gamma globulin (which some say helps, but studies say *doesn't*); antiviral and antiretroviral drugs, which are still under study but of questionable value and have potential side effects; and peculiar-sounding potions like one called kutapressin, a porcine liver extract that some say is helpful and others say isn't. One leading researcher pointed out to me that for every positive discovery we've seen about CFS, we've seen an equally persuasive *negative* finding about the same "remedy." Frustrating, to say the least. And to make matters even more complicated, somewhere between 25% and 40% get better when given a placebo—a simple sugar pill, that is—so medication studies are complicated further by the question, "*Would this person have gotten better anyway?*"

Psychotherapy or psychological counseling—in the form of support groups, group therapy or individual therapy—can be quite helpful for CFS patients. The goal is to alleviate fears and boost the emotional strength needed to go forward each day. Patricia Prinz notes that people with no support tend to have weaker immune systems and other poor signs of health compared to those with support systems in place. Even one or two people you can turn to for love or advice can make you feel significantly better. Sometimes it's easier to talk to a formal group that is in place to help you with your problems than to feel like you're always burdening the same people in your personal life.

It's also important to treat or eliminate any additional, confounding health problems that might be making you feel worse.

Finally, be as realistic as possible about the extent of your condition. Before you jump to the conclusion (as many with CFS do) that you cannot concentrate or remember things, try actually *testing* those skills. When doctors test memory and concentration skills, they find that most patients do *well* even when they believe they can't. Your condition is bad enough without making it worse with false fears.

Choosing a Doctor for CFS

There is a growing number of CFS treatment centers around the country; however, there is still a big problem with *lack* of knowledge about CFS among doctors and other health care professionals. The "it's all in your head" stigma still abounds, as does a simple ignorance of the symptoms that distinguish CFS from other problems. In your effort to relieve the individual symptoms you are feeling, you may go from expert to expert—say, a rheumatologist for your joint and muscle pain, a psychiatrist for your depression, a general internist for your fevers. This is okay, Dr. Straus asserts, *only* if you have a *conductor* or *director* for *all* of your care: someone who oversees all of the medications and other treatments that these various clinicians are prescribing. The best care always comes from a *global* perspective of your problem. The ideal person to do this, of course, is someone familiar with CFS. (*See* below for organizations that can point you in the right direction.)

FOR MORE INFORMATION ON SLEEP DISORDERS AND CHRONIC FATIGUE SYNDROME

FOR GENERAL SLEEP PROBLEMS

AMERICAN SLEEP DISORDERS ASSOCIATION
Rochester, MN
(There are 222 accredited sleep disorders centers in the U.S.)

BETTER SLEEP COUNCIL
P.O. Box 13
Washington, DC 20044

WAKEFULNESS-SLEEP EDUCATION AND RESEARCH FOUNDATION (W-SERF)
4820 Rancho Drive
Del Mar, CA 92014

NATIONAL SLEEP FOUNDATION
(public information source for the American Sleep Disorders Association)
1367 Connecticut Ave. NW
Washington, DC 20036
202-785-2300

FOR CHRONIC FATIGUE SYNDROME

CENTERS FOR DISEASE CONTROL AND PREVENTION DIVISION OF VIRAL DISEASES
Building 6, Room 120
Atlanta, GA 30333
404-639-1388

CHRONIC FATIGUE AND IMMUNE DYSFUNCTION SYNDROME ASSOCIATION
P.O. Box 220398
Charlotte, NC 28222
800-442-3437

NATIONAL CHRONIC FATIGUE SYNDROME AND FIBROMYALGIA ASSOCIATION
3521 Broadway, Suite 222
Kansas City, MO 64111
816-931-4777

CLINICAL CENTER COMMUNICATIONS,
The National Institutes of Health
Building 10, Room 1C255
Bethesda, MD 20892
301-496-2563

Chapter Nineteen

Substance Use and Abuse

It is so much more exciting to be sober,
to be exact and concentrated and sober.

—Gertrude Stein *in* John Malcom Brinnin, *The Third Rose*

The main body of this chapter will focus on alcohol and cigarette abuse, since these are extremely common and, sadly, more socially accepted habits than other substance abuse. Furthermore, there is more consensus on the best ways to recognize and treat alcohol and cigarette addictions. We will briefly discuss other forms of substance abuse at the end of this chapter. The causes of all substance abuse are multidimensional, including both social/environmental stressors and genetic susceptibility. No one, however, is doomed to abuse drugs. We all have within us the power to resist even multiple predispositions. Together, all substance abuse—including alcohol, cigarette and illegal drug use—causes over 500,000 deaths a year, according to the Robert Wood Johnson Foundation. This makes substance abuse the leading preventable cause of death in the U.S.

Women and Alcohol Abuse

The fact that some popular screening tests for alcohol abuse still pose the question, "Does your *wife* notice your drinking?" should give you an idea of how much attention has been paid to alcoholism among *women.* (Not much.) From basic research to clinical practice, experts have focused on men. While in reality alcoholism strikes both sexes, popular lore has held it up as a man's problem, depriving women of needed diagnoses and care. Alcohol-abusing men have traditionally been seen as facing a problem worth treatment: alcohol-abusing women have been viewed as shameful, "loose," aberrant creatures worthy of contempt. Happily, times are changing and with increased awareness of the frequency of alcoholism in women, plus advances in treating alcoholic women, we've come a long way toward giving women who abuse alcohol the support they need.

But we had a *long* way to come. Dr. Robert Millman, director of the drug and alcohol abuse programs at the New York Hospital/ Cornell Medical Center, notes that in the late 1700s, people called for the deaths or sterilization of women who were publicly drunk! Today, he notes, society seems to indicate that it's okay for women to drink, and even for women to get drunk, but *not* for women to have alcohol problems.

To keep things complicated even in the 1990s, women face discrimination on the basis of other inaccurate stereotypes *beyond* gender, such as the ridiculous image of alcoholics as slovenly bums. Many women alcoholics sport tidy suits and work in respectable jobs and don't arouse even the suspicion of alcoholism among many doctors, says Dr. Sheila Blume, medical director of the Alcoholism, Chemical Dependency and Compulsive Gambling Programs at South Oaks Hospital in Amityville, New York. Furthermore, Blume adds, family members tend to hide alcoholism among women because of the stigma so long attached to it.

ALCOHOLISM: WHAT YOU HAD TO SAY ABOUT IT

Susan, 53 years old
I come from an alcoholic family. My mother was an alcoholic and my father was an alcoholic. Children don't understand. I subsequently found

out. I didn't drink until I was 38 years old. I think there are a lot more women alcoholics than we know, it's easier for women to get away with it.

Once I started to drink, I was a daily drinker within months. I didn't drink as a party girl, in bars and so on. I drank at home. I didn't use it to be attractive, the life of the party. I had plenty of friends, I had a life until I started drinking. I drank because of fear, confusion and anger that I didn't know how to deal with. When I drank, I drank for oblivion, for the anesthetic effect of the alcohol. I used it to cope. I felt that it calmed my fears. I found the ultimate best friend. What I wanted was to erase myself, I simply wanted to cease to be. When you knocked on my door, there was no one home. We come in all shapes and sizes, as many alcoholics as you meet, that's how many reasons you find for it.

I was a blackout drinker, I didn't even remember the night before. Occasionally in the evening I would vomit before going to sleep so I wouldn't get the spins. I gave up movies, bridge, needlepoint, friends because they all interfered with my drinking. I drank bourbon. I was drinking a liter of bourbon a night. I had an incredible tolerance for alcohol, I could drink you and anyone else under the table and that reassured me. I thought I was too old to be an alcoholic. If I picked up the first drink, I'd drink to get drunk. I didn't understand a person who ordered a glass of wine and left half of it.

I was bloated, I don't know what damage I did to my esophagus, my liver, my pancreas. I'm very fortunate, I didn't have bleeding and shakes and liver damage. I was one of the lucky ones. I drank for about six years. I didn't see that I wasn't tired, I was drunk. I was divorced, I didn't have children, I was single in New York. The littany is just incredible. I never saw the reason my life was so tough was I was drinking. I had a business, I was working 6 days a week at least. I needed to relax, I didn't want you to call me after 9 p.m. because I needed sleep. I didn't see that I didn't want you to call me after 9 p.m. because it interfered with my drinking.

I became suicidal. Very tidy, very neat, and I wrote a will. I'm a good, nice little girl and did what good nice little girls do—at 49 I went for my annual physical. The doctor asked "how are you?" and I said "fine," and the tears just started rolling. I said, "I'm fine but I'm going to commit suicide." He walked me around the corner to a psychiatrist who understood I was not neurotic, not psychotic.

With antabuse (a medication) I stopped drinking for a while, two years. Then my mother died, and that night I uncorked the bottle. I couldn't get drunk, and I couldn't be sober. About two months later I bumped into a woman who had been a friend of my mother's, and I don't know why, but when she asked me how I was, I said, "I think I have a problem with alcohol." She said she was going to an AA meeting and I should come Wednesday, but I was busy, and she said you can come any Wednesday. I went, and identified not only with the speaker but with everyone else who was there. It's almost like I was born without an instruction manual and for me AA has done that for me, given me a road map and I get to lead it for the rest of my life. What AA has done for me is given me a bridge to life, I have a spiritual life, I have a personal life. I'm just so grateful to be sober, and alive, and to have a chance to live.

The twelve steps saved my life. Now I can live with happiness, with humor. It works one day at a time: I don't have to *never* have a drink the rest of my life. I just have to not have a drink *today.* People say "Would you like a drink?" I say "Yes— I would like a drink. A Coke, an iced tea".

THE HARD FACTS ABOUT ALCOHOL ABUSE

Women make up about one-third of all alcoholics—a much larger proportion than once assumed. And the disease doesn't come for free: women will spend 30 billion dollars on alcohol in 1994, versus 20 billion in 1984, according to the National Council on Alcoholism and Drug Dependence (NCADD). According to the American Psychiatric Association, 4.5 million women abuse or are dependent on alcohol. The severe physical and psychological damage that can result from alcoholism occurs faster and with less alcohol intake in women than in men (*see* "Symptoms of Alcoholism," below). A pregnant women who abuses alcohol can seriously and permanently damage her fetus—again, both physically and intellectually. According to a recent paper in the *Journal of the American Medical Association,* alcoholic women have a four-times greater mortality rate than nonalcoholic women and lose on average 15 years of life! Women account for more than a third of AA membership. According to the National Council on Alcohol Abuse and Alcoholism (NCAAA), women alcoholics have a 50–100% higher death rate than male alcoholics. The risk of breast cancer jumps with alcohol abuse, too (*see* chapter 25).

Because we often trivialize the existence or the severity of alcoholism in women, we ignore the fact that it is a "disease of losses," to steal Dr. Blume's expression. Abusing alcohol leads to a loss of self-esteem, of hobbies, of time, of intimacy with others, of jobs, cars, friends and spouses. Few of us can afford *any* of these losses, let alone *all* of them.

There are several important features that separate female alcohol abusers from their male counterparts. For instance, women react more intensely to a given dose of alcohol than men do. Women are widely known to develop higher blood alcohol levels than men for the same amount of alcohol consumed: in fact, after drinking the same amount of alcohol, a given woman the same size and weight as a given man will absorb 30% more alcohol into her blood-stream. One explanation is that women have less body water than men for the same body mass; another is that women might metabolize alcohol differently than men, due to relatively less of an enzyme called alcohol dehydrogenase in their gastric tracks. The bottom line, Dr. Millman notes, is that women absorb less alcohol in their guts and let more flow into their blood *as alcohol,* rather than as a metabolized version of alcohol.

While the scientific data is mixed on this topic, some women say they drink more before their menstrual periods or use more alcohol or drugs *during* their periods to relieve tension or depression. This "self-medicating" can be quite dangerous, especially since alcohol may mask pain temporarily but overall is an addictive depressant that makes many negative symptoms worse.

WHO IS AT RISK FOR ALCOHOLISM?

Recent trends point to younger women drinking more and developing more alcohol-related problems, according to Dr. Robert Millman. It's not surprising to see heavy-drinking adolescent girls, especially when certain alcoholic beverages are made to look so appealing to them. For instance, fruity wine coolers or breezers are appealing drinks for young people who aren't yet accustomed to the taste of "hard" alcohol—

their taste and pretty colors and packaging give the illusion that they're harmless. In fact, they contain as much alcohol as the equivalent amount of beer or even a shot of hard liquor!

Among women aged 35 to 49, Millman notes, those who are divorced or separated or in some other way suffer from a "lost role," are more likely to have drinking problems than women in stable marriages. In general, those who are unmarried, unemployed or partially employed are at greater risk of alcohol abuse. Women in the 50 to 64 range may be more prone to abuse alcohol if they have problems dealing with a so-called "empty nest," he adds, or find themselves with little to do to expand their horizons.

Among all women, Dr. Blume notes that women who abuse alcohol tend to be depressed (which alcohol worsens) and have low self-esteem; many have endured sexual or other abuse. Interestingly, while alcoholism precedes depression in men, it's often the other way around with women. Blume also finds that women who abuse alcohol are more likely to have insomnia, and trouble concentrating or functioning—although the chicken-egg syndrome gets in the way here. Also, while women tend to start abusing alcohol later in life than men, they present for treatment at about the same time as men, which Blume believes further illustrates the fact that alcohol has a faster, more devastating impact on women.

Women who abuse other substances are more likely to abuse alcohol. For instance, abusing prescription drugs like Xanax or Valium is associated with alcohol abuse. Sadly, these prescription drugs are often given to women for the wrong reasons in the first place and then lead to a chain of substance abuse.

Dr. Anne Geller, director of the Smithers Alcoholism Treatment and Training Center at St. Luke's-Roosevelt Hospital in New York, notes that women alcoholics are more likely to come from families of substance abusers (particularly families with alcohol abuse, which is in part hereditary). She also notes that women alcohol abusers have more gynecological problems than other women—again, watch for the chicken-egg problem here.

SYMPTOMS OF ALCOHOLISM: KNOWING WHEN TO WORRY

Part of knowing when to worry about alcohol intake is coming to understand what constitutes "normal" or "moderate" drinking. According to Dr. Blume, moderate drinking for women means no more than one drink a day. A drink equals a 12-ounce beer, a 5-ounce glass of wine, or a shot of whiskey, for example. The NCADD states that among women 18 and older, 55% drink moderately (which *they* define as less than 60 drinks per month), 5% drink heavily (more than 60 drinks per month) and 40% do not drink at all.

There are ways to recognize alcoholism in someone else: what's trickier is recognizing it in yourself. In others, alcoholism might show itself as someone "needing" to have a drink around at most functions (a friend who asks you, "Will there be drinks?"), or you may notice chronic sadness, brooding and/or explosions of anger. Does your friend tend to forget what happened the night before? This is a common sign of alcohol abuse. Contrary to popular belief, raucous behavior is *not* often part of alcoholism.

You might notice that women start out drinking with company, but often *limit* their public drinking to a reasonable amount and then *continue* drinking at home (sometimes secretly). Another typical female drinking pattern, according to Dr. Geller, is to work all day with little or nothing to drink, and then come home to get plastered—and drink oneself into oblivion in front of the TV-set. Women often don't *know* or *acknowledge* that they have drinking problems, so confronting them can be especially difficult.

DEALING WITH A LOVED ONE'S ALCOHOLISM

Those who live with alcoholics know all too well that the unpredictability is the hardest thing to accept. Children of alcoholic mothers come to know embarrassment and chronic worrying far beyond their years. Spouses know what helplessness, anger and betrayal feel like—and what it's like to see constant basic reasoning *fail*.

DO YOU HAVE A PROBLEM?

As with any kind of substance abuse, facing the fact that you have a drinking problem is the first, and most important, step en route to recovery. How can you tell if you have a problem? Various experts have put together lists of questions that at least give you a clue, if not a diagnosis, of a problem. I've chosen two of those lists—read through them and see if they ring any bells.

List #1.
Dr. Blume's suggested questions for every

woman to ask herself *every* year (almost like getting an annual Pap smear to detect cervical cancer). These questions will give you an idea if you are heading toward a drinking problem, or if you're already there:

1. Am I drinking more than I was a year ago? Why?

2. Do I ever feel like I *need* a drink?

3. Do I ever drink more than I intend to?

4. Do I ever decide to cut down on drinking? Why?

5. If prescribed tranquilizers, do I take them as dispensed or as I *feel* like taking them?

6. Do I mix these drugs with alcohol?

7. Would I worry if I had a daughter drinking like I do?

8. Has someone *said* something to me regarding my drinking?

9. Do I need a drink to get going in the day?

If you said "yes" to any of Dr. Blume's questions, you should talk to a trained alcohol abuse counselor. You may not have a drinking problem yet, but you could be on course to getting one.

List #2.

The following questions are from the National Council on Alcoholism and Drug Dependence, and should give you a sense of whether you're drinking to "manage" (that is, drown or avoid) problems, or if you're starting to hide a drinking problem:

1. Do you drink when you feel depressed, hoping that it will make you feel better?

2. Do you regularly use alcohol as medicine to relieve menstrual cramps, help you sleep, or calm your nerves?

3. Do you talk a lot about drinking?

4. Do you feel sociable only when you drink?

5. Do you drink when you are under pressure or after an argument?

6. Do you try to get someone to buy liquor for you because you are too ashamed to buy it yourself?

7. Do you hide the empty bottles and dispose of them secretly?

8. Do you buy liquor at different places so no one will know how much you purchase?

9. Do you plan in advance to reward yourself with several drinks after you've worked hard in the house or on the job?

10. Do you have blackouts—periods about which you remember nothing?

11. Do you ever wonder if anyone knows how much you drink?

12. Do you ever carry liquor in your purse?

13. Do you worry about hurting your child when you have been drinking?

14. Do you drink to make your husband less angry at you?

15. If you only drink occasionally, do you have a lot of drinks at one time?

16. Do you drink more when you have been emotionally or physically abused?

17. Do you feel panicky when faced with non-drinking days or when you are without money to buy alcohol?

18. Do you become defensive when anyone mentions your drinking?

19. Do you try to cover up when you can't remember promises and feel ashamed when you misplace or lose things?

20. Do you drive your car or operate machinery after you've been drinking?

21. Do you take sleeping pills or tranquilizers together with alcohol?

22. Do you use alcohol to have or to avoid sexual activity?

23. Do you think that drinks at home are okay but drinks in a bar are not?

24. Have you fallen down or hurt yourself as a result of drinking?

25. Are you absent or late for work more often after you drink?

26. Do you suffer from indigestion, nausea or diarrhea due to drinking?

According to the NCADD, answering *yes* to five or more questions could indicate an alcohol problem. (Answering yes to fewer than five might also suggest a problem.) *See* the information box at the end of this chapter for suggested places to call or write for help.

Other Signs of a Drinking Problem

A truly classic sign of a drinking problem, says Alan Budney of the University of Vermont, is *thinking* you may have a problem, trying to control it, planning not to drink—and ending up drinking anyway. This kind of attention to and subsequent failure to manage a possible problem is a worrisome sign, and one you should discuss with your doctor or a substance abuse expert.

Physical Signs of Alcoholism

The physical signs of alcoholism cover nearly all body systems, from irritation of the stomach and esophagus (with vomiting and upset stomach), brain and heart problems, liver abnormalities or cirrhosis of the liver, menstrual irregularities and trouble conceiving, early miscarriage and other complications of pregnancy, physical injury like bruises, bone breaks and drownings. Hypertension and breast cancer risks increase with excessive drinking. The effect of alcohol on cardiovascular health is still uncertain. While some studies suggest that *light* or *moderate* drinking is beneficial to cardiovascular health (perhaps in part by raising the "good" cholesterol or HDL), *excessive* drinking is harmful to the heart and to just about every other body part as well.

Fetal Alcohol Syndrome (FAS)

Fetal alcohol syndrome (FAS) or fetal alcohol effects (FAE), a milder version, can occur when a pregnant woman consumes alcohol. Alcohol affects the fetus both mentally and physically, causing certain facial abnormalities (which can be fairly subtle), and various levels of mental retardation. It is estimated that about 1 to 3 cases occur per 1000 live births, which ranks it with Down's syndrome and spina bifida for the top three causes of birth defects. The disorder has been around for centuries—perhaps for as long as alcohol has been around. Barbara Morse, director of the Fetal Alcohol Education Program at the Boston University School of Medicine, has two favorite quotes she uses when she lectures on FAS. The first is attributed to Aristotle (384–322 B.C.): "Drunken, hare-brain women most part bring forth children like unto themselves: *morosus et languidus.*" The second is from an 1834 select committee on drunkenness in the House of Commons: "Infants of alcoholic mothers have a starved, shriveled and imperfect look." Morse notes that this description holds fairly true to the look of FAS today.

The three key symptoms of FAS include: (1) pre- or postnatal growth retardation; (2) a wide range of brain impairment or mental retardation—spanning learning disabilities and neurobehavioral disorders; and (3) changes in facial structure than can even be hard for a specialist to detect. Some experts feel the FAS "look" is overplayed—that in fact the facial abnormalities of the syndrome are relatively subtle. The long-term impact of alcohol on older children who were exposed to alcohol in utero is less certain, but for many, the learning disabilities can be permanent. Still other research points to motor development delays in children whose mothers drank alcohol while breast-feeding.

It is believed that the effects of alcohol on the fetus are different at different stages of pregnancy. For instance, during the first trimester of pregnancy, when most organ systems are developing, alcohol can cause malformations of these systems. Such problems are thought to be rare. During the second trimester, alcohol can impair the baby's overall growth and metabolism. And in the third trimester, when the fetus is thought to be most vulnerable to alcohol, the rapidly developing brain can be adversely affected. This is an important message for women—especially those with alcohol abuse problems—to take home. If you have made the mistake of drinking heavily during the first several months of your pregnancy, there's still a lot to gain from quitting in the later months. Don't give up and say you've already done the damage. This might be the best possible time to get help for your alcohol problem. Animal studies show that your baby can do some catch-up developing late in the pregnancy and possibly avoid some of the detrimental effects of alcohol exposure. You also may save *yourself* irreparable physical and mental harm if you stop abusing alcohol..

Dr. Geller notes that detoxification during pregnancy should be done with extreme caution, with careful monitoring of blood pressure, pulse and any sign that detoxification might be getting out of control for the mother. If the mother is in trouble, chances are the baby is too. Most feel that during pregnancy, the best way to detoxify an alcohol-abusing woman is *in the hospital,* by means of *weaning,* not treatment with drugs.

Because there is little data on just how much alcohol can harm an unborn baby, many practitioners simply say, "Don't drink at all during pregnancy." Many experts on FAS feel that this advice is excessive and not based on scientific fact. The vast majority of cases of FAS occur in babies of chronic alcohol drinkers—those who "binge drink" several alcoholic beverages at a time or during a short time span while pregnant. They defy their colleagues to find a true case of FAS from a mother who drank an occasional glass of wine. However, the *inability* to show something does *not* mean it isn't true, and other researchers believe that small amounts of maternal alcohol intake can cause fetal problems as well. Dr. Richard Johnston, medical director for the March of Dimes Birth Defects Foundation, firmly states that alcohol should be avoided 100% during pregnancy. Ideally, he says, women should abstain *before* conception, but of course that's not always possible.

To quell a common fear: if you drank alcohol during the couple of weeks when you did not know you were pregnant, don't berate yourself or think that you have done your baby irreparable harm. Just stop drinking now and you should be okay. Barbara Morse remembers getting a call from one women who had eaten Kahlúa-flavored ice cream before she knew she was pregnant and was considering *terminating* the pregnancy to avoid having a baby with FAS! This is the outcome of a lack of data and alarming media "advice," Morse laments. Women simply become terrified, and loaded with guilt.

Here's what we *do* know about alcohol and the potential harm it poses to a fetus. Having several drinks at one "sitting" is worse than having the same number of drinks over a several hour period. Having a single drink a day, though *not* recommended, is not as dangerous as having seven drinks on one day each week. Hence, *binge* drinking is the worst thing you can do to your unborn baby. One major criticism of current research on FAS is that much of it is vague about the amount of alcohol consumed. For example, a study might say that a woman had twelve drinks in a week, but will *not* say whether she had a couple of drinks a day or drank it all on Friday and Saturday nights. Therefore we're limited in our knowl-

edge of what drinking behavior is most dangerous. When you break the studies down, Morse notes, having four or more drinks per day seems to be the riskiest behavior. The only known way to *prevent* FAS is to abstain from alcohol 100% while pregnant.

TREATING ALCOHOLISM IN WOMEN

Getting to treatment in the first place is a hurdle for many women. Employers are less likely to refer women than men to alcohol treatment, so women are more reliant on family and friends to encourage them. This can be tricky, since family members often hide women's drinking problems. General practitioners often *miss* alcoholism in otherwise "normal"-seeming women, adding to the problem. Add to these issues the fact that women often drink secretly and therefore take longer to be "rescued," and you have a complicated treatment situation. The NCADD states that women make up fewer than 25% of the patients in publicly funded alcohol treatment programs.

Dr. Millman feels strongly that alcoholism treatment for women should *focus* on women's drinking issues—at least to some degree. For example, the program doesn't *have* to be women-only (although there are some advantages to this), but it would be good to have a women-only track or group *within* the program. These tracks are becoming increasingly available throughout the country. For some women, all-female programs might be essential in order to let them comfortably address the private social, sexual or other issues surrounding their drinking problem. Sometimes a history of private or "embarrassing" problems connected to drinking will result in women's "clamming up" in mixed-sex therapy sessions. Dr. Geller echoes this idea, noting that treatment and discussion of issues such as incest require a tremendously *safe* environment for women, and that only single-sex programs can provide that safety. Another way to help insure proper attention to women's concerns in treatment for alcoholism is to select programs with female therapists and other female health professionals.

In general, however, there are many barriers to treatment for women. For instance, many alcohol and other substance abuse treatment programs fail to provide child care of any kind, making it impossible for women to enter them without risking temporary (or even permanent) loss of their children.

The first thing you must decide in choosing a treatment plan for alcoholism is whether you will need to be treated as an *inpatient* (in a hospital or clinic setting) or as an *outpatient* (living at home and visiting your doctor regularly). Dr. Judy Ann Bigby of Brigham and Women's Hospital in Boston, suggests the following guidelines:

Best for outpatient treatment. If your at-home social situation is intact (for example, your marriage is relatively healthy), you have not failed at *previous* treatment for alcoholism, your doctor finds that you have no *major* physical complications of alcoholism yet, and you have no history of major withdrawal, outpatient treatment may be right for you.

Best for inpatient treatment. If your at-home social situation is poor (for example, your marriage is failing or you have no supportive friends), you are on the verge of a life crisis (for instance, divorce or unemployment), your doctor finds that you have major physical or psychological problems from drinking, you have suffered a previous episode of withdrawal, you previously failed at outpatient treatment, or you are in a significant state of denial about your substance abuse (or lack insight into your problem), inpatient treatment might be right for you.

Both in- and outpatient treatment for alcoholism provide many treatment style options. For example, couples therapy, individual therapy, and family therapy are among the possibilities, and all of them have advantages. Sometimes a combination of two or three forms of therapy is useful. The well-known group Al-Anon gets widespread praise for its ability to *educate* family members or close friends of alcoholics about the meaning and impact of the disease. Sometimes, medication that causes vomiting when combined with alcohol is used as a deterrent to drinking. Drugs are also usually used during detoxification. Medication is *not* used for pregnant alcoholics, however.

Because women who drink excessively often have deep feelings of low self-esteem and inadequacy, the most effective treatment programs deal with these underlying feelings and build inner strength so that women won't need to build artificial strength with alcohol.

Another important feature of treatment programs for alcoholic women is attention to *other* addictions, such as sedatives or illicit drugs. Since women's addictions often multiply, it's important to treat *all* addictions, not just alcoholism, in order to bring a woman back to health. Dr. Millman adds that women whose sexual relations are connected to excessive drinking should abstain from sex until they're *off* alcohol completely. Then, they will be free to relearn sexual relationships *without* alcohol.

WOMEN AND SMOKING

Smoking is suicide for women. It's hard to find any type of women's health problem that's not exacerbated or caused by smoking. Of course, this isn't news. Far from it. We've known about the hazards of smoking for decades, but knowledge hasn't translated into common sense behavior. Ellen Gritz, professor and chair of the department of behavioral science at Houston's M.D. Anderson Cancer Center, says that women who smoke are at even greater risk than men, since we're not only subject to gender-neutral diseases (lung cancer, heart disease) but we also have gender-specific vulnerabilities across our life span (with smoking, fertility drops, menopause starts earlier, and bone loss accelerates, just to name a few).

Part of the problem is we've heard so *much* about how bad smoking is for us, the information has become background noise. It goes in one ear and out the other. The fact that we cannot face our mortality, and tend to think of risks and statistics as pertaining to someone *else,* but never to us, only makes the problem worse.

Of course, there are also those who point to their 90-year-old grandmothers who have smoked for decades and are doing fine, and argue that smoking doesn't hurt *everyone.* The remarkably powerful smoking lobby feeds this denial, saying (absurdly) that you can't *prove* that smoking causes disease. Of course you can prove it, and that 90-year-old grandmother is quite the exception, not the rule. The sooner we stop pretending that we are immune from the lethal effects of smoking, the sooner we can access the help we need to quit. We'll talk about how to quit later in this chapter.

Nonsmokers are quick to judge, question and ridicule smokers. Not only are they disgusted by the habit, and sensitive to the risks *others'* smoking pose to *them* (more on this later), but nonsmokers simply tend to look *down* on smokers in general. They speak of smokers as weak, stupid or ignorant. In some ways, it's similar to the way in which thin people regard fat people—wondering why they can't control themselves. These days, in certain parts of the country, smokers feel ashamed—as if they're second-class citizens. Before we heap blame or ridicule on everyone who smokes, keep this in mind: smoking is a powerful addiction. A recent surgeon general's report compares the addictive power of nicotine to that of heroin. Many of those who started smoking before they knew any better—or who assumed they could quit when they wanted to—now find themselves trapped in their fatal habit.

Many smokers have tried repeatedly to quit, and have failed. It's the rare smoker who is pleased about or proud of what she is doing to her body. If you are a heavy smoker, take heart: there *is* a way out—even the most entrenched smokers can quit. If you don't smoke, but care about someone who does, the best you can do is to encourage, support and exhort the smoker to quit—not by abusing them, chastising them or complaining about the habit, but by offering support in any way possible. We'll discuss some of the ways in which nonsmokers can help smokers to quit later in this section.

WOMEN AND SMOKING: THE UGLY STATISTICS

While overall, the incidence of smoking has been declining in this country, the decline has been slower among women than among men, and a remarkable number of Americans—about 50 million—still smoke. Cigarettes kill over 140,000 women per year in the U.S., says Dr. Corinne Husten, medical officer for the office on smoking and health at the Centers for Disease Control and Prevention. According to the American Lung Association, each year more Americans die from smoking-related illness than from car accidents, homicide, AIDS and drug abuse combined. The ALA also reports that the health care costs and lost productivity associated with smoking run an estimated *65 billion dollars a year*. The Centers for Disease Control and Prevention reports that by the year 2000, more women will smoke than men (not exactly the best arena in which to make a feminist mark).

There has been some progress in smoking cessation—but less for women than for men. In 1965, 31.9% of American women smoked; in 1987, that number stood at 26.8%. For men, the percentage of smokers was at 50.2% in 1965, and at 31.7% in 1987 (a bigger percentage decline). The hard numbers, as opposed to the percentages, look even gloomier for women: 22 million women smoked in 1965, 25.3 million women smoked in 1985.

HEALTH RISKS

Smoking causes a laundry list of diseases, and to go through them all would require a tome, not a chapter. I'll discuss a few of the biggies. The best known, of course, and the most feared, is lung cancer, which has reached epidemic proportions among American women. In 1987, lung cancer surpassed breast cancer as the leading cancer killer of white women; in 1990, it did so among African-American women as well. If you have ever seen advanced lung cancer close-up, you won't forget the image. I did a story on the epidemic of lung cancer among women for CBS in 1990, and met a woman in her early 40s in Lexington, Kentucky, who had been smoking since she was seven years old. Kentucky, one of the main tobacco-growing states, is among the women's smoking capitals of America: cigarettes are so prevalent, girls often start smoking there around the time they learn to spell. The woman I met had just undergone her first brain surgery for tumors that had spread from her lung. Her head was shaved, her face pale, bluish, and gaunt. She struggled just to breathe. It was a chore for her to walk from one side of her mobile home to the other. Doctors predicted she had just months to live. Her daughter, in her early 20s, was smoking away on the back porch. It is an image that will stick with me for the rest of my life.

According to a Yale University study, dose-for-dose, women are at higher risk of lung cancer than are men. This parallels women's particular vulnerability to alcohol, dose for dose, compared to men, as discussed above. Think about that the next time you've got a drink in one hand and a cigarette in the other.

A frightening fact about lung cancer is that while its effects are powerful and debilitatating once it has advanced, it often starts out with no symptoms at all. While some victims cough, or find blood in their sputum, these signs often don't appear until lung cancer has spread and the chance of cure is drastically reduced.

Apart from lung cancer, smoking causes a vast range of other respiratory diseases, including emphysema and bronchitis. According to the American Lung Association, current female smokers aged 35-plus are ten and one-half times more likely to *die* from emphysema or chronic bronchitis than are nonsmoking women of the same age. Also, smoking more than two packs a day gives you a five-times-greater risk of heart attack than non-smokers.

Smoking causes heart disease including heart attacks, stroke and diseased arteries throughout the body. Just *one to four* cigarettes a day doubles a woman's risk of heart attack, according to the Harvard Nurses' Health Study! Think of how many women who just "bum" a cigarette or two each day don't consider themselves at risk. Many of these light smokers don't even consider themselves "real smokers" in the first place, yet their risk of disease is significant.

For the pregnant woman, smoking is even more lethal, putting her fetus at risk of disease and death as well. Low birthweight, miscarriage, stillbirth and other tragic complications of pregnancy are all triggered by smoking. Quitting before you become pregnant could be lifesaving to you and your future child.

The health risks of smoking are powerfully amplified by oral contraceptives. Women who smoke and take the Pill are at increased risk of cardiovascular problems, including fatal blood clots.

Which Women Smoke?

According to a recent report from the Centers for Disease Control and Prevention, women who are older, and those who have less than high school education are more likely to smoke.

According to Dr. Corinne Husten, women *start* smoking at a younger age, and therefore have a greater risk of addiction, than do men. This could partially account for the large numbers of older women who have failed to kick the habit. Dr. Michael Fiore, director of the center for tobacco research and intervention at the University of Wisconsin at Madison, is alarmed that teenage girls are now smoking at the same rate as teenage boys, and have been doing so for about ten years. He notes that Caucasian teen girls seem to be smoking significantly more than African-American teens.

Tobacco Companies Targeting Women

Nearly every smoking expert I interviewed railed against the tobacco industry for aggressively targeting—and capturing—women. Ads from Virginia Slims to Ultra Lights are said to promise women coveted qualities from slimness to coolness. These are especially appealing to teenage girls, who are smoking at alarming rates: in a study of high school seniors, 4.9% of black teenage girls and 23.3% of white teenage girls were smoking. According to a recently published study from the University of California at San Diego (UCSD), smoking initiation among teenaged girls climbed and peaked in precise correlation with peak advertising rates in the 1970s. Women who did not attend college were found to be most vulnerable to the influences of tobacco advertising.

Research shows that women are more likely than men to use cigarettes to control both their weight and their emotions: ads that promote thinness and a cool, mellow, independent lifestyle feed into this image. Former Surgeon

General Dr. Joycelyn Elders coined a catchy, if depressing, theme that has been promoted by advertisers. She called it "the five S's": sexiness, slimness, successful, social and sophisticated. Young women in particular buy into each and every S—choosing smoking as one route to all of them. It seems logical to add a sixth S. After years of smoking, it's likely to be *sick*.

Young people in general are also being targeted by cigarette advertisers: the cartoon-style ads (for Camels, as an example) tug at a youthful audience, experts say. Since young women are especially at risk, this double whammy of advertising—to women, and to kids—hits us hardest.

Ironically, while we spend billions of dollars on smoking-related health problems each year, companies that manufacture cigarettes made after-tax profits of over $7 billion in 1989, according to the CDC. Eight hundred and forty packs of cigarettes are sold each second in the U.S. The ads that encourage us to smoke cost tobacco companies $4 billion a year. It's a very expensive way to die.

PASSIVE SMOKE, SIDESTREAM SMOKE, OR ENVIRONMENTAL TOBACCO SMOKE

The smoke we get secondhand, when others are smoking, causes cancer and many other respiratory diseases. This so-called "passive" or "sidestream" smoke has received a tremendous amount of attention lately, ever since the Environmental Protection Agency labeled passive smoke a "class A carcinogen"—ranking it with asbestos and radon as major cancer threats. The discovery that passive smoke can be lethal has given a major push to antismoking legislation and has created a new, vigorous backlash against smokers in many cities.

According to the American Heart Association, mothers who smoke ten or more cigarettes a day can cause as many as 26,000 new cases of asthma every year among their children! The same group says that infants are three times more likely to die of sudden infant death syndrome if their mothers smoke during pregnancy. I was horrified to read a recent study from Toronto that appeared in the *Journal of the American Medical Association* showing that nicotine and cotinine appear in the hair of fetuses whose mothers smoke. Since 18–20% of pregnant women smoke, this is a major women's and children's health crisis.

The Centers for Disease Control and Prevention recently put out a collection of passive smoke facts that raised a lot of eyebrows. Here's just a sampling: 3000 Americans will die because of passive smoke this year; passive smoke causes between 150,000 and 300,000 cases of lower respiratory infection a year in babies under the age of one and a half; between 7500 and 15,000 babies under one and a half years of age are hospitalized for pneumonia and bronchitis each year because of passive smoke; secondhand smoke causes 30-times as many lung cancer deaths as all regulated air pollutants combined; and for everyone who's ever tried to get a coworker to blow smoke the other way, here's a good piece of ammunition: nonsmokers at work are 34% more likely to get lung cancer than those in smoke-free offices.

QUITTING: A GOAL ANYONE CAN MEET

We know that many women are *trying* to quit these days. The quit rate (that is, the percentage of women who have ever smoked who have quit) rose from 19.1% in 1965 to 44.7% in 1991. With millions of women still smoking, how-ever—and lots failing in their attempts to quit—it's hard to celebrate. The fact is, most smokers relapse at least once when trying to quit. The average number of quit attempts is between three and four. The Centers for Disease Control and Prevention report that women aged 35–44 are substantially less likely to have tried to quit in the last year than are younger women.

Research shows that many teenagers believe they won't be smoking several years down the road, but lots of them still are. Somewhere between the intentions and the promises, addiction takes hold, and many smoke well into adulthood, when their risk of smoking-related diseases peaks.

Now here's the good news: over 37 million Americans are ex-smokers. Do you really believe that there is something 37 million other people can accomplish that you cannot? According to the American Lung Association, 1.5 million Americans join the quit ranks each year. You can be one of them.

You may have seen or heard in the lay media that men have a better quit rate than women. In fact, Dr. Husten says, this is a misinterpretation of the data. If you adjust the study results to show that many men who quit move on to other tobacco products, like pipes and chewing tobacco, you see that women do not in fact have poorer quit rates than men.

Most smokers (about 95%), including women, quit on their own. A smaller number attend smoking cessation programs, of which there are many different types. Some research suggests that women are slightly more likely to use smoking cessation programs than are men.

OBSTACLES TO QUITTING—FOR WOMEN

There may be unique, gender-related obstacles to smoking cessation. Judith Ockene, director of the division of preventive and behavioral medicine at the University of Massachusetts Medical School at Worcester, says that women use cigarettes more for stress and weight management than men do. Beyond the physical addiction, women's emotional dependence on cigarettes may be greater because of these two concerns. Ockene notes that the actual behavior of smoking—breathing in deeply, taking time out from the job or some other obligation—makes the whole process of having a cigarette seem relaxing. The solution, Ockene says, is to find *other* ways to take deep breaths and to take time out, such as exercise.

Many women admit that they smoke because it keeps their weight down—or because they fear that quitting will send their weight sky-rocketing. According to Dr. Ronald Davis, Chief Medical officer for the Michigan Department of Public Health and former director of the Office on Smoking and Health at the Centers for Disease Control and Prevention, it is true that women gain a bit more weight than men do when they quit smoking. But the amount gained is minimal (about six pounds on aver-age—a dress size at most). Some women don't gain any weight at all when they quit. And Dr. Davis stresses that the health impact of this weight gain is minimal or negligible compared to the risks of continuing smoking. Of course, most women aren't concerned about the health impact of those six pounds: they're worried about the *cosmetic* effect. This is one more rea-son why starting an exercise program while trying to quit smoking can offer significant benefits, offsetting weight gain, making your body look and feel better, *and* helping replace a bad habit with a good one.

Ellen Gritz adds that women often use cigarettes to mark time, which can be quite addictive in itself. If you use a cigarette to mark time away from the children, or breaks at work, the habit can become as much a part of your day as the alarm clock ringing, or catching the bus home.

QUITTING WITH THE NICOTINE PATCH

Some smoking cessation programs use the nicotine patch as a temporary replacement to the nicotine addiction in cigarettes. The idea is to gradually wean you off of your nicotine addiction and break the cigarette habit at the same time. If you've heard quite disparate reports about the effectiveness of this quitting tool, it's because success depends largely on how the patch is used. Most experts agree that without a complete behavior modification program in which you learn other skills to stay off cigarettes, the patch doesn't work as well. In fact, makers of the patch recommend that they be used in conjunction with more complete smoking cessation regimen.

A recent study by Susan Kenford and Dr. Michael Fiore of the University of Wisconsin Medical School found that the first two weeks after starting a smoking cessation program with the nicotine patch are especially critical. They found that quitters who had completely abstained from cigarettes for the first two weeks of treatment were much more likely to still be abstaining six months later than were those

who had broken down and had a cigarette during those first couple of weeks. Another study by Dr. Fiore published in the *Journal of the American Medical Association* in June of 1994 found that the nicotine patch is twice as effective as a placebo in getting patients to quit smoking, even when the patch is worn for a shorter time than manufacturers recommend. In this study, which was a review of 17 well-controlled studies on the subject, 22% of those who used the patch were still abstaining from cigarettes six months afterwards, while only 9% of those who quit with a placebo were still smoke-free.

Other forms of nicotine replacement include nicotine gum, and coming down the pike, nicotine nasal sprays. There are minor side effects with each type of nicotine replacement: the patch may cause skin irritations if you don't move it around enough, and the gum can cause minor oral problems. An extremely small number of people will become addicted to the nicotine replacement itself.

Talk to your doctor about whether you are even a candidate for nicotine replacement. Some people, because of past or present health problems (including hypertension) are advised to avoid these methods.

GENERAL QUITTING TIPS—FROM THE EXPERTS

Dr. Pamela Douglas, director of noninvasive cardiology at Boston's Beth Israel Hospital, says that there is an optimal window for quitting smoking, called the "action stage." At this stage, women can admit that they have a problem and are open to the idea of trying to quit, or at least to reduce the number of cigarettes they smoke. According to the Harvard Nurses Health Study, the health effects of smoking are dose-related, and while smoking even a few cigarettes per day can boost your risk of heart attack and heart disease, the less you smoke, the smaller your risk. So cutting down, while not as ideal as quitting, is an excellent idea. During this "action stage," women are advised to start making tangible changes in their smoking habits, such as buying fewer cigarettes, switching to less potent brands, and avoiding situations where they smoke most.

Should you do it on your own, or choose a cessation program? That's a highly personal decision. As I mentioned, most people quit on their own. But according to Dr. Fiore, those who smoke more than 25 cigarettes per day are more likely to use assisted smoking cessation programs. While those who used cessation programs were less likely to succeed than those who quit on their own (23.6% versus 47.5% in Fiore's study), this could be related to the fact that the heaviest smokers, who used formal programs, were the most severely addicted to nicotine. Fiore also found that those who use nicotine substitutes fail more, compared to those who quit cold turkey. Again, the severity of the smoking problem or addiction might contribute to these findings—if more addicted people use nicotine substitutes, they may be tougher quit candidates to begin with.

When should you quit? Anytime is a good time to quit, but the sooner the better. While you still reap tremendous health benefits from quitting later in life, a University of Michigan study found that smokers who quit before age 40 run half the risk of dying of lung cancer as those who quit after age 55. The researchers theorize that younger bodies repair themselves better. So don't delay—but if you're already older, know that quitting will bring many health benefits. Experts do note that for women, pregnancy is an excellent window in which to try smoking cessation. The incentive of protecting her baby is a powerful one for many women. The key, experts say, is not to let women relapse after delivery—which many women do. Perhaps the newest evidence about passive smoke's powerful negative impact on babies and children will provide new incentive for women to stay off cigarettes after delivery.

Whether you're trying to quit on your own or with a formal group, the American Lung Association has assembled the following tips that can make the process much easier:

- Set a quit date and stick to it
- Remove cigarettes, ashtrays, matches and lighters from your home, office and car
- Keep low-calorie snacks handy at all times
- Spend more time in places that do not allow smoking
- Tell everyone you're going to stop smoking
- Call a friend if you need help

Virginia Ernster, professor and former chair of the department of epidemiology and biostatistics at the University of California at San Francisco School of Medicine, advises aspiring quitters to find alternative activities for *both* their mouths and their hands: for example, chew gum or ice, crunch on a carrot (long thin foods resembling cigarettes), or knit. She also recommends finding good windows of opportunity for quitting, such as pregnancy, or while you're raising small children who are especially vulnerable to passive smoke. Other experts recommend brushing your teeth when you feel the urge to smoke, avoiding lingering after meals, rewarding yourself with saved money that you didn't spend on cigarettes, avoiding alcohol (which can be a trigger for many smokers) and keeping a journal of the things that trigger your smoking urges so you can redesign your schedule to avoid them.

Finally, Judith Ockene urges women to ask themselves, "What will I get out of quitting?" The answers are highly personal, different for every woman. Maybe you'll enjoy not smelling like cigarettes. Or you'll be able to run up a flight of stairs without stopping to gasp. Maybe you'll be welcomed more by hosts, or not feel ostracized in restaurants. Experts used to insist that the positive reinforcement should be *internal*—that is, you'll have to feel better about *yourself* for it to really count. But since many women are concerned about how *others* in their life perceive them, external reinforcement can be an important motivator, too (for example, will your children feel better about you if you quit?).

HOW YOU MIGHT FEEL WHEN YOU'RE QUITTING

The truth of the matter is that quitting doesn't feel very good at first for most long-term smokers. Breaking a habit, and an addiction, takes some work. For that reason, when you succeed, you should be very proud of yourself. Mark the date of your last cigarette and celebrate it at any interval you choose (weekly, monthly, yearly). According to the National Institute on Aging, the most common withdrawal symptoms are anxiety, restlessness, drowsiness, difficulty concentrating, and problems with digestion. Some just suffer with the craving for a cigarette, and

become terribly irritable and hard to be around. Others have few withdrawal symptoms, if any. It's impossible to predict how *you're* going to feel.

The good news is that when those bad feelings start to wear off (and even *before* they fade), some dramatic and positive things begin to happen in your body. The American Cancer Society breaks the effects down into the following time line, which I find to be one of the most motivational lists I've seen on the subject:

Within 20 minutes of quitting: Your blood pressure and pulse drop to normal, the temperature of your extremities drops to normal

8 hours after quitting: Blood levels of carbon monoxide drop to normal, blood oxygen rises to normal

24 hours after quitting: Your risk of heart attack drops

48 hours after quitting: Your nerve endings start re-growing, your senses of smell and taste are enhanced

72 hours after quitting: Your bronchial tubes relax, making it easier to breathe; your lung capacity rises 30%

2 weeks to 3 months after quitting: Your circulation improves, walking becomes easier, your lung function increases up to 30%

9 months after quitting: Coughing, sinus congestion, shortness of breath all recede; the hair-like cleaning cells, called cilia, regrow in your lungs; your ability to handle mucus, clear out your lungs, and ward off infection increase; your energy level goes up

5–10 years after quitting: Your risk of lung cancer is significantly down, your death rate is almost that of a nonsmoker, your risk of cancers of the mouth, pancreas, larynx and many other body organs drops and some precancerous cells are replaced by healthy ones

The bottom line: when you quit smoking, your body stops fighting for its life.

IN BRIEF: OTHER LEGAL AND ILLEGAL DRUG ABUSE AMONG WOMEN

According to the National Institute on Drug Abuse, 5% of women report having used illegal drugs in the past 30 days. That's about three million women—and some say the number is a lot larger—putting potentially harmful and uncontrolled substances into their bodies in a given month. According to the U.S. Department of Health and Human Services, over 500,000 women used cocaine in this time period; 3.9 million used marijuana. About one in four girls aged 12–17 have tried an illegal drug, says the National Council on Alcoholism and Drug Dependence. The total cost of drug abuse (*not* including alcohol) in 1990, according to the Robert Wood Johnson Foundation: $66.9 billion.

Sadly, pregnant women aren't immune to drug use, which means millions of children are at risk of hazardous effects from drugs, too. According to the NCADD, 11% of pregnant women use at least one of the following groups of drugs: heroin, methadone, amphetamines, PCP, marijuana, or cocaine. Add to this the fetal exposure to alcohol and cigarette smoke, discussed above, and you've got a tremendously high potential for permanent fetal damage. Apart from promoting permanent problems for these children, drug abuse can cause miscarriage, premature delivery, sudden infant death syndrome (SIDS) and other serious chronic health problems.

While we tend to focus on the abuse of illegal drugs, we often overlook the significant amount of abuse of *legal* substances, particularly psychoactive drugs like tranquilizers (including the popular benzodiazepines Valium and Librium), barbiturates (highly addictive drugs often used to treat anxiety) and others. These drugs are prescribed for a number of reasons, including to "relax" women, relieve anxiety, promote sleep and so on. Many experts feel they are overprescribed, too quickly refilled and that patients aren't monitored carefully while taking them. Sometimes, these drugs are prescribed over the telephone without even a proper evaluation by a mental health professional. And too often, women think that if one pill helps, another could only be better. The result: addiction, overdose and other tragic consequences. Certainly, these drugs have appropriate uses when properly monitored, and can be both helpful and safe. But because of their high potential for abuse, women should be extremely cautious when starting them. Insist on careful monitoring and regular reevaluation of your use of these drugs by your doctor. Ask for a good explanation of why you've been prescribed these drugs, what your problem is, what exactly the medication will do for you, what side effects to be aware of, and for how long you are expected to remain on the medication. If you are concerned that you may be addicted to or having some other problems with these medications, call your doctor immediately.

Some Signs You May Be Addicted to or Having Problems with a Drug

- You're worried you may have a problem, and find yourself wishing you didn't have to take a given drug
- Your function is in some way impaired by use of the drug—you're tired at work, or cannot care for your children properly
- You ask yourself *why* you're taking the drug, but take it anyway
- You are depriving yourself or your family of something needed as a result of your taking the drug, or spending money on the drug
- You can't stop taking the drug on your own

Treatment for Different Kinds of Substance Abuse

There are several different approaches to substance abuse treatment. Above all, they differ by philosophy. For instance, according to Alan Budney of the University of Vermont in Burlington, there is the classic Alcoholics Anonoymous "chronic disease" approach: that is, "Once a problem, always a problem." Then there is the more time-limited approach to addiction problems (which holds, that you *have* a problem, but you can be "cured" of it). The chronic disease model, while popular in this country, has its drawbacks, Budney says. For some it's so negative, it turns them away. Budney prefers a more positive, motivational, "You-can-get-past-this" approach to substance abuse treatment. But on the plus side, he notes, the A.A. idea that you're battling a chronic

problem can add an important spiritual component to treatment, since you bond with others in striving to reach a common, lifelong goal. Individuals must choose which treatment model works best for them.

If you have a substance abuse problem, there are several kinds of treatment centers/practitioners from which to choose. A relatively small percentage of substance abusers become inpatients at specialized substance abuse centers. Most, however, are outpatients, living at home and coming for treatment at a variety of venues, including special substance abuse clinics (most common), as well as individual doctors' offices (both psychiatrists *and* non-mental health practitioners). According to the Robert Wood Johnson Foundation, the most common substances for which patients seek treatment are alcohol and cocaine, followed by heroin and other opiates.

Women can be hard to treat, Budney says, since often their addictions are so-called "co-dependencies," connected to the drug abuse of their spouse or partner. He worries that there may be an increase in drug use among young women—and notes that women are catching up with men in various areas of substance abuse.

Some experts recommend treatment with medication to help overcome addictions (depending on the substance being abused), while others prefer behavioral treatments and support group therapy that focuses on finding alternatives to drug use, learning about the triggers to drug abuse, providing positive motivational feedback, and teaching skills like more effective parenting and/or self-esteem and coping strategies. Since women, more than men, often come to substance abuse treatment with multiple burdens—lack of money, childcare responsibilities, spousal abuse—finding programs that meet women's special needs is important. Unfortunately, that can be difficult. Often, substance abuse programs fail to provide childcare, making it impossible for women to attend or stay committed. If you can't find an appropriate substance abuse clinic near you, at least consider some part-time or outpatient treatment from a local practitioner: *something* is better than nothing at all. Sometimes, a combination of treatment with medication and individual or group therapy is the most effective approach of all. For instance, in the case of heroin addiction, most recommend giving the drug methadone, but since this causes an addiction all its own (albeit a safer, more controlled addiction), adding behavioral treatment to the regime can help patients get off medication altogether. Antidepressant medications have been used to treat cocaine abuse, with mixed results.

If you are experimenting with illegal drugs, at least become informed of both the risks to your body, and the risks of addiction. Cocaine can wreak havoc on your cardiovascular system, for example. Who can forget the case of basketball player Len Bias, who dropped dead on the court after using cocaine? Heroin is powerfully addictive: Alan Budney sees light users become hooked. This is also true of other opiates and various legal painkillers as well. Even after a few days' heavy use, Budney says, trouble signs like irritability, teariness and goose bumps can set in. Because the damaging effects and addiction can take hold quickly, the sooner you seek help, the more likely you will protect yourself and the ones you love from serious harm.

For More Information on Alcohol Abuse

Alcoholics Anonymous (AA)
World Headquarters
475 Riverside Drive
New York, NY 10115
212-870-3400

National Clearinghouse for Alcohol and Drug Abuse Information
P.O. Box 2345
Rockville, MD 20847-2345
800-729-6686

National Council on Alcoholism and Drug Dependence, Inc.
12 West 21st Street
New York, NY 10010
800-475-HOPE
212-206-6770

Adult Children of Alcoholics
World Service Organization
P.O. Box 3216
Torrance, CA 90510
310-534-1815

Al-anon Family Group Headquarters
P.O. Box 862
Midtown Station
New York, NY 10018-0862
800-344-2666

NATIONAL ORGANIZATION ON FETAL
   ALCOHOL SYNDROME
1815 H Street NW, Suite 1000
Washington, DC 20006
202-785-4585

WOMEN FOR SOBRIETY
P.O. Box 618
Quakertown, PA 18951
800-333-1606

WORLD SERVICE ORGANIZATION
P.O. Box 3216
Torrance, CA 90510
310-534-1815

DRUG ABUSE

SUBSTANCE ABUSE AND MENTAL
   HEALTH SERVICE
Center for Substance Abuse Treatment
11426 Rockville Pike, Suite 410
Rockville, MD 20852
800-662-HELP (English)
800-662-AYUDA (Spanish)

NARCOTICS ANONYMOUS
P.O. Box 9999
Van Nuys, CA 91409
818-780-3951

COCAINE HOTLINE
A Phoenix House service
800-COCAINE

COCAINE ANONYMOUS
9100 Sepulveda Blvd., Suite 216
Los Angeles, CA 90045
310-216-4444

SMOKING

AMERICAN CANCER SOCIETY
1599 Clifton Road
Atlanta, GA 30329
800-ACS-2345
or write your local ACS office as listed in the
phone book

AMERICAN HEART ASSOCIATION
7320 Greenville Ave.
Dallas, TX 75231
214-373-6300
800-AHA-USA-1
or write your local AHA office as listed in the
phone book

AMERICAN LUNG ASSOCIATION
1740 Broadway, P.O. Box 596
New York, NY 10019-4374
212-315-8700
800-LUNG-USA
or write your local ALA office as listed in the
phone book

NATIONAL CANCER INSTITUTE
Office of Cancer Communications
9000 Rockville Pike, Room 10A16
Bethesda, MD 20892
800-4-CANCER

ENVIRONMENTAL PROTECTION AGENCY
Indoor Air Quality Information Clearinghouse
P.O. Box 37133
Washington, DC 20013-7133
800-438-4318

OFFICE ON SMOKING AND HEALTH
   HOTLINE
Centers for Disease Control and Prevention
Mailstop K-50
4770 Buford Highway NE
Atlanta, GA 30341-3724
404-488-5705 (live person)
800-CDC-1311 (taped message)

PART SEVEN

Fitness and Diet

CHAPTER TWENTY

NUTRITION

We are indeed much more than what we eat, but what we eat can nevertheless help us to be much more than what we are.

—Adelle Davis, *Let's Get Well*

There's a simple bottom line about nutrition and your body: without the right fuel, your body will *never* perform up to its potential. That means your thinking potential, your energy potential, your friendliness potential, possibly even your life span will all be reduced if you continue to deprive your body of essential nutrients. You would never think of putting the wrong kind of gas into your car—after all, it could break the finely tuned machine. Why then are we so cavalier about eating unhealthful foods or, even more important, skipping the right ones? When you eat poorly, the machine that is your body *does* in fact break. Every part of you, from your brain and heart to your skin and bones, is compromised when it doesn't get the materials it needs to survive and thrive. The signs of compromise might be subtle; for instance, you might be a little more tired than usual, or have trouble concentrating on your work, or find yourself being irritable with people for no good reason. Sound familiar? Sometimes, there are physical signs that you're not eating well, such as a worsening complexion or something far more serious, like brittle bones or chronic fatigue. However it manifests itself, in some way or other you are damaging your body every day when you don't eat well. Believe it or not, at the extreme, people who chronically fail to get enough calories and nutrients actually *shrink* their brains!

Oddly enough, while most women know that they need healthful foods in order to be well, few of us eat the foods we need. Whether it's because we're always on the run or worrying about what other family members eat, or because we're concerned about gaining weight, or simply because we just don't understand what it takes to eat well, we tend to fall short on a number of essential nutrients. Few of us live the 1950s sitcom dream of eating three square meals at the table with our families, and registered dietician Bettye Nowlin blames much of our nutritional failure on this fact. We rely on convenience foods, takeout has replaced homemade, and if we do cook we often "plan" our meals minutes before we make them or simply grab something out of the freezer and toss it into the microwave oven. This kind of living might not have an immediate effect but there's no doubt it takes a long-term toll on our bodies. You might think you're getting away with something but your heart and bones know better. The fact is, modern American eating—especially for women—means getting too little of what we do need and too much of what we don't need.

MAKING CHANGES

The good news is it doesn't have to be this way. It is possible, I have learned, to eat quickly *and* well. (Of course the ideal would be to take your time, but let's be realistic!) It takes a little more planning—mostly on your shopping list, not your cooking time—but it can be done. Women I've spoken to who have made the relatively easy switch from thoughtless to thoughtful eating have seen immediate benefits not only in their energy and mood but in their bodies. What they don't yet know is how major a difference healthful eating will make years down the road, providing energy and vitality, fortifying their bodies against disease, and helping to transform the meaning of old age.

FOOD VERSUS DISEASE

It's no news that certain foods or individual nutrients can help prevent life-threatening disease, from cancer and diabetes to heart disease and beyond. Every day researchers learn something new about how the foods we eat can boost our immune systems, create anticancer chemicals in our bodies, or help keep our arteries clear and open so blood flows normally. On the flip side, there's just as much negative information about how the wrong foods can do just the opposite, fighting our bodies' ability to function properly. What most people don't know is how powerful food can be at determining the health of entire populations. In countries where fiber intake is high and fat intake is low (quite the opposite of the American diet), there are dramatically lower rates of heart disease and certain cancers. Carolyn Clifford, chief of the diet and cancer branch at the National Cancer Institute, compares the U.S., where we consume about 38% of our total calories from fat, to Japan, where the diet contains about 15% of calories from fat. Our breast cancer rate is five times theirs, in part because of this enormous difference in fat intake, Dr. Clifford says.

Even in subpopulations of the U.S., it's been found that people who eat lots of fiber have significantly lower rates of many cancers and other diseases. Of course no one can change her habits overnight, and it's unrealistic to advise American women to turn their diets upside down all at once in an attempt to stay healthy. What we must do instead is learn to find the foods we like from the long list of foods that protect us from illness, and gradually incorporate them into our daily diets. I'll help you do that in this chapter.

A WOMAN'S GUIDE TO HEALTHY EATING

Despite the fact that we've been deluged with information about nutrition and health, the information has always been given in a vague or spotty fashion. For instance, every women's magazine tells us to eat more calcium, and usually they list the foods that have calcium, but we're seldom told how *much* of these foods to eat each day and *when* to eat them. Surveys show that many women think that just one glass of milk a day will provide them with all the calcium they need to protect their bones. In fact, that's only about a third of what most women need! That first glass of milk is a good start—but it's only a start.

In this chapter, I'll give you a clear picture of how much food, and what kinds of foods, you need to eat to be a healthy woman. I'll emphasize the foods for which *women* have special needs, but keep in mind that the only way for any person to eat well, regardless of sex or age, is to eat a wide variety of fresh, wholesome foods.

You'll have to make me one promise—that you'll try not to think of food as medicine. Never lose sight of the fact that food is one of the great sensual pleasures in life. Food can be nurturing, it can be delicious, it can even be a work of art in the right hands; we should never medicalize it to the point at which it becomes simply a means to an end. Learning to eat properly should be not only healthful, but fun.

When we learn to have fun with food *and* to harness its potential to keep us healthy, we'll finally be on the right track.

WHERE WOMEN FALL SHORT

CALCIUM

At the top of the list of important nutrients for women is calcium, says Dr. Richard Rivlin, program director of the clinical nutrition research unit at The New York Hospital. We get too little calcium at all ages, he says, but older women especially have inadequate calcium in their diets. I'll spend a lot of time talking about calcium, not only because it's one of the greatest areas of failure in women's nutrition, but also because researchers have found that if you're low on calcium, you're likely to be low on other essential nutrients, too. Dr. Robert Heaney, a leading expert on calcium and bone at the Creighton University School of Medicine, says that women who lack sufficient calcium often have poor intake of magnesium, iron and vitamin B_6 as well.

Without calcium, which makes up most of our bones, we'd all be cripples. In addition, calcium helps regulate a vast array of other body functions, like our heartbeat, muscle contraction and nerve transmission. Women are starting to get the message about calcium's importance, but we don't yet understand what it takes to get enough calcium in our diets. One national hotline with calcium information gets about four thousand calls each month from women who are confused in one way or another about how to include adequate calcium in their diets.

You may have noticed a great deal of argument played out in the media in recent years over how much calcium women need, and whether or not it's useful for *older* women. These arguments, (mostly fought out among scientists who agree that we need calcium but continue to fight over a few hundred extra milligrams), fail to address one important fact: American women barely get *half* of the current RDA for calcium in the first place! Bonnie Liebman, director of nutrition for the Center for Science in the Public Interest, worries that people have stopped appreciating the importance of calcium because there has been so much focus on the role of hormone therapy in protecting bone. We must not make the mistake of getting caught up in battles over what helps bone *more,* when clearly there are several important factors. And what's the use of arguing over whether we should get *more* when we aren't even getting the *minimum* amount of calcium we need! It's time to get moving and just bring our diets up to at least the minimum standard for good health. One important study showed that just by bringing your calcium intake up to the current RDA—that is, the minimum standard—women had a reduction in bone loss.

Starting around adolescence when many girls make the unfortunate switch from milk to soft drinks, we fall into a downward spiral in which we get less and less calcium just when our bones need it the most. By the time we're older and many of us have fallen into a "tea and toast"-style diet, many of us hardly get any calcium at all. Keep this one fact in mind: calcium deprivation has serious consequences. One in four American women will break her hip at some point in her lifetime because her bones are too weak, too thin, too porous. Many of these fractures could be prevented with adequate calcium in the diet, along with a few other healthy lifestyle changes. (For more on calcium and bones, *see* chapter 4, "Bone Health.")

GETTING STARTED

The RDAs for calcium are as follows: 1200 mg for women aged 11–24; 800 mg for women aged 25–51; 1200 mg for pregnant or lactating women; and 1200 mg for women over 51. The 1994 NIH Consensus Development Conference on Optimal Calcium Intake recommends much more: 1000 mg/day for premenopausal women aged 25–49; 1000 mg for postmenopausal women aged 50–64 who are taking estrogen; 1500 mg for postmenopausal women aged 50–64 who are *not* taking estrogen; and 1500 mg for all women 65 and over.

CALCIUM SOURCES

Now that you have the numbers, let's take a look at how you can be sure to get enough calcium in your diet. The best source of calcium is dairy foods, such as milk, yogurt, cheese and, to a lesser degree, ice cream and cottage cheese. There's a piece of good news here: nonfat dairy foods have as much or more calcium than fatty versions of the same foods. For instance, skim or low-fat milk have at least as much calcium as whole milk. So if you, like many people, are trying to cut down on fats, you can still load up on calcium quite easily. If you have trouble eating dairy products because you are lactose-intolerant, there are several products in your local supermarket that supply lactase, the enzyme that you need to help you digest dairy foods. Finally, if you simply don't like or don't want to eat lots of dairy foods, calcium can be found in a variety of dark green vegetables and other sources. However, experts caution that it's hard to get more than half of your daily calcium from nondairy food sources.

The following chart gives some good calcium sources and tells you how many milligrams of calcium is in each food. A good frame of reference is a cup of milk—an excellent calcium source—which has about 300 milligrams of calcium. Take a look at how a single serving of other foods compares to a cup of milk. If you choose the foods that have the highest amount of calcium per serving, like milk, yogurt, hard cheese, collard greens, sardines with bones, and so on, you're likely to be able to fill your total daily calcium requirement with just a couple of foods. Also, take note of the fact that higher-fat foods often fall short on calcium—for instance, softer, fattier Brie cheese has only one-quarter the calcium of harder, leaner Swiss cheese.

Calcium-Rich Foods

Milk

- buttermilk: 285 mg/cup
- nonfat milk: 302 mg/cup
- whole milk: 291 mg/cup

Yogurt:

- nonfat yogurt: 450 mg/cup

Cheese

- American: 174 mg/ounce
- Brie: 51.9 mg/ounce
- cheddar: 204 mg/ounce

- cottage, low-fat: 155 mg/cup
- cream: 23.2 mg/ounce
- Gruyere: 308 mg/ounce
- parmesan, grated: 390 mg/ounce
- Swiss: 272 mg/ounce

Fish

- salmon with bones: 3 oz., 167 mg
- sardines w/bones, canned: 3oz., approx. 354 mg
- shrimp, canned: 3 oz., 98 mg

Fruit

- figs, dried, 10 figs, 269 mg
- rhubarb, cooked, sugar added, 1 cup 348 mg

Ice cream: Caution! It takes a bigger serving of ice cream to get as much calcium as lower-fat dairy foods like yogurt.

- hard: 88 mg/half cup
- soft: 118 mg/half cup

Vegetables: Caution! The dark green veggies listed below are calcium-rich and pretty well absorbed. For certain other dark greens, like spinach, the calcium has been found to be poorly absorbed.

- broccoli, boiled from raw: 136 mg/cup
- broccoli, boiled from frozen: 100 mg/cup
- collard greens, boiled from frozen: 357 mg/cup

- kale, boiled from frozen: 179 mg/cup
- mustard greens, boiled from frozen: 150 mg/cup
- turnip greens: 252 mg/cup
- soybeans: 131 mg/cup
- tofu: 4 oz., 152 mg (with calcium salts, up to 300 mg)

COMBINATION FOODS

- Pancakes: two 4-inch: 114 mg
- Pizza, ¼ of a 14-inch pie: 332 mg

MISCELLANEOUS

- Blackstrap molasses: 2 tbsp., 274 mg

Here are some examples of how to get a full day's worth of calcium. Let's say you're a 35-year-old woman and you're not pregnant or breast-feeding, so your RDA for calcium is 800 milligrams. Only one in four women your age gets enough calcium every day! Since milk has about 300 milligrams per cup, you'd need to have a little less than three 8-ounce glasses of skim milk *every day* to meet your calcium requirement. If you're a milk lover, lucky you. If you're not, you might try blending fruit into your milk or blending it with yogurt for a delicious low-fat shake. Many women find it more palatable, *and* more fun, to go with the "variety is the spice of life" theory when it comes to getting enough calcium. They prefer to get a broader mix of calcium-rich foods. Here are some ways to do that: a one-ounce piece of cheddar cheese has about 200 milligrams of calcium, and a cup of nonfat yogurt has about 450 milligrams of calcium. That means the same 35-year-old woman could have a piece of cheese with her morning toast, a

cup of yogurt along with lunch and a half-cup of milk with a snack at some point during the day—and she'd fulfill her calcium requirement without overdosing on a single food. Finally, here's an example for someone who prefers to *limit* her dairy intake: collard greens, one of the most calcium-laden vegetables, have about 350 milligrams of calcium per cup; sardines *with bones* have about 354 milligrams per average serving (the bones are essential); two 4-inch pancakes have about 114 milligrams of calcium. That means pancakes for breakfast, a sardine sandwich for lunch and collards as a side dish at dinner will bring our same woman up to her daily calcium requirement.

Some Tips to Go with Your Calcium.
It's been observed that when you eat your calcium along with foods rich in vitamin D, the calcium is better absorbed by your body. If you're drinking a few glasses of *fortified* milk each day, you're probably getting close to the vitamin D you need. If you drink skim milk, it's especially important that it reads "fortified" on the label because vitamins D and A are removed from milk when its fat is skimmed. If you're not drinking much fortified milk, you might want to consider a multivitamin supplement (*see* more on vitamin D later). There are also some things to *avoid* if you're trying to boost your calcium intake; says Barbara Levine, director of the Calcium Information Center at New York Hospital/Cornell Medical Center; for instance, excessive caffeine, sodium and protein can cause you to lose calcium, and *excessive* amounts of fat and fiber will interfere with your calcium absorption (milk in your fiber-rich cereal each morning, however, is *fine*). But before you get too hung up on remembering

these extra guidelines, keep in mind that in general, most rules about nutrition fit in with the old saying, "Everything in moderation." If you're in general good health, get enough calcium and don't overdose on any single food or nutrient, you're already ahead of the game.

Calcium Supplements: When and Which Ones?

Almost every expert I've interviewed on this topic feels that *real food,* not pills, is the best source not only for calcium but for other essential nutrients as well. The reason: calcium from foods tends to be best absorbed, plus foods have other essential nutrients, calories and hidden ingredients that the body needs.

However, while getting all of your calcium from foods is an *ideal,* we don't live in an ideal world. In the real world, many women fail to get calcium from their diets alone, and if you've done your best and are still falling short, calcium supplements may be the best option for you. (Millions of women are coming to that conclusion, to the benefit of supplement-makers: scores of millions of dollars are spent on calcium supplements each year in the U.S.) The key is to learn how to select the best pill, since there are so many on the shelves these days.

Choosing a Supplement.

The experts point to four key features of a good calcium supplement: first, it should have a high percentage of calcium; second, it should be easily absorbed; third, it should be reasonably priced; and fourth, it should have no toxic substances in it. The following table lists, in order from highest to lowest, the amount of calcium by weight in the different types of calcium supplement:

CALCIUM SUPPLEMENTS

CALCIUM SOURCE	CALCIUM BY WEIGHT (%)
• Calcium carbonate	40
• Calcium chloride	36
• Bonemeal	33 (AVG.)
• Di-calcium phosphate	30
• Calcium citrate	24 (AVG.)
• Dolomite	22 (AVG.)
• Calcium lactate	13
• Calcium gluconate	9

Caution: Bonemeal and dolomite should not *be used. They may be contaminated. Adapted with permission from* The Orthopedic Clinics of North America, Vol. 21, No. 1, January 1990.

Let's take a look at the calcium supplement table and get a better understanding of how these supplements work. You probably noticed that calcium carbonate, at the top of the list, has a significantly higher amount of calcium than most other forms of supplements. For this reason, it's one of the top supplement choices for American women, and it's highly recommended by experts. But there are a few caveats: calcium carbonate requires a pretty good deal of stomach acid to be well absorbed. That means it's best to take this kind of calcium supplement with meals, particularly with acidic items such as orange juice. Because we have less acid in our stomachs as we age, calcium carbonate can be a little difficult for older women to absorb. In fact, some women complain of stomach upset with this and other calcium supplements, and these pills have been known to cause constipation as well. To get around this problem, you might want to go down the list a ways and consider calcium citrate. Calcium citrate has less calcium by weight than some calcium supplements higher on the list, but it tends to be very well absorbed and does *not* require much stomach acid, so it can be taken without food—which may be more convenient for some women. (This also makes it a good choice for older women, who have less stomach acid in general.) At a recent women's health conference I attended, doctors were reporting anecdotally that their patients taking calcium citrate tended to have less constipation than patients taking other kinds of calcium supplements. Another solution to stomach upset caused by calcium supplements is to take the pills at bedtime, advises Kathleen Zelman, director of the dietetic internship program at Ochsner Medical Institution.

As for the price of calcium supplements, there's a broad range, from as little as a few dollars a month to more like $20 a month—so if your budget is tight, it's important to shop and compare. (See table below.) Once you've chosen a form of supplement that agrees with your stomach, has a pretty good level of calcium in it and no contaminants, shop and compare prices at your pharmacy and elsewhere.

Cost of Calcium Supplements

	CALCIUM PER PILL	TABLETS PER DAY	$ COST TO PHARM. FOR 30 DAYS
Carbonate:			
Generic USP (Roxane)	500 mg	1	2.07
Biocal 500 (Miles)	500 mg	1	2.14
Tums (Norcliff Thayer)	200 mg	3	2.25
Os-Cal 500 Chewable (Marion)	500 mg	1	3.03
Citrate:			
Citracal (Mission)	200 mg	3	6.03
Gluconate:			
Generic (Roxane)	45 mg	12	18.25
Generic (Upjohn)	87.75 mg	6	16.98
Lactate USP:			
Generic (Warner Chilcott)	84.5 mg	6	3.65
Generic (Upjohn)	84.5 mg	6	6.84
Generic (Lilly)	84.5 mg	6	9.94

Adapted with permission from The Medical Letter, Inc.

Checking If It Works: The At-Home Acid Test.

Nutritionists urge us to do our own at-home acid tests on calcium supplements to see if they'll be well absorbed. It's quite simple. Just pour 4 ounces of vinegar into a glass, then drop one calcium supplement into it. If the tablet dissolves within 30 to 45 minutes, it's likely to be well absorbed by your body. That's because vinegar closely resembles the acid your stomach makes to dissolve foods. If the tablet is still sitting intact in the glass after an hour or more, it will probably be poorly absorbed by your body, too.

Count 'Em.

One final consideration in choosing a calcium pill: take a look at how many milligrams of calcium you get from a single tablet (*see* table above). Some women find it annoying to have to take several pills a day, which is necessary if you choose a supplement with only a small amount of calcium per pill. Furthermore, some experts find that stomachaches are more common when you're taking more tablets per day. Calcium citrate, for example, has only about 200 to 250 milligrams of calcium per pill (although it *does* offer other significant advantages as discussed earlier). Other types of calcium have 500 or 600 milligram per pill. If you're getting a significant amount of calcium from your diet and using a supplement just to make up the last bit, a single 250 milligram pill might be all you need. If you're using supplements almost exclusively to fill your calcium requirement, one pill—even a calcium-rich one—just isn't enough. Also keep in mind that it's not a good idea to pop several calcium pills at once to get it over with for the day. Experts do *not* recommend taking more than about 600

milligrams in one sitting, since a lot of the calcium will go to waste—unabsorbed.

Antacids and Calcium Supplementation.

You may have heard that some over-the-counter antacids contain large amounts of calcium—and they do. The key is in choosing the right kind. Tums are good, well-absorbed, inexpensive sources of calcium, and even experts who hate to use brand names admit that they're a good choice for supplementation. However, antacids that contain *aluminum* are *not* good choices for calcium supplementation, since their calcium is less well-absorbed. Read the labels.

OTHER NUTRIENTS WE'RE MISSING AND WHERE TO FIND THEM

Iron.

Many younger, menstruating women are iron deficient. Each month, a significant amount of iron is lost through the one and one-half fluid ounces of menstrual blood, and few women get enough iron in their diets to replace it. The RDA for iron is 15 milligrams (although Wahida Karmally, director of clinical nutrition at the Irving Center for Clinical Research at Columbia Presbyterian Medical Center, feels that women who have stopped menstruating could get by just fine on 10 milligrams). The best-absorbed sources of iron are red meats, chicken, fish and liver. Spinach and other leafy green vegetables are also good sources of iron, but registered dietician Mona Sutnick of Philadelphia points to evidence suggesting that it's best to eat vitamin C rich foods *along with* the greens to improve iron absorption. Other good sources of iron include enriched whole grain breads and cereals, prunes and prune juice, and pinto or kidney beans. Flesh sources of iron are not only well absorbed but tend to help your body absorb iron from other sources as well. Add up the amount you're currently getting from your diet; if you're not getting enough and don't feel you can boost these iron-rich foods enough to meet your daily requirement, consider a multivitamin supplement with iron. (An extra iron tip: Experts advise doing your cooking in cast-iron pots and pans—believe it or not, your food will absorb iron from them!)

Folic Acid.

Most women get far less folic acid than we need, and if we have the potential to become pregnant, that can be serious. Experts have found a link between birth defects called neural tube defects and the mother's inadequate intake of folic acid. Johanna Dwyer, director of Frances Stern Nutrition Center at New England Medical Center, recommends that women eat more folic-acid-rich foods like dark-green leafy vegetables, dry beans, wheat germ and whole grains, peanuts and liver. But it's hard to get enough folic acid from food. This is one area where most experts recommend supplementation. You'll need 400 micrograms (which equals 0.4 milligram) of folic acid. If you've had a child with a neural tube defect in the past, you might need to double that amount.

Vitamin D.

If you eat large amounts of vitamin D-fortified foods like milk or cereals, you're probably okay. Vitamin D is also found in egg yolks and fish oil. But many women don't get enough vitamin D, and that can interfere with our bodies' ability to absorb calcium, says Dr. Bess Dawson-Hughes of Tufts University. Older women are especially prone to vitamin D deficiency, perhaps because they don't *absorb* the vitamin as well, but also because (a) they don't eat enough of it and (b) they don't go out in the sunlight as much. Sound strange? Our skin can actually synthesize vitamin D on its own with exposure to ultraviolet light. But these days, with many of us avoiding excessive sun exposure, we might be losing out on an important source of vitamin D. Women who live in northern climates are at especially high risk of vitamin D deficiency during the winter months. Dr. Dawson-Hughes stresses that vitamin D helps combat *winter* bone loss. If you aren't getting enough vitamin D, try a standard multivitamin with 100% of the recommended daily allowance for this vitamin. *Do not* take extra vitamin D—it can be toxic, because it builds up inside fat in the body.

Fiber.

American women get about half of the fiber we need, according to the National Cancer Institute (NCI). We get about 11 to 12 grams of fiber a day, and we need 20 to 30 grams! I could fill volumes with the impressive data on how a high-fiber diet can protect against colon, lung and other cancers, as well as reducing risk factors for heart disease. There are lots of theories on how fiber protects us—from the length of time it takes to get through our digestive tract to the vitamins and other elements these foods contain—but we don't need to worry about all that. What we need to worry about is learning how to get more fiber into our diets, since experts at the NCI and other institutes have recommended a 3 to 5-a-day *minimum* of fruits and vegetable servings to boost health. What's a serving? A medium-sized piece of fresh fruit, a half-cup of canned fruit, a half-cup of cooked vegetables or a cup of fresh salad, as examples. How many grams of fiber are in the foods you eat? Dr. Carolyn Clifford gives a few examples you can use as guidelines: an apple with peel has about 3.5 grams of fiber; ½ cup of kidney beans has 7.5 grams; ½ cup of broccoli has 2.2 grams; ½ cup of cooked carrots has 2.3 grams. Beans and legumes tend to be high in fiber; strawberries are big scorers on the list of high-fiber fruits. The more overcooked and canned foods you eat, the less valuable fiber you get. Shoot for fresh, whole fruits and vegetables and avoid fatty dressings and toppings if possible. Worried about the cost? Buy fruits and veggies when they're in season and seek out local farmer's markets if they exist in your area—it will make a big difference in your grocery bill.

FAT

Can we ever say enough about fat and its impact on health? A decade after fat and cholesterol hit the American consciousness, does the average consumer even know the difference between the two—or which foods contain them? Rather than try to cover the mountains of data on this subject, try to keep this simple idea in mind: American women eat *much* too much fat (about 36–42% of our total calories, instead of the recommended under-30% rule) and the result is more heart disease, more obesity and related illnesses, and more cancer than we'd have if everyone cut down on the amount of fat they eat.

You've probably seen headlines in the paper saying that dietary fat *does not* promote breast cancer, and a week later you'll see a headline that says it *does*. You've been told to avoid saturated fat in butter and to replace it with corn oil margarine, and then you've been slapped with the news that the margarine you're proudly spreading on your toast *also* boosts your risk of heart disease. No doubt there are fascinating research questions that have to be answered about the ability of fat to promote cancers in the first place or to accelerate their growth once they exist. And no doubt it's frustrating when a number of studies show that eating a diet low in fat will protect you from cancer . . . only to see them all refuted by a high-profile study from Harvard that *seems* to debunk the whole fat-breast cancer theory. So what's a woman to do? I have a suggestion. While we wait for the scientists to hash out the fine points of exactly how fat affects our bodies and which kinds are worse than others, let's seize the opportunity to cut down on *all fats now*—since we do know for sure that too much fat promotes diseases which kill hundreds of thousands of women each year. We'll also take a brief look at certain kinds of fat that may actually be *good* for us.

The Guidelines.

Experts say to reduce your intake of fat from the current 40% or so of total calories that American women eat to 30% or less of total calories. That's what the American Heart Association tells us, and what the National Heart, Lung, and Blood Institute tells us—in fact it's what almost every leading body of experts in this field tells us *on paper*. That's because it's good, reasonable public health policy. *However:* off the record, they always say that 30% is really *more* than most women should eat—and that 25% would go much further in cutting the risk of heart disease, obesity and cancer. They don't say it often on television or in the paper because (a) they don't want to confuse everyone and (b) they think it may be too much to ask of the general public, but they're certainly advising their loved ones to cut fat even lower than official guidelines suggest, so you should be aware of it too! I say let's be realistic: if you're eating 40% of your total calories from fat, let's begin with trying to get your intake down *one step at a time:*

Stop cooking with fat. If you do, you'll eliminate an enormous amount of the fat in your diet. Get nonstick pans and stop dropping butter into the skillet every time you cook. Another approach: use non-stick cooking sprays like Pam instead of butter, margarine or cooking oil. If you must use fat for cooking, make the switch from saturated fats like lard and butter to polyunsaturated fats like peanut or corn oil or, best of all, to monounsaturated fats like olive and canola oil. The reason it's important to reduce *all* oils, however, is that researchers simply don't know for sure which ones are harmful. Dr. Lee Wattenberg of the University of Minnesota and Dr. Rowan Chlebowski of the American Society of Clinical Oncology both point to research suggesting that corn oil promotes breast cancer in animals. It's still preliminary, they say, but it's intriguing. And to make matters even more confusing, monounsaturated fats may in fact be *good* for us to eat: Much research is being done on the subject. *No oil at all* is best for cooking—vegetables are just wonderful steamed—but if you aren't ready for that leap yet, at least make the move to better types of fat. Coconut and palm oils, plus hydrogenated fats, are among the worst choices. Discover broiling, boiling, poaching, roasting and baking as healthy, delicious alternatives to frying.

Avoid processed foods. Fat is hidden in many of the foods we eat. Most of us know that it's in fried donuts and processed cakes, but you'd be surprised to find it in seemingly harmless crackers as well. Just read the label and if you see lots of grams of fat or tropical oils on the ingredient list (palm oil, coconut oil, etc.), be strong and move on down the supermarket aisle. Thanks to new-and-improved labeling system designed by the Food and Drug Administration, you can now trust most products that say "low-fat" or "no-fat". This is far more valuable than a "no-cholesterol" promise.

Give up, or limit, toppings and dressings. Broccoli may be great for you but if you top it with fatty dressing, you offset its benefits. A lot of this may be habit. You might not even know how good a potato tastes with just some chopped scallions on it. Or if you're simply addicted to sour cream, try the nonfat version—*you'll* hardly know the difference, but your heart will.

Choose low-fat versions of dairy and other foods. Just switching from whole milk and high-fat yogurts and cheeses to the nonfat versions of these foods will dramatically lower the amount of fat you eat each day, notes Dr. Rivlin. If you used to think that low-fat foods tasted terrible, it's time for a trip back to the grocery store. Manufacturers have come a long, long way—many nonfat treats are actually tasty!

Trim the fat off meats and chicken. When you tug the skin off chicken, you turn it from a fatty to a healthy food. Choose cuts of beef like flank and round that have less fat to begin with, and when you use fattier cuts of meat (which should be *rarely!*) trim off as much visible fat both before and after cooking as possible. Women eat too much meat in the first place, says Dr. Walter Willett of the Harvard School of Public Health. And that means not only too much fat, but also excessive animal protein which leeches calcium from our bones, he says. The goal should be to move from meats to fruits, vegetables and grains. But when you *do* choose meat, be sure to cook it in such a way that excess fat can run off, (on grills, on slotted pans under the broiler, etc.).

Be fat-savvy at the salad bar. You may think that because it's a salad, it's low-fat. Not true. Many salad bar items, such as avocado, chopped eggs, cheese and so on are loaded with fat. Go for the simple, fresh vegetables and the beans (watching for too many calories and for oils on premade bean salads).

These changes alone may be enough to take you from the unhealthy average fat intake level to the under-30% goal. Keep these same points in mind when you're ordering in restaurants or even in fast-food eateries; if it's grilled or baked, it's better than fried, so the grilled chicken sandwich with a baked potato will be much better than the fried burger with french fries. Be tough and tell them to hold the mayo; just as a fatty salad dressing can ruin the health benefits of a pile of leafy greens, so the secret sauces on many fast food sandwiches can transform a healthy grilled treat into yet another plateful of fat. If you make these small changes in all areas of your diet—eliminating a bit of fat here and there all day long—before you know it, your habits will be changed and your overall fat intake cut dramatically.

LIMITING SALT

Americans eat too much salt. For most of us, it isn't a big health problem. For others with salt-sensitive hypertension or fluid retention (as we discuss further in chapter 24, "Heart Disease, Heart Health") it can be dangerous. Cutting salt in the diet is much easier, and tastier, than you think.

Eliminate Salt from Cooking.

When I first visited my in-laws in Portland, Oregon and heard that they cook with no salt at all, I wondered what the food was going to taste like. I was in for a great surprise, and a learning experience. For the first time, I enjoyed foods *without* salt that I had never liked *with it.* Pacific Northwestern cooking, known for its liberal use of fresh herbs and spices, lemon and other salt alternatives, is as or more flavorful than most other styles of cooking I've tried. Fresh herbs are the best choice, but if you don't have them, dried versions are delicious too. When your food is suffused with rosemary, thyme, different kinds of pepper, lemon and lime, flavorful vinegars, oregano, garlic and onion, various seeds, curries and myriad other spices, you will *never* miss the salt. For the most part, salt is a matter of habit. Replace it with tastier, healthier habits and you'll never look back. Cooking creatively with herbs and spices is also a good way to move away from fatty, oily foods.

If you're worried about the cost of using fresh foods with fresh herbs, become a season-sensitive shopper. Buy what's in season and you'll keep the price down. Also, something as inexpensive as baking chicken with orange juice is better than cooking it with salt and butter.

Eliminate Table Salt.

You may have the bad habit, as many Americans do, of shaking salt onto foods even before you taste them. Try taking a bite of your new salt-free or salt-light foods *before* adding table salt. Get the salt shaker off the table to begin with. Replace it with a pepper grinder. With time, you'll stop noticing the salt isn't there.

Watch For Heavily Salted Condiments.

Some mustards, ketchup, picked relishes and so on are loaded with salt. Replace them with low-salt versions (they're widely available in supermarkets) or try fresh vegetables instead: a slice of fresh tomato tastes better than ketchup on a burger.

Limit Prepared and Canned Foods.

Frozen prepared foods and canned foods are often loaded with salt you can't even taste. The amount in even some prepared diet foods, which you probably assume are very good for you, can be quite high. Cooking foods yourself is the best idea, but if you don't have time, start reading labels carefully. Choose low- or no-salt versions of canned and prepared foods (and limit the use of these non-fresh items as much as possible).

WONDERING IF YOU NEED A DAILY NUTRITION SUPPLEMENT?

You might, and you might not. You've probably heard a lot about certain kinds of nutrients, like antioxidants (vitamins C, E and beta carotene, a precursor to vitamin A) which may help fight diseases like cancer and heart disease. And we've already discussed the impact of calcium supplementation on bone health. Indeed there is a fascinating proliferation of research to suggest that foods, or nutrients, can be used to prevent disease. We're at a major crossroad in our understanding and belief about the role of nutrition not just to preserve life, but to actively prevent illness, or even reverse its early signs. The field, nutritional medicine, may represent the future of health maintenance in a world where high-tech medicine is breaking the bank. Supplements, not just real foods, clearly will play a meaningful role in this movement—but how great that role will or should be is still uncertain.

It's not all that surprising to think that nutrients might protect us from illness when you consider that many of the great lifesaving medications we use today were derived from plants. The key questions are which nutrients protect us, how much of them to take, and can we be *hurt* by large amounts of the very same vitamins that protect us in small quantities? You've probably noticed a proliferation of vitamin stores, suggesting that the best way to be healthy is to get your nutrients in tablet form. For most of us, this just isn't the case. If we eat a balanced diet, we don't need pills to prevent deficiencies. But since so many women fall short on basic nutrients, it's not a bad idea to take a single, one-tablet-a-day multivitamin for nutrient coverage. It is subject to scientific debate whether we should add specialized nutrients, like antioxidants, on top of that single pill. At this point, I suggest you talk to your individual doctor about what might be best for you. One thing most nutrition experts agree on is that you *do not* need, and may be harmed by, excessive doses of so-called megavitamins—especially those that contain vitamins that are stored in the fat of our bodies and can become toxic, like vitamins A and D. Other megavitamin tablets have a mythical effect in the first place, since we urinate the excess vitamin content out of our bodies, rather than using it!

The focus of diet and nutrition should always be on foods, not pills. Pills don't contain many of the macronutrients—bulky fiber, for example—that your body needs for fuel. We were built to chew, to taste, to experience and live on whole foods, not nutritional tablets. Make the foundation of your diet real, whole, fresh foods, and fill in the gaps, if you wish, with supplements. Jeffrey Blumberg, associate director of the human nutrition research center on aging at Tufts University, urges women to remember that vitamin pills are called "supplements" for a reason: they *supplement,* rather than *substitute,* for foods.

NUTRITION NOTES FOR OLDER WOMEN

As we age it becomes more difficult to keep a healthy nutrient balance for two reasons: first, we tend to absorb the nutrients from foods less efficiently than we used to; and second, we often have formed limited, poor eating habits (experts call it the "tea and toast" problem) for a variety of reasons (perhaps we don't eat enough total calories because we're less active these days and don't want to become overweight; maybe we are alone and can't or won't cook well-balanced meals for ourselves). Whatever the many reasons for it, we must reverse

this trend, since it sets up a vicious cycle of nutrient loss, weakness, inactivity and poor health. The old myth that older people are less active and therefore *need* fewer nutrients is being replaced, Jeffrey Blumberg says, by a new and more aggressive theory, in which we acknowledge that many older people have *greater* nutritional needs than younger people.

There are many experts who feel that older women absolutely need a multivitamin supplement each day, plus calcium supplementation to get the nutrients they need. If you choose the supplement route, be careful about the kind you choose and don't overdo any single nutrient (*See* section on supplementation below). Others feel that older women, like younger ones, can succeed in getting what they need from foods alone—with some extra effort. Here are some areas to focus on (for each nutrient, find the food sources listed earlier in this chapter):

Calcium. Shortly before and after menopause, we need as much calcium as possible to offset the tremendous loss of bone (about 15% of our total bone!) that occurs around this time. (*See* page 404 for your recommended calcium intake.)

Vitamin D. Many older women are vitamin D deficient. You must be careful to get enough of this vitamin because it helps calcium absorption at this vulnerable time for your bones. One reason older women fall short on this vitamin is they're less likely to spend time outside, where sunlight is used to synthesize vitamin D in our skin. While younger bodies increase their absorption of vitamin D to make up for less sun exposure, older people often don't have this compensatory ability.

THE PILL BOX

Enjoy reading telephone books? That's what a chart listing all the nutrients in all the multi-vitamin-and-mineral supplements would look like.

Following is a list of supplements compiled by the Center for Science in the Public Interest. They have rated the pills by their nutrient coverage, antioxidant content (a nice way to get some of these protective nutrients without a separate pill), cost, and so on.

The chart tells you which supplements met our criteria (+) for antioxidants ("Antiox") or calcium and magnesium ("Ca/Mg"). You can take what's missing (—) separately. It also lists about how much a month's supply costs ("$/Month"), as well as how many IUs of its vitamin A come from beta-carotene ("Beta-C").

The number in parentheses following some products' names is the daily dose if it's more than one pill.

SUPPLEMENT	ANTIOX[1]	CA/MG[2]	BETA-C	$/MONTH	COMMENTS
AARP Formulas #131, #195, or #196*	—	—	0	1.26	Standard multis. No chromium. #196 has no iron.
AARP Formula #222 (6)*	+	—	25,000	1.83	Chromium is a tad low (40 mcg). High in magnesium.
American Drug Stores Osco Multiple	—	—	5,000	0.90	Standard multi with some extra beta-carotene. Low in chromium.
Amway Nutrilite Double X (6)*	—	+	2,500	46.95	High in C (500 mg), but not other antioxidants. Low in chromium.
Barth's Ceropure Silver SF*	—	—	6,000	2.18	Same as Centrum Silver.
Bronson Daily Nutritional Packets (2)*	+	—	25,000	14.93	High in C (1,000 mg), E (400 IU), and beta-carotene, but not selenium.
Bronson Peak Performance Formula (6)*	+	—	10,000	17.35	Low in D and calcium (but not magnesium or chromium). Okay for men.
Centrum	—	—	1,000	2.01	Standard multi. Low in chromium. Has many imitators.

1. Antiox. criteria—Has two or more of the following: At least 250 mg of vitamin C, 100 IU of vitamin E, 10,000 IU of beta-carotene, or 50 mcg of selenium.
2. Ca/Mg criteria—Has at least 500 mg of calcium and 200 mg of magnesium.
*Available only by mail order. Most have 800 numbers.

SUPPLEMENT	ANTIOX[1]	CA/MG[2]	BETA-C	$/MONTH	COMMENTS
Centrum Silver	—	—	2,000	3.03	Low in iron and folic acid. High in chromium. Good for seniors.
Country Life Daily Action 75	+	—	5,000	4.48	High in C (250 mg) and E (150 IU), but not beta-carotene or selenium.
Futurebiotics Vegetarian Super Multi	+	—	15,000	2.99	Low in calcium and magnesium. High in chromium. Okay for men.
Geritol Complete	—	—	6,000	3.03	Too high in iron. Low in chromium.
GNC Mega-One (2)	+	—	5,000	10.00	High in C (300 mg) and E (300 IU), but not beta-carotene or selenium.
GNC Solotron	—	—	5,000	3.50	Low in copper and chromium. Some extra C (200 mg) and beta-carotene.
KAL High Potency Soft Multiple (2)	+	—	10,000	11.98	Selenium is the only antioxidant missing. Low in chromium.
KAL Mega Vita-min	+	—	15,000	6.49	Too much A from fish oil. Low in copper and selenium. High in chromium.
Myadec	—	—	1,250	2.88	Standard multi with extra iron. Low in chromium.
Natrol My Favorite Multiple (4)	+	+	10,000	18.39	One of the most complete we found . . . but expensive.
Nature Made Essential Balance	—	—	1,200	1.62	Standard multi with a bit extra C (120 mg). Low in chromium.
Nature's Bounty Natural Ultra Vita-Time	—	—	5,000	3.45	Low in E, copper, zinc, and selenium. No chromium.
Nature's Plus Ultra Two (2)	+	—	15,000	16.65	No copper. Not high in selenium or C (100 mg). Too much A. High in iron.
One-A-Day Maximum Formula Tablets	—	—	2,500	2.61	Standard multi. Low in chromium.
Puritan's Pride Mega Vita-gels*	—	—	2,000	5.38	High in C (300 mg) and E (300 IU), but not beta-carotene or selenium.

SUPPLEMENT	ANTIOX[1]	CA/MG[2]	BETA-C	$/MONTH	COMMENTS
Puritan's Pride One*	—	—	5,000	4.55	Vitamin C is 250 mg, but other antioxidants are low. High in chromium.
Rite-Aid One Daily + Minerals	—	—	5,000	1.35	Standard multi with some extra beta-carotene. Low in chromium.
Safeway One Tablet Daily & Minerals	—	—	5,000	1.98	Standard multi with some extra beta-carotene. Low in chromium.
Schiff All RDA (4)	—	+	5,000	7.96	Standard multi with some extra beta-carotene. No chromium.
Schiff Mega Hi II	+	—	2,000	4.68	No selenium or chromium.
Shaklee Vita-Lea (2)*	—	+	0	6.73	Standard multi with calcium. No beta-carotene or chromium.
Solgar Multi II Caps (2)	—	—	2,000	11.35	High in C (300 mg) and E (150 IU), but not beta-carotene or selenium.
Solgar Formula VM-75 Tablets	+	—	7,500	6.06	Low in selenium and chromium. No copper.
Theragran-M	—	—	1,000	2.91	High in iron. Low in chromium. Has many imitators.
Twinlab Dualtabs (4)	+	+	15,000	24.60	One of the most complete we found . . . but expensive. Low in iron.
Twinlab SuperTwin	+	—	17,500	11.88	Low in calcium and magnesium. High in chromium. Okay for men.
Unicap M or T	—	—	0	2.45	Standard multi. "T" is high in C (500 mg). No chromium.
Your Life Daily Pak for Women (5)	+	+	0	7.89	Low in beta-carotene, selenium, magnesium, and folic acid. No chromium.

All information obtained from manufacturers. ■ The use of information from this article for commercial purposes is prohibited without written permission from CSPI. ■ Information compiled by David Huang and Juliann Goldman.

Vitamin B$_{12}$. Many older people are found to be vitamin B$_{12}$ deficient because they're unable to absorb this important nutrient. The scary thing is, B$_{12}$ deficiency causes symptoms that resemble senility or dementia—forgetfulness, confusion, etc. Often these problems in older people are written off as Alzheimer's disease or just plain aging, when several months of B$_{12}$ injections in the hospital could cure the entire problem. Vitamin B$_{12}$ is a good one to get from a daily multivitamin, but if you're having problems with clear thinking or memory, talk to your doctor about it and make sure your absorption is okay and that there is no nutritional explanation for your problems.

Riboflavin. Some say the RDA for riboflavin is too low for older people. Milk is a good source, especially if it's in a cardboard container; some of the riboflavin is destroyed when it's in plastic containers under bright lights.

Folate and chromium. Many older women fall short on chromium and folate intake. A well-balanced diet filled with grains and vegetables will help, but some experts think supplementation is needed here. Things may improve if foods like cereal, bread and flour become folate-enriched, which is now under consideration.

Total Calories.

Make sure you don't fall into the trap of eating less when you need to eat more. If you stay active, your caloric intake needn't change. The reason so many older people need fewer and fewer calories is they're becoming more and more sedentary. If you remain active, which you absolutely should, you need to eat like an active person. Eating less predisposes you to the kinds of nutrient deficiencies we've been talking about.

What Older Women Should Watch Out For.

Be careful not to get too much vitamin A or D since these vitamins are stored in your body fat. Your liver isn't as efficient at clearing them out of the body as it used to be—and these vitamins can become toxic at high levels.

It's also worth noting that there a few nutrients women need *less* of as we age. Iron is one of them. When you stop menstruating, your iron needs drop. There's rarely a need for iron supplementation in postmenopausal women.

DIET CHANGES COMBINED: MAKING IT ALL HANG TOGETHER

Are you worried that you'll never be able to incorporate the information on fat, fiber, calcium, salt and so on into your real-life eating habits—especially if you're a busy person and don't have time to calculate percentages and grams of this and that? You're not alone. I've heard from many women who complain that unless you keep a pocket calculator on your body at all times, it's next to impossible to make *all* of the recommended diet changes at once. Your mind may be rattling with numbers: less than 30% fat; 1200 milligrams of calcium; and wait, how many grams of fiber was it?

Well I have some good news for you. The diet changes we've been discussing throughout this chapter *complement* one another: they don't conflict. To prove it, I enlisted the help of Dr. Johanna Dwyer, director of the Frances Stern Nutrition Center at Tufts University. She developed a weeklong menu of meals and snacks, which incorporates all of the bone-healthy, heart-healthy, anticancer diet recommendations for women we've discussed in this chapter (and all within an average weight-maintaining calorie range). (*See* Appendix.) With time and experience, you'll learn to make substitutions to this diet while keeping the nutritional content stable: for instance, you may want to replace one calcium-rich food with another; switch one citrus fruit for another; replace tuna fish with canned salmon; and so on. The revisions you make probably won't *precisely* match this diet, but they'll bring you pretty close to a well-balanced meal plan, with the fat level in check. Over time, with this weeklong diet as a guide, your healthy food selections will become more automatic.

OTHER WAYS TO MAKE HEALTHY FOOD CHOICES

If you don't like following meal plans, and prefer to choose from a wide variety of foods, a couple of expert groups have put together information that makes it all much simpler than it used to be. First, there's the new FDA Food Label. While it came under some criticism for not being simple *enough,* I think it's quite useful, and certainly will help protect you from false health claims (like "lite," and "low-fat," which now have regulated meanings). The best thing about the label is it gives you the total number of grams of fat (and saturated fat), cholesterol, fiber and sodium you should get in a day—and it gives you this information for both a 2000-calorie-a-day diet and a 2500-calorie-a-day diet (this is all at the bottom of the food label). Up top, the food label gives you the

number of grams of fiber, fat and so on in one serving of this particular food. So all you need to do is match the information at the bottom of the label (a full-day's needs) with the information at the top of the label (this single food item's values). If you know you need about 25 grams of fiber each day, and your bowl of cereal has about 5 grams of dietary fiber, you know you're a fifth of the way there—not much in the way of math. Or let's say you want no more than 30% of your total calories from fat in a given day, and you find that this one food has 40% of calories from fat; you'll want the *next* food you eat to have *less*—say 10% or 15% of calories from fat, to keep things evened out. The label helps you watch total calories, too, which gives you an idea of how much of your daily allotment you've consumed. The only caveat about calories is the FDA food label gives you a slightly higher caloric intake than some women actually get. For instance, if you eat 1700 calories a day (and *not* 2000), you'll need to adjust the information on the label a bit to get the right information for *you.* So if a given food provides 20% of the recommended calories from fat in a 2000-calorie diet, it actually provides over 23% for a 1700-calorie-a-day diet.

Another extremely useful chart is the USDA food pyramid, which gives you the basic outline of healthy eating.

As you can see, the old "four basic food groups" concept has gone out the window in favor of a stepped eating plan. Foods at the bottom of the pyramid (covering the largest space) are grains, pastas, breads, cereals and other healthy complex carbohydrate/fiber foods. Moving all the way to the top you see fatty foods, which take up the least space on the pyramid, just as they should take up the least

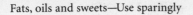
Fats, oils and sweets—Use sparingly

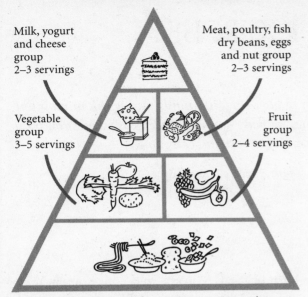

Milk, yogurt
and cheese
group
2–3 servings

Meat, poultry, fish
dry beans, eggs
and nut group
2–3 servings

Vegetable
group
3–5 servings

Fruit
group
2–4 servings

Bread, cereal, rice and pasta group 6–11 servings

Source: U.S. Department of Agriculture

space in your diet.

We've gone over the fact that it isn't hard to make healthy changes in your diet. But the most important question is: How can you get motivated to implement those changes in the first place? One answer comes from Jacqueline Whitted, a public health analyst at the National Cancer Institute. She has found that people make changes when the motivators are "culturally relevant" to them. For instance, in her work with women in African-American communities, she has discovered that by focusing on the matriarchal society (influencing the grandmother and in turn the family as a whole) she can create a domino effect of healthy behaviors that affects all generations in a family. The process of choosing, buying and preparing foods thus becomes a supportive, interactive

one—which reinforces women's ability to stick with their new healthy habits. Try to create healthy support systems within your own immediate community—with friends, family or colleagues. Don't allow people to undermine your new efforts to eat right, and ignore naysayers who claim you can't do it. Make your new healthy habits a part of your greater social network and they are more likely to endure.

FOR MORE INFORMATION ON NUTRITION AND DIET

AMERICAN DIETETIC ASSOCIATION
216 West Jackson Blvd., Suite 800
Chicago, IL 60606
800-366-1655

FOOD AND NUTRITION INFORMATION CENTER
National Agricultural Library
10301 Baltimore Blvd., Room 304
Beltsville, MD 20705-2351
301-504-5719

CENTER FOR SCIENCE IN THE PUBLIC INTEREST/NUTRITION ACTION HEALTH LETTER
1875 Connecticut Ave. NW, Suite 300
Washington, DC 20009
202-332-9110

NATIONAL DIGESTIVE DISEASES INFORMATION CLEARINGHOUSE
2 Information Way
Bethesda, MD 20892-3570
301-654-3810

CHAPTER TWENTY-ONE

EXERCISE

Sedentary people are apt to have sluggish minds. A sluggish mind is apt to be reflected in flabbiness of body and in a dullness of expression that invites no interest and gets none.

—Rose Fitzgerald Kennedy

For those of us who were born in the U.S. in the mid-20th century, there should have been a sign posted in the delivery room: "Welcome to the couch potato generation." For more reasons than you can count, including the proliferation of telephones, automobiles, television sets and desk jobs in front of computers, many of us have been shifted from our feet to our bottoms. As a result we're overweight, have poor strength, lots of obesity and weakness-associated illnesses, chronic aches and pains, and excessive pent-up tension.

Women are thought to be at greatest risk of many of these problems. Partly because we are not socialized around sports to the same degree men are, we've traditionally spent more time at home where couch life is readily available. And these days, because so many of us fill multiple life roles that leave little time for recreational, let alone physical activity, we're even more likely to be sedentary. The result? Starting at 25 years of age, experts say we will replace one pound of muscle with one pound of fat *each year!*

No more excuses. Women have to become more active if we want to improve the way we feel, the quality and possibly the length of our lives, and our overall health. We live longer than men on average: but we're undermining our health and strength before we get to a ripe old age. Diana McNab, a sports psychologist at Seton Hall University, feels that society has made women so "sewn up" and repressed that exercise is more vital than ever. As she puts it, we need to get sweaty, greasy, earthy, dirty, smelly and crazy—exercise must pull us out of ourselves so we can really start living. Most of us know that we have to become more active to be healthier. The trouble is, we don't know how or where to start, what it takes to be fit, and how to make time for it in our complicated lives.

Many of us are afraid to start exercising after months or even years of inactivity. If we're weak or overweight, we may be embarrassed to get out there and expose ourselves to the fit world. If we're sick or frail, we may not want to risk harming ourselves. The fact is, almost *any* woman can become more active—and safely. In this chapter, we'll go through some of the specifics on *how* to become more fit no matter what your starting point is. There's advice for women who have fallen out of shape and want to get back into it, for those who have never been fit in their lives, and for those who want to boost their current level of fitness. We'll take a look at some of the weaknesses unique to women, and how to reverse them. And we'll see the vast number of health benefits, both physical and emotional, that can result from getting in shape.

EXERCISE: WHAT YOU HAD TO SAY ABOUT IT

Barbara, 45 years old
I hate exercise more than anything in the world! I have severe pain from arthritis in both knees and bursitis in my hip. I'm walking because it's good for me, it's a way to be healthier. I enjoy walking when I can and swimming in a pool.

I'm six feet tall and over 200 pounds, I'm a large person. Unfortunately I guess I was the largest one in the [exercise] class and the other women were very fit and that was discouraging. At 45 when I see women my age who are very fit it's very discouraging to me, and it does hurt like hell, so I didn't go. I walk where no one knows me. I don't have to answer to anyone, I do it on my own. I go as often as I can, if I can go three times, great, if I can go five times a week, great. And I do feel that's my time for me, that's important.

Danielle, 21 years old
I play Division One soccer. Being unfit is the worst feeling, when you're unfit your performance goes down, other players beat you, you can't perform. When you're fit your whole attitude and body feels great, you're able to do more, you feel better about yourself, instead of walking with your head down you walk with your head up.

I want to be a coach: now that I'm in college, I try to teach the kids I coach how to be fit. I run, I lift, [my coach] keeps me on a nutrition program, a low-fat diet. She has let me realize that the food you eat can either hinder or help your performance. I wish someone had told me earlier.

Patty, 51 years old
I decided to go to school to be certified in aerobic health fitness and circuit training at age 49. [Before that] I played tennis mostly, and paddle tennis. I played on teams. Exercise was not really part of my life until my mid-30s. I grew up in a home where there wasn't much opportunity for women, my brothers were tremendous athletes, I was a spectator.

It's a whole fullness of life, you wake up every morning so happy, the day is here and I attribute it to this feeling of well-being. It's definitely being in shape. There aren't enough hours in the day. Some is psychological I'm sure. You know the saying, "Another day, another chance to be healthy"? It's like I can bike, I can swim or walk or play tennis or run. Now is the time to do everything. It's hard to remember back in my 20s, I feel better in my 50s than I did five years ago.

Another saying I love is "As I see it, today couldn't possibly have grown out of yesterday as I remember it."

Fitness Goals

The first thing you have to ask yourself is why you want to start an exercise program. Is it because you want to look better? Fit into a certain type of clothing? Flatten your stomach after pregnancy? Feel better when you run up a flight of stairs? All of these things can result from better fitness. But the smartest goals you can have are (1) to improve the health of your heart, lungs and other body systems; (2) to improve your strength and flexibility so that every task you perform in life feels easier, and you can do them all better; (3) to improve your mood and self-esteem. These are the basic health and functioning improvements that come with fitness. They require you to make exercise a lifetime commitment, not just a brief means to an end. As we discuss in chapter 22, just as the concept of weight *loss* should be replaced by the goal of healthy weight *maintenance* over a lifetime, so the pursuit of short-term exercise for a specific goal (getting into a bathing suit for summer) should be replaced by the goal of lifetime activity and vigor. Throughout this chapter, we'll focus on both strength and cardiovascular fitness. The additional benefits you can expect, including weight loss, maintenance of bone health, firming and toning

your body and so on, will also happen when you follow this plan. But our underlying focus will be exercising for health and well-being.

What It Takes to Become Fit

Diana McNab likes to say that becoming fit requires one key word: GOYA (Get off your ass). Others are more formal in their recommendations. In 1990, the American College of Sports Medicine (ACSM) issued a position statement on physical fitness for adults. It outlined the three key features of a successful fitness plan for the average person. Naturally, if you have particular health problems, you'll want to talk to your doctor about tailoring these recommendations to your needs. Anyone over 35 or with medical problems who is starting an exercise program, or changing one's activities to a significant degree, should seek doctor approval beforehand. At the other end of the spectrum, if you're in very good shape and want to get *more* fit, you'll want to aim for the tougher end of these recommendations.

The three key elements of exercise that you must consider for your plan are *frequency*, *intensity* and *duration*. The ACSM recommends the following basic plan for healthy adults:

Frequency: 3–5 Days a Week.

Exercising fewer than three days a week doesn't provide much fitness benefit (though it may be fun). On the other hand, exercising *too often* may predispose some of us to injuries (although many fitness experts, such as Christine Wells, professor of exercise science and physical education at Arizona State University, feel that *moderate* exercise such as walking every day of the week is a great idea).

Intensity: 60–90% of Your Maximum Heart Rate or 50–85% of Your Maximum Oxygen Uptake.

Since you'll need a sophisticated sports lab to tell you your maximum oxygen uptake, most of us should rely on the first figure, our maximum heart rate, when planning a fitness program. Here's how you can compute it. Subtract your age from 220. Let's say you're 40 years old. That means your maximum heart rate is 180. Take 60% of that and you get 108 beats per minute. Take 90% of 180 and you get 162. According to this plan, in order to achieve the best cardiovascular benefits from exercise, you should shoot for a heart rate of between 108 and 162 for the duration of your exercise. While you're exercising, to be sure you're in the right range, take your pulse once in a while (look at the second hand on your watch for ten seconds and count the number of beats you feel, then multiply that number by six. If things are going according to plan, the number you get will fall into your so-called "target range").

How fast should you go? That varies. A light stroll won't do much for your heart and lungs, though it very well may improve your mood, reduce pain from arthritic or just "rusty" joints, and start you on your way to a more vigorous fitness plan. To boost your heart and lung health, you need a little more speed: the exact amount will vary from person to person, but for walking, figure on a pretty good clip with your arms pumping forward and back, and some good breathing in and out, to get cardiovascular benefits. Follow the prescription above to see how your heart rate is doing: that's really the best way to measure that you're exercising at an appropriate level. If you want an exact speed prescription for *your* body type and overall health, ask for a fitness evaluation by a local coach (from the gym or Y, e.g.), or perhaps from your family doctor.

Duration: 20–60 Minutes of Continuous Aerobic Activity.

Most fitness experts feel that the longer you exercise, up to a point, the better—particularly for goals like weight loss or maintenance and cardiovascular health. Obviously, since you want this to be fun and you don't want to hurt yourself, you should consider dropping the intensity of your exercise when you increase the duration. Working out for an hour at 60% of your maximum heart rate is probably healthier, for the average person, than exercising for 20 minutes at 90% of your maximum heart rate.

These are the ACSM's recommendations for aerobic activity. They also made recommendations for so-called resistance training, or strength training. Weight lifting is the classic resistance training sport. The ACSM recommends that adults do some form of resistance training at least two times a week, with a minimum of eight to ten different exercises that work the major muscle groups of the body, doing at least one "set" of eight to twelve repetitions of each exercise.

WOMEN AND STRENGTH TRAINING

Strength training is very important for women in particular, since we have particular problems with upper body weakness. According to Cedric Bryant, former strength and conditioning coach at Penn State University and one-time strength coordinator at the United States Military Academy at West Point, women have enormous potential for increasing strength and endurance.

Those who can not do a single pull-up —and that includes most American women—can do ten of them after a couple of months of proper training. If you're not the type to go to a gym, fill a couple of milk containers with water or sand, he suggests, and start lifting them slowly at home. (Canned food can work, too.) You might want to ask someone with knowledge about weight lifting for the proper positioning and exercises to choose so you don't hurt yourself. You'll want to try a variety of exercises, including holding the cartons out in front of you and pulling your arms up and down, toward the floor and then toward the ceiling; opening your arms to the side and pulling the cartons toward your shoulders as if you were making muscles like Popeye; and many others.

If you're worried that weight lifting will turn you into a muscle woman, don't be concerned: if you use light weights and do multiple repetitions, you'll tone and strengthen your muscles, rather than building them up. If on the other hand you *want* to build muscle bulk, you can do so by increasing the amount of weight you're lifting and doing fewer repetitions per set. It's a good idea to talk to a weight training specialist at least once before starting a routine. First, you need advice on how to lift weights properly, since doing it wrong can lead to injuries, including overextension of vulnerable joints. Second, by seeking expert opinion, you can set up a plan that's tailored to your strength and functioning needs. If, for instance, you have a painful lower back, you may need extra abdominal exercises to strengthen that area. If your shoulders are aching from overuse and underdevelopment, you can focus on these areas. The key is to lift slowly and rhythmically, and to breathe in and out smoothly, experts say.

Afraid you're too old to start weight lifting? Unless you're over 110, you're probably wrong. I'll never forget a shoot I did for CBS on weight lifting for older people. A researcher at Stanford University was training people in their 70s, 80s and older to lift weights and improve their overall strength and flexibility. One woman in her 70s who had pretty much given up gardening and said she'd reached a point where she couldn't even pick up a bag of groceries, told me that after the strength training she was able to climb a tree in her backyard to do pruning! That was after just several months of weight training. Certainly when you're older—or more important, when you're out of shape and haven't used your muscles in years—you want to start any program slowly. But around the country there are more and more programs for strength training among older people, and they don't have age limits. After getting clearance from your doctor, look into programs like this one near you. Your local hospital, Y, health club, senior center or other group may offer something appropriate. The potential benefits are enormous, including everything from getting out of a chair more easily to walking up stairs, carrying groceries, picking up grandchildren and, who knows, maybe even winning a few bodybuilding contests. The independence you'll gain with strength training leads to better self-esteem and a sense of well-being at *any* age.

CHOOSING EXERCISE ACTIVITIES: A GUIDE FOR WOMEN

There is no limit to the number of activities from which women can choose. Gone are the days when there were "male" sports and "female" sports. Whether you like running, walking, cross-country skiing, rowing, swimming, biking, playing organized sports like squash, tennis or basketball, skating, dancing, doing dance aerobics, hiking or anything else, you'll get benefits from all of them. Most fitness experts say the more you mix up your workouts, the better. This is called cross training—a program in which you might walk one day, swim another, and bike on a third. Cross training is great for you because it reduces the constant stress and strain on the same set of muscles and joints, and helps you become strong all over your body—not just in your legs with cycling, for example.

Since women are vulnerable to bone loss (osteoporosis) at the time of menopause, certain exercises that help retain bone density are especially good for us. These include all so-called weight-bearing exercises. They include any exercise for which you have to carry your own weight—such as walking, running and dancing. Sports where your weight is buoyed, like swimming, aren't as good for bone protection. Cycling falls somewhere in the middle, depending on how hard you're working your body (pedaling uphill is better, for example). Weight lifting itself is great for maintaining bone density. Barbara Drinkwater of The Pacific Medical Center in Seattle, a leading national expert on exercise and its impact on bone, says that at *all ages,* those who exercise have greater bone density (as much as 10% greater) than those who are sedentary. She points to frightening research done on people who were put to bed for long periods of time and lost as much as 1% of their bone density each week! Furthermore, Drinkwater notes that since exercise builds better strength, coordination and flexibility, we're less likely to fall and break our

bones as we age if we stay fit.

Weight-bearing exercise helps more with weight loss than does non-weight-bearing exercise. Since many American women are overweight, activities where we have to lug our bodies around may be especially helpful.

LIKING YOUR CHOICE OF ACTIVITY

When trying to decide which exercise(s) is right for you, keep one key thing in mind: you have to *like* it. You'll never keep doing it if you don't, and since the goal is a lifetime of movement, you have to find something you'll stick with and enjoy. There has to be *some* activity out there that you will enjoy. If you haven't found it yet, keep trying different ones. Maybe if you can't find an exercise that you like per se, you may be able to find one that makes sense for other reasons—such as the fact that your neighbor, spouse or best friend will do it with you, or the fact that it takes you to a beautiful place (walking in a park, in the woods, or down streets with interesting shops and people-watching). Diana McNab says to choose an activity that's suited to your personality. For instance, if you're a perfectionist, end-result oriented, successful and "type A," your activity should be *fun* and playful. If on the other hand you're a light, playful person, you should consider a more formal exercise class with a beginning, middle and an end. Sound unusual? McNab has found that women are more likely to enjoy and stick with activities that are different from (and thus more refreshing than) their regular routine.

You might also try mixing up your activities to keep from getting bored. Walk one day, go dancing the next, and jump rope the third. At least you won't suffer from the monotony of it. Most people will stumble upon something they actually find fun, in spite of themselves!

ATHLETIC WEAKNESSES COMMON IN WOMEN

I mentioned that women tend to have poor upper body strength—and, as we discuss somewhat in chapter 4 on bone health, that can result in chronic upper body aches and pains. A combination of strength and flexibility training can make up for these weaknesses in a relatively short period of time. Some experts worry that with the increase in walking as a favorite form of aerobic, weight-bearing exercise for women (and it *is* an excellent choice), the arms and other upper-body muscles are being neglected further. If you're only doing a lower-body exercise, be absolutely sure to try some of the upper-body strength training we spoke of earlier. Also, when you're walking (or running, or dancing, or skating) *use* your upper body as much as possible. Flex and swing your arms, pump your fists in front of you; keep your upper body moving and working. This boosts the cardiovascular benefits of exercise as well.

Dr. Mona Shangold, co-author of *The Complete Sports Medicine Book for Women,* says that one of the biggest problems for women is not knowing how *much,* and what types, of activities are needed for fitness. As a result, Shangold finds many women still believe that doing toe-touches will tone their bodies. While stretching is certainly important, it does little for cardiovascular health or building muscle strength. You must combine stretching, aerobic activity and strength training to reap meaningful benefits.

Other vulnerabilities that have received attention in women include knee troubles due to a wide variety of problems, ranging from weak leg muscles to occasional problems with hip-knee alignment, (called the Q-angle). According to Christine Wells, this has been overplayed—not *all* women have problematic Q-angles. But many experts say that for those who do, special training of the leg muscles that support the knee can reduce the risk of pain and injury. Most knee problems in women result from long disuse followed by quick reentry into exercise without proper strength and flexibility preparation. Dr. Kimberly Fagan, director of the medical aspects of sports medicine at the University of Alabama, Birmingham, notes that many overuse injuries in women occur when we try to get back in shape after childbirth, or when we reach our 30s after fairly sedentary 20s, and we jump in too fast. The best way to protect knees is to strengthen the quadriceps, as well as the other major muscles in both the front and the back of the legs. The stronger these support muscles are, the less stress you'll place on your knee. Most important, says Dr. Fagan, is to start out slowly (5 minutes on a bike is fine) and build up gradually.

According to Dr. Carol Otis, director of specialty clinics at UCLA's student health services and chairperson of the American College of Sports Medicine Task Force on Women's Issues In Sports Medicine, there are three muscle groups that tend to be particularly weakened in women in their 30s (or older) who have been working behind desks, wearing high heels and being sedentary for a period of time. These weak areas are the abdominal muscles, the anterior thigh muscles (that is, the muscles in front of the thighs) and the anterior tibial muscles (the ones that cause shin splints). Dr. Otis advises all women who have been out of the world of sports and activity for a significant period of time to work on these muscle groups *before* getting into a new exercise program, in order to reduce the risk of injury and pain. You want to enter your new program feeling relatively strong and flexible to reduce the chance that you'll be forced to—or *want* to—drop out because of discomforts.

Because we have smaller total blood volume than men on average, we may have to be a bit more careful when exercising in extremely dry heat. The reason: we sweat a little less than men, and therefore run a greater risk of overheating. The solution is to drink plenty of water, more than you think you need (don't wait until you're thirsty), and use common sense: when the temperature is extremely high and the humidity low, watch your activity level, unless you're a top endurance athlete and you're acclimatized to this type of setting. (We may be at a competitive *advantage* compared to men when in humid athletic settings, Cedric Bryant points out—for the very same reasons listed above.)

There are some myths about women's athletic weakness that must be dispelled. One is that menstruation gets in the way of physical activity. It doesn't. You aren't weaker, or more vulnerable, when you menstruate. You can run, swim, jump or spin when you're menstruating, so don't use it as an excuse—or let anyone else use it as an excuse for why you can't participate in any athletic activity. In fact, some research shows that women who work out regularly—and continue to do so while experiencing menstrual discomfort—can *reduce* physical and emotional symptoms associated with menstruation.

TIMES WHEN WOMEN ARE AT RISK FOR INACTIVITY

Researchers have noted certain times of life when women are vulnerable either to giving up exercise or not doing it altogether. Two notable times are puberty (the beginning of adolescence) and mid-adulthood (around the mid-30s). According to Marcia Ory, a medical sociologist at the National Institute on Aging, the reason these periods of inactivity are so risky is that we do *not* have fitness "banks" in our bodies: it's *not* enough to do a certain amount of activity when we're young and expect it to hold over into adulthood. Fitness must be continuous throughout our lifetimes.

During puberty, while boys are growing taller, more muscular and more physically geared for athleticism, women experience changes in their bodies that move us *away* from the athletic ideal. We grow breasts, our hips widen, we develop more fat on our bodies and we often stop growing. Our bodies make a move toward childbearing, not exercising. But you don't have to look at it this way. There's *no* good reason we can't participate in and enjoy sports of all kinds with our new adult female bodies, and while many girls who excelled in particular sports like gymnastics or ballet will start to drop out—or be pushed out—at this time, there are countless other sports and activities that may be more suited to our developing frames. Unfortunately, social factors quickly come into play at this time as well, says Dr. Carol Otis. While boys are encouraged, even pressured to play sports as part of their normal socialization process, girls get much more peer pressure to engage in nonathletic endeavors—many of which are aimed at pleasing the opposite sex. Teenage girls are pushed to shop in malls more than they're pushed to sweat on tracks and in gyms. This is a shame, for many talented athletes and physically fit young women drop out of athletics at a time when they could be building the best possible habits for a lifetime of good health. If you have daughters, remember this destructive pattern as they reach their teen years, and stress the value of regular exercise for *both* sexes at *all* ages.

For women in their 30s and 40s who have both young children and careers, exercise may be the last thing in the world they have time for, or even interest in. When you're burned out at the end of the day, the last thing you can imagine yourself doing is changing into sweats and sneakers and going to work out. Even if you wish you *could*, you may have nowhere to leave your children—or perhaps you don't even get home until it's too dark to exercise outside and too late to go to a gym. Women in this age group should realize that it is absolutely critical to become physically fit, since menopause is shortly around the corner. We've reached our peak bone mass, and may be starting to lose bone; our risk for heart disease will climb in the next couple of decades. This is the time when exercise is most critical as *preventive medicine*. So despite whatever effort it takes (*see* "Getting Started," below) put movement back into your life before it gets *physically* hard to do so.

There is a piece of good news for sedentary *older* women, however. It's never too late to get started. Women in their 70s and beyond have been shown in studies, to be successful at making exercise a part of their lives after long periods of inactivity. According to Dr. Shanold, exercise can release older women from the vicious cycle of having little muscle, a slowed metabolism, trouble losing fat and even developing dietary deficiencies from trying to keep weight in check through calorie restrictions alone. When older women exercise and build muscle, they can eat more, develop greater energy, and in turn exercise more often and more vigorously.

IN BRIEF: MANAGING ARTHRITIS

Why discuss arthritis in a chapter on exercise? Because many women are unaware that physical activity is among the most effective treatments for this debilitating disease. Arthritis, in its many forms, causes pain and often immobility for millions of women. If you have painful arthritis, you may want nothing more than to lie in bed and never get up. But being sedentary only makes your problem worse. Moderate exercise—carefully controlled, and ideally designed by a physical therapist—can dramatically relieve your discomfort and disability. Whatever your age, and however extensive your arthritis may be, a customized exercise plan can help you to both feel *and* function better.

Before we talk about the role of exercise in treating arthritis, let's briefly discuss two common forms of arthritis in women. While we don't have the space for a lengthy discussion of the many different types of arthritis, the treatments for most forms of the disease are similar.

First, osteoarthritis, often called "wear and tear" arthritis because it develops over time and involves the breakdown of the cushiony cartilage in our joints and consequent painful rubbing of bone on bone, is quite common in *older* women. Signs of osteoarthritis include knobby finger joints (this is far more common in women than in men), as well as the loss of flexibility in joints and sensitivity to weather fluctuations. Often starting in one knee or hip, osteoarthritis moves to the back and neck as well. If you have osteoarthritis, you may feel like you *can't* exercise—that you're just too stiff, uncomfortable or in too much pain. In fact, exercises that increase the range of motion of your joints, increase the strength of your surrounding muscles and improve your balance all can improve your physical condition and sense of well-being. Swimming, weight training and walking are among the activities recommended for people with arthritis. But with your doctor's approval and careful attention to the progression (or regression!) of your disease, there are few activities you cannot enjoy.

Second, rheumatoid arthritis, which affects about three times as many women as men, is marked by pain, swelling, stiffness, redness and warmth in many affected joints. This form of arthritis is an autoimmune disease, in which the body's disease-fighting system turns on its own cells. As a result, other so-called systemic problems can develop (affecting the heart and lungs, for example), along with generalized symptoms such as fever and weakness. Blood tests help distinguish this especially virulent form of arthritis from other types. Again, carefully controlled physical exercise for strength, balance and flexibility can reduce discomfort caused by this disease. Experts say it's especially important, with this kind of arthritis, to find a proper balance between rest and exertion so as to avoid over-taxing your system. Physical therapists and arthritis experts can work together to offer you a customized exercise plan. In addition to formal exercise, just learning to sit, walk and stand with the right posture (again with the help of a trained physical therapist), can help reduce pain. Losing excessive weight takes stress off your joints and can greatly relieve arthritis pain and cut down the burden on your entire skeleton.

Of course, exercise alone is not adequate treatment for more severe cases of arthritis. Anti-inflammatory drugs (such as aspirin and ibuprofen) are quite useful in the treatment of arthritis; both over-the-counter and prescribed forms can be helpful. More powerful medications including steroids and other potent chemotherapeutic drugs play an important role in treating arthritis, but the "bigger guns," as they're called, should be used with caution and under the careful supervision of doctors watching for complications. In extreme cases where the knee or hip joint is destroyed, joint replacement is now an excellent surgical option for many women. I know of people who ski and play regular tennis on artificial hips.

Low-tech solutions such as heating pads, hot baths and other "home style" remedies also help beat arthritis pain. I met a terrific Texan woman in her late 70s who had a severe case of arthritis. At one point, she could not dress herself or get up out of her chair without assistance. She made a dramatic comeback using a combination of hot wax treatments for her sore hands, daily strength and flexibility exercises to keep her arms and fingers from stiffening, proper medication and sheer will. With the combined therapies she was soon able to rake the leaves in her backyard, drive a car, play outside with her dog and revive her social life.

GETTING STARTED WITH AN EXERCISE PROGRAM—AND FITTING IT INTO YOUR LIFE

The Centers for Disease Control and Prevention, along with the American College of Sports

Medicine, recently made an important announcement. Research showed, they said, that moderate exercise at short intervals throughout the day conferred some of the same benefits as planned, formal exercise for longer periods of time. Walking or running up and down stairs for ten minutes, three times a day, offered some of the same effects as the 30-minute work-out that's so often recommended by fitness experts.

The news is extremely important for anyone who is trying to build exercise into their lives for the first time—or for the first time in a while. It's also great news for those who are so overburdened that they cannot find 30 straight minutes in a day for exercise. This information tells us that the most mundane changes in your behavior—even before you start a more formal exercise regimen—can give you significant health benefits. For example, if you start walking up and down the stairs at work, instead of taking the elevator; walking to pick up your kids at school or to pick up groceries instead of driving; getting off the bus one stop early and walking the rest of the way to your destination; taking a short bike ride with your kids instead of watching TV with them while the water for dinner is getting ready to boil; walking up the street from work to grab lunch at a place with no waiting line, instead of standing still in a cafeteria line—and so on and so on and so on—all of these little ten-minute bursts of activity will make you a healthier person. This is so much less threatening, especially to the busy woman, than the concept of formal exercise. Christine Wells practices what she preaches: she actually *chose* an office on the second floor so she would have to walk the 16 steps up and down each day at work.

Sure, working out for a longer duration and intensity—as discussed earlier—is the best way to boost health and fitness. But for starters, especially for those who are getting going after a period of inactivity—these small changes can make a significant difference over time.

Dr. Otis urges women to set realistic goals when beginning exercise. In addition to getting unused muscles back in shape, she suggests giving yourself a short-term target to get yourself motivated. While it might be hard to imagine exercising every single day for the rest of your life, if you tell yourself that you're starting with just a week or a month, you're more likely to have the strength to begin. After a month, you may just have a new, healthy habit. And then you're on your way to a lifetime of fitness.

Working out with a partner is also helpful for women starting an exercise program. Abby King, a clinical psychologist and assistant professor of health research and policy at Stanford University's Center for Research in Disease Prevention, has found that women in particular are more likely to stick with and enjoy an exercise program if it involves social support and interaction. When you're committed to someone else—so they count on you not to drop out—you're more likely to keep it up. Your exercise partner can be your spouse, your neighbor—or your dog, for that matter.

If you're busy, try using your new exercise plan not as one more activity in your day, but as a substitute for less important—or time-wasting—activities. For instance, if you usually sit at your desk with your sandwich and try, unsuccessfully, to get work done at the same time, get outside and take a walk with your lunch instead. Bonnie Berger, associate dean of the College of Health Sciences at the University of

Wyoming in Laramie, says the more stressed you are, the harder you work, and the less time you have for exercise, the more you *need* to exercise. You'll think more clearly and perform better under pressure if you're physically active. So find a way to weave it into your day.

Barbara Drinkwater tells older women or those who have been inactive for long periods of time to get going slowly; you can't undo 30 years of sloth in a week or a month, she warns. Make up your mind that you are not going to be an old lady in a rocker, she says; say it out loud, to yourself and to your doctor. Then choose a slow-going plan of both aerobic and strength training that will give you some of your lost years back. Even if you begin with just a few minutes of movement a day, with time you'll build up to levels you never expected.

Whatever type of exercise program you begin, stick with it as consistently as possible. First, you want to create new, healthy habits, and the more consistent you are, the greater the chance you'll make this part of your life. But even more important, research shows that if you haven't been exercising for long, even two weeks of inactivity can rob you of many of the benefits you've accrued. The more years you work out consistently, the longer you'll be able to get away with respites from exercise (unavoidable ones, such as illness) without losing everything you worked so hard to gain.

The Psychological Benefits of Exercise

We've been talking about the physical benefits of exercise, and there are many. But there are also significant emotional benefits to physical activity, and it's these benefits that may keep you exercising for the rest of your life.

According to Bonnie Berger, both aerobic *and* nonaerobic exercise can bring about better moods, more vigor, better self-esteem, clearer thinking, stress reduction, and decreased levels of depression, tension and anxiety. And according to Dr. Larry Gibbons, president and medical director of the Cooper Clinic at The Cooper Aerobics Center in Dallas, many women *start* exercising to lose weight and look better, but end up *sticking with it* because they develop higher energy levels, less fatigue in the evening, greater ability to perform work and overall less tension.

The best exercises for emotional health are repetitive, noncompetitive and involve deep breathing, Berger says. There are immediate psychological benefits to exercise—possibly due in part to the release of feel-good brain chemicals called endorphins—and there are also longer-term improvements in your sense of happiness and well-being. Part of the long-term effect may be the sense that you're looking and feeling better, that you're taking care of yourself and that you're doing something that releases tension *and* promotes fun in your life.

People who exercise regularly say they feel terrible when they are forced to be inactive. Exercise is recommended as part of treatment for depression and other mood disorders, and it's a great stress-relieving alternative to bad habits like overeating or abusing cigarettes or other substances. When you need a quick "fix" of some kind, try getting outside and working your body. Dr. Gibbons believes that a major cause of depression and fatigue among women (particularly the 60% of women who are almost totally sedentary) is chronic lack of exercise. We *believe* we can't get out and become fit because we're tired: in fact, it's the exact opposite; we're tired because we don't exercise, Gibbons says.

Don't overdo it, however. Just as excessive exercise can have adverse physiological effects on your body (for more on this, *see* "When You're Overdoing It," below), so too much exercise can hurt your psychological health, making you fatigued and boosting tension.

When You're Overdoing It

If you can't talk while you're exercising, you're probably working too hard. Take it down a peg, and when you can speak a few sentences without gasping for air, you're back in the right range. Usually, watching your pulse and staying within the target range discussed earlier is a good safety guideline, too. If at any point you feel dizzy or weak, or feel chest or other pain, stop exercising and seek help right away. Signs of overheating include suddenly dry skin (you stop sweating) and dizziness. Get plenty of fluids into your body and rest in a cool place with someone else to help you.

The Health Risks of Exercise Addiction

You *can* have too much of a good thing. When it comes to excessive exercise, many of the benefits we've talked about—from improved bone density to better overall body health and strenth— start to unravel. There are serious physiological signs of excessive exercise which only show up when your body is already in the danger zone. These trouble signs include loss of menstrual periods (amenorrhea), a history of bone stress fractures, and chronic pain or injuries that just don't go away. There is an important syndrome,

the "Female Athlete Triad" (defined in 1992 by the American College of Sports Medicine Task Force on Women's Issues), in which women who exercise and diet have disordered eating or take in too few calories for their level of activity, disrupt the hormone balance in their bodies, lose their ability to ovulate and to menstruate, and finally lose bone at a rapid rate. Dr. Carol Otis warns that bone loss in young women who stop menstruating can mimic the osteoporosis of menopause. While research hasn't pinpointed the exact rate of bone loss in these young women, she says, we have lots of studies showing that the bones of 30-year-old female athletes can resemble those of an 80-year-old. It's terrifying to see the toll excessive exercise and dieting can take on a young healthy body—and how fast it can take that toll. Dr. Otis urges caution for women who exercise for more than two hours a day (if they aren't professional or team athletes), for those who use exercise not for fun but to compensate for other behaviors like overeating, for those who have missed three periods in a row, or for those who have repeat injuries and fractures. These women should seek help immediately from an educated fitness and/or health professional. Like other forms of addiction and abuse, exercise abuse requires professional treatment. (*See* the information section at the end of this chapter for resources—and read more about eating disorders in chapter 23.)

Fitness "Experts"—Finding Someone to Guide You

Some of us will be able to get in shape without assistance. Others will need or just prefer the guidance of someone who can help make sure we're doing activities properly, protecting our joints with weight lifting, and so on. If you're looking for a coach, trainer or just someone to consult at a local gym or club, be sure to find someone with the right credentials. Christine Wells worries that there are a lot people out there calling themselves "fitness experts" who really don't have the training or information to guide you. You *can* ask about credentials, and there are several you can rely on. If they were trained by the American College on Exercise, or the American College of Sports Medicine, these are two of the best. You'll want to be careful about working with someone who is trained in the use of just one type of machine or equipment. They may tell you they've been through an accreditation program with company X, but that doesn't tell you anything about their knowledge in other types of workout machinery or fitness health in general.

CHOOSING AND USING THE RIGHT ATHLETIC EQUIPMENT

One sure way to get yourself out of an exercise program faster than you got into it is to use the wrong equipment. When you wear the wrong shoes, for example, you're more prone to hurting yourself—and to just feeling crummy when you do your chosen activity. This is *not* to say that you have to wear fancy or expensive clothing when you exercise, or find the most costly pair of exercise shoes around. It just means you should use equipment designed for your sport. According to Dr. Otis, you should use aerobics shoes for aerobics, since they're more cushioned than many other types of athletic shoes. Running shoes, on the other hand, have better support, and should be used for running and jogging. Cross-training shoes, which many salespeople will tell you are

fine for *all* sports, really aren't great for much more than shopping, Dr. Otis jokes. They aren't supportive enough for running, cushioned enough for aerobics, or properly designed for other specialized sports.

Also, wear a proper bra when exercising. About 40% of women have breast discomfort when exercising. Some may drop out of activities because of the pain. Instead, try on some special exercise bras that give more support. There are several kinds, with more and less flexibility. Find one that's comfortable for you. You might want to jump around in the dressing room a little, to get an idea of how it works.

As for clothing, comfort is all you have to worry about. A cheap T-shirt and sweats are just as good as a fancy exercise outfit. Go with what's comfortable (generally, fabrics that breathe, like cotton, are best) and whatever fits your budget. I was amazed to learn that many women, particularly those who are older and/or overweight, will avoid exercise simply because they don't want to be seen looking frumpy or "not put together" in the gym or on the street. Abby King's research at the Stanford University School of Medicine reveals that many women are intimidated by skintight, spandex workout garb, and by the super-fit clientele at some athletic clubs. Just working out in *public* is unacceptable to many women, particularly if they're out of shape. If this is holding you back, think twice: not only will you start to have a body that looks more like theirs *if* you get out and exercise, but it's time to start being realistic and stop being vain. People who look that way are looking at themselves and at each other, not at you! Put your hair in a ponytail, lace up those sneakers, get out and do this for *yourself*—and no one else.

FOR MORE INFORMATION ON EXERCISE

PRESIDENT'S COUNCIL ON PHYSICAL FITNESS AND SPORTS
701 Pennsylvania Ave. NW, Suite 250
Washington, DC 20004
202-272-3421

WOMEN'S SPORTS FOUNDATION
Eisenhower Park
East Meadow, NY 11554
800-227-3988

AMERICAN COLLEGE OF SPORTS MEDICINE
P.O. Box 1440
Indianapolis, Indiana 46206-1440
317-637-9200

AEROBICS AND FITNESS ASSOCIATION OF AMERICA
15250 Ventura Blvd., Suite 200
Sherman Oaks, CA 91403
800-225-2322 (National except California)
800-446-2322 (California only)

ARTHRITIS

NATIONAL ARTHRITIS AND MUSCULOSKELETAL AND SKIN DISEASES INFORMATION CLEARINGHOUSE
Box AMS
9000 Rockville Pike
Bethesda, MD 20892
301-495-4484

ARTHRITIS FOUNDATION
1314 Spring St., NW
Atlanta, GA 30309
800-283-7800

CHAPTER TWENTY-TWO

WEIGHT LOSS, WEIGHT MAINTENANCE

*I had to face the facts, I was pear-shaped. I was a bit
depressed because I hate pears.*

—Charlotte Bingham, *Coronet Among the Weeds*

If you've heard it once, you've heard it a thousand times: Diets don't work. About 95% of dieters gain the weight back. Yo-yo dieting, gaining and losing, is bad for your health. Losing weight is easy, keeping it off is hard—or impossible. These are the messages we've been given by the media about dieting. And in fact, a number of scientific studies support the idea that dieting "doesn't work." The question is, what does that really mean?

If you lose weight, the diet worked, right? And millions of Americans diet—and lose weight—every year. Women lead the dieting pack, outnumbering men seven to one in weight-loss programs. Three out of four women try to lose weight at some point in their lives; another quarter of those who have *never been overweight* do the same, says Rena Wing, director of the obesity/nutrition research center at the University of Pittsburgh's Western Psychiatric Institute and Clinic. Thousands of pounds are lost each year—and thousands more are regained. Does that mean that dieting "doesn't work?" I'm not convinced of that. What you need to ask yourself is, *What was your goal in dieting?* Most people would say their goal was to lose weight. And therein lies the problem. If your dieting goal is to lose weight, and you lose it, your diet was a success. If you gain it back, that doesn't mean the original diet failed. In this section, we're going to focus on *reorienting our goals* not to losing weight, but to (1) getting healthier on a number of physiological scales (including blood pressure, cholesterol levels and so on), (2) permanently changing our body weight (quite different from "losing weight") and (3) changing our eating habits. Certainly, if these were the focused goals of most dieters, we could safely say that diets don't work.

Dr. Albert Stunkard, an authority on obesity at the University of Pennsylvania, calls this approach the "obesity as chronic disease" perspective. Being overweight is not a temporary problem. It is a lifelong problem. We should think about excessive weight the way we think about high blood pressure—that is, as something to reduce permanently, not just once or sporadically. And that requires a lifetime of new habits and commitment. The goal is not thinness, but good health.

Why the American obsession with weight loss, and thinness? Need I ask? Right now, go to your coffee table and grab a copy of a popular magazine. Any one. Look at the ads. For cars, for perfume, for beer, for cigarettes. Do you see anyone fat in those ads? Do you see anyone even slightly pudgy in those ads? Probably not. What you do see is a lot of bone. Perhaps the models have eating disorders, perhaps they don't. They may live on lettuce leaves, run ten miles a day, or they may be genetically programmed to be skinny. Whatever their story, they sure don't look much like the average American woman. Our obsession with weight is evident the moment a child is born in the U.S., says obesity expert Wayne Callaway of George Washington University Medical School. Immediately after asking the sex, we ask about the baby's weight! This is not true in many other societies, he adds. And 80% of 5th-grade girls think they're fat, notes Callaway.

Meanwhile, the average American woman, whoever she may be, spends an awful lot of time trying to look like the skinny women on magazine covers. And considering that slightly more than one in three middle-aged Caucasian women is significantly overweight, clearly the effort has been a losing one. The most recent report from the National Health and Nutrition Examination Survey (NHANES III) reports an 8% increase in the number of overweight Americans in the last decade.

Keep in mind that the advice in this chapter is intended for people who are actually overweight, and whose health may be compromised because of it. For those who are of normal, healthy weight, and who have good eating habits (*see* chapter 20 on nutrition), but feel compelled to get thinner for cosmetic or other reasons, there is another chapter in this section on eating disorders (chapter 23). If you are of normal weight (according to the parameters discussed below), look inside yourself and ask *why* you want to be thinner than you are. The reasons are apt not to be healthy ones. And there's lots of help for the many people like you.

WEIGHT LOSS: WHAT YOU HAD TO SAY ABOUT IT

Irene, 62 Years Old

I loathe heaviness. I love thinness. If you're thin, as far as I'm concerned nothing else matters, you can be sloppy, and so on. I weighed much more than I had ever weighed, I thought if I didn't lose it, I would become obese. I don't respect myself when I'm obese. All my clothes were too tight, I was unhappy. I feel that when I gain weight, it's because I'm trying to be self-destructive. Even worse than obese is that plump look.

I went on [a formal weight loss program]. My goal was to lose a significant amount of weight and I didn't feel I could lose it on my own. I'd been trying. One makes bargains with oneself, like "I'll have a big breakfast and then no lunch"—and then you have a big lunch! Dieting lasts, but one must have the realization that one can only have a certain number of calories per day, and as soon as you break that, you will gain weight. Portion control is very important. I do diet well if I have a plan, and have nothing else.

I like my diet because it gives me enough variety, and I can eat regular foods. I don't like to go shopping for special items. I walk every day, two miles—maybe it helped me lose it faster, or helped me keep it down. It doesn't make you lose the weight. I feel much better, but I'm very worried I'll gain it back. I'm worried about being on vacation. I'm a snacker, that's how I gain weight. I'm glad I look thin. I can wear things I haven't worn in years. I feel much better about myself.

Shannon, 38 years old

I'm seven pounds fatter than pre-pregnancy. Everything's fitting differently. I have to start dieting to get into my clothing. When you see me naked, you can see I have problems now, maybe because post-pregnancy you need to exercise. I have quite a large bottom, I put on weight in that area. People have remarked on it when I'm heavier. I'm careful about what I wear. The way I did stay thin in the past was to eat much less protein, and much more vegetables. And really important is the elimination of fat from the diet—it's amazing what happens. You can get accustomed to not eating fat.

I firmly believe that exercise makes you look better even if you weigh more, but it makes you hungry and you eat more. When I was pregnant I deliberately ate more high fat things, and now I'm addicted to chips—it's terrible. Another thing that helps keep you thin is a fear of being fat, a

tremendous dislike of it. I have a real problem with it for me, leftover from childhood. I was a chubby little kid, and I was quite heavy as a 13-year-old. I can remember from early childhood being mortified by the rolls on my stomach.

Sally, 36 years old

I've been fat all my life. I went on my first diet at seven years of age. I've spent my whole life yo-yo dieting. Dieting was so painful, and the result was self-loathing, self-hatred. People like my parents, my doctor, my weight loss programs were always telling me "If you wanted to, you could be thin."

There's a $33 billion diet industry telling us this every time we turn on the TV, every time we open a magazine. The message is "If you can't be thin, you're a moral failure, your life is meaningless." Society places these values on me, external pressure and external values. But they *don't* have to be *mine.*

The most severe yo-yoing I did was I lost 140 pounds and gained 180. I was totally freaked out, I hated myself, I was frustrated, in tears, in enormous emotional pain with the weight gain. I went to an all-girls high school which was good for me, I was student body president, I got opportunities fat kids didn't always have because there wasn't the sex thing. I was given leadership roles. But I never had a date in high school or in college.

There's this whole blame the victim thing around weight. I am now five foot, five inches tall and weigh about 325 pounds. It hit me—"Hey, I'm not a bad person." I always worked for human rights, I worked for the ACLU, so on a professional level I was defending others' rights—I thought it was time to defend my own rights. I always identified with oppression as a woman, but when I really experienced size oppression was when I was working in construction, there was another woman there who looked like she could be in *Playboy,* and she rode with the fore-man in the truck, while I worked with the jack-hammer.

I decided it was easier to change society than to change my size. This whole self acceptance is a continuing process. You don't wake up and say "I'm okay." Now I date, I've had partners, I was married and divorced. I love my body, its abun-dance, its softness and its curves. It might sound strange to an average-size woman, but I love my large breasts, my large belly, the folds and the rolls. And there's a sizeable proportion of men in society who prefer large women, although many of them are still in the closet. They think I'm the most gorgeous thing in the world!

My main message is don't put your life on hold waiting until you're thin. This isn't a dress rehearsal. Live life to the fullest and love yourself regardless.

Judith, 60 years old
My point of view is that calories count. Having been in periods of illness so depressed that I did-n't exercise and lost interest in food, my weight automatically went down. And periods where I exercised three hours a day and ate 2000 calo-ries a day, I didn't lose weight. Exercise makes me very hungry, it sets in and I am ravenous. When I don't go to the gym, a carrot or banana is okay for lunch. When I go to the gym, I want a big lunch. Maybe it's mental, you feel you deserve it. You think exercise gives you a license to eat. But most exercise only burns 350 calories, one dessert!

Clothes are very important to me. It would kill me to buy an expensive suit and not be able to wear it. And my image, because I'm tall, has

always been to look modelly. With the height, I'm five-ten, if I got heavy I'd be this huge person. I was very fat as a little girl. I lost it by the time I was twelve. As an adult woman I like the way I look thin. It has a lot to do with not feeling old, I haven't given up on youth or attractiveness. Also, over the last 30 years I've stayed thin to insure that my husband finds me attractive.

I don't feel deprived: when I take a bite of steak, I say, "Okay steak, I've had you before—okay potato, I've had you before." A taste seems to do it most of the time. But I have certain trigger foods—peanuts, peanut butter, peanut brittle, roasted salted almonds. I can't take one bite of them, because I cannot just eat one bite.

It's better to wear Italian than to eat Italian. I look at the pasta and think of an Armani suit. I'd rather feel a little nervous looking at the food at a cocktail party than feel nervous crazy the next day trying to lose it.

THE RISKS OF BEING OVERWEIGHT

The vast majority of us are worried about our weight for cosmetic reasons. Will I fit into that dress for the wedding? Will I be able to get into a bathing suit this summer? Will I ever put those blue jeans on again? These should be the least of our worries. Excessive weight is associated with a great number of health problems, including the very ones most associated with death and chronic disease in older women. High blood pressure, high blood cholesterol, high triglyceride levels, diabetes, arthritis, skin problems—the list of health problems associated with obesity goes on and on. When you are obese, which is usually defined as being about 20% over your ideal body weight (not hard to do: if your ideal weight is 135, and you weigh

161, you're there), your overall chance of dying is significantly greater than that for people of normal weight. Being fat kills you. Forget about that bathing suit, and start thinking about your heart.

How Do You Define "Overweight"?

There are lots of charts out there with "normal" weight, "ideal" weight and so on. Interestingly, some of the top experts in the weight-loss field think the simplest measures are the best ones. For instance, Dr. George Blackburn, chief of the nutrition/metabolism laboratory at the New England Deaconess Hospital in Boston, thinks the old standby of 100 pounds at five feet, plus five pounds for every inch over five feet, plus or minus 10%, is a healthy goal for women. That would mean a woman who is 5 feet 4 inches tall would be in the right range if she weighed 120 pounds, plus or minus 10% (as little as 108, or as much as 132). Other experts prefer to use charts such as the well-known Metropolitan Life company's height and weight tables, which have been modified (to include higher weights) over the years. Below is a comparison of the 1959 and 1983 Met Life tables, alongside the U.S. Department of Agriculture Guidelines from 1989.

While these charts are useful in defining a healthy weight *range,* you can see that they're hard to use for targeting a *personal* healthy weight goal, since a spread of more than 30 pounds in a given category is quite large.

HEIGHT (FT IN)	MET TABLES (WT. LBS.)		U.S. DEPT. AGRIC. (WT. LBS.)	
	1959	**1983**	**1989** age 19–34	35+
4' 9"	94–106	106–118		
4' 10"	97–109	106–120		
4' 11"	100–112	110–123		
5'	103–115	112–126	97–128	108–138
5' 1"	106–118	115–129	101–132	111–143
5' 2"	109–122	118–132	104–137	115–148
5' 3"	112–126	121–135	107–141	119–152
5' 4"	116–131	124–138	111–146	122–157
5' 5"	120–135	127–141	114–150	126–162
5' 6"	124–139	130–144	125–164	138–178
5' 7"	128–143	133–147	129–169	142–183
5' 8"	132–147	136–150	132–174	146–188
5' 9"	136–151	139–153	136–179	151–194
5' 10"	140–155	142–156	140–184	155–199

Naturally, women with smaller bones and frames should strive for the lower end of each spectrum, and larger-frame women should focus more on the higher end—but still, these are broad generalizations.

The *best* ways to measure healthy weight for height take a little computing. One important measure is your body fat. The ideal body fat measurement for women falls somewhere between 20% and 25% of total body mass. One of the better ways to determine that is with a test in which you're submerged in water (called hydrodensitometry) and your percentage of body fat is measured with special techniques. Some upscale health clubs and weight loss centers employ this technique, but most use cheaper, simpler methods of body fat measurement. However, Dr. Theodore VanItallie, founder of the Obesity Research Center at St. Luke's-Roosevelt Hospital, notes that even this relatively accurate method of body-fat measurement has its problems: since its results are affected by the mass of your skeleton, women who have lost bone may not get an accurate reading.

Another, less accurate way to measure body fat is with calipers that pinch fat in various places, such as the back of your arm or your belly. These are useful, but not as reliable as the underwater test.

A tool *you* can use to determine if you're overweight is called the BMI, or body mass index which I'll describe in a moment. Rena Wing recommends this, along with height/weight charts, for women who cannot access water immersion and other more precise body-fat measurement techniques. You calculate your BMI by dividing your weight in kilograms by your height in meters squared. (Weight specialists believe that a BMI of about 27 to 28 is a health hazard for women. This corresponds to being about 20% overweight.) It takes a little doing, but finding out your BMI really isn't that hard. Just follow the formula below. Let's say you weigh 150 pounds. First, you have to translate that into kilograms: the result is about 68.18 kilograms (you just divide your weight by 2.2). Now, let's say you're 5 feet 5 inches tall, or 65 inches tall. That translates into about 1.64 meters (to get that, you just divide your total inches, 65, by 39.6, which is the number of inches in a meter). Then multiply the number you get—in this case, 1.64—by itself: $1.64 \times 1.64 = 2.68$ (this is your height in meters squared). Now, for your last step, divide your weight in kilograms by your height in meters squared to get your BMI: for our example, the equation is $68.18 \div 2.68 = 25.4$. This person's BMI is 25.4: *not* considered obese.

Just for interest's sake, let's take a look at one of the charts above and look at a person who's 5 feet 5 inches tall: you can see that at 150 pounds, this person is considered too heavy by the Met Life charts, but in the reasonable range for the Agriculture Department charts. This is the type of person—and many American women fit this category—who should discuss what might be a healthy weight *for her* with her doctor. She does not seem to be at high risk for weight-related disease, but she may be borderline—that is, heading to trouble with further weight gain. If she has other major risk factors for heart disease or diabetes, her doctor may want her to lose a few pounds to get into the Met Life chart range. Or, this weight might be just fine for her if she's able to keep it this way.

Another useful measurement you can do at home is that of your healthy body *shape*; it's called your waist-hip ratio, or WHR. Getting your WHR is quite simple. Just divide your waist size by your hip size, and the result will tell you a lot about your weight-related risk of disease. For example, let's take a waist size of 28 inches, and a hip size of 38 inches. Divide 28 by 38 and you get about .7. Experts believe that for women, a WHR of greater than .8 is risky (for men, the cutoff point for an unhealthy WHR is different, at 1.0). So the example above is in the safe range. Let's look at two more examples. First, let's increase the waist size, but keep the hip size steady: so now we're talking about a waist size of 31 inches, and a hip size of 38 inches. Thirty-one divided by 38 is .81—just over the "safe" limit. Now let's keep the original waist size where it was at 28 inches, and increase the hip size to 43 inches. Twenty-eight divided by 43 is about .6—well in the safe range. There's an extremely important message here: Notice that a bigger waist, which usually means more fat in the belly, sends your risk of disease up quickly—while bigger hips, which usually means more fat in the hips, bottom and thighs, usually does *not* increase risk. Body shape, as we'll discuss below, may be even more important to your health than how much you weigh.

Body Shape: "Apples Versus Pears"

The type of weight you carry is extremely important in predicting adverse health problems, as we illustrated above with the waist-hip ratio calculations. You've probably heard of the different body types called "apple-shape" and "pear-shape". "Apples," those who carry most of their fat in their torsos (as abdominal or waist fat) tend to have many more health problems than do "pears," who carry their weight in their bottoms, hips and thighs. Many women are concerned about thigh, hip and bottom fat—again, for cosmetic reasons. In fact, says Dr. Reubin Andres, clinical director at the National Institute on Aging, we should be thankful for that kind of fat! We adapted this kind of body shape for the purpose of pregnancy and lactation. We lay down more fat on our hips and thighs during pregnancy, and then burn it up when breast feeding, says Dr. Stunkard. Few if any health risks have been associated specifically with lower-body fat. Trunk or abdominal fat, on the other hand, is a different story. Those with fat in their middles have a greater risk of heart disease and many of the other health risks listed earlier. Add smoking to abdominal fat, says Dr. Andres, and you put yourself at exceptionally high risk of heart problems. In addition, smoking itself seems to predispose people to more abdominal fat distribution.

Smoking, being sedentary, and of course our genes (heredity) predispose us to abdominal body fat. If your whole family carries fat in the stomach region, you're likely to carry it there, too. The good news is, fat is easier to lose from the abdomen! Women with bottom and leg fat struggle much harder to lose weight from their "problem" areas than do women who try to lose belly fat. Hormones also play a role in fat distribution. Estrogens or female hormones tend to place fat in the lower body, while androgens (male hormones) place it in the belly. That's one reason why you see more men with belly fat, and more women with lower-body fat. But of course there are exceptions to both cases. Some believe that hormonal changes at the menopause, when estrogen levels drop, predispose women to gaining belly weight—and they theorize that this accounts for some of the increase in postmenopausal heart disease rates.

If you have lots of abdominal fat, you'll want to pay particular attention to the advice in this chapter. For you, losing weight is much more important than it is for the woman who wants to wear pin-straight skirts; your life and health are more threatened by your added weight.

What Makes Us Fat?

Put most simply, we gain weight when the number of calories we burn falls short of the number of calories we take in. The more calories you eat, and the fewer calories you work off through exercise, daily activities or your basic metabolism, the fatter you get. These days, however, weight specialists are paying special attention to three factors that keep us overweight: (1) excessive fat in the diet; (2) lack of exercise; and (3) our genetic makeup.

Eating Fat Makes Us Fat

Per gram, fat has more calories than protein or carbohydrates. A gram of fat has 9 calories, while a gram of carbohydrate or protein has just 4 calories. The body likes to store the fat you eat as fat in your body, while it is more apt to take carbohydrate foods and burn them up for fuel. So the more fat you eat, the more calories you get *and* the more your body gets the stuff it likes to lay down as fat on *you*. There is a growing consensus that fat intake is much more important than total calorie intake as far as weight gain *and* overall health are concerned.

American women eat way too much fat. This is *not* a moralistic statement: it's a health statement. High fat intake is not only associated with being overweight, it's also known to increase the rate of artery clogging and high blood fats that lead to heart disease. We eat, on average, somewhere between 36% and 42% of our total calories from fat. We *should* eat fewer than 30% of our total calories from fat, and ideally, some experts say, more like 25% of our total calories from fat. Saturated fats, like butter and animal fat, are the worst of all: they should make up less than 10% of our total calories (or as few as possible)—but we eat more than 13% of our total calories from saturated fat. (For more on the specifics of cutting fat, *see* chapter 20, "Nutrition.")

The basic goal in cutting fat from your diet is to replace fatty foods with leaner foods—especially high-fiber foods, which we don't get enough of in the first place. This means switching from bacon and eggs most mornings to cereal with skim milk, from a bologna and cheese sandwich at lunch to a big tossed salad and dish of pasta with vegetable sauce, from red meat at dinner to lean, broiled fish. It also means throwing out most of the condiments we slather on otherwise healthy foods: mayo on bread, oil on vegetables, and so on. You might think you're incapable of giving up the fatty foods you love. In fact, there is a pervasive myth that we become *addicted* to high-fat foods, and can't break the cycle. Dr. George Blackburn says this is pure hogwash: we are "addicted," if anything, to the foods we are accustomed to eating, he says. Since American women are used to eating lots of fat, we think these are the only foods we will ever crave. In fact, it takes just six to nine weeks on average to readjust our internal food clocks to want different kinds of foods. After just a couple of months, Blackburn says, you'll find yourself beginning to crave the new foods you've been eating—vegetables, fruit, whole-grain breads, and other high-fiber items. Sure, you may always love and crave that occasional piece of cheesecake, but you won't need fatty foods as your staples forever if you try to make the shift.

Being Inactive Makes Us Fat

Over and over it has been shown that people who exercise less, weigh more. Women are less likely to exercise than are men, says Dr. Stunkard, putting us at even greater risk of obesity. A recent study showed that fewer than one in ten Americans exercises three times a week to the degree needed for cardiovascular fitness! Sitting in front of desks, in cars, on buses, and in lounge chairs is a near-guaranteed prescription for obesity. Exercise, on the other hand, lifts our calorie-burning potential by boosting our metabolism and creating muscle that is a more dynamic calorie-burner than fat (and looks a lot better, too).

Inactivity not only makes us become fat, Rena Wing adds, but it's one of the single most important predictors of who will keep weight on. We are not talking about becoming a marathon runner, although if that's what you want to do, by all means go for it. We're talking about putting movement back into your life. Walking at a good pace for just half an hour each day will make a tremendous difference over the course of time. Whatever you choose, from exercise machines indoors to taking your movement out of the house, regular, brisk exercise that gets your heart rate up and uses the muscles of your body will help you lose weight and maintain weight loss. It will also help lower your blood pressure, improve your blood fat levels, and boost many other measures of health. (For specifics on exercise for women, especially how much to do and how vigorously to do it, see chapter 21.)

One of the reasons exercise is so important in terms of weight loss is it increases your percentage of muscle or lean body tissue. They say the rich get richer; well, sad as it is, the fat get fatter. The more fat you have in relation to your total body mass, the lower your so-called basal metabolic rate (BMR). On the flip side, the more lean muscle you have, the greater your BMR. That means exercise pays off for you almost like compound interest. You not only get the benefits of exercise while you're doing it—feeling better, burning calories, keeping weight off—but you also burn more calories throughout the day (even while you're sitting!) since your basic metabolism—your engine, so to speak—is constantly burning at a higher level. After years of dieting and being sedentary, research shows it can take a few months of exercise just to jump-start that engine and bring you back to normal.

There is another good physiological reason why exercise should help maintain weight loss. Our bodies are programmed in sophisticated ways to *stop* us from losing weight. After all, for the species to survive, we can't starve. The body is loaded with signals to protect us from starvation, so when we start to diet or cut calories, bells go off all over the place warning our systems that trouble may be afoot. Our bodies slow down and go into starvation mode, using less energy, to protect us from weight loss—the very thing we're trying to achieve! The less you eat, the less your body requires to get you through the day; it just keeps turning the volume down, so to speak. Exercise helps break this cycle. By boosting your activity level, you turn your body's engine back *up,* increasing the calories you burn all day long, and stopping your body from turning itself off.

Rena Wing points out that there's a lot we don't yet understand about how exercise promotes weight loss. Perhaps it helps not only by boosting muscle and burning calories, but also by improving our mood and decreasing our hunger. Whatever the reasons, we do know for sure that people who are thinner exercise more on average, that people who are fatter exercise less, and that people who exercise tend to keep off the weight they lose over the long haul.

GENETICS HELP MAKE US FAT

If your parents are fat, you're more likely—but not guaranteed—to be fat. There is some degree of genetic programming involved in the tendency to be overweight. Of course, it's clouded by environmental factors, such as the fact that families may eat the wrong foods, and too much food, together—*and* may be sedentary together. But beyond those issues of habit, it's clear that just as our genes can program us to get particular diseases, or have a certain hair or eye color, so they can predispose us to being overweight. Dr. Stunkard says that this is all the more reason young and adolescent children of obese people should be targeted for weight-management programs before *their* weight gets out of control.

Skeptics about weight loss love to point out the negative physiological aspects of weight gain and loss, such as the fact that fat cells cannot be eliminated once created, and that fat cells forever cry out to be "refed". True, you can't eliminate fat cells, and some combination

or our genetics and environment may predispose us to having more of them (and getting more of them) than we want. But the good news is you can shrink the fat cells you have in your body (they vary in size by about eightfold!), and with proper weight maintenance techniques you can keep them small. There is nothing inevitable about being fat, except for a very few people with extreme medical problems such as serious hormonal imbalances. Even those who say they eat very little but remain fat have been shown, in studies, to be eating a lot more calories than they admit to themselves—or realize.

GENDER DIFFERENCES IN WEIGHT LOSS PATTERNS AND ABILITY

Most women who have tried to diet with their husbands or male friends have been slapped with the realization that weight loss just ain't gender-neutral. One more sexist fact to contend with is men lose more weight, and lose weight faster, than do women. Dr. George Blackburn uses the analogy that while men are using a V-8 engine, women are using a V-6 engine. As we discussed earlier, the amount of lean body tissue (such as muscle) that you have in your body makes it easier or harder to lose weight and maintain weight loss. Men have more lean body mass than do women. and hence burn their engines at a higher level all the time. When they exercise, or cut back on calories, they lose weight quite rapidly. Women, who carry more fat on their bodies on average (for the healthy purpose of childbearing), lose weight more slowly for the same amount of exercise done and calories cut. So when it comes to weight loss, Jane must stop comparing herself to John.

It's a losing battle, and one that doesn't have a lot to do with *either* of you meeting your goals.

There are other interesting gender differences regarding weight loss. Among them, women and men report different *obstacles* to weight loss in the first place. Rena Wing interviewed 100 men and 100 women aged 25–45 about what gets in the way of their ability to lose weight. Men said that knowledge was the biggest obstacle—that is, knowing which lower-fat and lower-calorie foods to choose from, and so on. Women had the knowledge they needed, for the most part, but *emotions* were their biggest obstacle to weight loss. While they didn't specify the emotions that got in the way of weight loss, they did say that *handling* emotions was the problem. As we've heard before, food is what many people turn to for comfort, as a retreat from negative feelings. Women may be more vulnerable to this than are men.

Still another gender difference experts have found is that women respond better to one set of dieting patterns, and men respond better to another. For example, says Dr. George Blackburn, women tend to succeed in losing weight when they opt for a "grazing" style of dieting, eating several small meals over the course of the day. Men, on the other hand, lose weight better when they eat three strict meals a day and eliminate snacking. (Of course, if you're going to try to adopt the grazing style, you need to know what you're doing, since you don't want to snack all day on the wrong kinds of foods.) The reason grazing works better for women, Blackburn says, is it reduces feelings of hunger and deprivation that often lead women to overeat. Furthermore, adds Wayne Callaway, eating frequently throughout the day helps keep our metabolisms up, which means we burn

more calories all day long. The key, however, is to learn to choose low-fat foods all day: a piece of fruit here, a cup of low-fat yogurt there, a couple of slices of whole-grain toast there—rather than high-fat grazing, which will surely backfire.

Finally, our lifestyles have created gender differences in weight problems. Women traditionally have spent more time in the home, where food is constantly accessible, and we've spent more time preparing food for the entire family than have men. Food preparation is terribly risky behavior, since "tasting" often becomes eating—both before and during meals! As women more often move out of the home and into the workplace, some of these trends will reverse. But as sociologists have shown us, there are still some basic realities in our society, including the fact that while women may work out of the home all day, we still often are the ones to come home and throw together dinner. If this is your case, you might consider turning this into a *positive*: if you control the food that's brought into your home and that your family eats, you can switch to lower-fat, lower-calorie choices not just for you but for your entire family. Everyone will benefit from the change, including your children, whose weight-gain patterns are set quite early in life.

What Happens to Women's Weight Over Time

As a rule, unfortunately, women gain weight steadily throughout most of life—at least until about age 65. Researchers have tried to understand why women keep gaining weight, putting us at increasingly high risk of weight-related disease. Some theorize that hormonal changes at menopause are partially responsible. Actually, in a study by Rena Wing and colleagues, it was shown that while women do gain several pounds in the perimenopausal years, they do so *regardless* of whether they actually go through menopause. Aging, not menopause, seemed more predictive of weight gain for women. Women most likely to gain weight in this study were sedentary and lived alone; African-American women were more likely to gain than were Caucasian women, though both gained significant amounts of weight in in their middle and premenopausal years.

Another risk factor for women's gradual weight gain is pregnancy. Most women gain weight with pregnancy—it's healthy to do so. But too many of us fail to take it off afterwards, and a few extra pounds with each baby can add up to quite a few extra pounds later in life. This is yet another reason why constant, life-long weight-control habits, not sporadic diets, are the only way to achieve and maintain proper weight.

How to Lose and Maintain Weight Properly: Tips on Healthy Dieting

The following advice, assembled form interviews with many different diet and weight loss experts from around the country, applies to anyone who wants to lose weight in a healthy way and keep that weight off permanently. If you are severely obese, and your health is immediately threatened by your excessive weight, see page 451 for additional advice.

Lose Weight Gradually.

As a rule, aim to lose no more than a pound or two at the most per week. The American Dietetic Association is even more strict, urging you to lose no more than a half to three-quarters of a pound per week! Another way to guide yourself is to lose no more than about one percent of your total body weight per week. If you weigh 160 pounds, that means no more than 1.6 pounds per week. The more slowly you lose weight, the better the chance you'll keep it off, the easier the process will be on your body, and the less likely you'll be to send your body into the starvation mode we discussed earlier. Over time, you'll find that your weight loss will slow down a bit as you get closer to your healthy weight. That's normal. Some weeks you may not lose at all. Others, you may lose more than usual. Over the course of one year, a 10% change in your weight is a good reference point for the average woman with a moderate amount of weight to lose.

Exercise.

As often as possible (and at least a few times a week) get up and move your body. Walk, run, play a sport, ride a bike, use a machine—just *move,* for at least 20 or 30 minutes. Keep this up while you're reducing calories, as well as after you increase calories slightly to maintain your weight. The combination of calorie restriction and exercise makes for better weight loss and maintenance.

Choose a Diet That Allows You To Eat Your Own Foods.

If you're restricting calories on your own, this isn't a problem. But if you're going to use a weight-loss program of some kind, you're much better off using one that teaches you to work with regular foods you purchase than one that gives you premade or preassembled foods. The reason: if you're going to learn anything about the best foods to eat to stay lean and healthy, you've got to do it for yourself. Blindly eating prepared foods (which, by the way, are sometimes laden with salt) will teach you little or nothing. Learning to buy the right foods, preparing them the right way and serving appropriate portions is the best way to go.

Don't Say "I'm Going On a Diet."
Instead, say that you're going to change your habits. There should be no time limit, and ideally, no strict weight limits in your mind (a loose goal is good, however). If you decide to change your ways for the long haul, your chance of success is much greater.

Keep All Nutrients and Food Groups Balanced.
Any diet that pushes you to eat mostly from a single food group (or a single food) is *inappropriate*. You want to eat a complex, complete diet with foods from every group, including fiber, protein and even some fat (we need it to survive). All-fruit diets, for example, are not good for your body. You need many nutrients and food materials that come from a wide variety of sources in order to be healthy. Emphasize fiber-rich foods like vegetables, fruits, grains, breads and pastas over other foods—but not to the exclusion of other foods. (*See* chapter 20 for more specifics.) Experts know that it's possible to diet (cut calories) and still get the right amount of nutrients. Some say it's a good idea to take a single multivitamin when you're restricting calories, just to be on the safe side. This does not mean taking megavitamins—just a well-balanced one-a-day tablet (*see* page 416 for a list of some leading brands and how they stack up).

Eliminate or Limit "Empty" Calories.
Simple sugars, alcohol, excessive fats—these calories generally add nothing to your overall health and well-being but take up a good portion of your daily calorie allotment. If you get rid of them, or at least cut way back on them (just a single glass of wine at a sitting, for instance, on rare occasions), you'll have more room for the foods that will fill you up and make your body stronger.

Stay In Touch With Your Doctor.
If you're planning to restrict calories and lose weight, let your doctor know, and make sure it's a safe thing to do given your overall health profile. As you lose (or gain) significant amounts of weight (say, 10% of your body weight) let your doctor reassess your overall health.

Eat Enough Calories.
Don't starve yourself. Somewhere in the range of 1200–1500 calories per day, depending on how much you exercise, is a good range for weight-loss diets. You'll want to boost your caloric intake somewhat once you've met your weight-loss goal, however: don't get trapped into a downward spiral of more and more weight loss to meet an unhealthy, unrealistic "ideal." If you're worried that you're overdoing it, take a look at chapter 23, "Eating Disorders."

Eat Slowly, Chew Well.
It takes a little while for your brain to discover that you're full. If you eat fast, you get more food (and calories) into your body than you really want or need, but you don't find that out until it's too late and you feel stuffed. If you chew your food well, put your fork down between bites, talk to others during meals (or

read if you're alone), you'll discover you're full before you overdo it.

Balance Your Senses.

Here's an interesting concept: Dr. Blackburn reports that since women's triggers to weight gain are usually in the form of sights and smells of food, you need to tantalize *other* senses in order to offset those triggers. An example would be listening to music you especially enjoy, getting out of the house to look at cheerful sights you don't often get to see (as with a walk in the park, for instance) and other stimulants that have nothing to do with food or eating.

Drink Lots of Fluids While Restricting Calories.

The more you drink—ideally, water—the more full you'll feel (and the happier your kidneys will be). Beware of drinking too much in the ways of sugary or high-calories juices; you'd be amazed how many calories you can pack away in beverages alone. But you *need* water, and there's pretty much no limit to the amount you can have safely, so drink before, during and after meals. Don't wait until you're thirsty.

Choose Behaviorally Oriented Weight-Loss Programs.

If you're using a weight-loss program, choose one that deals with behavioral triggers to overeating. For instance, instead of making global promises like "I will never eat ice cream again," allow for some lapses, and learn what it is that makes you want or feel you need ice cream at certain times. Keeping a chart of food triggers, or your feelings at different times of the day, can help. Once you understand your personal triggers, see if you can replace them

with other activities, like calling a friend or going for a walk instead of having a snack.

Have Nonfat Snacks at Your Fingertips.

In your purse, in your fridge, in the cupboards, in your pockets, nonfat snacks should be readily available to you. You're likely to be hungry when you're cutting calories, and when you're hungry, you may make mistakes (breaking down and having a fatty cookie just because it's there). Make sure that cookie *isn't there* . . . and replace it with carrot and celery sticks, fruit, nonfat crackers or, if you must, nonfat deserts. As long as these healthy options are available to you, you're less likely to fall off the wagon and become discouraged.

Don't Skip Meals.

Remember that under our new "rules," dieting doesn't mean deprivation. It means good habits. Good habits include eating regular meals (or even more frequent smaller meals, as we discussed earlier). Depriving yourself of breakfast isn't going to do anything to lower your weight, but it certainly will lower your mood. Sit down and take a minute to enjoy something good for you at regular intervals throughout the day, and you won't feel hungry, angry or deprived.

Formal Weight-Loss Programs.

Are commercial weight-loss programs useful and safe? Insofar as they meet the criteria listed above, yes. Programs that advise slow weight loss with well-balanced nutrition and so on can be quite effective. The key is that you learn something about weight maintenance and your triggers to weight gain while in the program. If you're blindly following a weight loss plan and aren't absorbing new information about healthy eating, chances are you aren't going to keep up the good work after the program ends. In fact, a committe of weight-loss experts for the Institute of Medicine is pressing the diet industry to publish long-term success and drop-out rates so consumers can get a fair look at what they're getting into. Today, those important records are "trade secrets," Dr. Stunkard complains, which leaves consumers in the dark. Many commercial plans that promised quick, dramatic weight loss came under fire several years ago, with thousands of lawsuits for health problems and even sudden death allegedly caused by rapid, unsupervised weight reduction and poor nutrition. But in general, losing weight in a properly designed, structured program, at least at first, is often a good way to get going and to keep your motivation high (someone's watching you, monitoring you, and counting on you) and to teach you a few things about weight problems in general. In addition, there's the social aspect of a weight-loss plan: going with a friend, or meeting new people at weight-loss meetings who share both your obstacles and your goals, adds one more layer of motivation.

Dieting Advice for the Extremely Overweight.
There are diets called VLCDs, or very low calorie diets, in which patients consume about 400–800 calories per day (about a third of what weight-loss diets normally should provide). These VLCDs often involve liquid diet preparations plus occasional solid food. While these diets are not necessary for those who have small amounts of weight to lose, they can, *under a doctor's strict supervision,* be just fine for the very obese. The key is that you're monitored

closely by trained physicians to be sure your body can handle the rapid weight loss. The doctor must monitor your many body systems and be sure no damage is being caused either by malnutrition or dehydration. These very restrictive diets work best, finds Rena Wing, when accompanied by behavioral treatment and exercise (both discussed earlier) in addition to major calorie restriction. It's important to note that these extremely low calorie diets do not work indefinitely. At some point, when exposed to an extreme calorie deficit, the body slows its metabolism in an attempt to prevent starvation—which means your weight loss could slow down or even stop. If you reach this kind of "plateau" while on a VLCD, talk to your doctor; ironically, increasing both your calorie intake and your activity level may be needed in order to kick you back into the weight loss mode.

Using Medication to Lose Weight.
Some scientists, following in the pattern of treating other eating disorders with medication, have studied the use of antidepressant medication on obese people. This strategy seems to work in some patients, particularly with a class of drugs called serotonin re-uptake inhibitors (alone or in conjunction with other medication). Many questions remain as to the effectiveness of using medication to treat obesity, and the safety of using these drugs long-term. But the possibility remains that for a certain subset of overweight people, including those with mood disturbances that predispose them to dangerous periodic overeating, medication may play a role in treatment.

Weight Loss Goals.
There is a strong movement in the weight loss

community to shift away from unrealistic, stringent weight-loss goals (like getting to your optimal weight according to height/weight charts) and to choose, instead, more moderate, attainable goals. For instance, experts find that telling a woman who weighs 180 pounds that she has to get down to 120 pounds will create a situation in which her early achievements—say, a 10 or 15 pound loss—seem like nothing more than a drop in the bucket. If we focus on improving overall health, a 15-pound sustained weight loss might make a considerable difference in that woman's health—bringing her blood pressure down, lowering her cholesterol level, or taking some pain off of her joints. These gains should be applauded, not minimized. When weight-loss goals become good health and not thinness, we'll be on the right track.

Experts recommend reappraising one's weight-loss goals with each 10% drop in body weight. By testing for important measures of health, like diabetes and blood pressure, we can tell if we're accomplishing useful goals. We can also ask ourselves (a) if we *need* to lose more weight, and (b) if we *want* to do so, or if we want to settle for a consistently high (but lower than before) weight. Incremental end points are much better than massive, far-off ones. And since there is some data (albeit conflicting) showing that yo-yo dieting—going up and down in weight—is unsafe over the long term, you just may be better off settling on a higher permanent weight (called a "set point") rather than bouncing up and down year in, year out. Susan Nitzke of the University of Wisconsin-Madison points to animal studies suggesting that yo-yo dieting causes coronary artery disease and adult-onset diabetes. Dr. Stunkard feels that even if yo-yo dieting doesn't harm our physical health, it does harm our emotional health with chronic disappointment and low self-esteem.

The ultimate goal for all of us, of course, is to come to terms with our bodies as we are able and willing to maintain them. We cannot change our bones, and after a certain point (with exercise and diet) we cannot transform our shapes. Once we have attained the goal of better health, better fitness, better strength and functioning, and lowered the risk of the many obesity-related health problems, it's time to come to terms with who we are, and the fact that we don't all look alike—nor do we, or should we, all look like the mannequins in store windows and on magazine covers. When we fall into the trap of chronic self-criticism, comparing ourselves to unrealistic images created by a society fixed on a narrow definition of beauty, denying ourselves food we need to survive and thrive, we miss the point of weight control for health, and move toward destructive weight-loss behavior.

....

FOR MORE INFORMATION ON WEIGHT LOSS AND MAINTENANCE

SEE RESOURCES AT THE END OF THE CHAPTERS ON NUTRITION AND DIET (PAGE 421), EATING DISORDERS (PAGE 471), EXERCISE (PAGE 436) AND HEART HEALTH (PAGE 504).

....

CHAPTER TWENTY-THREE

EATING DISORDERS

*Everything from television to fashion ads have
made it seem wicked to cast a shadow.*

—Peg Bracken, *The I Hate to Cook Book*

Disordered eating, which eats at the soul as it does the body, is terribly common among young women. When food, one's weight, body image and eating become a painful obsession, an eating disorder is the frequent result. But it's important to understand that while food and weight become the focus in an eating disorder, these are only *symptoms* of more serious underlying emotional problems and issues. If you or someone you love suffers from an eating disorder, don't make the mistake of focusing on food alone. With professional help, dig beneath the weight obsession to learn about and solve the underlying problems that led to the eating disorder in the first place. As you will discover in this chapter, there are many, diverse causes of eating disorders, and they're not always simple to dissect from one another. Treatment can be painstakingly slow, with ups and downs, and the road to recovery extremely rocky.

Recently, experts have come to think of eating disorders not as bizarre or unique illnesses but rather as eating problems that lie at extreme ends of a normal eating continuum, with dieting and restraint on one end and massive overeating on the other. When you take a look at the three main kinds of eating disorders, you'll understand why.

ANOREXIA NERVOSA

Commonly called just "anorexia," this eating disorder often takes hold in adolescence or young adulthood and is characterized by self-starvation and dangerous weight loss. (For details, *see* symptoms section below.)

....

ANOREXIA NERVOSA: WHAT YOU HAD TO SAY ABOUT IT

Joan, 27 years old

I wasn't eating anything. I was to the point where I was having a cup of tea and a rice cake all day. I don't know what kept me alive. I was skin and bones. I didn't see it. I was a skeleton. An emaciated sick-looking person. I disregarded it. I had no energy. Just taking a shower and raising my arms to wash my hair was an effort, but the ironic thing was doing little things like that told me I was okay.

My husband saw a different body than I did. I saw fat thighs and chesty for my waist. I was 90 pounds, five foot seven. In the beginning I skipped breakfast. Then it was easy to skip lunch. My husband didn't know, our breakfast and lunch schedules were different. Then dinner got smaller and smaller. Dinner became a game—I'd say, "I caught something on the way home," or "I worked out and got back late." My husband lost track.

I totally avoided social situations. I got worse and worse looking, I never felt good. I was constantly freezing. I think when it really horrified him was when I couldn't get out of the tub. I had to call him for help, and he was horrified. I used to have bruises on the bottom of my butt from sitting all day. I used to take hot baths to get warm but I had to put towels on my spine because it hurt so much. I remember saying to my husband, "Shake me and make sure I wake up—just make sure I'm breathing." In my heart I was afraid I wouldn't wake up. When I was at my weakest, I couldn't even read. I mumbled my words. People

must've thought I was drunk. I would lose my train of thought mid-sentence. I just said I wasn't feeling well. They speculated, Did I have a drinking problem? Did I have cancer?

Being a perfectionist, I said "Calm down, I can make this all better." I look back to when I was a teenager and wonder, was I predisposed? No self-confidence, no self-esteem, a perfectionist. I lived my life to please other people. It was awful when I bottomed out. In the beginning it was slow. Then in the fall of last year I plummeted. I don't know if I have a strong enough adjective. I felt life was caving in on me, problems in my marriage, and my work, and it all got worse because I had no energy. I had control over nothing but my weight. I totally brushed off anything anybody said about my weight. I layered my clothing, wore four shirts, very baggy pants. Someone would say, "Joan, you've lost weight," and I'd say, "You think so?" and brush it off or say it's the clothes. I was like "I'm in complete control, I'm fine." I got mad at one friend who [said I had a problem], I brushed it off, and found myself avoiding her. We used to have lunch every day.

I went through hell to find the place [that could help me]. One big roadblock was my HMO, any doctor someone would toss out at me was not on my plan. [With one doctor] I remember walking out of there thinking I could die under this man's care.

I hoped I would be able to eat food when I walked into the hospital. It started with one bite of rice and I thought I'd be a blimp. Most of my nutrition came from a nutrition supplement. Right now everything is so concentrated on me, it has to be that way for me to stay well. I don't have the energy to work on the marital problems so part of me feels selfish, but I have to do it now. I think he's tired of watching me struggle. I've been in the hospital three months and I haven't heard from my boss. I'm hurt. I was his right hand, but I always knew he didn't care. Part of it was the look on my husband's and parents' faces. I lost a sibling to diabetes—the hurt in their eyes, I can't be responsible for that, for putting them through that.

A doctor, (a friend of a friend), called me every day, he was the one who got me to this place. I'm indebted to him forever. I gained 32 pounds now. I don't like it. I still obsess, even more, about my thighs or that I look fat. It didn't feel good at 90, it doesn't feel good now. I'm supposed to be discharged tomorrow. I'm scared. I'm scared as hell. I wanna try. The relapse rate is high. I have a lot of issues, my marriage, my job. I have to put my life together and eat. It's scary. I'm going to do the outpatient follow-up program to prevent relapse. I'm a very determined, motivated person. I'm motivated by a challenge. It was hard, it was really really hard. I was driven by the want to get out and get my life back. You gotta have the will, the will to live.

BULIMIA NERVOSA

Known by most as "bulimia," (from the Greek words for ox and hunger) this now highly publicized illness was called "Anorexia's sister ailment" by *Newsweek* magazine in 1981, when few had heard about it. It now stands on its own, making headlines in connection with Princess Diana and other celebrities ever since. Bulimia consists of cycles of overeating (binging) and purging by means of self-induced vomiting and the use of drugs like diuretics, laxatives and other unhealthy methods of cleaning out the body. (*See* symptoms section below.) Bulimics tend to be a bit older than anorectics, often in their later teens, 20s and older, and may be of close-to-normal weight.

BULIMIA NERVOSA: WHAT YOU HAD TO SAY ABOUT IT

Elizabeth, 31 years old
I realized I had a problem long before I sought treatment. I've been bulimic for over ten years, I sought treatment a little bit here and there and was easily discouraged. Only three months ago did I join a program that specializes in eating disorders. I feel a lot better. I'm less depressed about it. The problem is better but not cured. I think it's going to be a long time.

The program I'm in is a combination psychotherapy and medication. I don't know if I'm getting the medication because it's a study, but I think I am. It's becoming aware of the patterns. I feel a chemical change when I engage in this (binging)—it's soothing, akin to drug use. It's exaggerated by anxiety. My particular pattern is more purging than bingeing, I might eat something considered normal and then throw up. I used to go through periods when I'd binge three persons' meals worth at once. It might be a couple pieces of pizza, a sandwich and another thing.

Usually the way my disorder has been I've often done it out of the house, fast food in secret, because people were in the house. You get really good at your addictions over the years. I would enjoy being by myself, read in a restaurant. If I was eating with friends and wanted to throw up after it, it became a secret ritual. I felt a huge split between my inner self and my outer appearance. I was pretty desperate and didn't know where to go. I was squelching my anxiety through this thing. I had this productive exterior. I really crashed this year, there were so many things I didn't attend to psychologically, needs for ten years. I really fell apart and just realized it was time to get help.

A long time ago a friend took me aside and asked if it was a problem and I admitted it. It's just very recently that I told a couple of friends and my mother. I was relieved that they didn't know. I told my mother: we've had tremendous problems in our relationship. I asked her to read up on it to understand it better. She did and found some centers. I went to one of them. I'm making a concerted effort to pay attention to how I act and feelings I have. I do feel like I will be able to have the two combine. When I think about it, I see it working out. I have a feeling it will always be present in some form, in the form of something nagging at me when I feel bad. I remember feeling hungry always. I wish I could tweak the part of my brain that handles appetite. I think it's from when I was little this behavior worked for me. The worst it ever got was maybe eight purges a day. I'd go into automatic. I got very good at it. I'd drink a certain amount of fluid that made it very easy to do it, it didn't hurt. I was hitting rock bottom and I think I really wanted to move on in my life. It was totally in my way. I'm going to be able to overcome this, to build up my strength. It takes enormous strength and courage and self-love and seeing it as something against yourself. To love yourself, that's mostly what it is: the discipline of beating it is part of thinking you're worth it.

BINGE EATING DISORDER

Related to bulimia in that it involves binging on large quantities of food, binge eating disorder differs from other eating disorders in that there is no purge or deprivation of food in response to the overeating. Those who suffer from binge eating disorder are often obese and endure tremendous pain, guilt and embarrassment about their eating habits. (*See* symptoms section below.)

BINGE EATING DISORDER: WHAT YOU HAD TO SAY ABOUT IT

Rose, 43 years old
Excessive binging. The inability to stop. A dozen donuts, a half gallon of ice cream, four–five pieces of pizza. As I'm doing it, I'm thinking "I might as well get it all in now because this behavior has to stop." I'm such a total numbness and departed from reality: all that dominates is getting the next bite. I have the desire to live and feel and look normal, to exist without the extreme domination of the food ruling my life. I believe I have an eating disorder, and anything good or bad or happy or sad even if things are fine this disorder triggers itself in very irregular patterns.

I would have to say the age I was first aware of it was when I felt unhappy with my childhood obesity, age 10, I started yo-yo dieting. I'm 43 now and it has progressed worse in the last 20 years. I've been seeking attention for the problem. I was most desperate 11 years ago when I went to a self help group, had a couple of situations with therapists seven–eight years ago. I hit a new bottom, a relapse a year ago, and I was very self abusive with the binging so I did seek help again. I was pretty close to suicidal, there were thoughts. A lot of times the mind would say, "You're not string bean perfect, you might as well do a number and binge."

There is not adequate help out there in any way, shape or form. Only a handful that really understand. One cannot really understand the insanity of the addiction unless one has experienced it oneself. In many years of trying to seek help, going to dieting/motivation places, nowhere have I been allowed to forgive myself until Dr. X. I was able to look at the problem in a new light, a lot of self forgiveness. Cognitive therapy, a lot of different behavior modifications. Not eating very fast, not eating while standing, not eating in the car, not eating without tasting the food. It's about healthy choices. Today I don't want to eat foods that aren't healthy choices. I'm more aware. It's about keeping my mind and body inside and out healthy, it's about choices, it's about decision. I'm able to make these. In a relatively easy comfortable way I've lost approximately 30 pounds of the 45 I had put on during my relapse.

Seek help, do a lot of homework. There are some wonderful self-help groups out there but sometimes we need help outside what that has to offer. We need to be treated from the inside out, what triggers the food thoughts from a physical point of view, from an emotional point of view. Doctors today are "parts" doctors—we need to be treated for our *whole* bodies and minds. It's a very painful disorder where we tend to isolate and really hurt.

THE HARD FACTS

About seven million women suffer from eating disorders in the U.S. While there is some overlap among the different disorders (bulimic anorectics, for example), we'll discuss them as separate entities for now. While eating disorders are not exclusively female problems, women account for more than nine out of ten cases. Anorexia is thought to be the most rare, affecting perhaps 1% to 2% of women. The statistics

on bulimia vary more widely, usually ranging from 2% to 5% of adolescent and young adult women and one in four college age women. It was once thought that eating disorders were primarily diseases of Caucasian, upper middle class women. Kathleen Pike, chief psychologist on the eating disorders unit at the New York State Psychiatric Institute at Columbia Presbyterian Medical Center, says we *now* know that these disorders span all races and classes. The considerable health risks—even life risks—posed by eating disorders contribute to the hard facts about these diseases: one in five anorectics will die as a result of their illness, usually from cardiac arrest or suicide.

As you will see below, starvation and binge-purge cycles place an enormous burden on the body and mind and put most organ systems of the body at risk of destruction. Also, women with eating disorders are more likely to suffer from depression and anxiety disorders, which come with a host of their own risk factors (*see* chapter 17).

WHO'S AT RISK? THE CAUSES OF EATING DISORDERS

There are as many explanations of what causes eating disorders as there are researchers studying them. Some focus primarily on society's obsession with beauty, particularly when it comes to women, and the fact that scrawny, prepubescent models' bodies are constantly paraded in front of today's teenagers as a message of what *ought* to be. We've all seen the tiny mannequins in stores wearing bathing suits we couldn't even fit into when we were twelve years old. Well, experts argue that these omnipresent images serve as a constant reprimand to young women whose images in the mirror do not reflect that Madison Avenue ideal.

Others have argued that since thinness is equated with feminity, starving oneself is an attempt to be as "female" as possible. Thinness or ladylikeness becomes a goal to aspire to, for many young women—an accomplishment in and of itself. The message reaches girls so early these days that a number of studies have found eight-year-olds already dieting! By the time they reach high school or college (called "eating disorder breeding grounds" by some researchers) and start dating, the desire to be thin (read: beautiful) intensifies.

Another prominent theory for what *causes* eating disorders is an emotionally "disordered" family life. Many women with eating disorders have troubled families in which support, problem solving and approval are sorely lacking, particularly between mother and daughter. Kathleen Pike has found that many mothers of eating disordered women have eating problems *themselves,* and also have a tendency to be critical of their daughters' weight and overall appearance. A combination of what she calls behavior "modelling" (in which the mother silently instructs the daughter on her weight and eating habits) and outright pressuring of the daughter to be thinner can contribute to the development of an eating disorder.

Ruth Striegel-Moore of Wesleyan University, president-elect of the Academy for Eating Disorders, stresses that adolescence and the onset of puberty can push a vulnerable young girl over the top: since girls gain more body fat and naturally move *away* from the idealized, sticklike masculine frame when they reach puberty, they are in a sense biologically programmed to experience disappointment with

their bodies. She notes that girls who develop early—that is, develop breasts, start menstruating, and gain weight before their peers—might be even more vulnerable than others to developing an eating disorder. An extension of this theory is that anorexia, for example, is an unconscious attempt to hold back the aging process by holding back the development of a fuller, female body.

Another potential eating disorder trigger is some form of substance abuse in the family. Children of alcoholics or other substance addicts are more prone to developing both eating and exercise disorders than other people. Eating disorders have come to be seen, in part, as forms of addictions themselves.

Personalities of women with eating disorders have also received a great deal of attention and many researchers describe vulnerable "eating disorder personalities," including the inability to cope with stress, a profound sense of inadequacy and ineffectiveness, difficulty with personal relationships, a sense of perfectionism and unrealistically high goals paired with the conflicting qualities of low self-esteem, poor assertiveness and trouble with problem solving. Women with eating disorders are generally more concerned with others' opinions, perceptions and approval of them. They are often competitive and highly motivated to please others—at the same time, they're often quite dependent on these significant others. Combine these qualities with a skewed body image, outside pressure to be skinny and beautiful, chronic dieting and hunger, a hypercritical parent and chronic depression, and you can see a highly vulnerable individual.

One thing worth noting is that researchers have had a "chicken and egg" problem when it comes to figuring out the cause of eating disorders. For example, women with eating disorders are known to have higher levels of depression, anxiety, feelings of guilt, rage and grief than women who do not have eating disorders. The question is, Do these feelings *precede and/or cause* the eating disorder, or do they arise as a *result* of the eating disorder—in the form of guilt after binging or purging, for example? There are many unanswered questions about eating disorders, which makes it trickier to treat them than some other biopsychological illnesses. The fact that every woman's experience is different, and her reasons/compulsions to be thin take on different meanings and expressions, makes treatment even harder.

Yet another association with eating disorders is a history of sexual, physical and emotional abuse. While certainly not all women with eating disorders have been abused, a large number *have* been. Whenever this is a cause, it is vital that the issue of abuse be addressed directly and aggressively in therapy. As with any cause or trigger of an eating disorder, the underlying issues need tending to, over and above the symptoms of the eating problem. When underlying problems are resolved, often (though not always) the eating disorder follows suit.

Triggers or subtle encouragements to disordered eating pervade our society, affecting children and adults alike. Ruth Striegel-Moore relates a very telling story about her own daughter's grade-school class. The teacher was giving out reward stickers to children who did not eat dessert! Happily, after Striegel-Moore discussed the issue with the teacher, the reward system was stopped. We must teach young girls (and boys) not only about moderation in all forms of consumption, but also to focus on issues of substantially greater importance than eating and body shape.

Researchers are learning more all the time about both the biological and the psychological components of eating disorders. Often called "mental illnesses," these disorders are thought to have biochemical or physical causes as well. For one example, a research team at the University of Michigan found increased levels of a brain hormone called vasopression in bulimic patients. This hormone is related to feelings of thirst, learning, memory and blood pressure regulation. More work on this particular brain chemical and many others will hopefully yield tangible information about the chemical causes and results of eating disorders, with the ultimate goal of providing new avenues for drug treatment.

When digging for the cause of an eating disorder, it's important to distinguish *causes* from *triggers*. While the underlying cause of an eating disorder might be much more complex or hidden, the trigger can be quite simple and obvious. For instance, many women have had eating disorders set off by the negative comment of an athletic coach ("You sure got hefty over the summer, didn't you?") or a disapproving parent ("You don't need that piece of cake, honey"). But it's important not to blame the person who triggers a binge, purge or bout of anorexia for causing the problem. Clearly, there were significant vulnerabilities built into the person with the disorder. She was, in many ways, a stick of dynamite waiting to be lit.

So when we ask, "Who is at risk for an eating disorder?", we have to think about social, biological, psychological, familial and other issues. We must avoid falling into stereotypical explanations, and consider how *this individual person* might be vulnerable because of *her* life experiences. As you will see later in this chapter, when it comes to treating an eating disorder, these individual issues take on the utmost importance.

SYMPTOMS: KNOWING WHEN TO WORRY ABOUT AN EATING DISORDER

As I briefly mentioned above, the symptoms of the various eating disorders differ significantly. Let's take a look at the different types, one by one. In this section, the answer to the question "When should I worry" is "now." Because eating disorders are so terribly damaging, both physically and psychologically, it's important to seek help as soon as the first signs appear.

ANOREXIA NERVOSA: DO YOU SEE YOURSELF, OR A LOVED ONE, IN THE FOLLOWING DESCRIPTION?

The following lists of symptoms come from the Diagnostic and Statistical Manual of Mental Disorders of the American Psychiatric Association.

Refusal to maintain body weight at or above a minimally normal weight for age and height; weight loss leading to maintenance of body weight less than 85% of that expected; failure to make expected weight gain during a period of growth, leading to body weight less than 85% of that expected

Intense fear of gaining weight or becoming fat, even though underweight

Disturbance in the way one's body weight or shape is experienced, undue influence of body shape and weight on self-evaluation, or denial of the seriousness of current low body weight

In women who have already started menstruating, the absence of at least three consecutive periods

There are two different kinds of anorectics:

The restricting type: no binge eating or purging behavior

The binge-eating/purging type: with binge eating, purging, self-induced vomiting, misuse of laxatives or diuretics

OTHER THINGS YOU MIGHT NOTICE ABOUT SOMEONE WITH ANOREXIA NERVOSA

Intolerance of cold

A downy fuzz or hairiness on the face or arms

A preoccupation with cooking, food preparation for others; peculiar habits in handling food

Frequent weighing of themselves, perhaps before and after exercise

Complaints of feeling bloated or nauseated after eating normal amounts of food

Irritability, difficulty concentrating, withdrawal, turning inward, depression

Tendency to bruise easily

Fatigue

Eating miniscule portions of food at meals, if eating at all

Sometimes, trips to the bathroom to vomit after meals

Hiding thinness under large, bulky clothes

SOME SIGNS A DOCTOR MIGHT FIND IN A PERSON WITH ANOREXIA NERVOSA

Bone loss or fractures due to osteoporosis that sets in when periods stop as a result of excessive exercise and inadequate calcium intake (hard as it may be to believe, Barbara Drinkwater of Pacific Medical Center in Seattle has found that the bones of anorectic women even in their early '20s are as porous as those of normal women in their '70s. The hunchbacking and vertebral fractures we associate with old age have already set in for some of these young anorectic women)

Electrolyte imbalance, dehydration

Anemia

Heart arrhythmias

BULIMIA NERVOSA: DO YOU SEE YOURSELF, OR A LOVED ONE, IN THE FOLLOWING DESCRIPTION?

Recurrent episodes of binge eating

(a) Eating, in a discrete period of time (within any two-hour period, for example) an amount of food that is definitely larger than most people would eat during a similar period of time in similar circumstances

(b) A sense of lack of control over eating during the episode (feeling that one cannot stop eating or control what or how much one is eating)

Recurrent inappropriate compensatory behavior in order to prevent weight gain, such as self-induced vomiting, misuse of laxatives, diuretics or other medications, fasting, or excessive exercise

The binge eating and inappropriate compensatory behaviors both occur, on average, at least two times a week for three months

Self-evaluation is unduly influenced by body shape and weight

Disturbance does not occur exclusively during episodes of anorexia

There are two different kinds of bulimics:

The purging type: regular self-induced vomiting, misuse or laxatives or diuretics

The nonpurging type: person uses other inappropriate compensatory behaviors such as fasting or excessive exercise

OTHER THINGS YOU MIGHT NOTICE ABOUT SOMEONE WITH BULIMIA NERVOSA

Discolored teeth caused by acid from vomit eroding the enamel

Swollen face, swollen glands

Weight fluctuations, sometimes dramatic, sometimes several times in the course of a year

Calluses on fingers and knuckles due to acid from self-induced vomiting

A very extroverted personality—"I'm having fun and everything's fine"

Eat enormous meals but never seem to get obese

Abuse alcohol or other drugs

Strict diets followed by excessive eating

Secretive regarding binges—hidden food, hidden laxatives or diuretics

Often use the bathroom after meals to purge; after purging, often appear swollen, agitated

Depressive moods

Overeating in reaction to emotional stress

SOME SIGNS A DOCTOR MIGHT FIND IN A PERSON WITH BULIMIA

Damaged esophagus and throat from vomit acid

Damaged colon from laxative abuse

Dehydration, electrolyte imbalance

Weak bones

Heart rhythm problems

TWO TRENDS THAT OFTEN OCCUR WITH BULIMIA: DO THEY SOUND TOO FAMILIAR?

Low self-esteem leads to depression and in turn to binging; binging leads to guilt and self-loathing and in turn to purging. The cycle repeats.

Excessive dieting leads to hunger which leads to a loss of inhibition and in turn to binging; binging leads to guilt, self-loathing, purging and renewed dieting and hunger

BINGE-EATING DISORDER

Recurrent episodes of binge eating

(a) Eating in a discrete period of time (for example, within a two hour period) an amount of food that is definitely larger than most people would eat during a similar period of time in similar circumstances

(b) A sense of lack of control over eating during the episode (feeling that one can't stop eating or control what or how much one is eating)

The binge eating episodes are associated with at least three of the following:

(a)   eating much more rapidly than normal

(b)   eating until feeling uncomfortably full

(c)   eating large amounts of food when not feeling physically hungry

(d)   eating alone because of being embarrassed by how much one is eating

(e)   feeling disgusted with oneself, depressed or feeling very guilty after overeating

Marked distress regarding binge eating

Binge eating occurs on average at least two days a week for six months

Binge eating does not occur exclusively during the course of anorexia or bulimia

(NOTE: It's important to keep in mind that while health care professionals have developed these definitions of the three main eating disorders, it is possible to *have* an eating disorder but not meet every one of the characteristics listed above. If you have some variation of the symptoms of any eating disorder, seek help: you can still benefit from treatment.)

SOME OTHER QUALITIES YOU MIGHT NOTICE ABOUT A BINGE EATER

This list was adapted from Overeaters Anonymous:

- Binge eaters often eat when they're not hungry
- They binge for no apparent reason
- They have feelings of guilt and remorse after they overeat
- They spend an inordinate amount of time and thought on food
- They look forward with pleasure and anticipation to eating alone
- They plan secret binges ahead of time
- They eat sensibly before others and make up for it alone
- Their weight affects the way they live their lives
- They try to diet for a week or more and fall short of their goal
- They resent others who say "use willpower" to stop overeating
- Despite evidence to the contrary, they continue to assert that they can diet on their own whenever they wish
- They crave to eat at a definite time, day or night, other than mealtime
- They eat to escape from worries or trouble
- They have often been treated for obesity or another food related condition
- Their eating behavior makes them or others unhappy

EXERCISE ADDICTS

Compulsive exercising can be a part of an eating disorder or a disorder in and of itself. For bulimics, exercise serves as another means to purge after indulging. For anorectics, it's another way to restrict calorie intake, starving the body of energy. Ironically, while moderate exercise strengthens the body and mind, excessive exercise does just the opposite, causing menstrual periods to stop, bone loss to accelerate, weakness, dizziness, loss of muscle and fluid more than fat, drops in blood sugar, increase in fatigue and lack of concentration. Experts have measured decreased muscle strength, loss of endurance, a drop in oxygen use and aerobic strength and other important measures of failing athletic potential in people who starve themselves and overtrain.

Exercise addicts make major life decisions around fitting in a workout, letting life slip by them in their blind effort to become fit. One disturbing feature of compulsive exercise is that victims don't have to *hide* their "little secret"; since exercise is praised in our society, the more they work out, the more positive feedback they get. In fact, they're destroying their bodies and need help, not praise.

Certain sports are known to have a disproportionate number of compulsive exercisers and participants with eating disorders. These include gymnastics, figure skating, ballet and other forms of dance, and running. To a certain degree, leanness puts these athletes at a competitive advantage; for instance, it has been observed that judges like the look of slender bodies—and excess weight *can* slow you down. But if you find, as experts warn, that you are exercising only to burn calories, to stay thin, to get rid of negative feelings—or if you find you are organizing your life around exercising and measuring your happiness according to your fitness level—you might have a problem. Therapy similar to that for eating disorders (*see below*) can be quite helpful—as can getting some hard medical measures of what you're doing to your body (bone scans, blood tests, etc.).

Preventing Eating Disorders

Because there are so many potential causes of eating disorders, it's difficult if not impossible to prevent someone from getting one. However, experts believe that, certainly within families, certain types of behavior might make eating disorders less likely. For instance:

Educate your preadolescent daughters about the changes they can expect in their bodies. Teach them to appreciate the beauty of their new curves and shapes—this will help build their self-esteem as their bodies develop and gain fat and weight. Telling them that a certain amount of increased fat is a sign of a healthy female body will go a long way toward offsetting their fears of becoming obese.

Try to focus on young women's successes in areas other than their weight—such as their school work, their kindness, or their creativity.

Don't promote weight loss as a high-priority topic in your home. If you often complain about your own weight, or talk about dieting, your message will come through loud and clear to your daughter or women friends.

Model healthy eating and normal, regular exercise for yourself and for the entire family.

Following a healthy diet and lifestyle as outlined earlier in this part, and keeping the whole family active in a fun, noncompetitive way (group walks, hikes, bike rides, ball in the park, etc.) will put exercise and fitness in a healthy, noncompulsive framework.

Watch for any change in a child's or friend's behavior regarding food, secrecy, weight loss—and *talk about it* immediately. Be direct, caring and honest. Ask if there is a problem, a reason they aren't eating, a reason they're going straight to the bathroom after eating, and so on, and offer help if needed. Backing off because you're uncomfortable doesn't do them, or you, any good.

None of these methods can guarantee prevention of an eating disorder. But all of them can promote healthier thinking about eating and weight gain, and show a vulnerable person that you care about them and are available to help them in any way possible. That might not pay off immediately, but people with eating disorders often say that prolonged support and love from others ultimately gave them the push to seek professional help (or for those with more minor eating disturbances, to work the problem out on their own).

Because the different kinds of eating disorders are quite distinct in their symptoms and sometimes their causes, treatments differ as well. Interestingly, even though we've known about anorexia for a lot longer than we've known about bulimia, there are more effective treatments for bulimia. Let's take a brief look at the treatments for each problem.

Treating Anorexia Nervosa

The initial and primary goal in treating anorexia is to get the patient to gain weight. This can be an excruciatingly slow, painstaking process because nothing is more horrifying to this person than the idea of getting fat. Often, inpatient treatment is needed to guide—or sometimes, unfortunately, force—the person to take in nutrients to save their life. Several experts I interviewed said that even a miniscule amount of weight gain—say, 1/16 of a pound—is an achievement. Forcing an anorectic to gain too much weight at once can completely backfire. Adding a single bagel during the course of a week can be a major milestone. This is *not* how nutritionists favor treatment, but sometimes it is the only realistic option, and reality—solutions—are what you're after.

Inpatient Versus Outpatient Treatment

In many ways, the ideal in treating any eating disorder is to allow the patient to come to a treatment center but live at home. The reason: it allows them to learn to incorporate their new habits into a real-life setting, in face of all of the temptations, conflicts and interpersonal problems that real life has to offer. This theory holds that hospital settings are unrealistically controlled, safe environments (where food is prepared for you and can be carefully monitored, and where support systems are all around you 24-hours a day). The fear is that when inpatients go home and face old problems and old habits, they might relapse. However, if the anorectic simply will not or cannot learn to eat more on an outpatient basis, then inpatient care might be necessary and extremely helpful

at least as a way of helping the patient get on her feet and begin recovery. Kathleen Pike of Columbia University and the New York State Psychiatric Institute suggests the following rules of thumb: if the patient's condition is life-threatening, immediately begin *inpatient* care. If she is not in immediate danger, *start* with outpatient treatment and if it fails—if there is no weight gain and no change of habits—move treatment into a clinic or hospital.

Whether inpatient or outpatient treatment is chosen, there are several key characteristics to a good eating disorder treatment program. First, it should use a *team* approach to care. Depending on the age of the patient, this might mean either an adult physician or a pediatrician, a psychiatrist or psychologist, a nutritionist (ideally a registered dietician), and, if exercise obsession is part of her problem, a coach or trainer as well. Depending on his or her background, perhaps the gynecologist would be an effective member of the team—in other cases, the school nurse might help. It's vital that the patient *trust* all members of the team, or a single part of treatment can undermine the healing process. Because eating disorders are multi-faceted problems, no one "expert" can address all of the issues involved in recovery. Someone must attend to the physical damage incurred by the eating disorder, someone to the underlying emotional problems that led to the disorder in the first place, someone to the patient's complicated relationship with food. Think of treating an eating disorder as putting a person back together again, a piece at a time. The painter should do the painting, the carpenter the woodwork, and the electrician the wiring. Let experts do the jobs they're best at doing.

Keep in mind that there is relatively little

solid scientific information on the *best* ways to treat anorexia. Researchers and clinicians are still experimenting with the most effective combinations of therapy, medication and other methods of support. Results will also be highly individualized, since eating disorders are so diverse in cause and behavior. So while one woman might gain a great deal from group therapy, another might strongly prefer private, individual counseling. Still another might prefer a combination of the two. Once you are convinced you have found a competent, experienced treatment group, you might have to sit back and work with them while they experiment with the best treatment for *you*.

THERAPY

Psychotherapy is a central feature in the treatment of anorexia. There are many different kinds of therapy (chapter 17 discusses some of them), but one stands out as particularly useful with this disorder: CBT, or cognitive behavioral therapy. This form of therapy focuses on the faulty thinking and belief patterns that can lead to eating disorders. Ask a potential therapist what kind of therapy she specializes in, if any, and also ask if they have extensive experience dealing with anorexia patients. More than ever before, we're growing to understand that just as medications have specific indications for particular diseases, so therapy must also be customized to the particular problem at hand. A marital counselor might have as little to tell you about dealing with anorexia as a computer technician could tell you about your carburetor. Fit the treatment to the problem.

For some women, especially younger women who live with their families, family therapy can be extremely helpful with anorexia. Not only does it serve to educate loved ones about the underlying issues and pains that contribute to the problem in the first place, but it gives the patient a chance, in a controlled setting, to vent and confront family problems that might compound the eating disorder—or may have helped cause it in the first place. Because families are often ignorant about eating disorders and become angry, panicked, resentful or fearful for the life and health of the woman with the disorder, unmediated discussions about the problem can be heated or hysterical, full of accusations and blame. Remember, some of these families have watched their loved one literally waste away before their eyes, punish themselves with hours and hours of exercise, vomit or use drugs to rob their bodies of needed nutrients. It can be devastating to experience an eating disorder from the "outside," both because of the fear and heartache directed toward the person with the eating disorder and because of the sense of ineffectualness, helplessness and guilt it can bring on parents, siblings and close friends. In the presence of a trained counselor, on the other hand, these discussions can be controlled and directed toward *positive* goals and recovery—looking to the future rather than the past. When family therapy works, it benefits everyone who participates—not just the "patient"—by opening up new lines of communication and support that perhaps faded or never existed in the first place.

If you happen to live in an area where specialized mental health care is hard to come by, most experts agree that some form of therapy—by a reputable and caring counselor—is better than none at all. At least it's a start. Make sure your therapist is properly certified in his or her area of counseling—whether social work, psychology, family therapy, and so on.

Once you've begun therapy, you may discover that your problem is serious enough that it warrants traveling some distance to a more comprehensive and experienced treatment team. Some of the organizations listed at the end of this chapter can help you find nearby experts.

MEDICATION

Unfortunately, drug treatment for anorexia has been disappointing. Antipsychotic medications were tried, but the side effects were powerful and the effectiveness unclear at best. Antidepressant medications have also not proved especially useful except in the case of fluoxetine, which may be helpful in the prevention of a relapse after other therapies have brought about a remission. Other drugs, including something called a serotonin agonist (called cyproheptadine), seemed helpful to nonbulimic anorectics, but we need a better understanding of whom this drug might help. Some experts feel that more work should be done with the drug lithium (commonly used to treat manic depression) to determine if it might help some patients with anorexia.

You might be wondering why I'm listing medications that *don't* work. Well, there's an important reason. While drug treatment for anorexia has been disappointing, drug treatment for bulimia has been successful, therefore it's *vital* that you get a proper diagnosis for your eating disorder so you don't waste your time with inappropriate treatments. Just as it's useless to take an antidepressant drug when you have an anxiety disorder, so it's useless to take a drug that might help bulimia if your problem is anorexia. This is all the more reason to seek the advice of experts who specialize in eating disorders.

TREATING BULIMIA NERVOSA

A number of those I interviewed noted that bulimics often lack positive activities, interests and relationships outside of their eating disorder, so building a broader range of such involvements is an important part of treatment. Developing meaningful friendships and tighter family bonds, learning to participate in activities other than exercise and eating (going to movies, or the theater; taking casual walks) can be vital parts of moving toward a life beyond the eating disorder. Cognitive behavioral therapy (CBT) and interpersonal therapy (IPT) can be extremely helpful in guiding a person to healthier thoughts, activities and relationships. CBT helps boost awareness of the mental and other triggers to binge eating. IPT also facilitates the trigger discovery process, and teaches patients new, healthier coping skills for all of life's relationships (making demands of others, and learning to take criticism in a more constructive way, for example).

As with the treatment of anorexia, treatment of bulimia should be team-based, with experts from various fields (*see* "Treating Anorexia," above).

MEDICATION

A major difference between the treatment of anorexia and the treatment of bulimia is that medication can be extremely helpful with bulimia.

Antidepressant medication holds the greatest promise in the drug treatment of bulimia. All three types of antidepressants (the tricyclics, the MAO inhibitors, and the newer Prozac family of drugs, called serotonin re-uptake inhibitors) have been helpful in treating bulimia. While researchers at the NY State Psychiatric Institute have noted that there are some limitations with the way antidepressants have been used to treat bulimia (namely, treatment has been short-term, with a fixed single dose), the results have still been exciting. Interestingly, you don't have to be depressed in addition to being bulimic to get good results from these drugs.

Other drugs, like anticonvulsants, have been tried for bulimia with some limited success, but antidepressants right now are leading the pack as far as effectiveness goes.

How do you decide whether to go on medication, especially considering the fact that these drugs do have side effects? Some treatment teams recommend starting out with talk therapy and seeing how it goes. If, after a couple of months, you have not improved as much as you or your practitioner had hoped, try adding a single trial of a medication. If you don't respond well to that drug, try a different one (let your doctor guide you in getting off of one and onto another properly). There are plenty of patients out there who respond well to one medication and not at all to another. For many women, six months of comprehensive, committed treatment will cure bulimia: however, you may need long-term follow-up or a continued occasional relationship with a therapist to keep yourself on track.

A major question researchers are now asking about the treatment of bulimia is if psychotherapy alone is helpful, and medication alone is helpful, wouldn't the two *together* be the best treatment possible? There are some studies that suggest this is the case, so you might want to talk to your practitioner(s) about launching both treatments at once for the best possible shot at a faster recovery.

TREATMENT OF BINGE-EATING DISORDER

There is no established "correct" treatment for binge-eating disorder. Dr. Robert Spitzer, chief of biometrics research at Columbia University's New York State Psychiatric Institute, says that treatment should be tailored to the particular problems the binge eater is facing. For instance, since depression is more common among binge eaters than among others, proper management of depression can sometimes make a dent in the eating problem as well. Dr. Spitzer also says that treatment with cognitive behavioral therapy (therapy based on reversing negative thoughts and behaviors) can help combat the triggers to binge eating. Research also suggests that interpersonal therapy can be helpful for this problem.

Some feel that self-help groups, like Overeaters Anonymous, can be very helpful with this kind of problem. They're often based on the twelve-step approach common to substance abuse treatment, and have a religious thrust to them, which will be appealing to some, and a turn-off to others. They're relatively inexpensive, however, and offer tremendous support, particularly for those who feel isolated and humiliated by their problem.

Marsha Marcus, director of the outpatient eating disorders clinic and partial hospitalization program at Western Psychiatric Institute and Clinic in Pittsburgh runs a group that treats binge eating disorder from the perspective of empowering the patient to take control of her life, teaching her that she has the tools to care for herself. Marcus contrasts this to the idea of turning over your care to a higher power, as some self-help groups promote. She also recommends behavior modification as the mainstay of treating *all* eating disorders. With this approach, the patient gradually learns to change her unhealthy behaviors, eating one scoop of ice cream instead of the entire carton, changing meetings with her boss let's say, that always seem to result in binges, and setting limited, not excessive, goals (such as "I'll cut down my eating just *once* this week"). Other behavior modification techniques that can help with binge-eating disorder include replacing the binging behavior with a healthier "habit" like exercise.

Susan Bartlett, a consultant in the weight and eating disorders program at the University of Pennsylvania, stresses that treatment for binge eating disorder should focus on gaining *control over eating,* not on weight loss. Binge eaters often have no planned meal times, and are therefore ravenous when they do eat. Bartlett teaches patients to spread their calories evenly throughout the day to avoid hunger that might precipitate a binge.

Finally, while dieting has been implicated as a possible cause of some eating disorders (the domino effect we discussed earlier in this chapter), dieting may be an acceptable part of treatment for binge-eating disorder, according to Marsha Marcus. Since many binge eaters are overweight, reasonable, controlled weight management may be an important part of getting back on a generally healthy life track.

LOVED ONES: HOW TO DEAL WITH SOMEONE WHO HAS AN EATING DISORDER

According to Dr. Michael Pertschuk, medical director of the eating disorders clinic at Friends Hospital in Philadelphia, the first rule for families dealing with an eating disorder is *silence doesn't work.* Saying that you don't want to make waves, rock the boat, offend a loved one, or just pretending that the eating disorder is a short phase your loved one is going through is the wrong way to approach the problem. The first correct step, he says, is to address the problem directly: for example, say, "You don't seem to be eating much and you're losing a lot of weight: I'm concerned about what I'm seeing; is something wrong?" Or: "You're going to the bathroom after every meal, and it looks to me like you're vomiting. Is there a problem? Can I help you?" You'll have to expect the person to deny whatever you suggest, says Marcus. Your goal, she says, is to express your concern and let the person know that if there's a problem, help is available. You're planting an idea: this is just the first step.

Dr. Pertschuk recommends that you try to pose your concerns as *your* perceptions, rather than as accusations. If you simply say, "You're not eating," you're inviting them to say, "Yes I am" and close the subject. If, on the other hand, you speak from your perspective and concerns, saying "It seems like you're losing too much weight and I'm concerned about you," it's harder for the person with the problem to dismiss you outright.

If the disordered behavior continues, which it usually does, your job as a family member or friend becomes harder. You need to help bring the person to a doctor or some other medical attention. In most cases you can't drag someone to see a doctor, but you can be very persuasive. Don't give up. Dr. Pertschuk says that adolescents with eating disorders often report that they were waiting for someone to take charge and do something for them, because they felt powerless to help themselves. After initially resisting help, many are immediately relieved once help is at hand.

Without a medical emergency, you can't force an adult to see a doctor. Often you can force your young children to do so, however. Even a visit to their regular pediatrician (where they will be weighed) can be helpful, since the doctor, who is more objective than you are, can address the issue from a medical standpoint. But be warned, experts say, that children with eating disorders become very adept at faking their weight, lining their clothing with change or drinking lots of water before doctor visits.

There is a point at which you *can* force an adult to get medical attention. In some states, if you can prove that a person is at immediate risk to themselves (for example, their weight has dropped into the life-threatening danger zone at about 60% below normal), you can force them into the hospital and keep them there on intravenous fluids or tube feeding to save their lives.

Experts say the worst thing parents can do is contradict one another. If one parent says there's a problem and the other denies it, people with eating disorders are very good at playing one parent off the other, diverting attention from the problem itself and delaying getting help. Parents need to be on the same team to be

helpful. If they aren't, it can be helpful to see an expert as a couple first, before trying to bring the child.

Sometimes the best thing families or close friends can do is to join therapy with the troubled person. Since eating disorders are often tied to more complicated social interactions, working out dysfunctional relationships as a team can be very useful. The fact that you too are committed to working on the problem takes the burden off the person with the eating disorder, in part, and shows love and commitment that are sorely needed at this time.

Sometimes women with bulimia nervosa will leave clues for loved ones to discover, such as vomit in a garbage pail, or diuretics on a desk top. *Don't ignore the clues;* they're cries for help. This person wants to be found out, and wants to be helped. Again, be direct but caring, and offer support in getting help.

Binge-eating disorder, which is often quite hidden, can be very tricky for friends and family members to confront. First, those with the problem are often older and may not have family or roommates around to notice their troubled behavior. Second, our society doesn't consider it polite or comfortable to talk about excessive eating or obesity. Loved ones are loathe to raise the issue of binge eating for fear of insulting or embarrassing the person with the problem. Try to swallow your humility and speak up, however. Just as with other eating disorders, the sooner you confront the issue and offer to help, the sooner your friend will get well. This is no time for standing on ceremony or convention. It's a chance to do a friend some significant good.

FOR MORE INFORMATION ON EATING DISORDERS

AMERICAN ANOREXIA AND BULIMIA
ASSOCIATION (NEW JERSEY)
201-836-1800

AMERICAN ANOREXIA/BULIMIA
ASSOCIATION
418 East 76th Street
New York, NY 10021
212-734-1114

NATIONAL ASSOCIATION OF ANOREXIA
NERVOSA AND ASSOCIATED
DISORDERS
P.O. Box 7
Highland Park, IL 60035
708-831-3438

ANOREXIA NERVOSA AND RELATED
EATING DISORDERS, INC.
P.O. Box 5102
Eugene, OR 97405
503-344-1144

NATIONAL EATING DISORDERS
ORGANIZATION
445 E. Granville Rd.
Worthington, OH 43085-3195
614-436-1112

OVEREATERS ANONYMOUS, INC.
WORLD SERVICE OFFICE
P.O. Box 44020
Rio Rancho, NM 87174-4020
505-891-2664

ANOREXIA NERVOSA AND ASSOCIATED
DISORDERS (ILLINOIS)
312-831-3438

CENTER FOR THE STUDY OF ANOREXIA
AND BULIMIA (NEW YORK)
1 West 91st Street
New York, NY 10024
212-595-3449

ANOREXIA NERVOSA AND RELATED
EATING DISORDERS, INC. (OREGON)
503-344-1144

PART EIGHT

The Top Two:
Cancer and Heart Disease

CHAPTER TWENTY-FOUR

HEART DISEASE, HEART HEALTH

Thanks to the human heart by which we live,
Thanks to its tenderness, its joys, and fears
To me the meanest flower that blooms can give
Thoughts that do often lie too deep for tears.

—William Wordsworth, "Ode" (*Intimations of Immortality*) St. 11

WOMEN AND HEART DISEASE

There was a time not too long ago when even the medical community considered the words "women and heart disease" to be a contradiction in terms. Heart disease wasn't a woman's problem. It was the killer of *men.* Major heart associations ran public service announcements advising women to watch for signs of their *husbands'* heart disease.

Sadly, even today, we haven't come such a long way. While the word is starting to get out to physicians (and I mean *starting*) most women still pretty much ignore the signs and risk factors for heart disease—if they even know what they are in the first place. Most heart disease experts I interviewed expressed strong concern over the fact that women are far more worried about breast cancer than they are about heart disease. Statistically, that doesn't make much sense: far more women die of heart disease than of cancer—*all* cancers totaled, in fact.

About ten million American women have some cardiovascular problem. At the age of 65, one in three women has heart disease—a staggering figure. All cardiovascular diseases combined kill over 485,000 women each year—and surprise, surprise: that's *more* than the total number of men killed by these diseases, according to the American Heart Association. Heart attacks alone kill nearly 250,000 women a year. Still, we do little to reduce our risk.

Part of the reason it's so easy for women to ignore heart disease is it tends to strike us later in life than many other high-profile diseases. Women's heart disease rates tend to pick up after menopause (which occurs, on average at about 51 years of age) and the heart attack rate in women runs about 10–20 years behind that of men. One theory of why women ignore heart disease in favor of cancer is that we tend to think of cancer as snatching us out of the prime of our lives, while heart disease, like wrinkled skin, is simply something to *expect* if you're lucky enough to grow old. After all, one in three women will die of heart disease—it's just the way we tend to "go," right? It's this myth that must be dispelled. Heart disease is *not* a normal part of aging, nor is it unavoidable.

The good news is that with risk factor modification, new drugs and improved surgical techniques, the death rate from heart disease has dropped over the last few decades. The bad news is women haven't benefited as much as men, for a wide variety of reasons we'll discuss in this chapter. African-American women, who sustain particularly high rates of certain risk factors for heart disease (like hypertension and diabetes), have also had historically poorer access to lifesaving treatments.

It's not just *unfortunate* that women's heart disease risk has been ignored for so long. It's *tragic.* Numerous studies have shown that because of clinicians' skepticism about women's risk for heart disease, and their tendency to say that symptoms are "all in your head," women haven't been given the same kind of rigorous

screening for heart disease, and therefore become much sicker as their disease develops, undiagnosed. A terrible cycle has developed, in which most diagnostic tools and treatment modalities are tailored to *men's* needs, so they're not as effective in women, and less likely to be *given* to women in the first place. This means women are even *less* likely to have their heart disease diagnosed, and in turn less likely to be referred to a variety of lifesaving procedures than men. Finally, partly because of all of this delay, when women *are* finally sent for potentially lifesaving surgery, it's often in an emergency situation, when we tend to do much worse than men! Women have more second heart attacks, and are less likely to live through complicated heart surgery than men are. It's a deadly cycle that can only be beaten, as we'll discuss, when women and their doctors cooperate carefully in listening for signs of disease and investigating *aggressively* when something awry is suspected.

One good reason for women to start considering their risk of heart disease is there's now a lot we can do to reduce that risk. This is one area of disease where lifestyle changes can accomplish a significant amount, not only in the way you feel every day, but also in your risk of death. Throughout this chapter, we'll look at the many causes and types of heart disease— from clogged arteries to electrical problems to high blood pressure to valve disease—plus the changes you can make in your behavior to cut your risk. We'll also take a look at the various diagnostic tools for heart disease and how they can be better tailored to women's needs. If you are having symptoms that might be related to heart disease (*see* description below), ask your doctor for an immediate, thorough, gender-specific workup to determine if any type of heart disease is your problem—regardless of your age.

Heart Disease: What You Had to Say About It

Gertrude, 79 years old
I had no history of anything of any kind. I had irregular heart beats for a good part of my life; at one point they called it tachycardia. I had stress in my life, a mother who was very ill at one point, a son who was very ill at one point.

I'm not a phlegmatic person. I didn't know what was going on. We were on a trip to Australia, seated on a plane for ten hours. We arrived late at night. As I got out, I had to run to get a taxi while my husband got our bags. I ran up an incline and felt this pressure on my chest. It was like a horseshoe or horse pressing on my chest. I thought it was being out of shape. I didn't think about it, just thought this sure is a heavy thing on my chest and we continued on our trip to Bali.

I felt quite well, walked on the deck of the ship. It never occurred to me I could have a heart attack. My husband had one, but that was different. My son is a physician and is constantly sending us lots of notes on this and that, so I'm sort of au courant with a lot of things, but I felt women do not have heart attacks as frequently as men or are less likely to have them than men. It never occurred to me for one minute. I could think of a thousand other things I could get.

Back home my cardiologist determined that I had had a heart attack. By this time, I had begun to swell. My cardiologist put me on medication. I was shocked beyond belief. I always thought a heart attack was like "Ahhh!" There were clues,

but you think it was that medication that did it, or I would attribute it to the fact that all my life I'd had these irregular heart beats.

I smoked from the time I was 18 'til I was in my 70s. I *know*—I'm positive that the smoking had a lot to do with it. My cholesterol was over 200. I had a lot of stress in my life, and we traveled in great style and only ate things totally divine and full of fat. And I didn't do much exercise. I have always been a swimmer all my life, and did a certain amount of stretching exercise. I know the young women today do aerobic exercise—I didn't do that sort of thing.

Insofar as exercise is concerned I've done much more. I try to do 20 laps a day in a forty to sixty foot pool. I can't get on a bike because I have bad knees, but I do try to walk as much as possible. I have a hip replacement. I try to do a little every day. I try doing the stretching and that kind of thing. Now I read the label, I don't buy anything without reading the label. I don't buy anything until I read the contents, fat and cholesterol. Occasionally I cheat, "Okay, just *one* of those." I'm very much aware when we go to dinner, that's the tempting time, the desserts, I just resist.

My message would be to take advantage of every bit of information you can. There's so much more we know today regarding women being just as much at risk for heart disease as men, especially after menopause. Stop smoking, pay attention to exercise, what you eat, avoid fat. We are not immune to heart disease.

Julie, 52 years old
The basis for all my [heart] problems is Marfan's syndrome. I wasn't diagnosed until 1984 during emergency surgery for aortic dissection. I inherited this from my father who died of an aortic dis-

section at age 46. There is still too much of that—people walking around undiagnosed. People are still acting on old information—"Why tell the patient when there isn't a lot you can do?" Women are more often told it's all in their mind. But of course there is a *lot* you can do.

I was doing a lot of things a person with a dilated aorta shouldn't do—doing aerobic exercise. When it's ready to go, it's really ready: I turned off the shower and something was wrong. I didn't know what it was, I was white or green or some color I wasn't normally and my friend took me to the emergency room. I didn't even have a doctor then. They replaced my aorta—I'm almost entirely Dacron inside! They have to watch all the parts of my aorta that were replaced.

There are people who live in fear chronically because of chronic disease. I'm determined to enjoy life. Humor is important for me. I started doing humor and creativity workshops, people know that a positive attitude makes a difference, but they don't know how to get it. All of life is about choices, it's all about making a choice of how to deal with the circumstances. [Resisting your disease] is like saying "I didn't choose to be tall, there's nothing I can do about it." I can resist it, and say, "I hate this, I don't want to be tall." Or I can be resigned to it, and say, "I'll just have to put up with being this way." Or I can *choose* tallness, embrace it, say, "This is part of me." That kind of acceptance isn't like saying it's the most fabulous thing that I have it, but in a funny way I've learned a lot from [my disease]. It widened me, broadened me as a person. That doesn't mean I don't miss tap dancing, but you have to say, "Fine, well, replace it with something else." It's made me examine my life like I never would have before. The medical community says if you have a serious illness, you have to be serious. Of course we have to take our illness seriously, but without taking ourselves too seriously.

Marion, 82 years old
I had a pain that wouldn't leave, a pain in the throat, that little spoon where your neck meets your chest. Dull pressure sometimes went into my chest, cramplike in the chest, shooting down my left arm. I thought it might be a heart problem. I called the doctor. At one time my cholesterol was 280 or 300. We brought it down with a low-fat diet to about 210, 220, and then we had to go to medication because we wanted to bring it down further.

They did an angiogram and two arteries were blocked, and they did an angioplasty two days later. The ballooning didn't work so they sent up the roto-rooter thing. I saw all the plaque fall away, it was amazing. It's not half as scary as you think it is. I was very leery about angioplasty but he said you're in good general health. The system gets out of whack, it's a blow, but after that thank God it was okay. The difference is I can walk and not get out of breath, and I don't get the pain in my throat. Use some sense and have a doctor who really explains it to you. I'm so much better.

SYMPTOMS OF HEART DISEASE THAT YOU CAN WATCH FOR

In some ways, women experience the symptoms of heart disease differently than men. These differences have received more attention recently, but Dr. William Castelli, director of the Framingham Heart Study, warns that women often experience heart pain just as men do. We'll take a look at *many* heart disease symptoms in this chapter, in order to cover all of the bases.

While there are no hard and fast rules, there

are certain common threads in the way women feel when heart disease is developing, or has become serious. Dr. Marie Savard, director of the center for women's health at the University of Pennsylvania, notes that women's chest pain often goes on for a long time, even months or years, lingering in a vague, sometimes subtle way that women come to think of as normal. The pain slowly builds, she adds, and is less often sudden or extreme than is heart pain in men. Sylvia Fields, coordinator of the primary care and community programs at Jefferson Medical College in Philadelphia, adds that while heart pain in men tends to go up the left side of the body and down the arm, in women it can be much more esoteric—affecting just the elbows perhaps, or the neck, or occurring only after meals (dangerously mimicking indigestion). The pain tends to be less sharp in women, she adds. Trudy Bush, professor of epidemiology and preventive medicine at the University of Maryland School of Medicine in Baltimore, notes that women often feel chest pain radiating down the back and *both* arms. This is in contrast to "classic" chest pain which is described as a dull, deep pain under the breast bone or as a band across the chest that might radiate to the *left* arm, shoulder, neck, jaw, teeth and down the back, along with sweating, nausea and faintness. Women might be "lucky" enough to have these more telltale signs, too—but often, women's symptoms are harder to pinpoint.

Women often have chest pain during exertion—even minor "exercise" like climbing stairs. Again, don't assume this is normal. Sure, if you're simply out of shape, you're not going to feel great when you run up a flight of stairs—a sign that it's time to get more movement into your life (*see* chapter 21 for advice on exercise for women). But if you notice that your chest pain *only* appears when you're exerting yourself, or gets worse at these times and subsides afterward, talk to your doctor and consider some of the diagnostic tools we'll discuss later.

Another type of heart disease symptom more common among women is the strange sensation that sometimes accompanies heart valve problems—most commonly, mitral valve prolapse or MVP. While lots of women have a minor problem with the mitral valve in their heart and *no* symptoms whatsoever, others may feel a chronic sense of breathlessness, discomfort in the chest, fatigue or weakness. And women are more prone to other relatively rare cardiovascular problems, including periodic vessel spasms that cause a great deal of pain.

Dr. Paula Johnson, a cardiologist at the Brigham and Women's Hospital, warns that for women with diabetes, heart disease symptoms may be even more vague or subtle than for other women. Sometimes, diabetic women feel only shortness of breath and sweatiness, and no chest or other pain at all when heart disease is developing. For this reason, and because they are at high risk of heart problems to begin with, women with diabetes should be vigilant about regular screening for heart disease risk factors, and maintain as heart-healthy a lifestyle as possible. (More on this later.)

Heart failure, yet another form of heart disease, has a wide set of symptoms of its own, including weakness; swelling in the ankle or other parts of the lower body as blood and fluid pool in the lower extremities; leg pain; coughing; dizziness or light-headedness; and chest, jaw, tooth or arm pain. With severe heart failure, patients often have an overwhelming sense of exhaustion, almost like the kind that accompanies a devastating flu—but in this case it lasts and lasts.

Of course, women can experience so-called "classic" chest pain, too—particularly during a heart attack. Dr. Joanne Manson, coprincipal investigator of the cardiovascular section of the Harvard Nurses' Health Study, shares Dr. Castelli's concern that all the recent talk of women's *different* cardiovascular symptoms may steer women away from vigilance about classic heart pain. Pay attention to the following symptoms, and if you experience them, call your doctor and 911 for emergency assistance.

Signs of a Heart Attack

- Crushing pain in the chest that may radiate into the jaw, the neck, the arms, the shoulders or the back.
- A feeling of intense pressure or weight, more than pain, in the chest—but true sharp pain is possible, too.
- Nausea, dizziness, fainting, sweating, shortness of breath, weakness or exhaustion that may accompany the symptoms above. (Some say these signs are more common in women than in men, but Dr. Marian Limacher of the University of Florida at Gainesville feels they're more common in *older* heart patients—and since many women with heart disease are older, this skews the symptoms to women.)

Remember, one reason heart disease has been so trivialized in women is that often, when women report symptoms that mimic heart attacks or heart disease, diagnostic testing rules

it out. Don't be embarrassed if this happens to you; a sensitive physician shouldn't chide you for "crying wolf." You'll be a lot better off erring on the side of caution than leaving symptoms unattended. True, some chest pain or discomfort will turn out to be unexplainable—or minor, caused by anything from gastric reflux (a problem in the esophagus) to referred neck muscle pain. Do *not* accept a diagnosis of "anxiety," particularly if you know you're not anxious! Even if heart disease has been properly ruled out, move on to some other aggressive investigation with your general internist.

Detecting Heart Disease in Women

They say that 90% of diagnoses can be made from "history"—that is, the patient's description of pain, disability, and so on. What you don't tell your doctor, he/she can't guess. Keep track of your bothersome symptoms—when they occur, what they feel like, what makes them come and go. Sylvia Fields notes that with the future of medicine moving toward shorter office visits, you may not have much time to explain your condition to your doctor. She feels this will be a particular disadvantage to women patients, since we tend to ask more questions and take more time in the doctor's office than men do. Bringing a few notes with details on how you've been feeling can help make short appointments more efficient.

The better your reported history is, the better the chance your doctor will receive information that could lead her/him to an accurate diagnosis. So, when you go to your doctor appointment, make sure you offer the following information:

- Your family history of heart disease—any parent, grandparent or other relative who had a heart attack, known heart disease or heart failure, hypertension, heart rhythm problems, etc.
- A profile of your symptoms written on paper: when and how it hurts most, what it feels like, how long it lasts, what kinds of activities bring it on, etc.
- If you smoke, or did in the past, confess.
- Give the doctor a good idea of your fitness level—how often, if at all, you exercise. This includes general activity that you don't think of as "exercise"—like walking to work, or picking up groceries.
- Tell about your risk factors for heart disease. If you don't know them—your cholesterol level, your blood pressure, etc.—that's one of the first things you'll want to have taken care of at this visit.

It's also vital that you find the right clinician, one who takes your concerns and symptoms seriously. If you're told that chest pain is probably "all in your head," or that "young women don't get heart disease," it's probably time to move on to a more enlightened physician. You want your caretaker to be not only attuned to your feelings and fears, but also one who will communicate openly with you when it comes time to explain diagnostic tools, medications and other treatments.

THE DIAGNOSIS

As I mentioned earlier, the classic tools used for detecting heart problems are notoriously inaccurate in women. However, many experts I interviewed noted that even these tools can be used more effectively in women by making small adjustments either in the way the tests are done, or in the standards by which the test results are measured afterwards. Dr. Richard Devereaux, head of echocardiography for The New York Hospital/Cornell Medical Center, finds that more and more centers across the country are learning "tricks" to make standard screening tests more effective in women. Things that can get in the way of effective imaging, he notes, such as breast tissue or the build of a woman's ribs, can be accounted for when tests are evaluated. Ask your doctor what kinds of adjustments he/she makes to boost the accuracy of heart testing in women. And remember, no doctor is a magician—he/she *cannot* tell you your heart is healthy by listening to a stethoscope, giving you a physical exam and sending you home.

If you have chest pain that indicates coronary artery disease—that is, the kind of chest

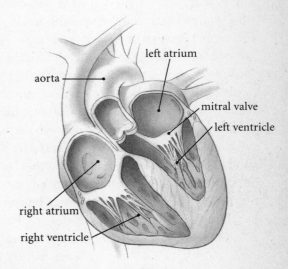

Normal human heart

pain mentioned earlier, which is a sign of heart disease that's related to clogged arteries—here's the kind of workup you should expect:

Heart Tests

1. First, you may be given an office *EKG test*—the electrocardiogram that's used to measure the electrical activity in several areas of the heart, and to determine if the heart is getting enough blood or if it's injured in some way. This test is not particularly effective in women, *but* if it shows serious abnormalities, you should be given a more thorough investigation immediately. One reason you can get lots of false results in women is that mitral valve prolapse, a fairly common problem in women, can skew the test results. If the results are questionable or even if they're normal, you should be given an exercise stress test.

2. The *exercise stress test* is an EKG test done while you're exercising on a treadmill. Or, if you can't exercise this way, you may be given drugs that make the heart think it's exercising. This test will show how the heart performs while you're under physical stress. Again (you're going to hear this a lot), this test is often inaccurate in women, who tend to have many so-called "false positives." False positives mean the test shows an abnormality, but the woman does *not* turn out to have heart disease, and may be subjected to further testing unnecessarily. (This is less likely to be a problem in older women with more risk factors for heart disease.) Subtle differences in the way the exercise

EKG is interpreted can help to insure better accuracy in women. Dr. Richard Devereaux finds that when he compares the heart's electrical activity to the heart rate, he gets a more accurate picture of disease in women. A negative test result—that is, one that says the heart is okay—is pretty reliable. On the other hand, if this test shows a serious abnormality, you might be put in an ambulance and taken to a hospital for treatment. If it shows *some* abnormality, or isn't clear, doctors will want to determine (a) if there really is a problem and (b) how bad the problem is. So . . .

3. They'll try a *stress thallium test.* What this means is that you'll do the same type of test again—exercising on a treadmill with doctors monitoring your heart—but this time, the doctors will inject a safe dye with a radioisotope into your veins which will travel to your heart, where it will "light up" any areas where the heart is damaged and not getting the oxygen it needs. This test, while still not perfect in women (or men), is much better than tests with no dye at all. If this test comes back abnormal, doctors will know that you have a problem—and they'll have a pretty good idea of the extent of the problem. Dr. Nanette Wenger of the Emory University School of Medicine worries that women's breast tissue can get in the way of a good image with this and other heart tests, interfering with doctors' ability to get a clear result. This interference should be taken into careful consideration, particularly when evaluating test results. If doctors know there is a problem, but not how bad it is, there's only one way to find out *exactly*

what's going on in the arteries—and you and your doctor together will have to decide whether to do it:

4. An *angiogram.* This is an invasive test, and carries risk. About one in a thousand cases have serious complications. There are some things beyond your control, but choosing an experienced doctor helps keep the odds of trouble down. Doctors snake a catheter into your arteries (usually through the groin), inject a dye into it, and are literally able to take a look at your arteries using X rays to see if and where they are blocked or damaged. This test is the "gold standard" diagnostic test—it gives good, clear answers—but no one rushes into it because of the risks it entails, and because it's costly. Furthermore, as Trudy Bush notes, even among women who have been prescreened and brought to angiography, half will turn out to have normal arteries after going through this risky and stressful routine. And women may do a little bit worse than men with this test because they have smaller arteries, which are more vulnerable to damage. On the whole, however, this test is quite accurate and useful. After looking at the results, doctors can determine if medication alone might control your problem (meaning that you don't have terribly bad blockages in your arteries) or if you'll need surgery.

These are the tests normally used for coronary heart disease. But as we mentioned earlier, there are many different types of heart disease, and chest pain can be a sign of several of them. If your stress tests were all normal, you may be referred for a different kind of test, such as one that looks at your heart's structure and function:

5. An *echocardiogram.* This excellent, painless tool lets doctors see how your heart is performing—the movement of its valves, walls, and so on. It is the definitive diagnostic tool for mitral valve prolapse, for example, as well as for many other heart valve problems. It shows heart enlargement, which can be caused by a variety of problems. It might indicate signs of a past heart attack (silent heart attacks are more common in women than in men) or the results of high blood pressure. By bouncing sound waves off the heart's structures, the "echo," as it's usually called for short, shows how well the heart is pumping and *can,* with additional technology, show blood flow to the heart as well. Experts at the Arizona Heart Institute report that to avoid the interference of large breast tissue in women, the TEE (transesophageal echocardiogram) can be used in which a transducer is placed down the throat to get closer to the heart. It's a more invasive version of the test, and of course is done with mild anesthesia. Dr. Patricia Cole of the Washington University School of Medicine in St. Louis finds the echocardiogram *with exercise* to be quite useful in women, as well.

Testing for Other Heart Problems.
If you have fluttering in your heart, or for some other reason you or your doctor are concerned about a heart rhythm disturbance, you'll be given an entirely different round of testing. For instance, you might be given a Holter monitor to wear on your body, painlessly, for 24 hours to record your heart's rhythms. If your doctor suspects valve disease, the echocardiogram men-

tioned earlier is the best test for you. If coronary artery disease has been ruled out, and you're still having chest discomfort, funny-feeling rhythms in your chest or any other heart-suspicious symptoms, these various tests should be considered.

Low-tech Testing.

We've been speaking so far about high-tech (and high-priced) testing, which Americans tend to love. But don't forget, low-tech testing for heart disease risk factors can be every bit as important. Finding out your cholesterol level (both the "good cholesterol" and the "bad cholesterol") and your blood pressure is extremely important. These risk factors are every bit as important in women as they are in men, but women don't seem to take them as seriously.

WHAT TO DO WHEN YOU'VE FOUND YOUR SPECIFIC PROBLEMS

ACHIEVING NORMAL CHOLESTEROL LEVELS

A recent report from the National Cholesterol Education Program at the National Heart, Lung, and Blood Institute stressed the importance of cholesterol management in women. Dr. James Cleeman, coordinator of the program, highlights the following important points for women:

1. Women 20 years and older should have both their total cholesterol level and their "good" cholesterol level (HDL) checked by a health professional. You can think of HDL as a garbage truck that picks up the bad cholesterol (LDL) in your arteries and carts it away. Women tend to have higher HDL levels than men, which is good—it protects us. You can try to boost your level of HDL by reaching a normal body weight, exercising, and stopping smoking. Having a high level of "good" cholesterol or HDL is so important that the recent NIH report made it a "negative" risk factor. That is, if you have a high HDL level (over 60) you can *subtract* another risk factor (say, obesity) from your overall heart disease risk profile.

   Your total cholesterol level should be under 200—this is defined as "low risk." Between 200 and 239, you're at "borderline risk." Over 240, you're at "high risk" of heart disease.

2. If your total cholesterol is 240 or greater, and your HDL is under 35, *or* if your total cholesterol is borderline and you have two or more additional risk factors for heart disease (obesity, high blood pressure, diabetes, a family history of heart disease, etc.), you should have a complete "lipoprotein profile" done. This is a test that will look at all of your blood fats, including your good and bad cholesterol levels and your triglyceride level (discussed later). When you get the breakdown of your different types of cholesterol, you want to see an LDL below 130, an HDL over 35, and a triglyceride level of under 250.

3. If your cholesterol level is high, dietary therapy and exercise should be used to lower it. This is an important message for women, Dr. Cleeman stresses, since we have a national obesity problem among women. The main goal of dietary therapy is to lower fat and cholesterol consumption. And ac-

cording to Dr. Virgil Brown, past president of the American Heart Association, losing weight (especially fat) brings about a drop in "bad cholesterol" (LDL) and in triglycerides.

4. If diet and exercise don't lower your cholesterol enough to put you in the safe zone, you should consider cholesterol-lowering medication (or estrogen replacement therapy). But remember: taking these medications doesn't give you license to eat whatever you want, or to remain sedentary. You have to work along *with* the medication to reap the benefits of drug therapy. Dr. Cleeman notes that if you are a premenopausal woman with a high cholesterol level but no other significant risk factors for heart disease, you should use diet alone and hold off on drug therapy until you reach menopause. The only exceptions to this rule are women with a "bad" cholesterol (LDL) level of 220 or greater.

We discuss cholesterol-lowering drugs briefly later in this chapter. For a complete discussion of estrogen replacement, *see* chapter 10.

Quick tip: Don't get your cholesterol tested with a fast finger-stick test in a mall or other quick-test setting. These tests are often inaccurate. To get the best results from blood cholesterol testing, you should fast for 12 hours before the test, and have it evaluated in a laboratory. The new at-home cholesterol testing kit is thought to be pretty accurate, and a good way to monitor changes in your cholesterol level, but it's still a good idea to have your cholesterol level checked by your doctor and evaluated in a professional laboratory.

When Women's Cholesterol Levels Start to Change for the Worse.

After menopause, a woman's "lipid profile"—that is, the levels of cholesterol and other fats in her blood—often become much worse. When you no longer have lots of the hormone estrogen in your system, your cholesterol levels climb rapidly—which is one reason for the increase in heart disease rates in older women. This is also one of the arguments for taking estrogen replacement (which we'll discuss in more detail later on). Even if your cholesterol was normal before menopause, be sure to have it rechecked periodically after menstruation has stopped (either naturally or through surgical removal of your ovaries). From 1980 to 1991, nearly one in five women had high cholesterol levels—and one in *two* women over 55 had high cholesterol, according to a recent American Heart Association special report. But there's good news as well: Dr. Basil Rifkind, senior scientific advisor to the vascular research program at the National Heart, Lung, and Blood Institute notes that recent government surveys find women have been doing better than men at lowering cholesterol levels over the past several years. He suggests that women may now be understanding the needed diet changes better—or at least may be more willing to implement some of those changes for themselves.

Why Bother Lowering Your Cholesterol?

You might think that all this talk about cholesterol levels is trendy and not all that important. Well take a look at this statistic: for each 1% rise in your cholesterol level, there is about a 2 to 3% rise in heart attack risk. If that doesn't wake you up, I don't know what will. High cholesterol in the blood, which is determined *both* by what you eat *and* by your genes, is an important risk factor for heart disease and heart attack.

ACHIEVING A NORMAL CHOLESTEROL LEVEL

Another blood level that women should be aware of is triglycerides. Triglycerides, which are somewhat less predictive of heart disease in men, appear to be a more important risk factor for women. Normal triglyceride levels are somewhere between 30 and 200; 250 and over is thought to be high. Certain drugs, including oral contraceptives, a sedentary lifestyle, drinking large amounts of alcohol, and eating excessive simple sugars all boost triglyceride levels in susceptible individuals. While it can be tough to get your level of triglycerides down, becoming more active, cutting your alcohol intake and trying to switch from simple sugars to a balanced diet with complex carbohydrates can help. (For more on healthy diet choices. *See* chapter 20.)

ACHIEVING NORMAL BLOOD PRESSURE

Try to comprehend the enormity of this problem: according to the American Heart Association's 1994 statistics, as many as 50 million Americans have hypertension; half of them are women. Over 19,000 women died in 1990 as a result of high blood pressure. After age 45, 6 in 10 Caucasian women and nearly 8 in 10 African-American women have hypertension—startling figures. Also according to the AHA, more than a third of those who have high blood pressure don't know it—and therefore don't know they're at high risk of stroke and heart disease. That's especially troubling, since more

than 87,000 women die each year of strokes, many of which are caused by hypertension. African-Americans and people living in the so-called "stroke belt" region of the southeastern U.S. have especially high rates of both hypertension and stroke. Because high blood pressure is often controllable with lifestyle changes and proper medication, there is no reason for *anyone* to live with chronic hypertension. It is a powerful and *controllable* cause of organ disease particularly cardiovascular disease—throughout the body.

Normal blood pressure means a systolic or top number of 120 and a diastolic or bottom number of 70—that is, the classic 120/70. But as Dr. Tom Graboys of the Brigham and Women's Hospital and director of the Lown Cardiovascular Center in Boston points out, "normal" varies from person to person, and depends a great deal on age—so that an octogenarian might be just fine with a much higher blood pressure, while someone in their 40s could be at significant risk at higher levels. In general, "high blood pressure" is defined as systolic or top pressure of greater than or equal to 140, and diastolic or bottom pressure of greater than or equal to 90. Many Americans are considered "borderline" hypertensive, which means they aren't in the danger zone yet, but they're getting close. Borderline hypertensives can keep their blood pressure in check by adopting the lifestyle changes listed below:

1. Exercise as often as possible, following the guidelines in chapter 21. And keep the following in mind: it is believed that exercising for a longer period of time, at a lower intensity, is the best way to get blood pressure down. Over time, you can increase the

intensity of your exercise, but this should be done gradually. For example, let's say you've chosen to walk for 30 minutes, five times a week. After a few weeks, add a shallow hill or two. A few weeks after that, try walking with your hands in the air—it's a lot more tiring than you'd think. Or add some hand weights. Bit by bit, challenge yourself a little more. Never make a sudden, significant change in your exercise pattern—you're more likely to injure yourself, overdo it, or drop out the next day because of aches and pains. As always, talk to your doctor before starting *any* new exercise plan.

2. Watch your salt intake—but take this advice with a grain of salt! Not everyone who has high blood pressure is "salt-sensitive." According to Dr. John Laragh, director of the cardiovascular center and hypertension centers and chief of the department of cardiology at the New York Hospital/Cornell Medical Center, salt fears have been vastly exaggerated: probably eight out of ten hypertensives are *not* affected by salt in the diet. And chances are, he adds, the other two don't know who they are anyway! Traditionally, everyone with high blood pressure is advised to lower their dietary salt intake by cutting back on table salt, cooking salt, salted snacks, canned foods and so on. Dr. Vera Bittner of the division of cardiovascular disease at the University of Alabama-Birmingham advises staying away from heavily salted foods like pickles and salted pretzels, and urges you to check the portion size along with the salt content of packaged foods, so you won't be fooled.

The only way to find out if salt really affects your blood pressure, Dr. Laragh notes, is to do a test—have your blood pressure checked by a professional, then cut out salt almost entirely for about two weeks, and then have your pressure rechecked by a professional. If it goes down significantly, you are probably "salt-sensitive," and should avoid salt as much as possible. If not—and this is the more likely scenario—no one is saying you should go out and eat salt out of the shaker, but you certainly won't have to worry excessively about salt anymore.

3. Get your weight down. Being overweight puts you at risk for high blood pressure— and sometimes, losing weight is enough to take you out of the danger zone. (For details on losing weight, *see* chapter 22.)

4. Stop smoking. But let me make this clear: smoking doesn't *cause* high blood pressure, as people often claim. While you may have temporary blips in your blood pressure while you're smoking, no one thinks these small temporary increases are so dangerous. What smoking *does* do is create a poisonous combination with high blood pressure. The two risk factors *combined* put you at extremely high risk of heart disease.

5. Moderate your alcohol intake. Alcohol not only boosts blood pressure, it also interferes with the effectiveness of some hypertensive medications. Of course, this should be balanced with recent information that moderate alcohol consumption helps protect against heart disease in other ways, such as by raising "good cholesterol" levels (HDL). Talk to your doctor about how much alcohol, if any, would be appropriate for you.

6. Finally, always be aware of what your blood pressure level is. Dr. Suzanne Oparil, president of the American Heart Association, urges women to have their pressure checked every single year—even if it's normal. She notes that women tend to be more compliant and successful hypertension patients than do men (taking their medicine regularly, for example), so finding out about a blood pressure problem *early* and taking action can be very protective for women. If your pressure is found to be high—or even just borderline—boost your screening tests to twice a year, says Dr. Vera Bittner. Because you can't feel anything, you'll never know if your pressure is getting worse, she adds—a fact that makes many people ignore hypertension altogether.

Another lifestyle modification to consider is whether or not to take birth control pills. Oral contraceptives are associated with a slight increase in blood pressure for most women, but nothing worrisome. For a small number of other women, though, oral contraceptives cause a more significant increase in blood pressure. Having other risk factors for hypertension *along with* oral contraceptives seems to make matters worse (if you're overweight, or African-American, this might apply to you). Certain women shouldn't take the Pill at all—that is, those with a personal history of thromboembolic disease, or a strong family history of hypertension. On the whole, if you do take the birth control pill, opt for the lowest possible estrogen dose.

Pregnancy and High Blood Pressure.
Pregnancy can also trigger high blood pressure. If it's not *too* high, doctors will recommend lifestyle changes and they'll continue to watch your level closely over each visit. Some experts feel that temporary high blood pressure during pregnancy could be a red flag alerting you to the possibility that you'll develop hypertension later in life. Whether or not that's true, it can't hurt you to watch your hypertension risk factors and keep them all in check (*see* above).

If high blood pressure soars or is part of a larger complex of symptoms known as preeclampsia (or eclampsia) during pregnancy, you and your baby may be in danger, and need immediate attention. Sometimes treatment *during* pregnancy will be effective. In other cases, if you are nearing your due date, early delivery may be warranted. This is just one *more* good reason to start regular visits to your doctor as soon as you think you may be pregnant.

Other more serious heart problems can also be associated with or exacerbated by pregnancy. Dr. Patricia Cole of the University of Washington-St. Louis, who treats large numbers of pregnant women with heart disease, urges women to listen to and watch their bodies for signs of a *sudden change* at any point in pregnancy—such as unusual swelling in the ankles, extreme shortness of breath, chronic coughing or other unusual signs. While minor degrees of most of these symptoms are typical of even the healthiest pregnancies, extreme versions can signal problems—perhaps with the heart valves. Most problems can be handled during pregnancy without harming the fetus, and should not be left unattended.

We'll discuss medication for high blood pressure later in this chapter.

Stroke and High Blood Pressure.
One of the main reasons to watch your blood

pressure is to reduce your risk of stroke, an often devastating event which, if it doesn't kill you, can rob you of significant quality of life.

There are several types of stroke, and women are susceptible to all of them. Hypertension significantly promotes the risk of something called hemorrhagic stroke, and also increases your risk of ischemic stroke. Stroke, a devastating event, can often be prevented with significant lifestyle changes. First, as mentioned earlier, fight to keep your blood pressure down. Avoid excessive alcohol intake. Smoking can be deadly. Black women are twice as likely to suffer strokes as white women. Anticlotting drugs can help prevent some strokes, but they can *promote* hemorrhagic stroke by causing bleeding into the brain, so it is vital to be monitored closely when taking them, and to be sure they're appropriate for your condition and set of risks.

DIABETES: THE FORGOTTEN HEART DISEASE RISK FACTOR

While people certainly take diabetes seriously, we tend to overlook its importance as a risk factor for heart disease. Dr. John La Rosa, chancellor of Tulane University Medical Center, notes that diabetes is the single most important heart disease risk factor for women, wiping out the heart disease gender gap and interacting dangerously with other risk factors. If you are diabetic, it is essential that you keep your blood sugar in check as much as possible, for research indicates that by keeping blood sugar levels close to normal over the long haul, you may be able to prevent some of the long-term consequences of diabetes. Trudy Bush of the University of Maryland in Baltimore thinks diabetes is so serious a risk factor that even very

young diabetic women should assume that their risk for heart disease is just as great as a man's. If you have diabetes, she asserts, you must aggressively control your blood sugar, blood pressure, diet and exercise patterns over your entire lifetime.

Another fact women have ignored is that diabetes interacts in a lethal way with *other* heart disease risk factors, such as smoking, notes Dr. Donna Younger, assistant medical director at the Joslin Diabetes Center in Boston. And the bad news, she adds, is that some women with diabetes substitute cigarettes for candy, putting themselves at high risk of death from cardiovascular disease. If you have diabetes, it is imperative that you stop smoking, avoid fats as stringently as possible, and see a doctor immediately if you have any feeling of chest pain. Dr. Joanne Manson, principal investigator of the diabetes component of the Harvard Nurses' Health Study, likens smoking while you have diabetes to "putting a gun to your head."

Manson also points to some worrisome data from the Nurses' Health Study suggesting that diabetic women's dietary habits may be contributing to their high risk of heart disease. While they are cutting down on their sugar intake, as they should, some women with diabetes are replacing those sugary foods with *fatty* foods like hot dogs and sandwich meat. This goes against the American Diabetic Association's recommendations and contributes to a slew of other heart disease risk factors that these women don't need—obesity and high cholesterol among them. Don't fall into this trap. Sit down with a nutritionist and figure out how to make more sensible switches from sugary foods to healthy substitutes. The goal is to boost your intake of complex carbohydrates, like whole grains, pastas, vegetables and fruit.

General Advice on Fighting All Forms of Heart Disease

What You Can Do for Yourself

If you like to take a fatalisic view of life and your health, and believe there's little you can do to affect your chance of getting heart disease, you're selling yourself short. Listen to what the following experts have to say about it.

Dr. Meir Stampfer of the Harvard School of Public Health and the cardiovascular arm of the Nurses' Health Study takes a very strong stand on heart disease: *It doesn't have to exist.* The vast majority of cases, he says, are of our own making—through unhealthy behaviors. The disease would all but go away if we changed the way we live. He personally has made most of the changes he preaches, and still enjoys life!

Dr. Kenneth Epstein, associate director of the division of internal medicine at Jefferson Medical College in Philadelphia, calls behavior modification—risk reduction through lifestyle changes—"the mamography of heart disease"—that is, a tool guaranteed to save lives. Scare tactics don't work, he says; so many women just don't listen.

Dr. Joanne Manson, codirector of women's health at the Brigham and Women's Hospital and Harvard Medical School, says "heredity is not destiny—you have tremendous control over your risk of heart disease—use that power."

One of my favorite stories about women and heart disease comes from Trudy Bush, who notes that when she lectures in a room with 200 women in it, and asks how many are at risk for heart disease, only about 2 women raise their hands. When she asks how many women in the room smoke, have hypertension, a family history of heart disease, and so on, dozens raise their hands! They're all at high risk, but don't know it, she says.

Clearly, the message about women's risk—and risk factors—just hasn't come across loud and clear. And that can be deadly. Dr. Suzanne Oparil wants every woman to know that risk factors for heart disease aren't additive—that is, having two isn't twice as bad as having one; they are multiplicative—having two is *far* worse than having one.

Certain risk factors, like smoking and high cholesterol, are particularly lethal in combination with one another. Dr. Pamela Douglas of the Harvard Medical School, editor of the book *Cardiovascular Health and Disease in Women,* points out that women have two sets of risk factors: those that we share with men, and those that are unique to our gender. These include:

Risk Factors for Heart Disease Shared with Men

- smoking
- high cholesterol
- high blood pressure
- diabetes
- family history of heart disease (for women, the mother's side is most important, but the father's side matters, too)
- obesity
- sedentary lifestyle

Risk Factors Unique to Women

- taking oral contraceptives, particularly the

older kind with lots of estrogen
- natural menopause
- surgical removal of the ovaries

TAKING CHARGE OF YOUR HEART HEALTH: RISK FACTORS YOU CAN MANIPULATE

1. **You can stop smoking** (*see* chapter 19 for more information on smoking cessation). Keep in mind, the damage caused by smoking is dose-related: while your risk of heart disease is greater the more you smoke, even a single cigarette each day can double your risk, according to the Harvard Nurses' Health Study. So if you can't quit yet, at least cut back! Smoking is such a powerful risk factor for heart disease, it erases the gender gap in young people—that is, even a *young* woman who smokes carries as high a risk of heart disease as men. According to Dr. Meir Stampfer, smoking causes *half* of all heart attacks in middle-aged women. He especially worries that women are taking up smoking earlier, putting themselves at long-term risk.

2. **You can exercise more, and lose weight.** In fact, don't think about it as "exercise"—think about it as getting up and moving. Your body wasn't made to sit on a couch; it becomes sicker and sicker over time when it isn't used. As a nation, Dr. Stamfer says, we're getting fatter—not leaner—despite a vast amount of information about the dangers of being overweight. Because belly weight is thought to be riskier to the heart than fat on the hips and thighs, Mary O'Toole of the University of Tennessee in Memphis emphasizes that you want to strive for a waist-to-hip ratio of *under* 0.8. (For more on this, see page 445.) O'Toole notes that exercise can be customized to meet different goals. For instance, as mentioned earlier, if you're trying to get your blood pressure down, you should exercise at a lower intensity for a longer period of time. If on the other hand you're trying to cut your cholesterol level, you should choose a higher intensity exercise, starting with a shorter period of time and building up the length gradually. If you're trying to lose weight, very long duration is the key: the longer, the better—and low intensity is fine.

3. **You can take hormone replacement after menopause** (*see* the brief discussion later in this chapter; for more details *see* chapter 10).

BELIEVE IT: YOU CAN DO IT YOURSELF!

You can *dramatically* reduce your risk of heart disease and make your quality of life better at the same time by making a few changes in the way you live. You do *not* have to fall prey to chronic pain, medication or risky operations to save your life. In many cases, you can do it for yourself. If you're not motivated by the idea of down-the-road benefits, remember that when you make the move from an unhealthy to a healthy lifestyle—eating better, quitting smoking, losing weight and becoming less sedentary—you'll start to *feel* better *now*. Your chest pain might abate, you'll stop coughing, your chronic aches and pains are likely to lessen, you'll feel more energetic and cheerful as healthy chemicals are released in your body. Chances are people will notice more color in your face, more spring in your step, and a general air of well-being about you.

Dr. Dean Ornish, president and director of the Preventive Medicine Research Institute in California, who is considered something of a guru in the world of heart disease risk factor reduction, made a fascinating discovery. He showed that with lifestyle changes alone—that is, an extremely low-fat diet (bordering on vegetarian), exercise and stress reduction—you can actually *reverse* the plaque buildup inside your arteries. I'm a big fan of his, not only because his ideas are so sensible, but because I remember interviewing him for CBS News many years ago when people thought his "lifestyle modification" plan was flaky, out of the mainstream, and would never go anywhere. He believed in it, stuck with it, and today, Dr. Ornish's results are so impressive that certain major health insurance packages now pay for the program, which is a dramatic departure from their attitude to behavior modification programs in the past. His approach to beating heart disease, once on the fringe, is now more than mainstream—it's the way of the future.

The best part of the news for women, according to Dr. Ornish, is that several sophisticated tests show that women reverse heart disease more easily than men. When we make healthy lifestyle changes, our arteries actually clear out to a greater extent, and we report *feeling* better than men do.

You may doubt whether you and your family will be able to make the massive lifestyle changes that are required to reverse coronary artery disease and/or reduce heart disease risk. Actually, Dr. Ornish says, it's easier to make *major* lifestyle changes than minor ones. With moderate changes, he says, you get the worst of both worlds—you feel deprived of the unhealthy foods you love to eat and you don't get significant health benefits, so you're easily discouraged. Your chest pain probably sticks around, your cholesterol doesn't budge and you're missing those double cheeseburgers like crazy. This is why most doctors can't get their patients to change their behavior for much more than a couple of weeks at a stretch. If, on the other hand, you make major lifestyle changes—cooking differently, choosing different foods for the long haul, moving your body regularly and reducing stress in your life—you will reap such significant health benefits you'll soon become addicted to healthy living! Furthermore, you'll come to enjoy the new foods and activities you're doing (creative low-fat cooking, and so on), once you learn more about them.

Dr. Ornish finds with his own patients that the promise of living longer isn't a great motivator; the promise of feeling great, on the other hand, is the best encouragement you can find. With some education and a good measure of discipline, you can apply Dr. Ornish's principles in your own home (thousands of people have). See part 7 of this book for more details on cutting fat out of your diet, boosting your activity level and reducing stress. And consider reading his excellent books, *Eat More, Weigh Less,* and *Dr. Dean Ornish's Program for Reducing Heart Disease.*

While you're gearing up to make a change, keep this in mind: if your willpower is so great that you're able to make dramatic changes in your lifestyle, more power to you. But Dr. Basil Rifkind of the National Heart, Lung, and Blood

Institute worries that if we ask some people to do *too* much, they won't do anything at all. He admits that it would be better to get your cholesterol down to 170 than to aim for 200—and that yes, it would be nice if women got their total fat intake to 20% of total calories instead of 40%, where many American women are now. But better to do *something* than *nothing,* he argues—at least as a beginning. We're only human, and we have to be realistic about the changes we're capable of making. If you're trying to reduce the fat in your diet even a little, you're on the right road—and you'll probably get some payback in lower heart disease risk even with moderate change. Don't throw in the towel just because you aren't ready to turn your entire lifestyle upside down. But your goals should be greater than your immediate lifestyle changes, so you have something to aspire to.

How should you get motivated? After nearly 40 years in practice, Dr. Herbert Semler, a cardiologist at St. Vincent Hospital and Medical Center in Portland, Oregon, knows that one of the most important parts of his job is preparing patients to make the changes that will keep them alive. You can give the best care money can buy, save a patient's life with medicine and technology, he says, but ultimately they will go home and have to decide for themselves if they can make fundamental, healthy changes in the way they live. Dr. Semler has found that while men are often hesitant to admit that heart disease has an emotional component, women pick up very well on this concept and are both responsive to and motivated by stress management and other heart-healthy behavior changes. His female patients are better than men at picking up on exercise, meditation, music, visualization and other relaxation techniques for reducing stress. He motivates his patients to make these changes in their lives by practicing what he preaches (he meditates and exercises daily) *and* with a lecture on what he calls the "four Ds": desire, determination, dedication and discipline. Try asking yourself the questions he asks his patients:

1. Do you have the *desire* to be healthy? Is it meaningful to you, something you want to accomplish?

2. Are you *determined* to achieve good health? Is it something you're willing to work to gain, and are you willing to give something up to attain it?

3. Are you *dedicated* to good health? Are you ready not to cheat, since cheating is only fooling yourself, cheating your heart, and cheating the rest of your body?

4. Do you have the *discipline* to stick with these changes, making them a part of your life forever?

Only when you're ready to say yes to these four questions, Dr. Semler says, are you ready to lead a heart-healthy life. The motivation must be internal if it is to be permanent.

YOUR PERSONALITY AND THE RISK OF HEART DISEASE

They say the eyes are a mirror to the soul. Depending if your eyes are smiling or glaring, open or mistrustful, they may be a mirror to your heart, as well! A growing body of research points to certain personality traits that put one at greater risk of heart disease. The trouble with this data is that it's hard to pinpoint exactly what a potentially troublesome personality looks like. While lots of studies look at the relationship between anger and hostility and heart disease, the definitions of anger and hostility often differ from study to study. Sandra Thomas, director of the Center for Nursing Research at the University of Tennessee at Knoxville, makes the following distinction: outwardly expressed anger, which is associated with temporary frustration and a reaction to commonplace life obstacles, may *not* predispose you to heart problems. Chronic *suppressed* anger, on the other hand, along with long-term hostility and rage, may predispose you to health problems. Hostility, which she defines as a more pervasive, negative, cynical view of the world— going through life with a chip on your shoulder—*is* associated with heart disease. The famous Framingham Heart Study, a major ongoing Massachusetts-based study on which many current theories about heart disease are based, found similar results.

Carl Thoreson, director of the health psychology research program and a leader in this field at Stanford University, notes that most studies on personality and heart disease risk have been based on men and therefore cannot necessarily be applied to women. He and his colleagues are working on a broader study involving women that should bring important results in several years. For the time being, he says, we're forced to extrapolate information both from research on men *and* anecdotal reports about women. This less formal data suggests that hard-driving, "type A" women are at risk of heart and other health problems just as men are. The chronically harried, charging, competitive "superwoman" whose engine is always running should take a step back and think about her health, Thoreson says. These women have more headaches, sleep problems, aches and pains than those who take life more slowly, or more in stride. Not only can you be retrained to change your hostile, hurried attitude and behavior, he notes, but you may live longer and healthier if you do. Thoreson's own work on men has shown significant improvements in health (fewer repeat heart attacks, for example) in those who learned to roll with life, be more patient and smell the roses.

Recently Thoreson and his colleagues have been exploring the role of increased spirituality in both women's and men's lives, looking at the ways in which the calming force of spiritual (not religious) thoughts can benefit health. But no one will be able to help re-orient women away from hostility if we cannot admit that we're hostile in the first place, notes Susan Czajkowski of the National Heart, Lung, and Blood Institute. She is concerned that women identify themselves as less hostile than men because it is not socially acceptable for women to be outwardly hostile. Until we confront our true feelings and underlying tensions, we won't be able to exchange them for peaceful emotions and behaviors.

William Haskell, professor of medicine at the Stanford University Center for Research in Disease Prevention, says that when you are dominated by personality problems like depression and anxiety, it's even harder than normal to make healthy lifestyle changes. As we discuss in chapter 17, both depression and anxiety disorders are quite common among women. Add this to the basic biochemical problems that arise with chronic frustration, hostility and stress, Haskell says, and you're putting yourself at still higher risk of heart attack. Psychologist

Margaret Chesney echoes his concerns, pointing out that women under stress tend to cope in negative ways, such as smoking, gaining weight, being sedentary, consuming more caffeine and sleeping less—all of which contribute to heart disease risk.

Suzanne Haynes, chief of the health education section at the National Cancer Institute, says that your socioeconomic status and degree of life and job control are related to your risk of heart disease. While these aren't necessarily *personality* issues, they certainly can impact on even the most positive personalities. If week after week, month after month, you are subjected to chronic frustrations, low control, little blows to your self-esteem on the job—if you have a controlling, paternalistic boss and little or no room for creativity or support from others—your risk of heart disease may be climbing every day. The solution, some experts say, is to quit your job and look for something better. But it's pretty obvious that if you're stuck in this kind of job, it's not because you *choose* to be. Certainly, do everything you can do to change your situation. But if you're stuck, be practical. Build skills to leave. Even if it means taking a single course each semester—or each year—at a local school to develop new abilities that might be used in a higher-level job with your present employer or elsewhere, go for it. Rally support from coworkers in similar positions to you; perhaps you can learn from each other, come up with better systems for running your office, and so on.

Another issue receiving attention in health research these days is women's status as an oppressed minority in our culture. Millions of women are poor, or abused, or single, working, low-income parents. Chronic discrimination and position as an underclass is now being studied as a risk factor for heart disease, with even more serious implications for women of color, who have historically been subjected to great prejudice in American culture.

ESTROGEN REPLACEMENT THERAPY AND YOUR RISK OF HEART DISEASE

In chapter 10, "Menopausal Health," I discussed hormone replacement in much greater detail—the risks, the benefits, the different regimens available, and so on. In this section, I'll just briefly cover the role of hormone replacement in reducing heart disease risk.

To take or not to take estrogen has become one of the most pressing and confusing medical dilemmas for women today. The media hasn't helped, putting forth on-again, off-again recommendations on both sides of the risk-benefit coin. What's a woman to make of the fact that her local paper runs a story on the tremendous heart benefits of taking estrogen replacement on Monday, followed by a piece on estrogen causing breast cancer on Friday? Before you can make *any* decision about hormone replacement therapy, you must come to understand how and why hormones affect your heart (and general) health.

Let's first get some understanding of how and why estrogen might help protect us from heart disease. Around the time of menopause, estrogen levels begin to drop in our bodies. That's bad news for your heart, since estrogen, in many ways, is a powerful protector of heart health. In fact, it's the primary reason why many young women can eat higher levels of fat and retain lower cholesterol levels than older women can. Once your hormonal profile is more "masculine," your heart disease risk starts to mirror that of men.

To name just a few of the cardiovascular problems that accompany the drop in estrogen: your cholesterol level climbs, with the bad cholesterol rising and the good cholesterol falling; your arteries change, becoming more prone to constriction and plaque development; and your belly fat increases. These and many other complicated changes in your cardiovascular system make the risk of heart disease and heart attack jump considerably around the time of menopause.

Studies have suggested, however, that when you *replace* estrogen (taking it in pill, patch or injection form) after menopause, you restore cardiovascular health, cutting the chance of a heart attack by as much as 50%. This number has been disputed, since definitive studies aren't in yet (they're several years off), but most experts agree that there is at least some significant cardiovascular benefit to estrogen replacement. Add progesterone to the hormone regimen, and the heart benefits are thought to drop off a bit. One expert described it as driving a car with your foot on the brake. The question is, how much does progesterone (which is added to the hormone regimen to help protect your uterus from cancer) *reverse* the cardiological benefits created by estrogen? We don't have the answer to that 64,000-dollar question yet. Studies should yield those answers in the near future, greatly clarifying the risk-benefit questions for some women.

Of course, few health benefits of medication come without risk. The downside of estrogen replacement (as well as its other health *benefits*) are discussed in chapter 10.

OTHER KINDS OF HEART DISEASES

VALVE DISORDERS

Problems with the heart's valves make up another heart disease category. Certain valve problems, like mitral valve prolapse, are quite common in general and even more common in women than in men.

The problem tends to run in families. Your doctor might be able to *hear* a heart valve problem by listening to your chest with a stethoscope, but the only way she can confirm the diagnosis is with an echocardiogram (*see* "Heart Tests" above). In the vast majority of women, mitral valve prolapse is perfectly

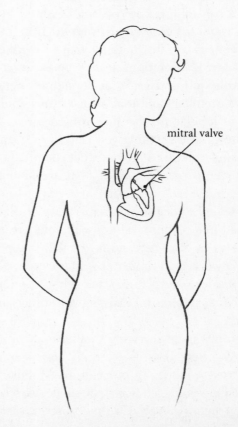

mitral valve

benign—in fact, you may not know you have it. In rare cases in which the mitral valve becomes leaky, you may develop symptoms including palpitations, breathlessness and rarely chest pain. This problem can be surgically repaired. Dr. Richard Devereaux of The New York Hospital/Cornell Medical Center theorizes that because the ratio of heart size to body size is lower in women than in men, women might be relatively protected.

Other common heart valve problems involve the aortic valve, which can be damaged or blocked by a variety of problems, including rheumatic fever—a disease you may think is obsolete, but actually made a comeback in parts of the country recently. Again, surgery can repair or replace most faulty valves. Dr. Delos Cosgrove, chairman of the department of thoracic and cardiovascular surgery at the Cleveland Clinic Foundation, notes that repair is often preferable to replacement, if it's surgically feasible. The key, as with other forms of heart disease, is to have the proper diagnosis made as early as possible.

Heart Rhythm Problems

Heart rhythm disturbances make up still another major category of heart problem. There are two main types: rhythm disruptions that originate in the atria or upper portions of the heart, and those that originate in the ventricles or lower part of the heart. Upper-heart rhythm problems tend to be less serious, causing occasional extra or skipped beats and other uncomfortable, but not life-threatening, problems. Ventricular arrhythmias, on the other hand, can be quite serious, causing symptoms like light-headedness or cardiac arrest. These lower-heart rhythm problems sometimes occur in patients with coronary artery disease.

Should you see a doctor if you feel your heart skip a beat? Dr. Debra Echt, director of the cardiac arrhythmia section at the Vanderbilt University School of Medicine, says *no*. Seek medical attention, she advises, only if your skipped beats are accompanied by other symptoms like shortness of breath, light-headedness, feeling like you might pass out or actually passing out, or continuous heart palpitations (and/or you measure your heart rate at more than 150 beats per minute).

If you *do* have these kinds of symptoms, you'll usually be given an electrocardiogram and an echocardiogram to check for both electrical and structural problems in the heart. You may be given a Holter monitor to wear for 24 hours: it reads your heart rhythms continuously. And you might also be given an exercise test to see if strenuous activity brings on your rhythm problems.

Upper-heart arrythmias are often treated with medication, and sometimes with a form of surgery that "zaps" the irregular rhythm back into sync. This curative surgery has recently become the first choice of treatment, over medication, for certain types of arrythmias. Talk to your doctor about whether you're a candidate for one of several antiarrhythmic surgeries. Lower-heart arrythmias, too, can be treated with either drugs or surgery. In some cases, though, with potentially lethal lower-heart rhythm problems, implantable defibrillators are used. These are tiny versions of the lifesaving chest paddles you're used to seeing on health-emergency TV shows. They're actually placed inside the chest surgically, where they react and kick the heart back into a normal rhythm pattern should it start beating dangerously. These tiny high-tech devices can save lives, and restore confidence to those who live in fear of fatal heart rhythm problems.

You may have heard some controversy about the use of antiarrhythmic drugs because of a study showing that in certain cases they can do more harm than good. In patients who were considered to be at high risk of lethal heart rhythm problems after a heart attack, certain antiarrhythmic drugs were used to try to *prevent* these life-threatening rhythm disturbances. It turned out that the drugs *caused* more deaths than they prevented! The moral of the story is that if you have a heart rhythm problem, you want a complete explanation of the location and type of disturbance, and a good reason why a certain drug or surgical procedure is being chosen. Not all heart rhythm problems are alike, not all treatments are alike, and the treatment you get can, in some cases, makes the difference between life and death.

HEART DISEASE MEDICATION

There are a vast array of drugs to treat just about every imaginable type of heart disease. Cholesterol-lowering drugs. Drugs to lower blood pressure. Drugs to control irregular heart rhythms. And so on. For too long, women have been prescribed antianxiety drugs in place of the proper heart disease medication. Avoid letting that happen to you by insisting on a full cardiovascular workup. Taking the right medication can help you avoid fatal outcomes of heart problems—and sometimes you can avoid costly, dangerous invasive treatments altogether.

When it comes to heart medications, we return to our original theme: most of these drugs were originally tested on and tailored to *male* patients. Because men have a totally different hormonal profile, tend to be larger and heavier than women, have different body-fat percentages and countless other biological differences, it's hard for many heart specialists to believe that drugs should work the same way—and as effectively—in women as in men. Unfortunately, that's how these drugs are prescribed. Fortunately, women do pretty well in spite of it.

Dr. Suzanne Oparil, president of the American Heart Association, points out that while we tend to hear a great deal about medication side effects in men—particularly when it comes to sexual function—we don't hear enough about these same problems in women. In fact, preliminary evidence suggests that certain heart drugs reduce women's sexual desire and ability to achieve orgasm. Drugs for hypertension often cause reduced sex drive and some mental impairment, depending on the class of medication. Whatever drug you're taking, listen to your body. If it responds badly, there are often alternatives that your doctor can prescribe. Don't ever stop a heart disease medication cold turkey without your doctor's consent, however.

Here are some examples of heart drugs you may hear about, and how they affect you:

Calcium Channel Blockers.

This class of drugs is used for a variety of heart ailments, including high blood pressure and rapid heart rhythms. Calcium channel blockers work by relaxing the blood vessels and cutting down on the squeezing force of the heart. They do have side effects (but these tend to be minor) including dizziness, flushing and constipation. Dr. Thomas Graboys, director of the

Lown Cardiovascular Center, finds that some women don't like these drugs because they dilate the blood vessels in the legs, often causing swelling that is cosmetically unpleasant. Since these drugs have the added benefit of helping with chest pain and rhythm problems in addition to hypertension, however, they're important options for women. Graboys says the solution to the side effect, sometimes, is to use low doses of calcium channel blockers in combination with other hypertension drugs. Combination therapy is quite useful with many heart medications, in that you may be able to reduce the side effects and enhance the benefits from each medication. This kind of sophisticated therapy requires a well-trained and experienced cardiologist, however, to be sure that the dosing is right, the drug interactions safe and the side effects tolerable.

Beta Blockers.

These drugs have some similar effects to calcium channel blockers, like lowering blood pressure and slowing the heart rate, thus reducing the output of the heart. After a heart attack, these drugs save lives. For both men and women, they cut the rate of overall mortality and the incidence of heart attack and sometimes stroke. The side effects can be bothersome, such as reduced sex drive, sluggishness and depression, and weight gain—but some experts find that women tolerate these drugs better than men do.

ACE Inhibitors.

Short for angiotensin converting enzyme inhibitors, these drugs keep blood vessels open and reduce fluid volume in the blood. They're quite effective at lowering blood pressure. Like

beta blockers, these drugs save lives if taken regularly after a heart attack. Side effects include weakness, fluid retention, palpitations, headaches, rash and others—mostly minor. In general, these drugs are quite well tolerated. Ace inhibitors have emerged as important tools in heart disease prevention and treatment for both men and women.

(**Note:** Both ACE inhibitors and beta blockers are less effective in African-Americans than in Caucasians.)

Antiarrhythmic Drugs.

These drugs affect the electrical system of the heart. They can cause stomach upset, fatigue, blurred vision, dizziness and other side effects. Anyone who is prescribed an antiarrhythmic drug should get a clear description of why she needs it. Short of a serious, life-threatening rhythm of the lower heart, there is less and less indication for these drugs, warns Dr. Thomas Graboys. (*See* "Heart Rhythm Problems" above for more information.)

Diuretics.

These commonly prescribed drugs (which have been around the longest, and are among the cheapest of heart medications) flush fluid from the body and were once the main treatment for hypertension. They are sometimes more effective in African-Americans than in Caucasians, for reasons that are only partially understood. Some experts think they're still a top choice for women, since we tend to retain more fluid due to estrogen and progesterone changes. Diuretics protect those with high blood pressure against stroke. They can be useful in combinations with other heart drugs, too; for instance, you may want to take a calcium channel blocker, but use a diuretic to help lessen the effects of blood vessel swelling. There are some metabolic drawbacks to the drugs, according to Dr. Thomas Pickering of the New York Hospital Cornell Medical Center: They can increase blood sugar, uric acid, and cholesterol (all bad), and they can reduce potassium in the body, predisposing the patient to heart rhythm disturbances. On the plus side, Dr. Pickering adds, is a *theoretical* possibility that diuretics may help protect against osteoporosis by decreasing calcium excretion from the body.

Anticoagulants.

These are drugs that prevent clotting, such as heparin. Also related are the so-called "clot-busting" drugs that are given in the event of a heart attack in progress, which can prevent some degree of permanent damage to the heart. Trudy Bush points out that even in the emergency room, women are less likely to be given these lifesaving drugs than are men. Evidence suggests that they save women's lives when they *are* used, but it's also been observed that women have more adverse reactions to them (like bleeding) than do men. More research is needed to explain why.

Aspirin.

Once considered a benign medication in most Americans' medicine cabinets, aspirin, one of the oldest blood-thinners, has turned out to be a potent and important heart drug. According to Dr. Charles Hennekens, chief of preventive medicine at the Brigham and Women's Hospital in Boston, aspirin plays several beneficial roles in cardiovascular care. First, for women who have already had heart attacks, strokes or other so-called "occlusive events" (problems involving clots in blood vessels), taking aspirin *afterwards* cuts the risk of repeat crises—and also reduces the risk of death. Second, aspirin can be lifesaving for women *during* a heart attack. For those who are currently having a heart attack or have had one within the past 24 hours, taking aspirin immediately and continuing to take it regularly thereafter can prevent subsequent heart attacks, strokes and death. Sadly, this word isn't out: Dr. Hennekens reports that about 5,000 more lives could be saved each year if all women were offered this vital and inexpensive treatment.

Finally, aspirin can *possibly* help women whom Dr. Hennekens calls the "walking well." These are women who are healthy and are considering taking aspirin to prevent a *first* heart attack. Will it work? Unfortunately, we won't have a firm answer to this question for a couple of years, when an important study will be completed. While we do know that taking regular aspirin cuts the risk of a first heart attack in *men,* we don't yet know if this is true for women. Dr. Hennekens and many of his colleagues predict that women, like men, *will* benefit from taking aspirin regularly (in lower doses than men take). But we'll have to wait for science to prove if they're right.

Digitalis.

One of the oldest heart drugs, digitalis has been around for two centuries. It slows the heart rate and strengthens the heart's pumping force. Its side effects include nausea, loss of appetite, visual problems and heart rhythm disturbances.

Nitroglycerin.

This drug, which comes in pill, patch and mouth spray forms, opens the coronary arteries when they shut down. There are few side effects, but some experience headaches or a drop in blood pressure when taking them.

Cholesterol-Lowering Drugs.

Often the first drug used to lower cholesterol is *niacin,* otherwise known as vitamin B$_3$. It is thought to be quite safe, causing some side effects like flushing of the skin, gastrointestinal upset and, in certain cases, irregular heart rhythms and liver trouble. Usually, if you start with a small dose and build up, you can minimize some of the side effects—particularly those that affect the skin. Niacin gets the "bad cholesterol" down and the "good cholesterol" up, which makes it a good all-around first choice. Sometimes it's given in conjunction with another drug called *colestipol*—but this can boost the chance of stomach upset. There are more effective drugs out there—but they're often much more costly, as well—such as *lovastatin,* which made headlines for its ability not only to cut cholesterol levels but to *reverse* the plaque buildup in the arteries that is so often associated with heart disease. The side effects of lovastatin are rarely significant, but experts are quick to point out that since it hasn't been around for long, we don't know about its long-term safety record. *Lopid* is another drug with a minor side effect profile that boosts the "good cholesterol," cuts the "bad cholesterol," and lowers the heart attack rate—an extremely desirable added benefit. There are several other cholesterol-lowering medications as well. The key in choosing the right one for *you* is to determine, as discussed earlier, your precise cholesterol problem. If, for example, you have very high triglycerides, which seems to be important in women, you'll want to seek a drug that additionally lowers triglycerides. Dr. Frederick Kuhn, director of preventive cardiology at St. Agnes Hospital in Baltimore, says a typical scenario for postmenopausal women is *both* a high "bad" cholesterol level and a high "good" cholesterol level. For this reason, it may be smarter to choose a drug that aggressively lowers "bad" cholesterol rather than one that raises "good" cholesterol, Dr. Kuhn notes. Select a drug that fits your needs. We have more information these days than we used to about how to tailor cholesterol-lowering medication to specific problems.

SURGERY FOR HEART DISEASE

You can pretty much go down the list of invasive heart procedures and find that women do relatively poorly compared to men. Whether we're talking about invasive screening tests, like the angiogram discussed earlier, or actual treatments, such as coronary bypass surgery (in which clogged coronary arteries are bypassed with a healthy artery from somewhere else in the body), or balloon angioplasty (in which a tube or catheter is snaked into the blocked artery and a balloon inflated to press the blockage out of the way), women are less likely to be referred to these procedures *and* do *worse* when they finally are. Women have greater operative mortality, greater relapse after most procedures, and more complications at every stage of the process, according to Dr. Katherine Detre, who evaluates treatments for coronary artery disease at the University of Pittsburgh Graduate School of Public Health.

Why do women do worse in heart surgery? There are many theories, and probably many reasons. First, women tend to be sicker, and older, when they have these procedures done. There is a bad reason for this: delay in treatment. There is also an inevitable reason for it: women get heart disease later than men do. In addition to often having more severe heart disease when we make it to surgery, women often have *additional* risk factors, such as diabetes, that make surgery more complicated.

But even after you allow for *these* disadvantages, the average woman has one more significant disadvantage when it comes to heart disease surgery. Our arteries—and our total body size—are smaller than men's, making surgery *technically* more difficult. One cardiologist pointed out to me that when larger women with larger arteries undergo heart surgery, their results are much closer to men's. Hopefully, with time, surgeons will develop newer and more appropriate tools to deal with women's different anatomy, boosting the success rate of surgical procedures. Dr. Detre suggests that with technology already better than it was when some earlier studies of heart surgery on women were performed, it's possible that women will start to do better *now*.

What Can You Do to Boost Your Chance of Success?

- First, listen to your body and tell your doctor about any symptoms *early,* before your heart disease has had a chance to become extensive.
- Have regular screening tests for blood pressure and cholesterol so you'll know if you're at high risk of heart disease *before* it develops.
- Choose the best, and most active, surgeon possible. In the case of coronary angioplasty, for example, you want a surgeon who does at *least* 75 procedures a year (at

a center that does at least 200 a year), according to the American Heart Association.
- Follow your doctor's advice *after* the surgery. This is vital. Women often fail to begin the new healthy behaviors, like regular exercise and stress reduction, that can reduce our chance of subsequent heart problems. You must understand that even if it is a success, heart surgery isn't a miracle cure. After surgery, we still must contend with the same problems and habits that led to heart disease in the first place. Only by battling those risk factors will we save our newly healthy hearts from relapse.

Valve Surgery

According to Dr. Delos Cosgrove of the Cleveland Clinic Foundation, much of the same advice you've heard about bypass and balloon angioplasty surgeries also applies to surgery to repair heart valves. Always choose a center that does a large number of procedures each year, he urges, and a surgeon who does at least 20 a year of *your* particular procedure. One of the more common valve problems in women, mitral valve prolapse, can often be *repaired,* he notes—whereas we used to believe that most of these valves needed to be completely *replaced.* Dr. Cosgrove, who is one of the country's leading valve surgeons, says he worries most about frail, older women patients who may do well *during* surgery but not have the strength to fight back *afterward.* With the number of surgeries on women increasing, (thanks in part to increased risk factors like smoking) this concern might become more prevalent. Again, the better the surgeon *and* the better your compliance with doctors' advice after the procedure, the greater your chance of survival.

MAKING A COMEBACK AFTER A HEART ATTACK

For many reasons, women are known to do worse than men after heart attacks. We're more likely to die soon afterward, and more likely to have subsequent attacks. We also seem to do worse at "bouncing back," taking longer to go back to work (if we go back at all). Dr. Pamela Douglas of the Beth Israel Hospital in Boston questions whether this is connected to the fact that women are less likely to participate in rehabilitation programs after heart attacks. And Dr. Marian Limacher of the University of Florida at Gainesville is concerned about older women with heart disease, who may find it hard to keep medical appointments because they're isolated, perhaps widowed and living alone, and not very mobile.

Dr. Nanette Wenger of Emory University cites a laundry list of emotional problems women are more likely to suffer after a heart attack, including anxiety, depression and sexual problems. Many women start leading a hermit-like existence to avoid risk. While it is absolutely normal to expect a period of depression and worry after a heart attack, you must start to fight back emotionally as early as possible. If you live alone, this process can be more difficult; in fact, research suggests that women who have little support in the way of friends or family tend to do worse in recovery (*and* are more prone to heart disease in the first place) than those with strong support systems in place. If you feel a need for greater support, consider joining a group of women who have been

through the same ordeal to discuss your feelings and coping strategies. Your doctor may be able to help you form such a group, if none exists in your area. Reach out to friends or neighbors who may have become more distant as your disease progressed; perhaps you've been avoiding social situations for some time because of your symptoms, or just out of inertia.

When you are sufficiently recovered, consider getting involved in projects that allow you to help others and step out of your own worries for a while each week. For example, read to the blind, cheer up young children in the hospital, volunteer at a local charity or become a contact person for other women with heart disease who have questions about what to expect in surgery. Suzanne Haynes believes that in the same way that group or social support has been shown to help in programs for smoking cessation, it can be harnessed to help women reduce *other* risk factors for heart disease and to build back the emotional strength to get well.

FIGHTING THE "DAMAGED GOODS" ATTITUDE

If some combination of good fortune, good habits, good genes and good willpower have helped you avoid heart disease to this point in your life—congratulations. Keep up what you're doing, and teach it to friends! If, on the other hand, you've already gone down the road to heart disease—or suffered a serious cardiovascular event—don't consider yourself "damaged goods." There is a lot you can do to protect yourself from further problems; the advice in this chapter pertains to you, too. It's never too late to start living a heart-healthy life. Step-by-step, even if it's a slow process, you can make a comeback to the level of confidence and enjoyment of life that seemed natural before you became ill. Always, when in doubt, grab onto support; no one can be expected to go it alone. Get in touch with one of the support groups or institutions listed below, and start making your comeback today.

Dr. Claude Lenfant, director of the National Heart, Lung and Blood Institute, puts it simply: be an aggressive consumer of heart health care. Go to your physician and do not allow him/her to brush you off or tell you not to worry about it, he advises. You must be insistent: say that you want your care to be "just so," the same as you would demand of another type of service provider. And if you're an older woman, adds Dr. Castelli, this message goes doubly for you: don't let sexism *and* ageism combine to keep you from the care you deserve. Too often, doctors say it isn't worth *bothering* to treat older people aggressively because they have so little time to live. Dr. Castelli counters this fallacy with the story of a woman in his Framingham Heart Study who had a heart attack at age ninety—and then went back to college!

There's no denying our past failure to focus on women's heart disease, Dr. Lenfant concludes. But complacency is a thing of the past. It was done not by design, but by default. Now let's do everything we have to do as scientists, as health care professionals, as women and as health care consumers to reverse the trend that landed us where we are today. Moving forward to good health is our only option, and it is a good one.

FOR MORE INFORMATION ON HEART HEALTH

HIGH BLOOD PRESSURE INFORMATION CENTER
120/80 National Institutes of Health
Box A.P.
Bethesda, MD 20205

YOUNG HEARTS SUPPORT GROUP
708-387-0918

AMERICAN HEART ASSOCIATION
800-AHA-USA-1 or write to your local AHA office as listed in the phone book

NATIONAL HEART, LUNG AND BLOOD INSTITUTE INFORMATION CENTER
P.O. Box 30105
Bethesda, MD 20824-0105
301-251-1222

NHLBI
For information on cholesterol and high blood pressure
800-575-WELL

AMERICAN DIABETES ASSOCIATION
1660 Duke Street
Alexandria, VA 22314
800-232-3472

CHAPTER TWENTY-FIVE

FIGHTING WOMEN'S CANCERS

Everyone who is born holds dual citizenship, in the kingdom of the well and in the kingdom of the sick. Although we all prefer only to use the good passport, sooner or later each of us is obliged, at least for a spell, to identify ourselves as citizens of that other place.

—Susan Sontag, *Illness as Metaphor*

Cancer is the number two killer of American women. Almost more important, though, it is the number one health *fear* of many women—often to the exclusion of our concern about other illnesses. It would be nice if we could say that all of the attention and worry we give to cancer translates into protective behaviors, like cancer screening or improved eating and other habits. But for most of us, it doesn't. We ignore the vast amount of solid medical information about how to prevent and detect cancer.

I am convinced that some of the reasons for this inaction are connected to the fact that few women know a) how valuable cancer screening can be, b) exactly which tests to have done, c) when, where and how often to have those tests, and d) the types of cancers that most often affect women (other than the obvious). We tend to get information about cancer piecemeal—a report about mammography on television, a friend being diagnosed with cancer, something about Pap smears in the local paper. As a result, we get the *general* message that there are things we can do to protect ourselves from cancer. But the *specifics* elude most of us, and the result can be deadly.

It's time to face the information that can save our lives. In this section, I will answer those basic questions about the most common cancers that affect women, and I'll give you a simple plan to follow year after year to greatly boost your chance of catching a cancer when it's still curable. We'll also discuss ways of *preventing* several cancers—since the best way to deal with cancer is *not* to deal with it at all. Prevention and early detection are the tools that can save your life. If you are destined to get cancer by your genes or some other cause, do yourself the service of letting doctors find it early when it can be fully eradicated.

According to the American Cancer Society, there are more than eight million Americans *living* with a history of cancer. That's right—*living* with it. Five million of them have been cancer-free for at least five years, which is an important survival marker for many cancers. Thanks to both early detection and new aggressive treatments, more and more people are living to tell about cancer. The following statistics, compiled by the American Cancer Society, give an impressive view of how far we've come in saving lives threatened by a wide variety of cancers:

FIVE-YEAR CANCER SURVIVORS

- 1930s: fewer than 1 in 5
- 1940s: 1 in 4
- 1960s: 1 in 3
- 1994: 4 in 10

An overall 40% survival rate over five years *for all cancer patients, regardless of the stage of their cancer,* is a lot better than most people assume—and *many* more survive if their cancers are caught in the earliest stages, before they have spread throughout the body.

Of course, the picture isn't all rosy. About 1.2 million people will be diagnosed with cancer in 1994 (excluding skin cancers) and almost half that many will die of cancer this same year. Too often, because of negligence in screening, or worse, because of faulty screening or plain bad luck, cancers are found late in their development, when they are either too large to remove surgically or too widespread in the body to kill with cancer drugs. To some degree, with proper medical care and consistent, careful screening, you can prevent this from happening to you. But there are no guarantees, and often it's no one's fault when you're found to have late-stage cancer. The ACS believes that nine out of ten cancers could be caught at a controllable stage with proper screening.

CANCER: WHAT YOU HAD TO SAY ABOUT IT

Betty, 68 years old
I smoked for 40 years, age 18–61. I started when I was in college. We didn't know. Peer pressure, everybody else smoked. I was the only one entering college who didn't smoke. I was addicted to nicotine. There were times I'd go 2–3 hours without a cigarette; I smoked a pack and a half a day.

In February of 1987 I developed a sore throat and a sinus infection; the sinus infection went away, and the sore throat didn't. They told me to drink hot tea. We [women] think we're impermeable to these diseases men get. I can't get through to women, it goes right over their heads; men listen. I had a hysterectomy because of cervical cancer due to smoking. I had lung cancer and throat cancer. You do it to yourself, you're a fool if you feel cheated. We all had a chance to quit, the information was out. The night before my surgery I had a cigarette. When I woke up with tubes coming out of my body I knew I'd never have another cigarette.

You can't swim with a hole in your throat. My body now has limitations, I had extensive surgery.

It was the most horrifying thing to wake up on the table and know you're speechless. The first thing to consider is the damage to the physical part of your body. Your breath, your stamina, and let's face it, you get wrinkles. And how dirty and smelly it is. Almost my whole entire life is dedicated to cancer survivors and getting kids not to start smoking. So far I've gotten four people to quit.

Rosemary, 57 years old
My lump was picked up by an insensitive general practitioner. I left his office stumbling in tears, he said he wouldn't permit reconstruction. This was in 1978. I was so traumatized by the doctor who wouldn't reconstruct that I refused to have the lump aspirated. Luckily it wasn't cancer [that time].

Then the next time I was told I had microscopic breast cancer. I was shocked when they recommended mastectomy. They were kind, but gave me no good answers. Two other physicians said, "We concur." I still said, "You're supposed to be my friends, you're supposed to save my breast!" But the statistics weren't great for lumpectomy for my type of cancer. I talked to a plastic surgeon and he suggested waiting six months for reconstruction. I couldn't bear the thought of waiting. I thought, "They'll take my breast and they won't give it back!" In the end I had reconstruction on both breasts, two gel-filled implants, and I can truthfully say that I don't know what it's like to lose two breasts—I got two different ones!

When I hold my grandchildren, I feel like a woman. Breast reconstruction with implants let me focus on optimal treatment, not on disfigurement. Slapping on external prostheses would be very hard for me. For some women, breasts are important sexually. I'm a very sexual person, I believe it's what you bring and how you feel about yourself in the relationship, and I just couldn't imagine being free and open like before without breasts. I enjoyed going out in evening dresses with cleavage showing and the beauty of it is, I can do that still, even better than before! I'm sitting here right now with a twinkle in my eye, I wish my 57-year-old face looked like my cleavage!

Jill, 45 years old
I was diagnosed two and a half years ago at 42½. It was found with my second mammogram. I had to get over the anger, there was tremendous anger. Death never occurred to me, mutilation of my body did. I had a bilateral mastectomy and no chemotherapy. I waited six months for reconstruction. I'm single, which is the reason I decided to have reconstruction. I had just seen augmentation, which is very different—in the back of my mind, I thought it would be good. I was very disappointed. My sister says they're beautiful, but it was not what I pictured.

I'm single, do I want to go out there again? I'm coming to terms with it. Cancer was the worst thing that ever happened to me and the best thing that ever happened to me. It empowered me. I was always strong, now I'm more easygoing, I stop and smell the flowers. I've learned to say no, I've learned to get angry, to speak up, not get depressed. It gave me permission to be what I wanna be, wear what I wanna wear, I don't care what people think. I love life and I never did before. I was holding off having my nipples done. Now I'm going to do it.

Elaine, 57 years old
It's been five years since my bilateral mastectomy. It was easy to give up my breasts for my life. The option of breast reconstruction was made

available to me, but I didn't want it, I didn't need it. I felt there were more important things to worry about. My husband supported me. I use external prostheses. I can be any size I want! I got two sizes. Nobody who looks at me can see my prostheses. I don't use them with a bathing suit, I feel perfectly comfortable, it doesn't bother me at the beach, there are plenty of women nearly flat as me. I was only a 32-A before; my husband says, "I must never have been a boob man." Anything I wanted to do he supported me. I encourage women who feel pushed to reconstruction to realize that there's an option.

Linda, 44 years old
I found my cancer during a regular breast self-exam, I was 40 at the time. I had a lumpectomy and chemotherapy. I never had a sense of devastation to my body, I never had a sense of loss over losing a breast. I have a faint scar and very natural-looking breast. My surgeon was excellent. I kept a sense of my wholeness, an ability to move forward and not have the constant reminder of having had breast cancer. There are days when I don't even think about having breast cancer. I don't think that's true of women with a mastectomy scar.

I entered chemotherapy with a very positive attitude feeling that I was securing my good health, I felt a sense of power by doing it. I had some typical side effects, nausea, weight gain, but I was able to deal with it because of medication my doctor gave me. I did have hair thinning and it was very hard for me. But I had no [major] hair loss and that too kept me from a sense of devastation to my body, losing part of my femininity.

Connie, 50 years old
My gynecologist examined me and said she wanted to put me in the hospital right away, she

thought I had a large cyst, she didn't say cancer. I never thought cancer until after my surgery, they told me it was cancer but they cleaned it all out. They never said everything would be okay, I'm a little annoyed about that, they don't let you know how it really is. Going through this terrible ordeal, chemotherapy, losing my hair, somehow I thought it would be okay.

I'm very close to God. Somehow I thought this is a chance to get close to God, a real shakening. I'm strong, I became stronger as I went on. My relationship with my husband and my children became stronger after the cancer. When I had to really fight for my life I became stronger. I'm struggling again, back on treatment, I've been on and off for ten years. I do have remissions, thank God, that gives me some breaks.

Chemotherapy is one of the worst—the worst thing is being so nauseous. I've lost my hair five times which really means nothing to me anymore. But the worst part is the weakness, being so tired all the time, preparing yourself physically and mentally for each treatment. I start getting nauseous and throwing up *before* I go for treatment, it gets to you, it's very psychological. I'm very ill right now, I know I'm very ill. I'm having a difficult time eating food and chewing, sometimes I have to take liquids. I was in the hospital a whole month, and now I'm going back in a week. I don't know if I'm ready.

I have a wonderful support group, we meet each week, it gives you a boost, and you're there to pick someone else up. My whole focus and my key is my relationship with God, this keeps me going. God is there to help me. I often say, "What am I doing here, what is my purpose on this earth? I'm trying to help people and live a Christian life. Why has all this stricken me?" But I'm not the only one struggling. Nobody knows what someone else has. I'm just gonna fight it. I don't wanna hear any diagnosis of how many years I have, I don't wanna hear it.

Frances, 59 years old
I was expecting nothing. I was one of these nuts that went every six months for a physical, I had mammograms, I did everything right. Nothing hurt, I just had a little pulling. The doctor couldn't see me for six months. They asked if it was an emergency, I said no. The worst part of women is we're so scared of making a fool of ourselves, so I said no. They don't take you seriously, they say it's nothing. Three months later I called again and said I really think the doctor should see me. They said the doctor is too busy. I asked to speak to the doctor. He said, "You don't still have your ovaries, do you? You've had a hysterectomy, right?" He didn't think it was anything.

I went through hundreds of tests, already six months later. It [the ovarian cancer] could've been caught six months earlier. I really blame him that he didn't find it sooner. I said how could you let me wait six months? He said the nurses tried to protect him. I said who tries to protect *us*? Doctors put themselves on a pedestal. People say everyone looks for a scapegoat. I know I would've had cancer anyway, but it would've been caught sooner.

I was operated on, it was a horrible operation. I was very sick for weeks. And when I got better they wanted me to go on chemotherapy. I switched doctors. She said you're gonna have the worst year of your life, but you'll have your life. She was right. I lost my hair, every stitch of my hair came out, I wasn't prepared. I guess the dose was so strong. I was very sick, I was throwing up for days. When I got the Zofran [antinausea drug] I got up and felt fine. Zofran is a miracle drug. I think it's almost cruel and unusual treat-

ment *not* to give it! I had a second operation after six months of chemo, a second-look operation. After the first chemotherapy I never had cancer again. They took 42 biopsies, the doctor was jumping up and down, there was none left. I was like someone from a war who's the only one who survived—I got depressed! When I look back I can't even remember what I looked like without hair. She made me go through three more chemotherapy sessions *after* that surgery. She called it life insurance. I don't go through a day where I don't think about it.

I play tennis, I travel, I do everything—but I don't do anything long-term anymore. I have to take a pill to sleep at night. A day doesn't go by without my thinking about it coming back. I don't think anyone who goes through this can go back to a normal life. Everytime I feel something I think it's back. If I can help one person, if I can save one person, not let a doctor tell them he has no time, it's worth my talking to you. Tell the doctor *now, today* you want to be seen.

WHAT EXACTLY IS CANCER?

A cancer, or cancerous tumor or growth, is one in which cells of the body multiply out of control. Two cells rapidly become four, then eight, then sixteen and so on. This madcap cell growth can be caused by a great number of factors, including environmental carcinogens (cancer-causers) like cigarette smoke or asbestos, our genes (family history), viruses, hormonal imbalances, and probably many habits and behaviors, including diet. Cancers take time to develop—sometimes many years, as in the case of certain cancers of the cervix. Sometimes tiny, early cancers go undetected even with the best screening techniques.

CANCERS THAT MOST AFFECT WOMEN

Women tend to fixate on cancers of the reproductive system, like ovarian cancer, breast cancer, cancer of the cervix and uterine cancer, as if these are the only cancers we have to worry about. In fact, the cancers that affect the greatest number of women are those in the lung, breast, colon, rectum and uterus. The other reproductive cancers are certainly important,

and merit attention—but it's vital that women wake up to the fact that other cancers that we think of as men's problem *do* affect us, too. Lung cancer recently surpassed breast cancer as the leading cancer killer of women—thanks above all to high smoking rates among women. The illustration below from the American Cancer Society gives cancer incidence rates for both genders at a glance, and points to the fact that cancer is, overall, gender blind.

Prostate 200,000	Breast 182,000	Lung 94,000	Lung 59,000
Lung 100,000	Colon & Rectum 74,000	Prostate 38,000	Breast 46,000
Colon & Rectum 75,000	Lung 72,000	Colon & Rectum 27,800	Colon & Rectum 28,200
Bladder 38,000	Uterus 46,000	Pancreas 12,400	Ovary 13,600
Lymphoma 29,400	Ovary 24,000	Lymphoma 12,100	Pancreas 13,500
Oral 19,800	Lymphoma 23,500	Leukemia 10,500	Lymphoma 10,650
Melanoma of the Skin 17,000	Melanoma of the Skin 15,000	Stomach 8,400	Uterus 10,500
Kidney 17,000	Pancreas 14,000	Esophagus 7,800	Leukemia 8,600
Leukemia 16,200	Bladder 13,200	Liver 7,200	Liver 6,000
Stomach 15,000	Leukemia 12,400	Bladder 7,000	Brain 5,800
Pancreas 13,000	Kidney 10,600	Brain 6,800	Stomach 5,600
Larynx 9,800	Oral 9,800	Kidney 6,800	Multiple Myeloma 4,800
All Sites 632,000	**All Sites 576,000**	**All Sites 283,000**	**All Sites 255,000**

Excluding basal and squamous cell skin cancer and carcinoma in situ.

Available on reproduction sheet (5005.94)

GENERAL ADVICE ABOUT CANCER DETECTION

Each cancer naturally has its own set of unique signs and symptoms that we'll discuss throughout this chapter. But there are some general signs that we should all be aware of that can indicate cancer is present. The American Cancer Society uses the following anagram to help you remember them: CAUTION. The letters stand for:

Change in bowel or bladder habits;

A sore that doesn't get better;

Unusual bleeding or discharge;

Thick spot or lump in breast or anywhere else;

Indigestion (bad, more than once in a while) and problems with swallowing;

Obvious change in a wart or mole;

Nagging cough or unusually hoarse voice.

Of course, it's not enough just to remember the letters. You have to make a habit of watching your body for these signs, on a regular basis. No, it doesn't mean you have to become neurotic, studying every nick or bruise for a sign of cancer. But it does mean paying attention to changes in your feelings, appearance or habits—and most important, not ignoring your instincts if you have the sense something strange is going on in your body, and that feeling or sign persists. Don't fall prey to what psychologists call "denial"— failing to get medical attention because deep down you don't want to discover bad news. The way you should come to look at cancer is that it's *good* news to catch it early. Be aggressive, and find a doctor who's aggressive, too.

WHO GETS CANCER?

Everyone and anyone can get cancer. Young, old, fat, thin, light skin or dark, cheerful or sullen. It's very important for everyone to consider herself at risk, and therefore take appropriate precautions. If your family is riddled with heart disease and no one has had cancer, that doesn't mean *you* won't get cancer. If your grandmother smoked for 40 years and never got lung cancer, consider her incredibly lucky, not immune—and realize that you might not have the same good fortune. We are all at risk, and the sooner we realize this as a whole population, the sooner we can make the changes that will reduce *all* of our risk of cancer.

You may have read or heard about the "type C"—the supposed cancer patient type, pleasant, suppressing emotions, overly amenable. While there is interesting data both to support and refute such a portrait, this kind of stereotype can be misleading and punitive. After all, if there is a cancer "personality," or set of "cancer behaviors," it seems we might be to blame for getting cancer. This is a terribly negative way to look at a problem that can arise through no fault of our own—even in *spite* of our best efforts. True, there is a great deal of information emerging about personality and mood and the risk of disease. But there is more we do *not* understand in this field of study than what we *do* understand. Don't get caught up worrying about the kind of personality you've had until now. Focus on today, and getting the fighter's personality to reduce your risk as much as possible, or battle cancer head-on. The one kind of personality you need if you *are* diagnosed with cancer is the strong kind. Later in this chapter, we'll discuss how you can take the strongest stand, choosing the most state-of-the-art treatments for your particular problem.

GENERIC CANCER PREVENTION: CAN WE AVOID CANCER IN THE FIRST PLACE?

There is no way to guarantee yourself protection from cancer. But when you look at all of the studies of cancer risk factors and how to prevent individual cancers, several approaches emerge. The biggest is smoking. Quit smoking—and quit other tobacco and "smokeless" tobacco products—and your risk for many cancers (including lung, cervix, bladder and esophageal cancer) will drop. Avoiding other known carcinogens, like asbestos and other environmental pollutants, can only help.

Another area to consider is diet. Diets rich in fruits, vegetables, beans and other high-fiber foods are associated with decreased risk of several cancers (not to mention a better heart disease profile, as well). The foods most associated with cancer reduction are those containing antioxidants—the now-famous vitamin group including beta-carotene, and vitamins C and E, notes Jeffrey Blumberg, associate director of the U.S.D.A. Human Nutrition Research Center on Aging at Tufts University. Antioxidants are believed to inhibit the action of carcinogenic free radicals in the body by turning them back into safe molecules. People who consume the greatest amount of antioxidants have lower rates of several cancers, including those of the esophagus, colon, lung and other gastric cancers. Foods in the antioxidant group include most yellow, green and orange fruits and vegetables (cantaloupe, squash, apricots and so on); vitamin C is in citrus fruits, broccoli, strawberries and tomatoes, to name a few; vitamin E is found in polyunsaturated vegetable oils, seeds, nuts, green leafy vegetables, asparagus, avocados, whole grains, berries and beans. There is evidence too that taking antioxidants in the form of *supplement* pills, and not just as foods, also confers some protection against a variety of cancers. According to Dr. Walter Willett of the Harvard School of Public Health, more research is needed in this hotly disputed area, to help determine the precise role of not only antioxidants, but also the hundreds of other chemicals, and bulky fiber itself, in *real* foods on cancer risk.

Overall, stick to fresh foods when you can. Salt- and nitrite-cured foods have been associated with increased rates of certain cancers. These foods can be tempting because their saltiness and fattiness make them tasty favorites for sandwiches (cured meats, etc.).

Dermatologists and oncologists alike plead with their patients to stay out of the sun—or to use sun protection when in it. Skin cancer has reached epidemic proportions in this country and is clearly associated with sun exposure: the more sun you get, the worse off you are.

Still another group of generic cancer-prevention tips fit together like a puzzle: they are 1) to avoid excessive fat in the diet, 2) to avoid excessive overall calories in the diet, and 3) to stay at a lean weight. Leaner people with lower-fat, lower-calorie intakes have a decreased risk of several cancers, notes Diane Birt of the Eppley Institute for Research in Cancer and Allied Diseases. And according to Michael Pariza, director of the food research institute at the University of Wisconsin at Madison, cutting calories in excess of biological need—even by 10%—causes a significant reduction in breast cancer in laboratory animals. Physical activity may also be connected to decreased cancer risk, but it could be part and parcel of the above-mentioned findings. Dr. Rachel Ballard-Barbash of the National Cancer Institute notes that especially in postmenopausal women, being overweight can contribute to the risk of breast cancer, and can block its detection. She theorizes that women with increased levels of fat, particularly in the abdominal region, metabolize the hormone estrogen differently, possibly predisposing them to breast cancer. As this case illustrates, researchers are becoming interested in the way one risk factor impacts on another, creating a domino-like effect in which our bodies become vulnerable to a variety of cancers through several different means.

New research suggests, too, that the *timing* of your weight gain may affect your risk of cancer. One study showed that women who gained more than 15 pounds between the ages of 16 and 30 were at greater risk of breast cancer than women who didn't put on that added weight. Women who carried 15 extra pounds at age 30 had a 37% greater risk of breast cancer than women of normal weight; those with 20 extra pounds had a 52% greater risk. More research must be done to confirm and explain these interesting findings.

Finally, just when you thought that there was *something* that exercise couldn't prevent or cure, new research from the University of Southern California suggests that exercise, particularly during the childbearing years (and especially in the years immediately following your first period) can significantly reduce your risk of breast cancer. Regardless of the activity chosen, women who exercised at least three hours per week in the early years of menstruation cut their risk of breast cancer by 30%, says

researcher Leslie Bernstein of U.S.C. She attributes the reduction in risk to the beneficial hormone profile (less estrogen) caused by vigorous exercise—but this has yet to be proved.

Of course, following recommended screening tests to detect cancer early is also a theme I will often raise in this chapter. Screening doesn't prevent cancer, but it does help prevent *advanced* cancer by letting you catch the disease early, when it can be cured.

As we have learned in recent years, there are some cancers we are just preprogrammed to get—by our genes. The task for the near future will be for scientists to locate the precise spot on which these genes reside, and to develop treatments to target those genes.

Where to Go for Cancer Treatment: General Advice

Dr. Max Wicha, director of the University of Michigan Comprehensive cancer center advises *all* women with cancer to seek comprehensive cancer care centers—ideally, those so designated by the National Cancer Insitute. Dr. Wicha and his colleagues from all over the country are sounding a theme that has become central to excellent cancer care: team treatment for cancer is the best treatment for cancer. Multidisciplinary cancer treatment, using not only combinations of several drugs, but many different treatment regimens (drugs, radiation and surgery) has proved *better* at curing many cancers than one approach alone. In the old days you might be shuttled between a medical oncologist, who specializes in drug therapy, and a radiation oncologist, who uses radiation to treat cancer, and a surgical oncologist, who cuts disease out of the body: and each specialist would extol the virtues of his or her approach. Today, cancer treatment has been revolution- ized into a team approach in which experts from the various specialties not only cooperate in treating patients, but actually map out the course of treatment together before any therapy is begun.

The reasons to seek care at a multidiscipli- nary center are twofold. First, these centers attract many of the most talented doctors from around the country, and because they are known for their state-of-the-art services, they are referred patients from all over the country. Therefore they often have wide experience in treating many types of cancer. Second, much of the cutting-edge research on new cancer treat- ments takes place at these centers, which means they're among the first to become aware of exciting new treatments, and you may have the opportunity to take part in studies that could offer more benefits than standard treatment (and could bring about better treatments for other women like you in the future). These studies are called clinical trials, and in many cases, participating in them reduces or elimi- nates your cost of treatment.

In the information section at the end of this chapter, you'll find out how to contact the NCI to find a designated cancer center near you. There are 28 such centers around the country, plus a number of less comprehensive, full-service cancer centers of different NCI designations.

What if you're particularly attached to, and confident about, your own local doctor? Often, you don't have to give up personal, familiar care in order to get the best new treatments. Sometimes your own doctor can implement plans set forth in more specialized cancer treat- ment centers. In other cases, you might get one form of treatment at a cancer center, and another form from your personal doctor.

Depending on where you live, you might have to travel for state-of-the-art cancer care. That can be costly and inconvenient, but it can also save your life. More and more comprehen- sive cancer care centers around the country have set up living quarters (like hospital-affili- ated hotels) for patients who have come from out of town for treatments that last several days, weeks or even months. While it isn't home, at least it's convenient to the hospital.

We'll begin this chapter with information about breast cancer. This section will be longer than the others, because it raises certain broad themes—early screening, treating cancer spread, multipart treatment, coping with emo- tional stress and managing cancer pain—that apply to *all* of the cancers discussed thereafter.

BREAST CANCER

The most-feared cancer among women is actu- ally the number two cancer killer of women: breast cancer. Over 180,000 cases will be diag- nosed, and 46,000 women will die of breast cancer in 1994. Much has been made of the fact that breast cancer rates have been climbing, spurring concern that something in the envi- ronment may be causing an explosion of cases. In fact, many experts believe that the greater part of this increase (which, by the way, has recently stabilized) is due to improved detec- tion methods—principally mammography.

Breast cancer statistics like the commonly quoted "one in eight" have grabbed headlines and misled women to believe that their chance of getting it is greater than it really is. One in eight women will get breast cancer *by the end of her lifetime.* Your risk each year, and each decade, is much lower on average. The following chart from the National Cancer Institute gives your average breast cancer risk at various ages:

Chances of Developing Breast Cancer

By age 25: 1 in 19,608
By age 30: 1 in 2,525
By age 35: 1 in 622
By age 40: 1 in 217
By age 45: 1 in 93
By age 50: 1 in 50
By age 55: 1 in 33
By age 60: 1 in 24
By age 65: 1 in 17
By age 70: 1 in 14
By age 75: 1 in 11
By age 80: 1 in 10
By age 85: 1 in 9

But low or high, average risk has little meaning to the individual. One way to help determine *your* risk of getting breast cancer is to look at *your personal* risk factors for the disease. This is far from an exact science, but it puts a dose of reality into your estimation of risk. Unfortunately, most cases of breast cancer occur in women who do not have these risk factors. And according to Dr. Maureen Henderson, head of the cancer prevention research program at the Fred Hutchinson Cancer Research Center in Seattle, since we cannot *control* most of these risk factors, they aren't as useful to women as we wish they were. With those caveats in mind, the risk factors for breast cancer are listed below.

Breast Cancer Risk Factors

Experts differ on the issue of "major" versus "minor" risk factors for breast cancer, partly because different studies assign different relative risks to each factor. The following grouping is common:

Major Risk Factors for Breast Cancer

- older age (risk climbs after age 40, but younger women get breast cancer, too)
- a personal or family history of breast cancer
- relatively young age at first menstruation: before 10
- relatively old age at menopause: after 55
- relatively old age at first pregnancy: after 30 or early 30s

Other Risk Factors for Breast Cancer

- certain kinds of noncancerous breast disease, such as atypical hyperplasia
- drinking more than one to two alcoholic beverages per day
- a deficiency of vitamin A (found in carrots and other orange and yellow vegetables and fruits)
- radiation exposure
- never having biological children
- excess body weight
- possibly hormone replacement therapy
- possibly diet—fat content, fiber, and so on.
- possibly exercise

Dr. Maureen Henderson urges women (who have the option) to do their childbearing as early as possible, ideally by age 30; to avoid excessive alcohol; and to keep their weight as close to normal as possible, especially after menopause, when added weight is thought to be riskier. She also asks women to determine, with adequate information, whether long-term use of oral contraceptives and/or hormone replacement would be risky or advisable for them (for more on hormone replacement and the possible risk of breast cancer, *see* chapter 10).

Above all, she urges, we must focus on so-called "secondary prevention"—that is, early detection of breast cancer. Breast cancer, like all cancers, is most effectively treated when it's caught early. Early means before it has spread to other parts of the breast, or to other parts of the body through the bloodstream. The good news is there are three useful tools for detecting breast cancer that can greatly boost your chance of catching it when it's still at an early stage. These tools are the breast self-exam (we show you exactly how to do it beginning on page 78), mammography and the physical breast exam by your doctor. Together, these screening tests save thousands of lives. Learn how to maximize your use of all of them. (For a complete discussion of the three tools every woman must use to catch breast cancer early, *see* chapter 6, "Your Breast Health.")

THE NEXT STEP: IF BREAST CANCER IS DETECTED

Not all breast cancers are equal. If your biopsy shows malignant cells, that can mean many things. There are many different kinds of breast cancers, and they're categorized in a wide variety of ways. Don't immediately assume that yours is life-threatening: many are not. For instance, some breast cancers are confined to particular parts of the breast, such as the ducts (*see* chapter 3, "Your Reproductive Anatomy"). If it's contained in the duct and hasn't spread, it may be called ductal carcinoma in situ (DCIS). Other breast cancers are found in the lobules: again, if they're fully contained in the lobules, they may be called LCIS (lobular carcinoma in situ). Still others are found in different parts of the breast tissue. Different kinds of cancers tend to have different cure rates, depending on other factors as well as their location.

Other factors that distinguish one breast cancer from another include the size of the tumor, and, according to several sophisticated tests, the cancer cells' aggressiveness. In addition, your doctor will want to determine if your cancer is hormone-sensitive or not; that is, is it estrogen-receptor positive or negative? This will tell if hormone treatment might be helpful, in addition to or instead of other drug therapy.

Another important piece of information will be whether your cancer is still contained in your breast, or if it has spread to other parts of your body. The first place surgeons will look is the lymph nodes under your armpits—called your axillary nodes. If there is cancer present in at least one node, your tumor has spread beyond the breast, and your treatment will be tailored to tackle it systemically. Breast cancers also can spread to other body organs, such as the liver or the bones. You will be given tests to see if the cancer is present in any of these locations.

IF YOUR BREAST CANCER IS CAUGHT EARLY

According to Dr. Monica Morrow, director of the Lynn Sage Comprehensive Breast Center at the Northwestern University School of

Medicine, three-quarters of breast cancers are caught early—that is, in what's known as stage 1 or stage 2. At this time, you have three main surgical options:

- **Modified radical mastectomy.** With this procedure, the surgeon will remove your entire breast and your lymph nodes from under your armpits. This procedure is less disfiguring than its predecessor, the radical mastectomy, in which the muscles of the chest wall that sit under the breast were removed as well. Full radical mastectomy is rarely done these days.

- **Modified radical mastectomy with reconstruction.** With this two-part procedure, you are given the modified radical mastectomy (as above) immediately followed by the rebuilding of a "new" simulated breast—while you're under the same anesthesia. This means you'll wake up from surgery with your new "breast(s)," which some women find helps the emotional healing process tremendously. (*See* more on breast reconstruction below.)

- **Breast conservation therapy with radiation to the remaining breast.** Breast conservation surgery is an option for women with early stage breast cancers. The procedure goes by many names, from lumpectomy to quadrantectomy to partial mastectomy and many others. What they all mean, essentially, is that your cancerous tumor will be removed, along with a margin of breast tissue around it—but the rest of your breast will be left intact. That remaining tissue is treated with radiation to kill any stray cancer cells.

Many women were recently terrified by news reports showing that one of the researchers in a major study on breast conservation plus radiation had falsified some of his data. Women naturally panicked, thinking that their choice could have been the wrong one. In fact, top scientists have determined that the study's original conclusions were correct; lumpectomy plus radiation is just as effective for treating early cancers as is mastectomy.

Some women have the gut sense that removing the entire breast (mastectomy) is a better way to get rid of breast cancer than just taking out a lump; they just assume that if a little surgery is good, a lot must be better. But gut feelings aren't always correct science. Dr. William Wood, codirector of Emory University's Winship Cancer Center, has observed

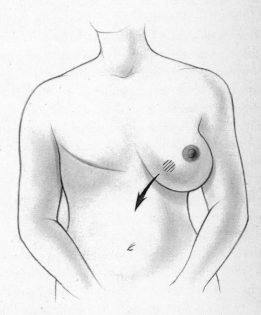

Lumpectomy

that women who have not done much reading about breast cancer have a tendency to tell their surgeons to "just take it off." In fact, experts find that some breast tumors, because they're so close to the breast bone, are *better off* treated with lumpectomy and radiation, since they're hard to remove entirely with mastectomy. Considering the psychological and physical benefits many women find in keeping their natural breasts, just having a *choice* is empowering.

The trouble is, not all doctors are spreading this important word. Despite strong scientific data, surgeons in certain parts of the country are not performing breast-conserving surgery in many cases where it would be appropriate. There is some suggestion that many of them aren't even giving women the option in the first place. A study published in the *New England Journal of Medicine* found that older, male doctors, and those in the Southeast and the Midwest, and in rural areas across the country, were significantly less likely to offer breast conservation to their patients than doctors in the Northeast. And sometimes when it is offered, says Dr. Mary Jane Houlihan of Beth Israel Hospital's BreastCare Center in Boston, the patients aren't given an unbiased choice; rather, they're told, "If it was my wife or daughter, I wouldn't recommend breast conservation."

Younger male doctors, female doctors, those who specialize in cancer treatment, and those at urban and academic medical centers are more likely to offer lumpectomy and radiation. It's pretty frightening to think that where you live in the country could have such a dramatic impact on the type of medical care you're *told about*—let alone given. But before you think you're in the clear if you live in the Northeast, Dr. Lori Goldstein, director of the breast evaluation center of Philadelphia's Fox Chase Cancer Center tells of a doctor in suburban Philadelphia who asked her recently, with great skepticism, if breast conservation is *really* an option for breast cancer patients. Ignorance is everywhere, she warns. Dr. Marc Lippman, director of the Lombardi Cancer Center at Georgetown University Medical Center, notes that three-fourths of women will choose lumpectomy over mastectomy if given a fair, informed choice in the matter.

How to Make Your Decision.

Choosing one type of breast cancer surgery can be extremely difficult, considering the fact that you are probably frightened and have little information on which to base your decision. The first thing you must do is get the survival data on *your particular cancer*. There is a great deal of literature out there, and your doctor can get his/her hands on it, showing the survival rates for particular types of cancers, at particular stages, with different treatment modalities.

Keep a few things in mind when you do make your choice, however. First, while you may want to keep your breasts, certain women are not good candidates for breast conservation therapy. For instance, if your breasts are small, and your cancer is relatively large (even if it hasn't spread at all), the result of breast conservation therapy can be pretty poor. Think about it: if you take a large mass out of a small mass, you aren't left with very much. Your breast(s) might look unusual after conservation therapy. In this case, you might be happier with a full mastectomy followed by breast reconstruction for the most natural-looking outcome. (On the other hand, if your breasts are large, and the cancer small, your result might look terrific with breast conservation.)

Another thing to keep in mind when making your choice is how much time you want or are able to commit to your treatment. Radiation therapy requires coming to a radiation center for several weeks at a stretch. For some women, this is either impossible (the center is too far from a rural area, perhaps) or undesirable. I remember when we covered Nancy Reagan's choice to have a modified mastectomy even though her cancer was caught early, this issue got a lot of attention: Mrs. Reagan said she did not want to take time away from her active life to have repeat treatments. A lot of women criticized her for what they thought was a "backward" decision. In fact, after being informed of all the options, her choice was a valid personal one.

Radiation therapy also *can* cause side effects that should not be overlooked, such as a reddening and sometimes scarring of the skin. The better the radiation therapist—and the more you comply with instructions at the time of treatment—the lower the chance of problems.

Sometimes, your decision will come down to a gut feeling—even if you're well informed of your options. If you simply feel you'd be more at ease to have your entire breast removed, which some women report, then by all means don't let anyone talk you out of it. In addition, if you are perfectly comfortable living without breasts at all, don't let anyone talk you into breast reconstruction. These choices are highly personal, and are bound up with issues that no one can fully understand but you—including how you have always felt about your breasts, what they mean to you now, how the breast cancer has made you feel about your future, and so on.

You'll also want to talk to your doctor about what the follow-up for each treatment entails. After lumpectomy and radiation, for example, you'll need more than the normal number of mammograms and doctor visits to make sure the treatment was successful and that the rest of the breast is clear of disease. If you have your lymph nodes removed surgically, you may have to deal with swelling, vascular or other problems in your armpits and arms. Each case has its own set of subsequent issues and concerns. Become informed about all of them before you make your choice.

Finally, if you're an older woman facing this decision, Dr. Susan Love urges you to stick to your guns in face of both the sexism and ageism that makes its way into some surgeons' offices. For example, many older women are told to have mastectomies because they "don't need their breasts anymore." No one but you can say if you "need" your breasts, and what you might need them for! If breast conservation is an appropriate *medical* option for you, *you* can decide if it's the *best* decision.

TIMING YOUR BREAST CANCER SURGERY

Ruby Senie, an epidemiologist at Memorial Sloane Kettering Cancer Center in New York, believes that the timing of your breast cancer surgery can affect your chance of long-term survival. Her research has noted that women with breast cancer that has spread to the lymph nodes who have breast cancer surgery during the first two weeks of their menstrual cycle (that is, *before* ovulation) are more likely to have a cancer recurrence and more likely to die than women who have their surgery *after* ovulation, at the end of their menstrual cycles. A possible explanation for this is that a few stray cancer cells are "freed" during surgery, let loose into the bloodstream, and the estrogen present at this stage of the hormonal cycle encourages the division of cells—thus leading to the development of more cancer. This is all theory at this point and far from conclusive. Other researchers have found, contrary to Senie's and other's research, that timing does *not* affect outcome. Part of the problem in sorting out this data is that different researchers have used different timing patterns for their studies, so it's a little like comparing apples and oranges.

For now, few experts would recommend changing the time of your scheduled surgery to fit a certain segment of your menstrual cycle— partly because most women can't pinpoint *exactly* where they are in their cycle at a given time. But this is an area of research to watch— and you might want to ask your particular surgeon's thoughts on the issue.

BREAST RECONSTRUCTION

Reconstruction of the breast can be done several ways. One option for rebuilding new breast is to use implants (both silicone-filled implants, which are quite controversial and will be discussed further in a moment, and saline-filled implants are options). Another way to reconstruct breasts is with fat and tissue from elsewhere in your body.

Dr. Bernard Chang, a surgeon who uses both techniques at the Johns Hopkins Hospital, says that the cosmetic result of this latter technique—called the TRAM flap procedure—is much better than the result with implants. Using the body's own tissue—taken from the fatty part of the abdomen—makes the new breasts feel more natural. They also don't run the risk of collapse, as implants do if they rupture. Using tissue from the patient's own body can be quite complicated, as it requires careful management of blood vessels to insure normal blood flow to the new breast tissue. Part of the issue, Dr. Chang notes, is picking the right patient in the first place; those with poor blood flow, for instance, might not be great candidates for the TRAM Flap procedure. When the procedure is a success, it kills two birds with one stone: not only are natural-looking breasts created, but a flabby tummy is eliminated as a side bonus! Many of his patients report being happier with their new figures than they ever were before, which surely helps the ultimate emotional recovery from breast cancer.

If you choose breast implants, which two million American women have done, there are several important issues to keep in mind. The hottest issue of all concerns the use of silicone-filled implants. You've probably heard that there is great controversy over the use of these implants. In response to a number of reports of *problems* with these implants, the FDA conducted an investigation and announced that there is an association between silicone breast implants and various autoimmune diseases such as scleroderma, lupus and others. While not conclusive, enough data emerged to scare the FDA into action before more women were put at alleged risk. Many surgeons spoke out against the FDA announcement, saying that it was grounded more in fear than in scientific data, but the agency stood its ground—and today, only women who are having reconstruction after breast cancer are permitted to get silicone breast implants (and that's only if they're willing to become part of a registry of cases to be monitored by the FDA). Women wishing to increase the size of their breasts for cosmetic or other reasons are *not* permitted to use these implants—they must use saline-filled implants instead. (We discuss this procedure in chapter 6.)

Just a few of the symptoms associated with silicone breast implants include vague joint and muscle pain, arthritis, tight puffy skin on the hands and elsewhere on the body, fever and rashes. The symptoms are usually treated with prescription pain relievers and various immunosupressive drugs. These signs of so-called autoimmune diseases occur in a very small percentage of the nearly two million women who have the implants, but according to Dr. Richard M. Silver of the Medical University of South Carolina, there is reason to believe that the association could be real *for some women*—and that there could be a subset of women at higher risk of problems which we haven't yet identified. Dr. Silver notes that an implant doesn't need to rupture in order for the silicone to makes its way into the bloodstream; in fact, these implants leak or ooze silicone in tiny amounts even when they're fully intact. He points to much older data showing that miners who were exposed to silica had a higher rate of certain autoimmune problems than others, noting that this is *not* a new concern.

Remember, the vast majority of women with these implants are doing just fine. But if you do develop an autoimmune disease that's associated with a breast implant—or if your implant ruptures, causing breast or chest pain, a lump or change in the position or shape or size of the implant/breast—you should have it removed. Dr. Wendie Berg, assistant professor of radiology at the Johns Hopkins School of Medicine, is trying to determine if symptoms are more likely to develop with complete rupture of the implant, or if just having the implant in your body is enough to trigger problems. About 15% of the 400-plus women she and her colleagues have scanned with MRI turn out to have had implant ruptures, but keep in mind that she is dealing with a *symptomatic* population, not the average woman with an implant. If you're feeling fine and your implants look and feel normal from the outside, chances are you don't have to worry.

A variety of imaging techniques can help determine if the implant has ruptured. About half of women do lose their autoimmune symptoms after the implants are removed—some significantly—Dr. Silver says. If on the other hand you have had no problems with the implant, and no unusual symptoms, you should not rush to have it removed; surgery has risks of its own. However, if you're suffering from so much anxiety over the issue that you can't live with the implants in your body, you too might be a good candidate for implant removal.

Saline filled implants—which, by the way, have silicone shells—are thought to be much safer, but they have risks of their own. First of all, they are more prone to rupture. Since saline (or saltwater) is safe, there's no concern about it spilling into your bloodstream; however, it's not fun to have surgery to remove and replace the device. Some women complain that saline implants look and feel less like real breasts than do silicone implants, and that they have a "sloshy" feeling. Another risk to *both* kinds of implants is something called "capsular contracture," in which the tissue surrounding the implant hardens and forms a nest of hard, knobby tissue, affecting the way the new breast feels (sometimes hard as a rock) and looks.

If you do choose breast implants, you will have to decide, after hearing your doctor's advice, whether to have the implant placed in *front* of your chest muscle or *behind* it: While the surgery to put the implant behind your chest muscle is more complicated, it is thought that if you have any of your original breast tissue left over after the surgery and need mammography screening, it's better to have the implant behind your chest muscles so it won't obscure the X-ray image.

Finally, some women will choose *not* to have breast reconstruction, but rather to leave their chests bare. If you are comfortable with this option, go for it: there are advantages, such as no more surgery, no pendulous breasts to get in the way of exercise or cause any type of discomfort, no need for bras, and so on. This choice may be easier for women who never particularly liked their breasts or, even more so, for women who were *bothered* by large or uncomfortable breasts.

CHEMOTHERAPY: DRUG TREATMENT FOR BREAST CANCER

If your cancer has spread to your lymph nodes or elsewhere in your body—*or* if it's large (usually larger than 2 centimeters)—you will be advised to have chemotherapy (or hormone treatment, to be discussed later) after your surgery. This means you will be given medication to fight your cancer *spread,* after the *local* disease (in the breast) has been treated with surgery and/or radiation. Cancer drugs are known to improve the survival rate for women whose cancer has spread to the lymph nodes or elsewhere.

Some experts think that even for the smallest cancers that have *not* spread out of the breast, giving chemotherapy could improve the already extremely high survival rate. This is still controversial, and must be weighed against the 1% chance of major complications from treatment.

Cancer drugs are almost always given in groups—usually three at a time. It has been found that several drugs together are more

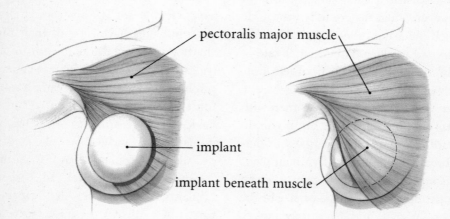

Breast implant in front of and behind chest muscle wall

effective than any one of them alone. The most common combinations are CA (which stands for cyclophosphamide and adriamycin), CAF (adding a third drug, 5-flurocracil) and CMF (substituting methotrexate for adriamycin in patients who may have cardiovascular problems and therefore can't take adriamycin). There are many other drugs that can be tried as well, including newer ones that have grabbed headlines, like Taxol—which seems to be a powerful addition to the breast cancer drug arsenal (more on Taxol in the section on ovarian cancer, below). The drugs can be given both intravenously (in the hospital) and by mouth in pill form. Some women will be given an injection every few weeks—others will go on and off the drugs every two weeks. The duration of treatment varies as well, ranging from several weeks or months to a year. If your cancer is found to be "estrogen-receptor-positive," you may be given the drug tamoxifen or another hormone treatment for a several-year stretch—and you might not take any of the other cancer drugs mentioned earlier. Just as there are many types and stages of breast cancer, so there are a wide variety of treatments with different risks and benefits.

Dr. Lori Goldstein of the Fox Chase Cancer Center in Philadelphia stresses that because there are so many "active" drugs for breast cancer (that is, so many drugs that kill breast cancer cells, at least in the short term) it's worth being aggressive and trying lots of options if the first drugs you try are ineffective. The goal is to get around cancer drug resistance, she adds, since after a period of time, even effective drugs can lose their potency as the body starts to resist their action. There's good news from laboratory research, Dr. Goldstein notes, wherein scientists have found several ways to reduce cancer drug resistance in the test tube. In patients, it's still a game of cat and mouse in which you must move from drug to drug as previous agents lose their effectiveness.

Chemotherapy stirs up a great deal of fear in women's minds because we think of the nausea, vomiting, hair loss and other debilitating images that have been put forth in the media. True, some forms of chemotherapy have these side effects, plus others like diarrhea or constipation, runny nose, and sexual problems. But other cancer drugs do *not* cause these effects. It's important for you to keep in mind that every woman is different, and even if a drug had a certain affect on your friend or relative, it might not affect you the same way. In addition, there are a variety of ways to control the side effects of chemotherapy. Here are just a few:

1. Having the right expectations can help, since as least some portion of the side effects from chemotherapy have to do with *anticipated* symptoms. So learn about the drugs you're going to be taking. Hormonal therapy tends to have minor side effects— hot flashes are the biggest problem with tamoxifen, for example—but nausea isn't usually a problem. The drug Cytoxan, on the other hand, often causes nausea. The drug Adriamycin almost always causes hair loss. Knowing what to expect will likely make your symptoms easier to manage, partly because you can plan ahead and try to reduce the symptoms commonly associated with your treatment.

2. Plan ahead: if your drug regimen is likely to cause nausea, some doctors recommend that you eat a *small* meal before your treat-

ment, and only very small meals afterward. Eating a great deal at once can make nausea worse. There are also medications to reduce nausea, like Zofran, which can be given by pill or intravenously *before* the chemotherapy regimen is started.

3. As much as possible, improve the environment in which you're having the chemotherapy done. If the hospital doesn't provide music in the chemotherapy room (this is actually becoming more common), then bring your own—with earphones, if the hospital requires them. Listening to a tape of your favorite, soothing music can help to distract you from the unpleasant side effects you may be anticipating, says Dr. Mary Costanza, medical oncologist at the University of Massachusetts Medical Center at Worcester.

4. Use at-home antinausea drugs *early,* as soon as you have the first sign of discomfort. Do *not* wait until you start vomiting, advises Dr. Costanza. That's already too late. Common antinausea drugs like Compazine and Norzine and others can help a great deal if taken early enough.

5. Studies differ over whether you can reduce hair loss due to chemotherapy. A drug like Adriamycin, which is one of the most effective anticancer drugs, causes hair loss in almost all patients. There have been some reports that by cooling the hair follicles, either with ice packs on the head or some other method, you can reduce the amount of the drug that reaches the hair follicles and thereby reduce hair loss. Some experts believe it helps, others say they've seen no indication that it's effective in adults (some of the studies were done in children who receive smaller doses of Adriamycin in the first place). One problem with the technique is you need to subject the patient to quite cold temperatures (about 75.2 degrees) to achieve a questionable benefit, which can be uncomfortable.

6. Anticipate hair loss (it might not happen, but you're better off expecting it and being pleasantly surprised) and, if you're uncomfortable having your baldness visible, or don't like wearing hats or scarves, purchase a wig *before* the chemotherapy begins. Experts recommend this so patients are prepared in the event that hair loss starts quickly. If you don't lose your hair, all the better. There are many excellent, natural-looking wigs available these days, especially those made from natural hair—but these tend to be more expensive than the synthetic kind.

More important than the visible side effects of chemotherapy are the internal complications. With proper management, these can be kept to a minimum. Complications of chemotherapy include a low blood count, liver problems and bleeding complications, among others. These are rare complications at small doses, however, and your doctors should be monitoring you closely during your treatment. There will be cases in which the drugs, at the dose they're needed to be effective, are just too toxic for your body. In that case, doctors need to try a different drug or combination of drugs. Tamoxifen or other hormone treatments for cancer have side effects of their own, including symptoms of menopause (hot flashes, vaginal dryness, etc.) *and* internal effects like increased blood clotting and a very slight increased risk of uterine and liver cancer. Again, if you are monitored closely while on any of these medications, problems will be detected early and you may be able to change your dose, or switch to another drug regimen.

BONE MARROW TRANSPLANTATION

You've probably heard of bone marrow transplantation as a treatment for breast cancer. One common misconception about this treatment is that the marrow transplant *itself* is some kind of treatment. In fact, the bone marrow isn't the "active ingredient": the purpose of this treatment is to allow doctors to give powerful doses of cancer drugs that would otherwise be too toxic for the body to handle. The transplanted bone marrow, full of protective fighter cells, can be thought of as a rescue team that comes to the aid of your body when it's struggling to tolerate toxic cancer drugs.

There are several ways to "harvest" bone marrow—the best being autologous (self-given) bone marrow. In this case, your own bone marrow is removed and stored, then given back to you as the rescue device described above. Bone marrow transplantation ordinarily requires several weeks in the hospital in a completely sanitized environment, and costs tens of thousands of dollars. But a way to shorten that stay *and* reduce the cost of this treatment is to use so-called "stem cells" (known as stem cell therapy) in which the precursors to bone marrow cells are taken directly from the patient's blood stream with an IV, and then treated with growth stimulants to produce even more disease-fighting cells, and again, given back to the patient to rescue them from toxic treatments. All of these procedures are experimental at this time, and while they show promise in that patients are able to tolerate much more powerful doses of drugs, we still don't have the bottom line information we need: that is, does bone marrow transplantation save lives? Studies are underway to give us the answer.

IF YOUR CANCER SPREADS TO OTHER ORGANS

If your cancer is found to have spread to other organs of your body, such as the liver or the bones, you will probably continue to be given drug therapy—but other kinds of cancer specialists may come back into the picture. For example, if the cancer spreads to your brain, or bones, a radiation therapist may try to control the cancer spread with radiation beams. Sophisticated cancer centers now have ways of narrowly targeting specific regions with high-potency beams, as a way of maximizing treatment to the area without harming nearby organs or tissues. Sometimes, if there is a large mass or masses in a new area, your surgeon will come back into the picture and remove the new tumor(s). This is yet another reason why it's so important to try to find a *team* of cancer specialists to treat you. When all of the experts are working together—the drug specialist, the radiation specialist and the surgeon—your chances are best that you'll get the ideal treatments at the right times.

REDUCING CANCER PAIN

In recent years there have been significant advances in managing cancer pain. But many cancer specialists are deeply concerned about the fact that the word hasn't spread around the country, and many patients are still suffering needlessly. Keep in mind that cancer pain doesn't always appear where you expect it. For example, a tumor in your neck can cause pain in your hand, and a tumor in your liver can cause pain in your shoulder. So if you're feeling discomfort *anywhere* in your body while you're being treated for cancer, discuss it with your doctor. There may be a good explanation—and a solution.

Dr. Kathleen Foley, chief of the pain service at Memorial Sloane Kettering Cancer Center, notes several advances in pain management that can make a big difference in patients' comfort levels. For example, if your disease is advanced and you can't take medication by mouth, you may be able to take it by means of a patch on your skin. Or perhaps you're a candidate for a self-administered pump that releases pain medication when you feel you need it (this is most useful for postoperative pain, Dr. Foley notes). She also recommends slow-release forms of many medications, which help prevent the problem of uneven pain control, in which medications reach sudden peak and trough levels. And to counter side effects in general, there are a variety of medications that can be taken along with pain medicine—such as psychostimulants to reverse drowsiness, or anticonstipation drugs. Older women should be especially careful with pain medication, Dr. Foley stresses, since it can exacerbate already-existing confusion or other problems. This *doesn't* mean they should suffer pain needlessly; it just means they should be watched closely for side effects and switch medication if one is causing problems.

Remember that no one can guess how you're feeling: You have to speak up in order to receive proper treatment for cancer pain. Don't try to be a hero or a martyr; try to feel as good emotionally and physically as possible at this taxing time. Explain exactly where you hurt, and when, and if your cancer specialist isn't offering helpful advice, seek the advice of a pain specialist. The goal is to be pain free, and functioning as well as possible.

BREAST CANCER PREVENTION

Until recently, what people called breast cancer "prevention" was really breast cancer early detection. We can prevent many deaths with early detection, but we can't prevent cancers from happening in the first place. Because, as we discussed earlier, many breast cancers occur in women with no apparent risk factors, changing your habits can't guarantee breast cancer prevention. For some women, that leaves one option: preventive surgery. Some women who are considered to be at high risk of breast cancer—particularly those with powerful family histories of the disease (mother, grandmother, sisters, etc.)—have opted to have their breasts removed *preventively*. The procedure, which is extremely controversial, is called prophylactic mastectomy. It is a highly personal decision—and also requires finding a surgeon willing to do the procedure. Since there's no guarantee you'll get breast cancer even if everyone else in your family has, it's a pretty drastic measure to take to prevent an "unknown." But for some women, it's all they can do to restore peace of mind. If you are considering this option, by all means get *all* of the data you can on the your particular risk of getting cancer, and weigh it against the emotional and physical toll of the surgery.

Today, there is another revolutionary option emerging for breast cancer prevention. A major trial is taking place through the National Institutes of Health to see if the drug tamoxifen can *prevent* breast cancer in women at high risk of the disease. This is a new concept: giving a drug to otherwise healthy women to try to prevent a disease. As mentioned earlier, tamoxifen is used to *treat* certain kinds of cancers—that is, cancers that are estrogen-receptor-positive (or "hormone sensitive"). The goal of this study, which will follow about 16,000–18,000 women in the U.S. and Canada, is to see if the drug can reduce the risk of breast cancer by blocking the action of the hormone estrogen in the breast. We already have data showing that tamoxifen can reduce the incidence of *repeat* breast cancers in women who had previous ones, and that it can reduce the rate of cancer *spread* in women with earlier cancers.

Some critics of the tamoxifen study complain that we're putting healthy women at unneeded risk. Others argue that the drug, which has been in use for many years, is known to be safe, and that the chance of preventing thousands of cancers is worth a small risk. The risks associated with tamoxifen use include blood clots in the legs (a very tiny incidence that can sometimes be predicted by leg pain) and, at a much higher dose than is being given in this trial, an increased risk of uterine cancer. Many women on tamoxifen experience hot flashes of the type associated with menopause; these are not medically worrisome, but can be uncomfortable. On the flip side, there may be benefits to taking tamoxifen, such as a reduced risk of heart disease—but this remains to be confirmed. Dr. Robert C. Young, president of the Fox Chase Cancer Center in Philadelphia, says that "life has some risks and side effects," and believes this study is one of the most important clinical trials ever done. He adds, "One day, we will call the prophylactic mastectomy [preventive removal of the breast] Neanderthal!"

Dr. Brian Henderson, president of the Salk Institute in La Jolla, California, and an expert in chemoprevention of cancer, points out that using tamoxifen to prevent breast cancer isn't really all that different from what we've been doing *accidentally* in the past. Oral contraceptives (the Pill) have been shown to greatly reduce the risk of both cancer of the ovaries and cancer of the lining of the uterus. Taking the Pill, therefore, is chemoprevention: it's not so revolutionary after all. The same goes for taking the hormone progesterone along with estrogen replacement therapy after menopause. The only reason to add progesterone, Henderson points out, is to reduce the risk of endometrial cancer that *would* have been promoted by estrogen alone. Again, chemoprevention. Henderson argues that we should look at tamoxifen in the same protective light that we've looked at these other drugs over many years.

If you have been told you're at high risk for breast cancer and want to consider joining the tamoxifen trial, call the National Cancer Institute at the number listed at the end of this section.

DETERMINING WHO WILL GET BREAST CANCER: THE FUTURE

In September of 1994 researchers at the University of Utah, the National Institute of

Environmental Health Sciences and others announced the discovery of a gene for breast cancer. This discovery holds great promise for the treatment—and someday the cure—of familial breast cancer. Soon, a blood test will reveal many of the women who are destined to get at least a *genetic* form of the disease—and these women can weigh their very tangible odds against the risks of preventive treatment.

There are a variety of other high-tech, futuristic treatments for cancer that are just around the corner—some of which are already being used experimentally. We'll discuss these at the end of this chapter.

(For a discussion of non cancerous problems of the breast, *see* chapter 6, "Your Breast Health.")

YOUR FEELINGS ABOUT CANCER: COPING

After being diagnosed with breast or any cancer, you are likely to take a ride on a roller coaster of emotions, including fear, rage and disbelief. These feelings are normal, expected, and usually get better with time—or with counseling. According to Dr. Jimmie Holland, chief of the psychiatry service at Memorial Sloane Kettering Cancer Center, cancers that have the potential to disfigure—such as head and neck cancers, breast cancers and others—are often the hardest to cope with because patients must face a different physical image of themselves. All cancers can take a serious emotional toll, however. If talking out your feelings with your loved ones isn't doing the trick—that is, it isn't making you feel gradually better with time—you may want to consider more formal counseling. And beyond counseling, there are many tech-

niques for stress reduction and relaxation that can help you restore your confidence, collect your thoughts and find strength to fight your disease. You can choose among several options.

First, there are support groups for breast cancer; if you feel you want to discuss your emotions with other women who are experiencing some of the same feelings, support groups are a good way to go (for references, *see* the information section at the end of this chapter). It's important to choose a support group that includes women at your stage of cancer, if possible. It can be unnecessarily draining and frightening to meet with women who are facing a poor prognosis if you happen to have a very good one, for example. It can also be discouraging to talk with women who are expected to get well, if you have been told your chances are not very good. According to Anne Coscarelli, director of the Rhonda Fleming Mann Resource Center for Women With Cancer at UCLA, it is absolutely vital to *individualize* emotional treatment for cancer. Just as each cancer is different in some way—whether by cancer type, stage, or some other characteristic—so each *person* is different *before* she becomes sick with cancer. Treatment that boosts cancer coping skills, just like drug or other medical treatment, must be tailored to *your* needs and concerns—so you don't end up, as Coscarelli warns, lumped together with women with totally disparate needs and concerns. You may be worried about how to face dating again after your breast has been removed; another woman may be focused on preparing to leave a husband and children behind. So groups are fine, Coscarelli says, as long as they are appropriately "grouped."

If groups aren't for you, individual counseling can be extremely helpful as well. According to Dr. Fawzy I. Fawzy, professor and deputy chair of the department of psychology and biobehavioral sciences at the UCLA School of Medicine, the goal is to move from "avoidance coping" to "active behavioral coping" and "active cognitive coping." For all their scientific names, this is quite practical advice. What it means, Dr. Fawzy explains, is that you must change from trying to ignore your problem—tucking it away in your mind and not facing it or talking about it—to actively dealing with the diagnosis of cancer head-on. When you face your problem, you can move from seeing it as a threat, to seeing it as a *challenge* that you can overcome. We can do this, he says, by breaking down the more global "threat" into individual pieces which you *can* conquer—such as first getting information about your cancer, then talking to experts and reading more about it, talking to others who have been in your position, making choices about treatment, sharing your advice with others, and so on. When you face your cancer and talk about it, you become more adept at asking others for support—something that women are often loathe to do, since so often we are the care*givers*, not the care receivers.

Facing the diagnosis of cancer aggressively and openly can be painful at first. Dr. Fawzy acknowledges that it can be distressing at first to look bad news in the face, and to talk to others openly about it. But soon thereafter, he says, you'll start to take hold of support systems and you will begin to feel stronger. If you bury your fears inside, refuse to face what you are going through or to let others help you face it, you will pay for it in the long term with sleeping problems, loss of appetite, feelings of stress, and other common side effects of repressed worry.

This is no way to fight a disease.

Julia Rowland, co-director of the psych-oncology program at the Georgetown University Medical School, has found that certain women are at relatively high risk of *severe* distress following the diagnosis of breast cancer. Those who have problems in their marriages, a poor relationship with their health care providers, low expectations of a good outcome from treatment, a weak overall support system (lack of supportive friends or family), as well as those who have a history of psychological problems, may fare worse than others who don't fit these categories. If you find yourself in one or more of these groups, you might do well to develop a counseling support team even *before* you start to feel depressed—a form of preventive psychological medicine. Certain vulnerable women can develop a syndrome that Julia Rowland likens to post-traumatic stress disorder (PTSD) after being diagnosed with breast cancer. PTSD is most commonly associated with traumatic events like war, earthquakes and other sudden unexpected disasters. Rowland and colleagues have seen similar patterns of behavior in breast cancer patients, including feelings of numbness, reliving past experiences of trauma, flashing forward to an image of oneself dying, and feeling dissociated from things happening around oneself. Both group and individual therapy can help a great deal with these symptoms.

Most women with cancer successfully move past their fear and on to something more productive. One doctor reported that many of her patients move from shock and anger to what she terms a "get-on-with-it" stage in which they even go through emotional *growth* as a result of the cancer and treatment. The value of life now in focus, many women move forward with a more active, positive outlook on life and a desire to squeeze every benefit from it. If you don't feel like you're reaching this stage on your own, by all means reach out and ask for help. Dr. Fawzy has heard the complaints of many a patient in his office, lamenting the fact that husbands, friends, siblings haven't "been there for them." He always asks, "Have you asked them for support?" The answer is usually "no". Only by asking for support graciously—and receiving it graciously—will you ever find the comfort you need, he insists. So go out and ask for it: from professionals, from loved ones, from anyone you trust.

PROBLEMS WITH SEX AFTER CANCER TREATMENT

Even those who recover emotionally and generally feel back to "normal" after cancer treatment can have one lingering problem: sex. Some women say their sex lives never rebound to the way they were before the diagnosis and treatment of cancer. There are several reasons for this common concern. First, there are some real physiological issues: sometimes cancer treatment can affect your sexual function—chemotherapy can bring on menopausal symptoms including vaginal dryness; radiation and chemotherapy can cause tremendous fatigue, which certainly hurts the libido. Beyond the physiological problems, though, are serious psychological issues that have to be addressed. According to Beth Meyerowitz, director of clinical psychology at the University of Southern California, many women experience profound body image changes after cancer treatment. If your breast was removed, or your uterus taken out, your sense of femininity and sexuality might be altered. Perhaps you are modest in a way you never were before—afraid to show scars, or the lack of a breast or breasts. If your sex life was less than passionate *before* treatment, it can be even harder to get back on track.

Finally, another serious impediment to healthy sexual function is your *partner's* attitude to you after cancer treatment. Often, partners are afraid of physically hurting you after surgery, Beth Meyerowitz finds. They may feel guilty about wanting sex when you have been through so much trauma—so they "lay off," and you feel rejected.

If your sexual problems are physical, consider lubricants to restore vaginal moisture (*see* list on pages 255–256), and get extra rest, a proper diet and some exercise to fight fatigue. For emotional problems surrounding sex, *talk to your partner*—and perhaps, talk to a sex counselor experienced in treating cancer patients. Your oncologist may be able to recommend someone; or, a local sex counselor may know who in the area focuses on post-cancer care. Often all your partner needs is a little encouragement from you and education from an expert on the fact that there's no risk of harming you with sex—especially if you've been cleared by your doctor. Think of sex as part of your recovery, part of getting back to who you were—and still are—before cancer entered your life.

WHEN YOU'RE NOT GETTING BETTER

How do you know when you're *not* coping with cancer adequately and it's time to get more help? Dr. Jimmie Holland says to seek professional help if you start questioning whether to bother going along with your treatment, if you're having trouble eating or sleeping, if you feel you're in such a dire situation that you can't see the light at the end of the tunnel, and so on. What kind of health professional should you seek? That depends. If you are physically and emotionally unable to function, you may need medication, so a physician is the way to go. If you're just looking for emotional support, Dr. Holland says many people benefit from returning to a spiritual support system, such as a church, mosque or synagogue leader. There is no "best" form of support.

Relaxation and stress reduction therapies are also quite valuable in coping with cancer. Dr. Anne Coscarelli describes cancer as a stressor that hits like a bomb on top of already stress-packed women's lives. It is so hard to manage the stress of cancer while dealing with other life demands that stress reduction techniques are sorely needed—and can make a big difference. Whether by focusing on relaxing images, listening to music you enjoy, resting in a comfortable chair, meditating or any other method you prefer, you can help your body and mind shed some of the fear and tension that make coping so much harder. Dr. Holland recommends progressive relaxation, in which patients are coaxed to relax each part of the body, eventually relaxing the *entire* body, while picturing themselves in a peaceful place. Dr. Holland says patients can make good use of the technique at bedtime if they're having trouble falling asleep, or at any time of day when anxiety and stress start to build.

Will relaxation and stress reduction help you fight cancer? That far Coscarelli and Holland—and many of their colleagues across the country—won't yet go. While Eastern philosophy and medicine suggest that the immune system actually becomes stronger when stressful forces are overcome, there isn't as much hard data as anyone would like on that score. But cancer specialists argue that it shouldn't matter if relaxation can save your life; you shouldn't have such a strict end point in mind. Why not reap the tangible benefits of feeling better, enjoying life more and coping with your fears—and if you *happen* to become more healthy while doing it, all the better. When you attach a goal to relaxation, such as getting rid of cancer, two problems can emerge: first, says Anne Coscarelli, if your cancer *does* return, you'll feel like a failure—which is preposterous; and second, if you are constantly looking to measure success, you're working against the very process of relaxation. So learn to think of healing in a broader sense: not just getting well according to laboratory tests, but feeling well while you're trying.

Colon and Rectal Cancer

Because women tend to focus so heavily on cancers of the reproductive system—linking our risk of cancer to our gender, and not to the fact that we are also generically *human*—we don't take cancers of the gastrointestinal tract seriously enough. This is quite tragic, considering that colorectal cancers, as colon and rectal cancers are collectively termed, are diagnosed in about 160,000 people each year, half of them women. According to the American Cancer Society, 28,200 women are expected to die from these cancers in 1994. Dr. Elin Sigurdson of the Fox Chase Cancer Center worries that because these cancers most often affect people over age 60, there is a sense of resignation among people at risk; they often *expect* bad health at this age, she says, and therefore don't aggressively fight to prevent it or catch it early. This is, for the most part, a preventable cancer—there's no reason to resign yourself to getting it at any age!

There is some good news about colorectal cancers—and that is that *screening works.* Thanks largely to better screening tests, which we'll discuss in a moment, the death rate among women due to colorectal cancers has dropped by about a third in the last three decades. With screening, these cancers are found early, before they have spread to distant parts of the body. At this early stage, they are quite curable and often cause little disruption of life. Found later, they can progress and cause all of the complications, disability and mortality risk of any cancer that moves throughout the body. Too few women are screened regularly, and as a result, many needless deaths occur.

Unfortunately, the highest-profile cases of colon cancer have given a weak message to women. While former president Ronald Reagan was treated early for precancers of the colon, and has fared quite well, the most notable *woman* to recently suffer from this form of cancer, actress Audrey Hepburn, died of the disease. We need more examples of high-profile women *saved* by early screening to get the important word across.

RISK FACTORS FOR COLON AND RECTAL CANCER

As with many types of cancer, having a family history of these diseases boosts your chance of getting them. In addition, if you have a family history of polyps in the colon or rectum—that is, benign or precancerous growths—your risk of colorectal cancers goes up. Other risk factors for these cancers include inflammatory bowel disease and certain lifestyle habits—namely eating a low-fiber, high-fat diet.

You'll notice I listed both high-fat *and* low-fiber diet together. The reason is, scientists aren't absolutely sure whether having a high-fat diet *alone* promotes colorectal cancers, or whether high-fat is just a substitute for low-fiber. It's well accepted that eating lots of fiber, particularly the so-called "insoluble" fiber found in vegetables, fruit, grains and many other complex carbohydrates, is protective against colon cancer. In fact, in vegetarian populations where dietary staples are high-fiber, colon cancer is quite rare; whereas in the U.S., where we eat loads of fat and nowhere near the fiber we need, the colon cancer rate is quite high. Some experts point to the situation in Japan, where colon cancer *used* to be quite rare, but is increasing at a fast pace as fat in the diet increases. (*See* chapter 20, "Nutrition," for advice on how to increase fiber in your diet.)

How does fiber protect us? There are theories, but no one knows for sure. We used to believe that since stool moved through the bowel faster with high-fiber diets, potential carcinogens weren't around long enough to have an impact. This theory is now fading in favor of the belief that fiber somehow affects cancer-causing "free radicals" in the body so they don't get into the bowel. However fiber works, it may be the most powerful preventive medicine we have against colon cancer.

Dr. Michael Thun, director of analytical epidemiology for the American Cancer Society, adds another interesting factor to the colon cancer prevention list: aspirin (and other aspirinlike drugs). In numerous animal studies, and in several studies of humans, aspirin and related drugs have been found to cut both the incidence of colorectal cancers *and* the death rate from these cancers. Dr. Thun's best guess about how aspirin might protect us—and it's still only a theory—is through the drug's inhibitory effect on something called prostaglandins, which are created by colorectal tumors. In other words, aspirin might be shutting off one type of colorectal cancer promotion. Unfortunately, we don't know the best dose of aspirin to prevent colon cancer, so no one is making widespread health policy out of the findings. Unlike the research on aspirin and cardiovascular disease, which was carefully controlled, the studies on aspirin's effect on colon cancer have looked at many different doses and regimens of aspirin over time. And because aspirin and its cousin drugs carry risks like gastrointestinal bleeding and stroke, it's not a good idea to try to treat yourself without a doctor's advice and supervision.

Screening for Cancers of the Colon and Rectum: The Tests You Need

There are three main tests for cancers of the colon and rectum. They are the digital rectal exam, the test for blood in the stool, and a test with a scope (flexible sigmoidoscopy). Let's discuss each one.

1. The *digital rectal exam* is the test in which your health care practitioner inserts his/her finger into your rectum and feels for abnormalities. Many people find this uncomfortable or awkward, but it should not be painful if done properly. You may feel a bit sweaty or dizzy if you're not comfortable with this test—in fact, some doctors avoid doing it because patients are so averse to it! The fact is, it takes only a few seconds; if you breathe in and out and relax it really shouldn't be a big deal at all. This exam should be done every year from the age of 40 onward.

2. The test for "occult blood" or hidden blood in the stool is an important cancer screening tool. Normally you will put a bit of your stool on a slide or two and send it (or give it) to a laboratory for investigation. This easy test saves lives. Just because you don't see blood in your stool doesn't mean you're cancer-free. The blood that might indicate cancer is invisible to the naked eye, and needs to be examined under a microscope. This simple, noninvasive test should be done every year starting at age 50.

How to Get the Best Results from the Occult Blood in Your Stool Test

The American Cancer Society recommends that you take the following steps for a couple of days before you give a stool sample:

A) avoid vitamin C or multivitamins with vitamin C in them

B) avoid iron

C) avoid broccoli, turnips, cantaloupes, cauliflower, radishes, parsnips and other foods in this group that have so-called "high peroxidase activity"

D) avoid red meat

E) avoid aspirin and nonsteroidal anti-inflammatory drugs

3. Sigmoidoscopy—ideally, "flexible sigmoidoscopy"—is a test in which the doctor uses a small scope to investigate further into your colon than she would be able to do with just her finger. While stiff scopes can be quite uncomfortable, the flexible sigmoidoscope is, as its name suggests, more pliable and therefore has the double advantage of seeing curvy areas better and causing less discomfort. Don't avoid this test just because it sounds unpleasant. It doesn't take long, is considered mildly uncomfortable, *not* painful, and, again, saves lives. The test should be done every three to five years after the age of 50. If you are at high risk of getting colorectal cancers or if you have suspicious regions that your doctor wants to follow more closely, you'll likely fall into the more frequent screening group.

If Something Unusual Is Found with These Screening Tests.

Just because something unusual turns up on these tests doesn't necessarily mean you have cancer. But it does mean you'll be referred for further testing, including things like deeper scopes into the colon, and X-ray testing.

Finding Colon and Rectal Cancer Yourself.

There are several signs of colorectal cancers that you may be able to detect yourself—but this is hardly the best way to screen for these diseases, since by the time you have symptoms, the cancer may be well-developed. This case can be likened to the case with breast cancers, in which often by the time you can *feel* a problem, it has been around for quite a while. These obvious signs of colorectal cancers, compiled by the American Cancer Society, include a change in bowel habits, abdominal cramping, rectal bleeding and visible blood in the stool.

TREATING COLON CANCER

If you do have cancer of the colon or rectum, and it is localized—that is, still confined to the colon—you may be offered conventional surgery alone to remove the growth, and possibly radiation therapy along with it. If you're vigilant about screening, you're much more likely to find a tiny cancer which, once removed, leaves you with an excellent chance of complete cure (between 80% and 90%) with surgery alone. There are studies ongoing to determine whether giving cancer drugs (chemotherapy), or other high-tech treatments, enhances the survival rate in those with colorectal cancers that have spread elsewhere in the body. It seems to be most useful when some tumor is left behind after surgery. As with all cancers, the farther it goes, the harder it is (though not always impossible) to control and cure.

Surgery to treat colon cancer is much better than it used to be, so the need to wear external bags for your bowel movements has gone down from 50% to 5%, according to Dr. Elin Sigurdson of Philadelphia's Fox Chase Cancer Center.

OVARIAN CANCER

When Gilda Radner, the famous comedienne of "Saturday Night Live" and Hollywood fame, died at 42 of ovarian cancer, this disease was put on the map of public consciousness and has remained there ever since, sometimes to a degree out of proportion with its incidence rates. But there's a good reason for the tremendous concern some women have about ovarian cancer. While 24,000 new cases will be diagnosed in 1994, the death rate is quite high: in the same year, over 13,000 women will die of ovarian cancer. To put this in some perspective, while the yearly incidence is one-ninth that of breast cancer, the yearly death toll is half that of breast cancer.

Why do so many people die of ovarian cancer? Because this cancer is *extremely* hard to detect. As a result, when it is detected, it has often spread beyond the ovaries, at which point it is hard to cure. Tucked inside the pelvis where they are hard to reach with conventional screening tests, ovarian cancers elude detection even by the best screening methods available. Furthermore, by the time you have any symptoms of ovarian cancer, the disease has often progressed to a dangerous point.

So what can be done about it? Certainly we must not resign ourselves to being "beaten" by this cancer. There is some indication that by using a number of screening tests together, we may boost the chance of catching these cancers earlier. More on this in a moment.

Risk Factors for Ovarian Cancer

The older you are, the greater your risk of ovarian cancer—but young women certainly get this disease as well, as Ms. Radner unfortunately proved. Other risk factors include not bearing biological children, having a family history of ovarian cancer (especially if two first-degree relatives had the disease), a personal history of breast cancer, and certain rare genetic disorders. There is thought to be a family pattern of both breast and ovarian cancers occurring together; some day the gene will be pinpointed and we will know who is at risk for this combination of cancers. In April of 1994 the National Institutes of Health issued a consensus panel report about ovarian cancer. In it they state that while women with no family history of ovarian cancer have just a 1 in 70 chance of getting the disease, women who have a first degree relative (mother, sister or daughter) with ovarian cancer have a 5% risk of getting it themselves, and women with two affected first degree relatives have a 7% chance. Those with one of the rare hereditary forms of the disease are urged to have aggressive screening, which we'll discuss more later.

Another *possible* risk factor for ovarian cancer is the use of talcum powder—but this is uncertain. Dr. Mary Daly of the Fox Chase Cancer Center suggests that talc may set off an inflammatory process in cells that is somehow connected to cancer. However, Dr. M. Steven Piver, chief of gynecologic oncology at the Roswell Park Cancer Institute in Buffalo, NY, cautions that the studies linking talc to ovarian cancer were done in the past, when talcum powder had bits of asbestos in it. We don't know for sure that there is any connection between talc and ovarian cancer *today,* Piver says.

On the flip side of the coin, some factors *protect* us against ovarian cancer. For example, oral contraceptives are strongly protective; the longer you take them, the lower your risk of getting ovarian cancer. This fact gets too little attention. Oral contraceptives may be among the oldest forms of chemoprevention for cancer.

DETECTING OVARIAN CANCER

As I mentioned earlier, it's hard to catch these cancers early. About 70% of cases are found in "stage 3" (in which the cancer has already spread out of the pelvis); at this stage, only one in three women will be disease-free five years later, according to the National Cancer Institute. Dr. Mace Rothenberg, executive officer of the Southwest Oncology Group in San Antonio, Texas, explains that because the symptoms of ovarian cancer often resemble simple constipation (bloating of the abdomen that doesn't disappear with bowel movement; abdominal discomfort), women wait an average of nine months to seek medical attention. Only half of women with ovarian cancer will have vaginal bleeding. The time that elapses between the first symptoms and the visit to the doctor can make the difference between catching a tumor before and after it has spread.

Generally, the only test most women have that *could* reveal ovarian cancer is a pelvic exam by their doctors, in which the hope is that he or she will feel a slight change in the size of the ovaries. But this is extremely subjective; you can't always count on a doctor's fingers detecting a problem early. Furthermore, because the cancer isn't common, it takes about ten thousand pelvic exams to pick up one ovarian cancer, says Dr. Carolyn Runowicz, director of the division of gynecologic oncology at New York's Albert Einstein College of Medicine. Once the visible signs of ovarian cancer have appeared, you may be given a test called an ultrasound in which sound waves are bounced off of the ovaries to try to reveal abnormalities. There is also a blood test for ovarian cancer, called CA-125, but it is unreliable as a sole screening test. According to Dr. Arthur Fleischer, chief of diag-

nostic sonography at the Vanderbilt University Medical Center, the blood test for CA-125 reveals only *half* of stage 1 ovarian cancers.

Dr. Robert C. Young, president of the Fox Chase Cancer Center in Philadelphia, points out that while all three tests are substantially less than perfect, the three tests together—with some refinement—may be quite helpful in high-risk women. Right now it's not appropriate to screen *all* women this way, he believes, since "it's like looking for a needle in a haystack"; of the 60–70 million women over 40 in this country, about 21,000 get ovarian cancer. Which ones will get it, we don't know—and without a great screening tool, we'd subject a lot of women to testing that yields no useful advice. In high-risk women (which of course will be easier to define when the gene(s) for ovarian cancer is found), more aggressive screening, at least in an experimental setting, makes more sense. Here's what they're attempting at Fox Chase and other top centers around the country to catch ovarian cancer earlier:

1. First, instead of doing conventional ultrasound tests in which the sound-wave-gathering probe is put on the patient's abdomen, they're using a technique called transvaginal ultrasound. With transvaginal ultrasound, the probe is placed inside the woman's vagina, bringing it much closer to the ovaries—therefore providing a much better image of potential problems. The transvaginal ultrasound is painless and available at many medical centers, but unfortunately it's still experimental and unproven as a screening test for ovarian cancer. If you are at high risk for ovarian cancer, however, you may be able to join a clinical trial using this screening method, in which case you won't

have to pay for it. There are some experts, such as Dr. Fleischer of Vanderbilt, who feel even today that all women should have a transvaginal ultrasound annually starting at age 40. It's the best test we've got, he argues: Why wait to use it?

Dr. Robert Ozols, senior vice president of medical science at the Fox Chase Cancer Center, urges women to keep in mind the downside of transvaginal ultrasound: while this test is pretty good at detecting *something* in the ovaries, it isn't great at telling *what* it has detected. It may show up benign ovarian cysts, for example, which then require further testing to rule out—or detect—cancer. The 1994 NIH consensus panel report warned that aggressive screening sometimes results in unnecessary surgeries which, of course, carry risk of their own. In some ways, it's similar to the situation with mammography, which detects *something* abnormal in the breast, but can't tell you if it's cancer or a benign lump. One possible solution in the case of the transvaginal ultrasound test is to use "color Doppler" technology to get more specific results. By indicating blood flow within the mass, this technique helps distinguish malignant from benign tumors.

2. In addition to the transvaginal ultrasound, they give the CA-125 blood test—which is useful to some extent, but much more so when done in combination with other screening tests.

3. Finally, some are giving pelvic exams—that is, a physical examination by your doctor—every *six* months, instead of every year as most women are advised to have them. If you and your doctor determine that you are at high risk of ovarian cancer (according to the parameters discussed earlier), this more vigilant screening could be appropriate for you.

Because this kind of aggressive screening is experimental, we don't yet know if it brings about important so-called "end points"—that is, catching earlier cancers or saving lives. As a result, aggressive screening is not covered by insurance, nor is it being recommended widely at this point. Also bear in mind the downside of screening, as discussed earlier: lots of unnecessary follow-up procedures may be done to confirm or rule out cancers. You'll have to find a balance, with your doctor's help, between seeking peace of mind and excessive meddling.

TREATING OVARIAN CANCER

Only one-third of ovarian cancers are confined to the ovary when they are detected. Two-thirds have spread beyond the ovaries and into nearby pelvic regions. In either case, your treatment usually starts with surgery to remove the ovaries (called oophorectomy), and may be more extensive, including removal of your uterus and fallopian tubes (hysterectomy and salpingectomy). If the cancer is caught very early in a young patient, and is confined to one ovary, surgeons may just remove the one affected ovary in an effort to preserve fertility.

Even if the ovarian cancer is large and bulky in the pelvis, a good surgeon can remove most of it. I met a woman who was diagnosed with advanced ovarian cancer on a story I did for CBS in Massachusetts. Her experience started out terribly—and unfortunately, her case is all too common. The surgeon opened her pelvis, saw the extent of her ovarian cancer, and, as she put it, "he closed me up and sent me home to die." He did not even *attempt* to remove the extensive cancer he saw. When she got to a more sophisticated cancer center in Boston, the Dana Farber Cancer Institute, skilled surgeons reopened her and were able to remove most of the visible cancer. She was then put on anti-cancer drugs, and went into a several-year remission. Not everyone will have such a happy ending, but clearly, going to a specialized cancer center will increase the chance of your getting proper care. (*See* the information section at the end of this chapter.)

Wherever you choose to get your care, Dr. Runowicz urges patients with ovarian cancer (or any gynecologic cancer) to seek the attention of a specialist—called a gynecologic oncologist. She worries that because patients don't know to ask for this kind of expert, they go into the operating room without the best support, and the wrong decisions can be made about diagnosis and treatment. Since there's little time to lose with this cancer, getting it right from the start is especially vital. You don't necessarily have to dump your trusted general doctor in favor of a new specialist, as many patients fear. Instead, ask your doctor if he/she would work *along with* a gynecologic cancer specialist, both in the operating room and during your subsequent care.

Additional Treatment for Ovarian Cancer

There are several drugs available for treating ovarian cancer, and in general, patients respond quite well to drugs *at first:* their cancers shrink or disappear, and patients feel well again. For the small number of women whose cancer is caught early (in stage 1 or stage 2), surgery plus drug treatment has a cure rate of over 90%. For cancers that have spread further, though, the cure rate is significantly lower. After a period of good response to treatment, many women with later-stage disease develop resistance to the drugs, and the cancer reappears. Recurrence is the biggest challenge in the drug treatment of ovarian cancer.

The most common drugs for ovarian cancer include platinum-based medications, like cisplatin and carboplatin, combined with other therapies. More recently, you may have heard of the drug Taxol, which is obtained from the bark of the Pacific yew tree. Recently, the trees (and hence the drug) were in short supply; it takes about 20,000 pounds of bark from 2000 yew trees to get 1 kilogram of Taxol, according to the American Cancer Society. That translates into four to six trees to get enough drug for one patient! As a result of the shortage, scientists have created a synthetic version of the drug.

Taxol has been promising in patients with advanced disease who have failed on other medications; it is thought to work by preventing the separation of cells into daughter cells—the hard-to-control cell division that leads to cancer spread. Dr. Ozols likens the drug to a "crazy glue" that interferes with the cells' ability to separate. Taxol is now being examined as a first-line treatment in combination with other standard drugs.

In addition to trying new drugs, and new combinations of drugs, oncologists are studying the best way of *giving* drugs to treat ovarian cancer. For example, there may be some advantages to administering drugs directly to the site of the tumor for certain patients.

Radiation treatment for ovarian cancer can

also be helpful in reducing pain, and treating fistulas that may have resulted from previous surgery, according to Dr. Ozols.

Other high-tech treatment strategies, including bone marrow transplantation (discussed briefly in the breast cancer section above), hormonal treatments and other so-called "biologic therapies" (discussed briefly at the end of this chapter) are being studied for use in ovarian cancer.

PREVENTIVE SURGERY FOR OVARIAN CANCER

Some women considered to be at extremely high risk for ovarian cancer (such as those with two first-degree relatives with the disease) are asking surgeons to perform preventive surgery—called prophylactic oophorectomy (preventive removal of the ovaries)—so they don't have to face the frightening risk of ovarian cancer. This, like the prophylactic breast removal discussed earlier in this chapter, is an extreme measure that would never be recommended widely, but may be appropriate in the highest-risk patient who has completed her childbearing and is living in terror of getting ovarian cancer. If you are considering this option, and have talked to your surgeon, be sure to ask about the importance of estrogen replacement therapy after the procedure, since losing your ovaries puts you into artificial menopause. Also keep in mind that preventive removal of the ovaries is no guarantee that you'll avoid ovarian cancer. There remains a tiny risk that other tissue similar to the ovaries, which will remain in your body, could develop ovarian cancer, says Dr. Piver. In his study, 6 out of 324 patients developed cancer in the abdomen despite having their ovaries removed.

CANCER OF THE CERVIX (CERVICAL CANCER)

If you'll refer to the illustration in the left column on page 35 in chapter 3 on reproductive anatomy, you'll see that the cervix lies at the mouth of the uterus. Cancer of the cervix, therefore, is one type of uterine cancer—but must be distinguished from endometrial cancer, which is cancer of the *lining* of the uterus. We'll start with a discussion of cervical cancer, and move on to discuss endometrial cancer next.

About 15,000 women are diagnosed with invasive cervical cancer each year, and many more (about 55,000) are diagnosed with so-called "cervical carcinoma in situ"—which means cancer that remains confined to the cervix, usually to its surface. Only about 4600 women will die of cervical cancer in 1994, thanks to effective screening with the Pap smear test. **But:** Although the number is small, those 4600 cases do *not* have to occur. According to Dr. Patricia Eifel, associate professor of radiotherapy at The University of Texas M.D. Anderson Cancer Center, most women who come to see her for *invasive* cervical cancer have had no Pap smear for 15 years or have ignored unusual symptoms for a long period of time. The death rate from cervical cancer is more than twice as high in African-American women as in caucasian women, suggesting that black women are in special need of better screening efforts.

RISK FACTORS FOR CERVICAL CANCER

The earlier the age at which you first have sexual intercourse, and the more sex partners you have thereafter (or the more sex partners your partners have), the greater your risk of cervical cancer. Other risk factors or potential triggers include cigarette smoking and having certain strains of the sexually transmitted virus HPV (human papillomavirus). Clearly, not all women who have HPV, nor all women with multiple sex partners, get cervical cancer. But the more of these risk factors you stack up, the greater your chance that you will get this disease.

SIGNS OF CERVICAL CANCER

Abnormal uterine bleeding (that is, bleeding outside of your normal menstrual period or after you have reached menopause), and abnormal vaginal discharge are two signs of cervical cancer. Pelvic pain can be a sign of *advanced* cervical cancer but is not usually how the disease is caught. Do not ignore these symptoms. Cervical cancer is highly curable if caught early enough, so don't delay in reporting abnormal signs to your doctor and getting in for a Pap smear.

DETECTING CERVICAL CANCER: THE PAP SMEAR

The Pap smear is the screening test for cancer of the cervix. With this test, your doctor takes a small sticklike instrument, puts it into your vagina and scrapes a few cells from the surface of your cervix. Some women find the test completely painless, while others who have more sensitive nerves in that area find it briefly painful or uncomfortable (like a pinch on the skin), but it's over in a matter of seconds. The cells are placed on a slide and reviewed by a pathologist in a lab for signs of changes. These changes are then reported to you in the form of a *grade* or *stage*—ranging from early, precancer-

ous abnormalities to full-blown cancer.

Certain groups of women are less likely to have Pap smears done—including women over 65, those who live in rural areas and those with low incomes. Insurance doesn't always cover the test, which can cost in the range of $15 to $30, and is done once a year. The test saves lives; every woman should have it.

You may have heard controversial reports about Pap smears in the news. In one major New York City case, thousands of Pap test results were lost and never reported to patients, some of whom had cancer and didn't know it. Other reports show that the Pap smear is not a perfect test, and that is true: because of misreading by pathologists, poor cell samples and other potential problems, there are potential false negatives in Pap smear tests. That means that a percentage of women who are told that they do not have cervical cancer in fact *do* have it. The false negative rate, which may be higher at unaccredited laboratories, is one excellent reason to have a Pap test every single year. If a problem is missed one year, it will be caught another. Often, cervical cancer is slow-growing, so the annual Pap test gives you a terrific chance of catching either precancerous cells or cancer early.

When to Have a Pap Smear Test.
The test should be done every single year in women who are sexually active, regardless of their age—and in women 18 and older even if they're not sexually active. If the test comes back normal three years in a row, you can have it done at longer intervals (at your doctor's discretion), unless you're thought to be at risk of new cervical infections, for example.

TREATING CERVICAL CANCER

If you have early precancerous changes on your cervix, or cancer that is contained on the surface cells of the cervix, you're in luck: treatment is almost always curative. You'll have a choice of several therapies if the abnormal cells are on the surface, including cryotherapy (freezing), electrocautery (burning with electric current), laser therapy or conventional surgery to remove surface cells. Often these surface procedures can be done on an outpatient basis in your doctor's office, and you'll go home the same day. After treatment, you'll be monitored with more frequent Pap smears than usual—perhaps every six months or so. After several years of normal Pap smears, you can revert to annual screening.

If the cancer has progressed into the cervix, beyond the surface, you'll need more extensive surgery to remove it. And if the cancer is very large or has moved beyond the cervix altogether—that is, invasive cervical cancer—you will need radiation treatment as well.

Radiation treatment for cervical cancer, which consists of putting radioactive treatment implants in the uterus and vagina, takes a good deal of clinical skill. Dr. Patricia Eifel, whose team does over 200 of these procedures a year, wants women to know how important it is to find a radiation oncologist who is experienced in this particular procedure. Even a well-trained radiation oncologist who is very experienced in other areas of radiation treatment can be less skilled than you'd hope, if he/she does only a few cases of this type a year. The goal is to find experienced doctors in order to keep side effects, such as bowel obstruction, bladder and bleeding problems to a minimum.

ENDOMETRIAL CANCER: CANCER OF THE LINING OF THE UTERUS

Each year there are more than 30,000 cancers detected in the body of the uterus (to be distinguished from the cervix, which is the opening of the uterus). Most of these are in the lining of the uterus, called the endometrium. According to the American Cancer Society, about 5900 women will die this year of endometrial cancer.

RISK FACTORS FOR ENDOMETRIAL CANCER

This tends to be a cancer of postmenopausal and/or obese women, although it can affect younger women too. It's also found more in women with diabetes and high blood pressure, which is only *partly* explained by the fact that these women are more likely to be overweight. There are some familial or inherited cancer syndromes in which women are at greater risk for clusters of cancers, including endometrial, ovarian, breast and colon cancers. Your doctor should take your family's cancer history and if there appears to be a cluster of these cancers (especially if they occur relatively early in your female relatives' lives) you should be watched more carefully for early signs of disease—particularly abnormal bleeding from the vagina.

You'll notice that other risk factors for endometrial cancer are connected to hormones in the body: for instance, early first menstruation; late menopause; a history of infertility; failure to ovulate; estrogen replacement therapy (*without* progesterone added); and possibly treatment with the drug tamoxifen.

Symptoms of Endometrial Cancer

The *good* news about endometrial cancer is that its main symptom, bleeding from the vagina, does often occur early in the disease. That means if you watch for abnormal bleeding and report it to your doctor immediately, you're likely to catch the disease in time for a cure. Dr. Richard Barakat, a surgeon at the Memorial Sloane Kettering Cancer Center in New York, finds that vaginal bleeding often brings women into the doctor's office *fast,* and that quick response can save the lives of women with endometrial cancer. This is one more reason to get to know your menstrual cycle; you'll be more attuned to changes in your bleeding pattern and you'll bring it to your health care provider's attention faster.

Naturally if you're postmenopausal and have vaginal bleeding after a long time without it, you should pay attention and see a doctor. And if you're taking hormone replacement, and find that you're bleeding *outside* the normal pattern your doctor told you to expect (or differently from the pattern you've had for a while), let your doctor know about it. You may be given an endometrial biopsy (more below) or a D & C— dilation and curettage—a surgical procedure requiring anesthesia, in which the lining of your uterus is removed for testing.

Detecting Endometrial Cancer

While the Pap smear usually detects cancer of the cervix (since the cervix lies at the opening of the uterus and is accessible through the vagina), Pap smears usually *do not* detect cancer of the lining of the uterus. The only way to detect this cancer is to do a biopsy of the uterine lining, which requires putting a thin tube through the cervix into the uterus and sucking out some tissue for study in a lab. This can be uncomfortable, causing cramping, but requires no anesthesia and can be done during your regular visit to the gynecologist. Endometrial biopsies are not routinely performed; they are recommended for women with symptoms of possible endometrial cancer, and they are recommended *annually* for women who fit particular risk categories, such as those who take estrogen replacement therapy *without* supplemental progesterone (estrogen alone can promote endometrial cancer; progesterone cuts that risk). If you can't tolerate an endometrial biopsy (perhaps because your cervix is very tightly closed, and it's too painful to force a catheter through), you may be given a D & C.

The annual pelvic exam, which is considered part of the yearly cancer screening regimen for all women, is also part of the general screening for endometrial cancer, but it is not a diagnostic tool.

Treating Endometrial Cancer

Surgery to remove the uterus (hysterectomy) is most often the treatment for endometrial cancer, and is the only sure way to *cure* the disease (if it hasn't spread out of the uterus). Depending on whether the cancer has spread, you may or may not be given further surgery for other pelvic organs. Hormone therapy (treatment with the hormone progesterone) has been used with some success for precancerous conditions of the uterine lining (called hyperplasia, or atypical hyperplasia), keeping these conditions from developing into cancer. In some especially complex or severe precancerous conditions, however, hysterectomy is still recommended to insure a cure.

In some cases, radiation therapy is also used to treat endometrial cancer—either *instead* of hysterectomy, or in addition to it. For instance, if you are too frail or sick to undergo major surgery and therefore can't have a hysterectomy (because of severe heart disease, let's say), radiation therapy can be used to help stave off your endometrial cancer. Radiation treatment alone is *sometimes* able to cure *very* early endometrial cancers. Radiation therapy is also used *after* hysterectomy for some insurance, in certain cases. Dr. Barakat says that if your cancer has spread *less* than halfway through the lining of your uterus (which doctors can tell you after removing your uterus), you may be given radiation therapy just to your vagina, which involves about three weeks of treatment, with two 30-minute sessions a week. If the cancer has spread *past* the halfway mark of your uterine lining, you will probably be given radiation treatment to both your vagina *and* pelvis, which takes a couple more sessions per week, and a couple more weeks of treatment than vaginal radiation therapy alone.

Chemotherapy is not normally part of the treatment for endometrial cancer, *unless* the cancer spreads out of the uterus and into other parts of the body (called metastatic disease). About 25% of endometrial cancers are found when they have spread beyond the uterine lining, Dr. Barakat notes. Endometrial cancer can spread to the lungs, liver and elsewhere in the body. Once the cancer has spread, cancer drugs can be used to help control the disease.

LUNG CANCER

The leading cancer killer of women, lung cancer rates have been dropping in men, but are still increasing in women. The reason, above all else, is smoking. If you've heard it once, you've heard it a thousand times. But that doesn't make it any less true. Since women's smoking rates took off later than men's, the rate of lung cancer incidence and death are later on the curve for women, so in recent years we've just begun to experience the horrifying effect this one bad habit can have on health. Sadly, American women are leaders in the trend. Dr. Michael Thun of the American Cancer Society points to the horrifying statistic that while American women make up just 5% of all women in the developed world, we make up 50% of the deaths from smoking. A depressing way in which to be trendsetters.

Even though lung cancer kills more women than breast cancer does—and has for the last seven years—it is nowhere near as high on the emotional radar scale for most women as breast cancer is. Again, this is partly because women tend to think of their cancer risk in terms of their gender, focusing on cancers of the reproductive tract far more than on other cancers in the body. Dr. Thun is concerned that women aren't even thinking about this cancer as an important risk in their lives, which only makes it less likely that the trend will reverse anytime soon.

OTHER RISK FACTORS FOR LUNG CANCER

Beyond active cigarette smoking, *passive* smoke—or sidestream smoke that you breathe when someone around you is smoking—is a significant cause of lung cancer. If you find it hard to tell a friend to stop smoking because it smells bad or bothers your eyes, try telling her to stop because she's *killing* you. If cigarette smoking were eliminated, we'd prevent 3000 lung cancer deaths *each year* from passive smoke alone, according to the American Lung Association. (For much more on smoking and tips on how to quit, *see* chapter 19.)

Beyond smoking, there are other causes of lung cancer in women: asbestos exposure; radiation; and possibly environmental radon, to name a few.

DETECTING LUNG CANCER

Chest X rays are the best way to detect lung cancer. In addition, when cancer is suspected, examination of the sputum and an exam in which a tube is put down into your bronchial passages will also be used.

There are also signs of lung cancer that you might notice yourself, such as:

- a persistent cough—the famous smoker's "hack"
- sputum with blood
- chest pain
- chronic pneumonia or bronchitis

The trouble is, these signs often show up after lung cancer has spread. As a result, lung cancer is often detected late—after it has moved out of the lungs into other body organs, like the brain. The overall survival rate at all stages is quite low—at 13%. After it has spread to the brain, the survival rate is 0%, according to Dr. Robert C. Young. If you're lucky and catch it while it's still in the lungs, surgery alone may be used. If it has spread, as we've discussed with other cancers in this chapter, drug therapy will be recommended along with surgery. Sometimes, drug therapy will be given *before* surgery to shrink the tumor so that surgery has a better

chance at being effective. Radiation therapy is also used to treat lung cancer, usually along with other treatment methods.

There are two general kinds of lung cancer: small cell and non-small cell. The prognosis for lung cancer depends on what type it is and how far it has spread. About 75% of lung cancer cases are in the non-small cell type (there are three types within this category); sadly, only one in ten patients with this diagnosis survives five years. These are appropriate cases for creative new and aggressive treatments that can sometimes be provided through clinical studies. The National Cancer Institute keeps a list of such trials throughout the country. *See* the information section at the end of this chapter for the number to call.

BLADDER CANCER

More than 13,000 women will be diagnosed with bladder cancer in 1994. Like ovarian cancer, bladder cancer often goes untreated because its symptoms are vague (sometimes imitating bladder infections). There are no regular screening tests for the disease.

RISK FACTORS FOR BLADDER CANCER

Smoking doubles your risk of bladder cancer; exposure to a number of occupational toxins like dye and rubber also seems to boost risk; and women in urban areas are, according to the American Cancer Society, at greater risk of bladder cancer.

DETECTING BLADDER CANCER

There is no simple screening test for bladder

cancer. The only way to detect it with certainty is to use the cystoscope, or bladder scope, a tool that is inserted through the urethra and into the bladder.

SIGNS OF BLADDER CANCER YOU MIGHT NOTICE

A fact that is quite worrisome to many doctors is that the symptoms of bladder cancer are quite common, and imitate other relatively benign bladder problems, such as urinary tract infections. The signs to watch for are blood in the urine and increased urinary frequency. Sometimes, women appear in their doctors' offices complaining of chronic urinary tract infection symptoms; they're treated with antibiotics and are told to drink a lot of water (neither of which has any impact on cancer), and their cancer goes undiagnosed until it spreads. If your symptoms don't abate after antibiotic treatment, return to your doctor for further testing.

TREATING BLADDER CANCER

The further along the cancer gets, the more drastic the treatment. Many women will have their bladders removed surgically and replaced with a plastic bag outside the body. As is often the case with cancers, if it has spread throughout the body, cancer drugs will be used—sometimes *before* surgery (similar to the use in lung cancer discussed above). Radiation therapy can help, sometimes before conventional surgery as well. Once bladder cancer has spread to distant parts of the body, the survival rate over five years is low, at about 9%. Don't ignore symptoms until it's too late for a cure.

SKIN CANCER

Skin cancer is discussed in chapter 5, "Your Skin Health."

HIGH-TECH, FUTURISTIC AND ALMOST-HERE TREATMENTS FOR CANCER

Ask almost any cancer specialist what's most exciting about cancer treatment and they launch into a lecture on gene therapy. As we are on the verge of numerous groundbreaking discoveries of precise cancer gene locations, research is already underway to develop treatments to "turn off" those genes, creating so-called "cancer vaccines" and other space-age technologies to make cancer cells turn on themselves.

Amazingly, a bit of the future is already here in some leading centers. For example, at the University of Michigan Comprehensive Cancer Center, experts are already targeting women who have the marker for the familial breast cancer gene for special prevention and treatment programs. Dr. Max Wicha, director of the cancer center, reports these exciting examples:

1. A woman who had stood by and witnessed breast cancer attack almost every woman in her family was about to have her breasts removed preventively because she was sure that she, too, would get the disease. Genetic testing showed that she did not have the marker for the gene, and therefore was at no increased risk. She *dropped* plans for the surgery.

2. Another woman with a strong family history of breast cancer was found to carry the breast cancer gene marker, and was sent for

mammography screening *years* before she would have been given it normally. An early cancer was caught; she was treated and is now fine. Genetic testing probably saved her life.

3. Several women who were found to have the gene marker for breast cancer were put into the revolutionary tamoxifen trial mentioned earlier in this chapter, to try to *prevent* these likely breast cancers from occurring.

These cases are only the beginning of what genetic testing can offer in the way of lives saved and fears calmed, but give you a glimpse into the vast power of genetic information.

Other high-tech cancer treatments that you may have heard about are in experimental use today. These include monoclonal antibodies, missile-like antibodies that are formed by joining both normal and cancer cells and which home in on cancer targets in the body, piggybacking radiation or other treatments directly to the site of a tumor. Another group of treatments getting a great deal of attention are the potent immunologic therapies called biologic response modifiers. These treatments, which include drugs like interferon and interleukin-2, are derived from the body's own disease-fighting cells and are harnessed and multiplied many times over to fight cancer more aggressively. Even the old standbys—conventional surgery, radiation treatment and drug therapy—

are being updated to treat cancer more effectively and aggressively. Top cancer centers are using machines that deliver radiation beams precisely to the tumor site, sparing nearby organs the damage that used to occur so often with radiation treatment. I have seen this treatment in action and it is truly phenomenal to witness how computerized three-dimensional mapping of the body can guide the radiation to its hidden targets in the body. With bone marrow transplantation, ever more powerful drug combinations are being used to treat drug-resistant cancers, and new drugs are being discovered all the time, as we uncover new ways to understand how cancer cells work.

But the best news for you today is that there is so much you can do to take action on your own behalf in fighting cancer. Through better information about screening tests and risk factors for all kinds of cancer, you are now armed with the information to protect yourself better than any generation before you. The lowest-tech method of all—prevention—is in your hands. Seize this exciting opportunity to care for your body, and if you are faced with cancer, fight back with the latest and the best available weapons. We are lucky to be living at the frontier of a new stage in the war against cancer, and can only hope we'll live to capitalize on the fruits that are sure to be borne even in the next decade. Perhaps we will then look back on the old days when cancer, now an arcane disease, actually made headlines.

FOR MORE INFORMATION ON FIGHTING CANCER

GENERAL
AMERICAN CANCER SOCIETY
800-ACS-2345
or find your local chapter listed in
the yellow pages

NATIONAL CANCER INSTITUTE
OFFICE OF CANCER
COMMUNICATIONS
Building 31, Room 10 A 16
9000 Rockville Pike
Bethesda, MD 20892
800-4-CANCER

SOCIETY OF GYNECOLOGIC ONCOLOGISTS
401 North Michigan Ave., Suite 2200
Chicago, IL 60611
800-444-4441
312-644-6610

NATIONAL COALITION FOR CANCER SURVIVORSHIP
1010 Wayne Ave.
Silver Spring, MD 20910
301-650-8868

LOOK GOOD, FEEL BETTER
800-395-LOOK

CHOICE IN DYING
200 Varick Street, 10th Floor
New York, NY 10014

COLLEGE OF AMERICAN PATHOLOGISTS
800-LAB-5678

NATIONAL WOMEN'S HEALTH NETWORK
1325 G St. NW
Washington, DC 20005

CONCERN FOR DYING
250 W. 57th Street
Rm 831
New York, NY 10107
212-246-6962

COLLEGE OF AMERICAN PATHOLOGISTS
325 Waukegan Rd.
Northfield, IL 60093-2750
708-446-8800

AMERICAN SOCIETY OF PLASTIC AND RECONSTRUCTIVE SURGEONS
444 E. Algonquin Rd.
Arlington Heights, IL 60005
800-635-0635

AMERICAN COLLEGE OF RADIOLOGY
1891 Preston White Drive
Reston, VA 22091
800-227-6440 (Mammography information)
703-648-8900

CANCER CARE, INC.
1180 Ave. of the Americas
New York, NY 10036
800-813-HOPE
212-221-3300

BREAST CANCER

NABCO (NATIONAL ALLIANCE OF BREAST CANCER ORGANIZATIONS)
9 E. 37th Street
New York, NY 10016
212-719-0154

NATIONAL HIGH-RISK REGISTRY, STRANG CANCER PREVENTION CENTER
428 E. 72nd Street, Suite 700
New York, NY 10021
800-521-9356

Y-ME NATIONAL BREAST CANCER ORGANIZATION
212 West Van Buren Street
Chicago, IL 60607
800-221-2141
312-986-8228 (24-hour hotline)

BREAST IMPLANTS

U.S. FOOD AND DRUG ADMINISTRATION OFFICE OF CONSUMER AFFAIRS
5600 Fishers Lane
Rockville, MD 20857
Breast Implant Information Line: 800-532-4400

SCREENING TESTS

The following screening tests will help you and your health care provider catch problems before they become serious. Experts and institutions vary in their recommendations: I have followed the advice of many of those I interviewed, plus some major organizations such as the American Cancer Society and the National Cholesterol Education Program of the National Heart, Lung, and Blood Institute. But these are only general guidelines for people who do not have signs or symptoms of disease. By all means see your doctor whenever you suspect something isn't right, such as a lump in your breast or a cough that won't go away: don't wait around for your next yearly visit.

Furthermore, your individual risk factors may warrant more or different testing. Always ask your personal health care provider which tests are best for you—and how often to have them. Then put the information on your calendar and follow through! Screening tests save tens of thousands of lives every year.

Keep in mind that not all insurance plans cover screening tests. Some cover certain tests and not others. Talk to your provider about which tests are covered and if you discover that you cannot afford some important exams, take further action before you skip them. For example, ask a doctor, nurse or local health department about programs in your area that periodically provide lower-cost health care screening for those in need.

Notice that the following screening tests are listed according to age categories. This means that if you are over 50, you must follow the guidelines leading all the way up to your age group. For example, the guidelines for those over 20 and those over 40 all apply to you, too! Circle each age category that pertains to you and follow all pertinent guidelines.

Age 18 (or whenever you become sexually active) to 40

Every Year

A Pap test for cancer of the cervix. If you have been diagnosed with abnormal cells on your cervix, you may be told to have this test even more often. If you have had a normal Pap test 3 or more years in a row, your doctor may say that it's okay to have the test less often.

Every 1 to 3 Years

A pelvic examination by your doctor. If you are sexually active, or have had pelvic problems in the past (such as pelvic inflammatory disease) many experts feel that every year is best.

Age 18 and Over

Every Year

Blood pressure measurement. Increase frequency according to your doctor's advice if your level is borderline high or high.

Weight check. It would be a good idea to weigh yourself far more often than once a year, to keep yourself aware of unhealthy increases or decreases in weight. But at *least* make sure you're weighed on a proper doctor's scale once a year, and ask your health care provider for an assessment of your weight and body shape.

Every 5 Years

Cholesterol test. Increase frequency according to your doctor's advice if your level is borderline high or high.

Age 20 and Over

Every Month

Breast self-exam. See page 78 for details on how to perform this important screening test.

Every 3 Years

Health counseling and cancer checkup, including tests for cancer of the thyroid, ovaries, lymph nodes, oral region and skin (according to the American Cancer Society).

Age 20 to 40

Every 3 Years

Breast examination by your health professional.

Age 40 and Over

Every Year

Digital rectal exam by your health care provider; that is, a physical examination of your rectum.

Breast examination by your health professional.

Pelvic examination by your health professional

Health counseling and cancer checkup, which for women includes tests for cancer of the thyroid, ovaries, lymph nodes, oral region and skin, according to the American Cancer Society.

Age 40 to 49

Every 1 to 2 Years

A mammogram or breast X ray.

Age 50 Plus

Every Year

A fecal occult blood test, or test for hidden blood in your stool. This is a screening test for cancers of the colon and rectum.

A mammogram or breast X ray.

Every 3 to 5 Years

Flexible sigmoidoscopy a screening test for cancers of the colon and rectum.

At Menopause

If you are considered at high risk for cancer of the lining of the uterus (endometrial cancer), you should have an endometrial biopsy at intervals determined by your doctor. One example: if you're taking estrogen replacement therapy without progesterone and still have your uterus, this test is recommended for you.

MENUS AND RECIPES

LOW-/NON-CALORIE BEVERAGES CAN INCLUDE:

tea (iced or hot)

coffee

seltzer (plain and fruit-flavored
but not sweetened)

spring water

diet soda

ABBREVIATION KEY

c = cup

tsp = teaspoon

Tb = tablespoon

oz = ounce

* Recipe for this dish provided in appendix.

MONDAY

BREAKFAST

1 1/2 c 40% bran flakes[1]

1 medium banana

1 slice pumpernickel toast with 1 Tb jam

1/2 c orange juice

1 c 1% milk

LUNCH

Salad in medium pita (2 c lettuce, 1/4 c green
pepper, 1/4 tomato, 1/4 medium carrot)

2 Tb low-fat salad dressing

2 oz lite cheese

2 fig bars

Non-calorie beverage

SNACK

2 medium plums

1 oz unsalted dry roasted peanuts

[1]Or any cereal with less than 2 g fat and greater
than 3 g fiber per serving

DINNER

Baked sole stuffed with spinach*

1 whole wheat roll with 2 tsp soft margarine

4 oz non-fat frozen yogurt with 2 Tb chocolate or multicolor sprinkles

Non-calorie beverage

ANALYSIS

Calories:	1730
Fat (g), (% calories from fat):	40 (20)
Saturated Fat (g), (% calories from saturated fat):	10 (5)
CHO (g), (% calories from CHO):	274 (61)
Protein (g), (% calories from protein):	81 (18)
Fiber (g):	31
Calcium (mg):	1240

TUESDAY

BREAKFAST

2 pieces whole wheat toast with 2 tsp jelly

1 medium fresh orange

1 c 1% milk
Coffee/tea

LUNCH

3 oz 95% fat free cold cuts, 1 Tb low-fat
  mayonnaise, lettuce and tomato on 2
  slices whole wheat bread
1 fresh apple
1 c low-fat fruit yogurt
Non-calorie beverage

SNACK

3 graham crackers
1 kiwi

DINNER

10 cheese raviolis or 3 pierogies
3/4 c tomato sauce[2] with 2 oz 90% lean
  ground beef or ground turkey
Salad with 2 Tb low-fat dressing (2 c lettuce,
  1/4 c green pepper, 1/2 tomato, 1/2
  medium carrot)
2 oatmeal raisin cookies, 2″ diameter
Non-calorie beverage

ANALYSIS

Calories:	1797
Fat (g), (% calories from fat):	41 (20)
Saturated Fat (g), (% calories from saturated fat):	13 (7)
CHO (g), (% calories from CHO):	275 (59)
Protein (g), (% calories from protein):	95 (21)
Fiber (g):	24
Calcium (mg):	1342

[2]Any bottled tomato sauce with less than 300 mg
sodium and less than 3 g fat per 1/2 cup serving.
When adding meat to a non-meat sauce, use a
ratio of 2 oz meat per 1 cup of sauce.

WEDNESDAY

BREAKFAST

1 c oatmeal with 1 tsp cinnamon-sugar
  and 1/4 c 1% milk
1/2 grapefruit
1 c 1% milk
Coffee/tea

LUNCH

1 c cooked tricolor corkscrew pasta with 3/4
  c meat sauce (see Tuesday dinner) and 2
  Tb Parmesan cheese
1 c fresh fruit salad (1/3 c grapes, 1/3 c
  melon, 1/3 c strawberries)
Non-calorie beverage

SNACK

1/2 c low- or non-fat pudding with 2 Tb lite,
  non-dairy topping

DINNER

Sweet and sour stir-fried chicken*
1 c white rice
1/2 c low-fat frozen yogurt with 1/3 c blue-
  berries
Non-calorie beverage

ANALYSIS

Calories:	1784
Fat (g), (% calories from fat):	34 (16)
Saturated Fat (g), (% calories from saturated fat):	10 (5)
CHO (g), (% calories from CHO):	286 (61)
Protein (g), (% calories from protein):	108 (23)
Fiber (g):	20
Calcium (mg):	990

THURSDAY

BREAKFAST

1 honey apricot muffin*
1/2 c low-fat cottage cheese
2 peach halves, canned
Coffee/tea

LUNCH

Sandwich on hard roll with 3 oz 95% low-fat
   cold cuts or 1/2 c tuna, with 1 Tb low-cal
   mayo, lettuce and tomato
1 medium pear
1 oz lite popcorn
1 c 1% milk

SNACK

1 c low-fat plain yogurt
1/4 c dried prunes
1 Tb wheat germ

DINNER

1/4 of a 12″ meatless pizza
Salad with 2 Tb low-fat dressing (2 c lettuce,
   1/4 c green pepper, 1/2 tomato, 1/2
   medium carrot)
1/2 c raspberry sorbet
4 vanilla wafers
Non-calorie beverage

ANALYSIS

Calories:	1744
Fat (g), (% calories from fat):	43 (22)
Saturated Fat (g), (% calories from saturated fat):	14 (7)
CHO (g), (% calories from CHO):	253 (57)
Protein (g), (% calories from protein):	96 (22)
Fiber (g):	25
Calcium (mg):	1273

FRIDAY

BREAKFAST

2 pieces whole wheat french toast
   (2 tsp soft margarine, 1/4 c egg substitute)
2 Tb lite pancake syrup
1 c 1% milk
Coffee/tea

LUNCH

3/4 c seafood salad (1/2 c fish based crab
   substitute, 1 Tb low-fat mayo, 2 Tb
   chopped celery) in medium whole wheat
   pita pocket
1 c prepared[3] vegetable soup
Fresh orange sections (1 medium orange)
Non-calorie beverage

SNACK

4 oz seltzer and 4 oz fruit juice
1 c fresh cherries

DINNER

Low-fat fried chicken*
1 c steamed broccoli with lemon and garlic
1 1/3 c brown rice
1 c fruit flavored gelatin
Non-calorie beverage

ANALYSIS

Calories:	1804
Fat (g), (% calories from fat):	33 (17)
Saturated Fat (g), (% calories from saturated fat):	7 (3)
CHO (g), (% calories from CHO):	288 (64)
Protein (g), (% calories from protein):	89 (20)

[3]Any prepared vegetable soup with less than 500
mg sodium per cup

Fiber (g):   22
Calcium (mg):   1377

SATURDAY

BREAKFAST

1 4″ diameter whole grain bagel, with 2 Tb
    lite cream cheese
1/2 fresh grapefruit
1 c 1% milk
Coffee/tea

LUNCH

Shrimp and pasta primavera*
2/3 c pineapple tidbits in own juice
1 c non-fat yogurt (i.e. lemon or vanilla)
    with 1/4 c wheat germ
Non-calorie beverage

SNACK

1 1/2 c fresh strawberries

DINNER

Hearty minestrone soup*
2 slices black bread with 2 tsp soft margarine
1 chocolate cupcake*
Non-calorie beverage

ANALYSIS

Calories:	1757
Fat (g), (% calories from fat):	36 (18)
Saturated Fat (g), (% calories from saturated fat):	9 (5)
CHO (g), (% calories from CHO):	287 (64)
Protein (g), (% calories from protein):	84 (19)
Fiber (g):	27
Calcium (mg):	1098

SUNDAY

BREAKFAST

Cheesy vegetable omelet*
1 honey apricot muffin*
1/2 fresh grapefruit
1 c 1% milk
Coffee/tea

LUNCH

Hamburger (3 oz lean beef) on bun, with 1
    tsp mustard, lettuce and tomato
1/2 c coleslaw
1 fresh peach or plum
Non-calorie beverage

SNACK

1 oz light tortilla chips with 1/4 c tomato
    salsa

DINNER

Pasta with white bean sauce*
1 Tb grated Parmesan cheese
Salad with 2 Tb low-fat dressing (1 c lettuce,
    1/4 c green pepper, 1/2 tomato, 1/2
    medium carrot)
1/12 angel food cake with 1/2 c fresh straw-
    berries
Non-calorie beverage

ANALYSIS

Calories:	1803
Fat (g), (% calories from fat):	52 (25)
Saturated Fat (g), (% calories from saturated fat):	18 (9)
CHO (g), (% calories from CHO):	246 (53)
Protein (g), (% calories from protein):	99 (21)
Fiber (g):	20
Calcium (mg):	1234

BAKED STUFFED SOLE
(for Monday Dinner)

Serves 4

   1 lb sole cut into 4 pieces
   juice from 1 lemon
   1 1/2 cups cooked rice
   1 lb cooked spinach
   1/8 tsp garlic (minced and dried)
   dash parsley
   2 tsp plain bread crumbs
   2 tsp melted margarine

1. Pour lemon juice over fish.
2. Combine remaining ingredients and put one quarter of the mixture over each filet.
3. Fold each filet into thirds and secure with a toothpick.
4. Sprinkle 1/2 tsp plain bread crumbs over each filet and a few drops of melted margarine.
5. Bake 10–15 minutes at 450°.

SWEET AND SOUR STIR-FRIED CHICKEN
(for Wednesday Dinner)

Serves 4

   1 lb cubed raw chicken
   1 red pepper, cut into strips
   1 green pepper, cut into strips
   1 small onion, sliced
   3 c raw broccoli, coarsely chopped
   2 c summer squash, sliced and quartered
   4 medium carrots, sliced
   8 oz drained pineapple chunks
   8 oz sliced and drained water chestnuts
   1 Tb olive oil
   1 cup sweet and sour sauce
   vegetable oil spray

1. Spray vegetable oil in non-stick skillet, and stir-fry chicken for 2 1/2 minutes.
2. Set chicken aside while cooking the vegetables.

3. Heat olive oil in skillet for sautéing vegetables. Add carrots and sauté for 1–2 minutes.
4. Add broccoli and summer squash, and add a small amount of water to steam the vegetables. Loosely cover the skillet with the lid (while stirring to prevent sticking) until broccoli has turned bright green.
5. Add onion and peppers.
6. Stir-fry for about a minute, then add chicken back to the mixture until warmed and until peppers are cooked but still crisp.
7. Add sauce and simmer 1–2 more minutes.
8. Serve over rice. (Shrimp or tofu may be substituted for chicken.)

HONEY APRICOT MUFFINS
From Sue Bee Honey
(for Thursday and Sunday Breakfast)

Makes 18 muffins
   1 1/2 c whole wheat flour
   1/2 c oatmeal
   1/2 c chopped pecans (optional)
   3 tsp baking powder
   1/2 tsp cinnamon
   1/2 tsp nutmeg
   1/2 c honey or sugar
   3 Tb melted margarine
   1 egg (or egg substitute)
   16 oz canned apricots, drained and chopped

1. Mix all dry ingredients.
2. In a separate bowl, hand-mix all other ingredients.
3. Mix liquid ingredients with dry ingredients, just enough to blend.
4. Pour into muffin cups with paper linings.
5. Bake at 350° for 25–30 minutes or until done.

LOW-FAT FRIED CHICKEN
(for Friday Dinner)

Serves 2
   8–10 oz boneless, skinless chicken breast
   1 c crushed cereal (corn flakes or other)

1/2 c fat free Italian salad dressing
1 Tb lime juice

1. Dip chicken in salad dressing and coat with cereal.
2   Pour lime juice over chicken and bake at 350° for 30–40 minutes, or until done.

SHRIMP AND PASTA PRIMAVERA
(for Saturday Lunch)
Serves 4

4 oz chicken broth (may substitute 4 oz water with 1 package instant soup mix)
1 Tb lite soy sauce
1 Tb canola oil
2 garlic cloves, minced
1 1/2 c broccoli flowerets
1 each red and yellow pepper, sliced
1 c zucchini, sliced and quartered
1/3 c scallions
1/2 lb large shrimp, raw, peeled and de-veined
1/2 lb angel hair or vermicelli pasta, uncooked
8 Tb reduced calorie creamy Italian dressing
2 Tb Parmesan cheese
fresh cracked black pepper

1. Cook pasta per package directions and reserve.
2. Heat canola oil in large skillet and brown garlic.
3. Heat half the chicken broth and soy sauce.
4. Add broccoli and peppers, stirring frequently.
5. When partially tender, add zucchini and scallions.
6. When tender, remove from skillet.
7. Using the same skillet, heat remaining broth and garlic.
8. Add shrimp and cook until pink.
9. In large bowl, combine shrimp, vegetable mixture and cooked pasta.
10. Toss with dressing and Parmesan cheese.
11. Serve warm or chilled, topped with cracked pepper.

Hearty Minestrone Soup

(for Saturday Dinner)

Makes 6 12-ounce servings

1 28 oz can canned tomatoes, including juice
2 c water
1/2 tsp salt
1/4 tsp pepper
3/4 tsp basil
1/4 tsp oregano
1/4 tsp thyme
1 1/2 c cooked kidney beans (or 19 oz can of kidney beans)
1 c sliced carrots
1 c sliced celery
1 medium onion, finely chopped
5 oz frozen cut green beans
1/2 c lima beans (frozen or canned)
1 8 3/4 oz can whole kernel corn, drained, or 1 1/2 c frozen whole kernel corn

1. Steam carrots, celery, onion in steamer for 3 minutes.
2. Steam cut green beans and lima beans in steamer for 2 minutes.
3. Combine all remaining ingredients in large saucepan. Add vegetables and simmer until tender.

Hint: A crock pot can help develop the flavor. Try cooking on medium heat for 4–6 hours.

Quick Chocolate Cupcakes

(for Saturday Dinner)

Makes about 1 dozen cupcakes

1 1/2 c all-purpose flour
1/2 c sugar
1/4 c baking cocoa
1 tsp baking soda
1 c water
1/4 c vegetable oil
1 Tb vinegar or lemon

1 tsp vanilla extract

1. Heat oven to 375°.
2. In a medium mixing bowl, combine flour, sugar, cocoa and baking soda.
3. Add water, oil, vinegar and vanilla.
4. Beat with a mixer, wire whisk or wooden spoon until batter is smooth and ingredients are well blended.
5. Pour batter into paper-lined muffin pans (2 1/2 inches in diameter), filling each 2/3 full.
6. Bake 16–18 minutes or until wooden pick inserted in center comes out clean.
7. Remove to wire rack; cool completely.
8. Apply topping as desired (powdered sugar, frosting, cocoa, etc.)

CHEESY VEGETABLE OMELET
(for Sunday Breakfast)

Serves 2

1 c egg substitute (equivalent of 4 eggs)
3 large mushrooms (optional)
1/2 red pepper
1/2 c broccoli flowerets
3 scallions
2 oz low fat cheddar cheese
2 Tb low fat cottage cheese
1 Tb Parmesan cheese
pepper
vegetable oil spray

1. Chop vegetables.
2. Cook mushrooms until slightly brown in vegetable oil-sprayed skillet over medium-high heat.
3. Add scallions, peppers and broccoli and cook 1 minute on medium-high. Remove from pan.
4. Spray skillet again with vegetable oil over medium heat and add egg substitute. When eggs become firm, push with spatula along center of pan to allow uncooked eggs to flow into the center.
5. When eggs are firm enough, flip them.
6. Place cooked vegetables, cottage and cheddar cheese on half of the

cooked eggs. Fold the other half over to cover the vegetables and cheese.
7. Top with a few extra scallion pieces and Parmesan cheese. Add pepper as desired.

PASTA WITH WHITE BEAN SAUCE
(for Sunday Dinner)

Serves 4

1/2 lb of short pasta, penne or rotelli, uncooked
2 Tb olive oil
3–4 cloves of garlic, minced
1 can cannellini beans and liquid, 16 ounces
freshly ground black pepper, to taste
1 tsp crushed red pepper
1 c sweet red pepper, diced
1/4 c fresh parsley
3/4 c of freshly grated Parmesan cheese

1. Cook pasta al dente, (tender, but still has some bite) drain and set aside.
2. In a large frying pan or wok, heat the oil and cook the garlic for about 30 seconds, be careful not to brown the garlic.
3. Add the beans and liquid, and all types of peppers, cook for 1–2 minutes.
4. Add the pasta and cook for another minute, to heat the pasta throughout.
5. Add the Parmesan cheese and stir to distribute ingredients.
6. Pile in a serving bowl, top with parsley and serve at once.

LIST OF EXPERTS INTERVIEWED

The following experts were interviewed for this book. I thank them all for their time and ideas.

WOMEN'S HEALTH CARE, YOUR HEALTH CARE

Elizabeth A. Alexander, M.D., M.S., Professor and Associate Chair, Clinical Services, Michigan State University, Department of Family Practice, College of Human Medicine, and Editorial Board Member; *Marcia Angell*, M.D., executive editor, The New England Journal of Medicine; *Karen Carlson*, M.D., Assistant in Medicine, and Director, Women's Health Associates, Medical Practices Evaluation Center at Massachusetts General Hospital; *Richard M. Frankel*, Ph.D., Associate Professor of Medicine, University of Rochester School of Medicine and Dentistry, and Residency Program Co-Director, internal medicine, Highland Hospital, Rochester, NY; *Judith A. Hall*, Ph.D., Professor of Psychology, Northeastern University, Boston; *Florence P. Haseltine*, M.D., Ph.D., Director, Center for Population Research, National Institute of Child Health and Human Development, National Institutes of Health, and Senior Editor, Women's Health Journal; *Thomas S. Inui*, M.D., Professor and Chairman, Department of Ambulatory Care and Prevention, Harvard Medical School and Harvard Community Health Plan Medical School; *Irwin H. Kaiser*, M.D., Ph.D., Professor Emeritus, Albert Einstein College of Medicine; *Sherrie H. Kaplan*, Ph.D., Senior Scientist, Co-Director, Primary Care Outcomes Research Institute, New England Medical Center; *Judith H. LaRosa*, Ph.D., Clinical Professor of Public Health, Tulane University School of Public Health and Tropical Medicine, and Former Deputy Director, Office of Research on Women's Health, National Institutes of Health; *Aaron Lazare*, M.D., Chancellor/Dean, University of Massachusetts Medical Center at Worcester; *Mary B. Mahowald*, professor in the department of obgyn and in the college of U. Chicago, an assistant director at the center for clinical medical ethics, U. Chicago; *Christina Malongo*, Family Nurse Practitioner, Feminist Women's Health Center, Portland, OR; *Ian McWhinney*, M.D., Professor Emeritus, Department of Family Medicine at the University of Western Ontario, London, Ontario; *Cindy Pearson*, Program Director, National Women's Health Network, Washington, DC; *Deborah L. Roter*, Dr.P.H., Professor, Department of Health Policy and Management, Johns Hopkins School of Hygiene and Public Health; *Susan E. Skochelak*, M.D., M.P.H., Associate Professor, Department of Family Medicine, and Special Assistant to the Dean for Primary Care Affairs, University of Wisconsin Medical School at Madison; *Moira A. Stewart*, Ph.D., Professor, Department of Family Medicine, Center for Studies in Family Medicine, University of Western Ontario, London, Ontario

YOUR SKIN, HAIR AND NAIL HEALTH CHAPTER

Joseph P. Bark, M.D., Immediate Past Chairman of Dermatology, St. Joseph Hospital, Lexington, KY, and author, "Retin-A and Other Youth Miracles"; *Diana Bihova*, M.D., Clinical Assistant Professor of Dermatology at NYU Medical Center; *D'Anne M. Kleinsmith*, M.D., dermatologist in private practice, West Bloomfield, MI, and affiliated with William

Beaumont Hospital, Royal Oaks, MI; *Jerome Z. Litt*, M.D., Assistant Clinical Professor of Dermatology, Case Western Reserve University School of Medicine, and author, "Your Skin: From Acne to Zits"; *Marianne O'Donoghue*, M.D., Associate Professor of Dermatology at Rush Presbyterian St. Luke's Medical Center, Chicago; *Neil Sadick*, M.D., Assistant Clinical Professor of Dermatology, Cornell University Medical College, and attending at both NY Hospital/Cornell Medical Center and Northshore University Hospital; *Rachelle A. Scott*, M.D., Associate Professor of Clinical Dermatology, The NY Hospital/Cornell Medical Center; *Nia K. Terezakis*, M.D., dermatologist in private practice, New Orleans, LA, and Clinical Professor of Dermatology at Tulane Medical School

YOUR BONE HEALTH CHAPTER

Susan H. Allen, M.D./Ph.D., Associate Professor of Medicine, Division of Endocrinology, Diabetes and Metabolism, Department of Internal Medicine, University of Missouri School of Medicine, Columbia; *Carol Frey*, M.D., Associate Clinical Professor of Orthopedic Surgery at the University of Southern California, and Director of the Orthopedic Foot and Ankle Center, Los Angeles, CA; *Howard S. Glazer*, DDS, President-Elect, Academy of General Dentistry, and Assistant Professor, Department of Dentistry, Albert Einstein College of Medicine; *Deborah T. Gold*, Ph.D., Assistant Professor of Psychiatry and Sociology, and Senior Fellow in the Aging Center at Duke University Medical Center; *Jo A. Hannafin*, M.D./Ph.D., Attending Orthopedic Surgeon, Hospital for Special Surgery, NY; *Paul J. Hirsch*, M.D., Chairman, Committee on Public Education, American Academy of Orthopedic Surgeons, and Clinical Associate Professor at New Jersey Medical School in Newark, NJ; *C. Conrad Johnston*, Jr., M.D., Professor of Medicine, and Former Director of the Division of Endocrinology and Metabolism in the Department of Medicine, Indiana University School of Medicine; *Betsy Love*, R.N., M.N., Associate Director for the Center for Metabolic Bone Disorders at Providence Medical Center, Portland, OR; *Gregory R. Mundy*, M.D., Chief, Division of Endocrinology and Metabolism in the Department of Medicine, and Professor of Medicine, University of Texas Health Science Center at San Antonio; *William J. Robb, III*, M.D., Senior Attending, Evanston/Glenbrook Hospitals, Clinical Instructor, Northwestern University Medical School, and President, Illinois Orthopedic Society; *Barbara J. Steinberg*, D.D.S., Professor of Dental Medicine, Medical College of Pennsylvania, and Clinical Associate Professor of Oral Medicine, University of Pennsylvania School of Dental Medicine; *John D. Termine*, Ph.D., Eli Lilly and Co., executive director of Lilly Research Laboratories; *Eboo Versi*, M.D., Ph.D., Chief of Urogynecology, Brigham and Women's Hospital in Boston, and Associate Professor of Obstetrics and Gynecology and Reproductive Biology at Harvard Medical School

EXERCISE CHAPTER

Bonnie G. Berger, Ed.D., Associate Dean, College of Health Sciences, University of Wyoming, Laramie; *Cedric X. Bryant*, Ph.D., Associate Director of Sports Medicine, StairMaster Sports/Medical Products, Inc.; *Barbara L. Drinkwater*, Ph.D., Research Physiologist, Department of Medicine, Pacific Medical Center, Seattle, WA; *Kimberly M. Fagan*, M.D., Director of Medical Aspects of Sports Medicine , U. of Alabama, Birmingham; *Larry W. Gibbons*, M.D., M.P.H., President and Medical Director, Cooper Clinic at the Cooper Aerobics Center, Dallas, TX; *Abby C. King*, Ph.D., Clinical Psychologist, Assistant Professor of Health Research and Policy, Stanford Center for Research in Disease Prevention, Stanford

University School of Medicine; *Diana I. McNab*, M. Ed., Adjunct Professor and Sports Psychologist, Seton Hall University; *Marcia G. Ory*, Ph.D., M.P.H., Medical Sociologist in Health and Illness, National Institute on Aging, National Institutes of Health; *Carol L. Otis*, M.D., Director, Specialty Clinics at U.C.L.A. Student Health Services; Chairperson, Ad Hoc Task Force on Women's Issues in Sports Medicine, American College of Sports Medicine; *Mary L. O'Toole*, cross list with heart disease; *Mona M. Shangold*, M.D., Professor of Obstetrics and Gynecology, Hahnemann University, Philadelphia; *Christine L. Wells*, Ph.D., Professor of Exercise Science and Physical Education, Arizona State University

NUTRITION CHAPTER

Jeffrey B. Blumberg, Ph.D., Associate Director and Professor, U.S.D.A. Human Nutrition Research Center on Aging, Tufts University; *Rowan Chlebowski*, M.D./Ph.D., Chair of the Cancer Prevention and Control Committee, American Society for Clinical Oncology, and Professor of Medicine, at UCLA School of Medicine, and Harbor-UCLA Medical Center; *Carolyn K. Clifford*, Ph.D., Chief, Diet and Cancer Branch, National Cancer Institute, National Institutes of Health; *Bess Dawson-Hughes*, M.D., Associate Professor of Medicine, Tufts University; *Johanna T. Dwyer*, D.Sc., R.D., Director, Frances Stern Nutrition Center, New England Medical Center, Professor of Medicine (Nutrition), and Professor of Community Health, Tufts University School of Medicine, and Professor of Nutrition, Tufts University School of Nutrition; *Robert P. Heaney*, M.D., John A. Creighton University Professor, and Profesor of Medicine, Creighton University, Omaha, NE; *Wahida Karmally*, M.S., R.D., Director of Nutrition, Irving Center for Clinical Research, Columbia Presbyterian Medical Center; *Barbara Levine*, Ph.D., R.D., Associate Professor of Nutrition in Medicine, Cornell University Medical College, Adjunct Faculty Member, Rockefeller University, Research Coordinator, Clinical Nutrition Research Unit, NY Hospital/Cornell Medical Center, Director, Strang Cancer Prevention Center, and Director, Calcium Information Center, Cornell University Medical Center; *Bonnie Liebman*, M.S., Director of Nutrition, Center for Science in the Public Interest; *Bettye J. Nowlin*, R.D., Manager, Public Affairs, Dairy Council of California; *Michael W. Pariza*, Ph.D., Director, Food Research Institute, Chair, Department of Food Microbiology and Toxicology, and Wisconsin Distinguished Professor, University of Wisconsin, Madison; *Richard S. Rivlin*, M.D., Program Director, Clinical Nutrition Research Unit, Memorial Sloane-Kettering Cancer Center; Chief, Nutrition Division, and Professor of Medicine, The New York Hospital/Cornell Medical Center; *Mona R. Sutnick*, R.D., Ed.D., spokesperson, American Dietetic Association; *Lee W. Wattenberg*, M.D., Professor of Laboratory Medicine and Pathology, University of Minnesota, and Member, Original National Research Council Group on Diet and Cancer; *Jacqueline Whitted*, Ph.D., Public Health Analyst, Division of Cancer Prevention and Control, National Cancer Institute, National Institutes of Health; *Walter C. Willett*, M.D., M.P.H., Dr.P.H., Chair, Department of Nutrition, and Fredrick Stare Professor of Epidemiology and Nutrition, Harvard School of Public Health, and Professor of Medicine, Harvard Medical School; *Kathleen Zelman*, M.P.H., R.D., Nutritionist in Private Practice, Atlanta, GA, and Spokesperson, American Dietetic Association

WEIGHT LOSS, WEIGHT MAINTENANCE CHAPTER

Reubin Andres, M.D., Clinical Director, National Institute on Aging, National Institutes of Health; *Diane F. Birt*, Ph.D., Professor of Biochemistry and Molecular Biology, University of

Nebraska Medical Center, and Professor, The Eppley Institute for Research in Cancer and Allied Diseases; *George L. Blackburn*, M.D./Ph.D., Associate Professor of Surgery, Harvard Medical School, and Chief, Nutrition/Metabolism Laboratory, The Deaconess Hospital, Boston; *C. Wayne Callaway*, M.D., Associate Clinical Professor of Medicine, George Washington University, former director, Center for Clinical Nutrition, George Washington University Medical Center, member, U.S.D.A./H.H.S. 1990 Dietary Guidelines Advisory Committee, and Chair, American Dietetic Association Dietary Recommendations for Women, 1986; *Susan Nitzke*, Ph.D., R.D., Associate Professor of Nutritional Sciences, University of Wisconsin-Madison, and University of Wisconsin-Extension; *Albert J. Stunkard*, M.D., Professor Emeritus of Psychiatry, University of Pennsylvania; *Theodore B. VanItallie*, Professor Emeritus of Medicine, Columbia University College of Physicians and Surgeons, and Founder, The Obesity Research Center, St. Luke's-Roosevelt Hospital; *Rena Wing*, Ph.D., Professor of Psychiatry, Psychology and Epidemiology, and Director, Obesity/Nutrition Research Center, University of Pittsburgh School of Medicine, Western Psychiatric Institute and Clinic

EATING DISORDERS CHAPTER

Susan J. Bartlett, M. Ed., Intern in Psychology, Friends Hospital, Philadelphia, and Consultant, Weight and Eating Disorders Program, University of Pennsylvania School of Medicine; *Simone A. French*, Research Associate in Epidemiology, division of epidemiology in the school of public health, U. Minnesota; *Paula Levine*, Ph.D., Director, The Agoraphobia Resource Center and The Anorexia and Bulimia Resource Center, and Psychologist in private practice, Coral Gables, FL; *Marsha D. Marcus*, Ph.D., Assistant Professor of Psychiatry and Psychology, University of Pittsburgh School of Medicine, and Director, Outpatient Eating Disorders Clinic and Partial Hospitalization Program, Western Psychiatric Institute and Clinic; *Michael Pertchuck*, M.D., Clinical Associate Professor of Psychiatry, University of Pennsylvania, and Medical Director, Eating Disorders Clinic, Friends Hospital, Philadelphia; *Kathleen M. Pike*, Ph.D., Assistant Professor of Clinical Psychology, and Chief Psychologist, Eating Disorders Unit, NY State Psychiatric Institute, Columbia Presbyterian Medical Center; *Robert L. Spitzer*, M.D., Professor of Psychiatry, Columbia University College of Physicians and Surgeons, and Chief, Biometrics Research Department, NY State Psychiatric Institute; *Ruth Striegel-Moore*, Ph.D., President-Elect, Academy for Eating Disorders, NY, and Associate Professor of Psychology, Wesleyan University

SUBSTANCE USE AND ABUSE CHAPTER

Sheila B. Blume, M.D., Medical Director, Alcoholism, Chemical Dependency and Compulsive Gambling Programs, South Oaks Hospital, Amityville, NY; Clinical Professor of Psychiatry, SUNY Stonybrook, Board Member and Past President, American Society of Addiction Medicine; *Alan J. Budney*, Ph.D., Assistant Professor, Department of Psychiatry and Psychology, University of Vermont, Burlington; *Ronald M. Davis*, M.D., Chief Medical Officer, Michigan Department of Public Health, Lansing, and Former Director, Office on Smoking and Health, Centers for Disease Control and Prevention; *Virginia L. Ernster*, Ph.D., Professor and Former Chair, Department of Epidemiology and Biostatistics, U.C.S.F. School of Medicine; *Michael C. Fiore*, M.D., Director, Center for Tobacco Research and Intervention, and Associate Professor, Department of Medicine, University of Wisconsin-Madison; *Anne Geller*, M.D., Chief, The Smithers Alcoholism, Treatment and Training Center, St. Luke's-

Roosevelt Hospital Center, and Associate Professor of Clinical Medicine, Columbia College of Physicians and Surgeons; *Ellen R. Gritz*, Ph.D., Professor and Chair, Department of Behavioral Science, University of Texas M.D. Anderson Cancer Center, Houston; *Corinne G. Husten*, M.D., M.P.H., Medical Officer, Office on Smoking and Health, National Center for Chronic Disease Prevention and Health Promotion, Centers for Disease Control and Prevention; *Robert B. Millman*, M.D., Saul P. Steinberg Distinguished Professor of Psychiatry and Public Health at Cornell University Medical College, and Director, Drug and Alcohol Abuse Programs, New York Hospital/Payne Whitney Clinic; *Barbara A. Morse*, Ph.D., Director, Fetal Alcohol Education Program, and Assistant Research Professor of Psychiatry, Boston University School of Medicine; *Judith K. Ockene*, Ph.D., Professor of Medicine and Director, Division of Preventive and Behavioral Medicine, University of Massachusetts Medical School, Worcester

FIGHTING CANCERS IN WOMEN CHAPTER

Susan M. Ascher, M.D., Assistant Professor of Radiology and Associate Director of Body M.R.I., Georgetown University Hospital; *Rachel Ballard-Barbash*, M.D., M.P.H., Research Epidemiologist, Applied Research Branch, Division of Cancer Prevention and Control, National Cancer Institute; *Richard R. Barakat*, M.D., Assistant Attending Surgeon, Memorial Sloane Kettering Hospital; *Arthur E. Baue*, M.D., Professor of Surgery and Former Vice President, St. Louis University Health Science Center, Medical Center; *Wendie A. Berg*, M.D./Ph.D., Assistant Professor of Radiology, Johns Hopkins School of Medicine; *Bernard Chang*, M.D., Assistant Professor, Division of Plastic, Reconstructive and Maxillofacial Surgery at Johns Hopkins Hospital; *Graham A. Colditz*, M.B.B.S., M.P.H., Dr.P.H., Associate Professor, Department of Epidemiology, Harvard School of Public Health, and Associate Professor of Medicine, Harvard Medical School; *Mary E. Costanza*, M.D., Professor of Medicine, Department of Hematology/Oncology, University of Massachusetts Medical Center at Worcester; *Anne Coscarelli*, Ph.D., Director, The Rhonda Fleming Mann Resource Center for Women with Cancer (U.C.L.A.); *Mary B. Daly*, M.D./Ph.D., Associate Director, Cancer Control Science Program, and Director, Margaret Dyson Family Risk Assessment Program, Fox Chase Cancer Center, Philadelphia, PA; *Eugene R. DeSombre*, Ph.D., Professor, Ben May Institute, University of Chicago; *Patricia J. Eifel*, M.D., Associate Professor of Radiotherapy, University of Texas M.D. Anderson Cancer Center, Houston, TX; *Fawzy I. Fawzy*, M.D., Professor and Deputy Chair, Department of Psychiatry and Biobehavioral Sciences, and Deputy Director, Neuropsychiatric Hospital, U.C.L.A.; *Arthur C. Fleischer*, M.D., Professor of Radiology and Radiological Sciences, Professor of Obstetrics and Gynecology, and Chief, Diagnostic Sonography, Vanderbilt University Medical Center; *Kathleen M. Foley*, M.D., Professor of Neurology, Neuroscience and Clinical Pharmacology, Cornell University School of Medicine, and Chief of the Pain Service, Department of Neurology, Memorial Sloane Kettering Cancer Center, New York; *Matthew T. Freedman*, M.D., Associate Professor of Radiology and Director of Resident Education, Georgetown University Medical School; *Lori Goldstein*, M.D., Director, Breast Evaluation Center, and Associate Member, Fox Chase Cancer Center; *Saul B. Gusberg*, M.D., Past President, American Cancer Society, and Distinguished Service Professor Emeritus, Mt. Sinai School of Medicine of C.U.N.Y; *Brian E. Henderson*, M.D., President, Salk Institute, La Jolla, CA., and Distinguished Adjunct Professor, U.S.C. School of Medicine; *Maureen M. Henderson*, M.D., Head, Cancer Prevention Research Program, Fred Hutchinson Cancer Research Center, and Professor of Epidemiology and Medicine, University of Washington, Seattle; *Jimmie C. Holland*, M.D., Professor of Psychiatry, Cornell University Medical College, and Chief of the

Psychiatry Service, Memorial Sloane Kettering Cancer Center, NY; *Anna Lee-Feldstein*, Ph.D., Assistant Professor, Department of Medicine, U.C. Irvine; *Wende W. Logan-Young*, M.D., Director, Elizabeth Wende Breast Clinic, Rochester, NY; *Mary H. McGrath*, M.D., M.P.H., Professor of Surgery and Chief, Division of Plastic and Reconstructive Surgery, George Washington University Medical Center; *Beth E. Meyerowitz*, Ph.D., Associate Professor and Director, Clinical Psychology, University of Southern California, Los Angeles; *Barbara S. Monsees*, M.D., Associate Professor of Radiology, and Chief, Breast Imaging Section, Mallinkrodt Institute of Radiology, Washington University School of Medicine, St. Louis, MO; *Monica Morrow*, M.D., Associate Professor of Surgery, and Director, Lynn Sage Comprehensive Breast Center, Northwestern University School of Medicine; *Funmi Olopade*, M.D., Assistant Professor of Medicine, and Director, Cancer Risk Clinic, University of Chicago Medical School; *C. Kent Osborne*, M.D., Professor of Medicine, and Interim Chief of Medical Oncology, University of Texas Health Science Center, San Antonio; *Robert F. Ozols*, M.D./Ph.D., Professor of Medicine, Temple University, and Senior Vice President of Medical Science, Fox Chase Cancer Center, Philadelphia; *M. Steven Piver*, M.D., Chief, Department of Gynecologic Oncology, and Director, The Gilda Radner Familial Ovarian Cancer Registry, Roswell Park Cancer Institute, Buffalo, NY; *Julia Rowland*, Ph.D., Co-Director, Psych-Oncology Program, and Staff Psychologist, Department of Psychiatry, Georgetown University Medical School; *Mace L. Rothenberg*, M.D., Assistant Professor of Medicine, University of Texas Health Science Center, and Executive Officer, Southwest Oncology Group, San Antonio, TX; *Carolyn D. Runowicz*, M.D., Associate Professor and Director, Division of Gynecologic Oncology, Albert Einstein College of Medicine and Montefiore Medical Center; *Ruby T. Senie*, Ph.D., Associate Attending Epidemiologist, Breast Service, Department of Surgery, Memorial Sloane Kettering Cancer Center, NY; *Richard M. Silver*, M.D., Professor of Medicine and Pediatrics, Division of Rheumatology and Immunology, Medical University of South Carolina in Charleston; *Elin R. Sigurdson*, M.D., Ph.D., Member, Department of Surgical Oncology, Fox Chase Cancer Center, and Associate Professor of Surgery, Temple University, Phildelphia; *Michael J. Thun*, M.D., Director, Analytical Epidemiology, American Cancer Society; *Nancy Toth*, R.N., B.S.N., Coordinator, The Breast Care Center, Hershey Medical Center; *Max Wicha*, M.D., Director, The University of Michigan Comprehensive Cancer Center, and Professor of Medicine, University of Michigan; *Stephanie F. Williams*, M.D., Associate Professor of Medicine, Section of Hematology/Oncology, and Co-Director, Bone Marrow Transplant Program, University of Chicago Medical Center; *William C. Wood*, M.D., Joseph Brown Whitehead Professor and Chairman, Department of Surgery, Emory University School of Medicine; *Robert C. Young*, M.D., President, Fox Chase Cancer Center, Phildelphia; *Rebecca A. Zuurbier*, M.D., Director, Breast Imaging, and Assistant Professor of Radiotherapy, Georgetown University Medical Center

YOUR GYNECOLOGICAL HEALTH CHAPTER

G. David Adamson, M.D., Associate Professor of Reproductive Endocrinology, Stanford University School of Medicine; *Mary Lou Ballweg*, President and Executive Director, Endometriosis Association; *Tamara G. Bavendam*, M.D., Director, Female Urology, and Assistant Professor of Urology, University of Washington School of Medicine, Seattle; *Kathryn L. Burgio*, Ph.D., Director, the University of Alabama Continence Program, and Associate Professor of Medicine, Division of Gerontology and Geriatric Medicine, University of Alabama at Birmingham; *David S. Chapin*, M.D., Senior Obstetrician and Gynecologist,

Beth Israel Hospital, Boston; *Nora Coffey*, President, Hysterectomy Educational Resources and Services, Bala Cynwyd, PA; *J. Andrew Fantl*, M.D., Professor of Obstetrics and Gynecology, and Director, Benign Gynecology and the Continence Program for Women, Medical College of Virginia, Virginia Commonwealth University; *Bruce L. Flamm*, M.D., Area Research Chairman, Kaiser Permanente Medical Center, Riverside, CA, and Associate Clinical Professor, U.C. Irvine Medical School; *Cheryle B. Gartley*, President and Founder, Simon Foundation for Continence; *Eileen Hilton*, M.D., Infectious Disease Consultant, Associate Professor of Medicine, and Director, Lyme Disease Center, Albert Einstein College of Medicine; *Connie A. Jackson*, M.D., Staff Obstetrican/Gynecologist, Beth Isreal Hospital, Boston, Clinical Instructor, Obstetrics and Gynecology, Harvard Medical School, and Attending Physician, Southborough Medical Group, Southborough, MA; *Robert G. Lahita*, M.D./Ph.D., Chief, Division of Rheumatology and Connective Tissue Diseases, St. Luke's-Roosevelt Hospital, NY, and Chairman, Board of Directors, Lupus Foundation of America, and Associate Professor, Department of Medicine, Columbia University College of Physicians and Surgeons; *John W. Larsen*, M.D., Director, Wilson Genetic Center, Acting Chairman, Obstetrics and Gynecology, and Professor of Obstetrics and Gynecology and Genetics, George Washington University Medical Center; *Barbara S. Levy*, M.D., President, American Association of Gynecologic Laparoscopists, and Assistant Clinical Professor of Obstetrics and Gynecology, The University of Washington, Seattle; *Jane L. Marks*, R.N., Clinical Coordinator, Comprehensive Continence Program, Johns Hopkins Geriatric Center; *David L. Olive*, M.D., Chief, Section on Reproductive Endocrinology, Department of Obstetrics and Gynecology, Yale University School of Medicine; *Margaret R. Punch*, M.D., Assistant Professor, Department of Obstetrics and Gynecology, University of Michigan Medical Center, Ann Arbor; *Vicki C. Ratner*, M.D., President, Interstitial Cystitis Association; *Neil M. Resnick*, M.D., Chief, Division of Gerontology, Brigham and Women's Hospital, Boston, and Associate Professor of Medicine, Harvard University Medical School; *David H. Sherman*, M.D., Assistant Clinical Professor of Obstetrics and Gynecology, Mt. Sinai School of Medicine, NY; *Deborah Slade*, M.A., Executive Director, Interstitial Cystitis Association; *Sara E. Walker*, M.D., Professor of Internal Medicine, Division of Immunology and Rheumatology, University of Missouri-Columbia, and Chief, Rheumatology at Harry S. Truman Memorial Veterans' Hospital

YOUR BREAST HEALTH CHAPTER

Stephen A. Feig, M.D., Professor of Radiology, Jefferson Medical College, and Director of the Breast Imaging Center, Thomas Jefferson University Hospital, Philadelphia, PA; *Suzanne W. Fletcher*, M.D., M.Sc., Professor of Ambulatory Care and Prevention, Harvard Medical School; *Diane L. Gerber*, M.D., Plastic and Reconstructive Surgeon, Flossmoor, IL; *Roxanne J. Guy*, M.D., Plastic and Reconstructive Surgeon, Attending Physician, Holmes Regional Medical Center, Melbourne, FL; *Mary Jane Houlihan*, M.D., Surgical Oncologist, Beth Israel BreastCare Center, and Instructor, Harvard Medical School; *Daniel B. Kopans*, M.D., Director of Breast Imaging, Massachusetts General Hospital, and Associate Professor of Radiology, Harvard Medical School; *Marc E. Lippman*, M.D., Physician/Scientist, Director, Lombardi Cancer Center, Georgetown University Medical Center; *Susan M. Love*, M.D., Director, U.C.L.A. Breast Center, and Associate Professor of Clinical Surgery, U.C.L.A. School of Medicine; *Debra L. Monticciolo*, M.D., Director, Division of Breast Imaging, Emory Clinic, and Assistant Professor, Department of Radiology, Emory University School of Medicine; *Richard H. Patt*, M.D., Chief, Magnetic Resonance Imaging Section, and Director,

Body Magnetic Resonance Imaging Section, Georgetown University Medical School; *Henry S. Pennypacker*, Ph.D., President, Mammatech Corporation, and Professor of Psychology, University of Florida, Gainesville; *Petra R. Schneider*, M.D., Plastic and Reconstructive Surgeon, Attending Physician, Holmes Regional Medical Center, Melbourne, FL; *Yvonne S. Thornton*, M.D., Director, Perinatal Diagnostic Testing, Morristown Memorial Hospital, NJ; *Linda J. Warren*, M.D., Executive Director, Screening Mammography Program, British Columbia (Canada), and Clinical Professor, Department of Radiology, University of British Columbia, Vancouver, Canada

MENSTRUAL HEALTH CHAPTER

Jay L. Daskal, M.D., Vice Chairman, Obstetrics and Gynecology Department, Illinois Masonic Medical Center, and Clinical Associate Professor of Obstetrics and Gynecology, University of Illinois College of Medicine; *Charles H. Debrovner*, M.D., Associate Professor of Obstetrics and Gynecology, New York University and Roosevelt Hospital, and Attending Physician, Beth Israel North, NY; *Jill M. Rabin*, M.D., Chief, Ambulatory and Urogynecologic Care, Department of Obstetrics and Gynecology, Long Island Jewish Medical Center, New Hyde Park, NY, and Assistant Professor of Obstetrics and Gynecology, Albert Einstein College of Medicine; *Michelle P. Warren*, M.D., Head of Reproductive Endocrinology, St. Luke's-Roosevelt Hospital, NY, and Associate Professor of Obstetrics and Gynecology and Clinical Medicine, Columbia College of Physicians and Surgeons

PREMENSTRUAL SYNDROME CHAPTER

Stephanie DeGraff Bender, M.A., Director, PMS Clinic, Boulder, CO; *Jean Endicott*, Ph.D., Professor of Clinical Psychology, Department of Psychiatry, College of Physicians and Surgeons, Columbia University, and Chief, Department of Research Assessment and Training, NY State Psychiatric Institute, and Director, Premenstrual Evaluation Unit, Columbia Presbyterian Medical Center; *Michelle Harrison*, M.D., Director, Medical Affairs, Johnson & Johnson Worldwide Absorbant Products and Materials Research, and Clinical Associate Professor of Family Medicine, Robert Wood Johnson Medical School/UMDNJ; *Jane A. Harrison-Hohner*, M.S.N., R.N.P., R.N.D., Director of the Menstrual Disorders Program, and Assistant Professor, School of Nursing, Oregon Health Sciences University; *Joseph F. Mortola*, M.D., Director, Division of Reproductive Endocrinology, Beth Israel Hospital, Boston, and Associate Professor of Psychiatry, Obstetrics and Gynecology and Reproductive Biology, Harvard Medical School; *Ana Rivera-Tovar*, Ph.D., clinical psychologist and director of the P.M.S. program at Western Psychiatric Institute and clinic

MENOPAUSAL HEALTH CHAPTER

John C. Arpels, M.D., Founding Member, North American Menopause Society, and Associate Clinical Professor, Department of Obstetrics and Gynecology, UCSF Medical Center School of Medicine; *Steven Austad*, Ph.D., Associate Professor of Zoology, University of Idaho, and Affiliate Associate Professor, Department of Pathology, University of Washington; *Lonnie Barbach*, Ph.D., Psychologist, Clinical Faculty, UCSF Medical School, author of "The Pause: Positive Approaches to Menopause" and "For Yourself"; *Elizabeth Barrett-Connor*, M.D., Professor and Chair, Department of Family and Preventive Medicine, U.C.S.D.; *Laura D. Bookman*, Director, Menopause Wellness Center, Beth Israel Hospital, Boston; *Vivien K. Burt*,

M.D./Ph.D., Director, U.C.L.A. Neuropsychiatric Institute/Women's Life Center; *Janice Green Douglas*, M.D., Director, Division of Hypertension, and Professor of Medicine, and Physiology, & Biophysics, Case Western Reserve University School of Medicine, Cleveland; *J.C. Gallagher*, M.D., Professor of Medicine, Department of Bone Metabolism, Creighton University School of Medicine; *Patricia A. Ganz*, M.D., Director, Division of Cancer Prevention and Control Research, and Professor, Schools of Medicine and Public Health, U.C.L.A.; *Judith S. Gavaler*, Ph.D., Chief, Department of Women's Health Research, Oklahoma Medical Research Foundation; *Deborah Grady*, M.D., M.P.H., Associate Professor of Medicine, Epidemiology and Biostatistics, U.C.S.F. School of Medicine, and Director, Women Veterans' Comprehensive Health Center, San Francisco Veterans Affairs Medical Center; *Dr. Kathleen Hutchinson*, Assistant Clinical Professor, Yale University School of Medicine; *Howard L. Judd*, M.D., Chairman, Department of Obstetrics and Gynecology, Oliveview-UCLA Medical Center, and Professor, Obstetrics and Gynecology, UCLA School of Medicine; *Patricia A. Kaufert*, Ph.D., Professor of Community Health Sciences, University of Manitoba, Canada; *Bruce Kessel*, M.D., Director, Menopause Research, Beth Israel Hospital, and Assistant Professor of Obstetrics, Gynecology and Reproductive Biology, Harvard Medical School; *Fredi Kronenberg*, Ph.D., Director, Richard and Hinda Rosenthal Center for Alternative/Complementary Medicine, and Associate Professor of Physiology in Rehabilitation Medicine, Columbia College of Physicians and Surgeons; *Margaret Lock*, Ph.D., Professor of Medical Anthropology, McGill University, Montreal, Canada; *Marjorie M. Luckey*, M.D., Co-Director, The Osteoporosis and Metabolic Bone Disorders Program, and Assistant Professor, Department of Obstetrics, Gynecology and Reproductive Science, Mt. Sinai Medical Center, NY; *Kathleen I. MacPherson*, R.N./Ph.D., Professor in Women's Studies and in the School of Nursing, University of Southern Maine, Portland; *Bruce S. McEwen*, Ph.D., Professor and Head, Laboratory of Neuroendocrinology, Rockefeller University, New York; *Sonja M. McKinlay*, Ph.D., President, New England Research Institutes, Watertown, MA; *Diane E. Meier*, M.D., Co-Director, The Osteoporosis and Metabolic Bone Disorders Program, Associate Professor, Department of Geriatrics and Adult Development, and Associate Professor, Department of Medicine, Mt. Sinai Medical Center, NY; *Richard D. Moss*, M.D., Associate Clinical Professor, Department of Obstetrics, Gynecology and Reproductive Science, Mt. Sinai School of Medicine; *Frederick Naftolin*, M.D., Director, Yale University Center for Research on Reproductive Biology, Chief, Obstetrics and Gynecology, Yale-New Haven Hospital, and Chairman, Obstetrics and Gynecology, Yale University School of Medicine; *Veronica A. Ravnikar*, M.D., Professor of Obstetrics and Gynecology, and Director, Reproductive Endocrinology, Infertility and Menopause, University of Massachusetts Medical Center at Worcester; *Marilyn L. Rothert*, Ph.D., R.N., Acting Dean, The College of Nursing, and Professor, Michigan State University, East Lansing; *Joan L.F. Shaver*, Ph.D., R.N., Professor and Chair, Department of Physiological Nursing, University of Washington, Seattle; *Barbara B. Sherwin*, Ph.D., Professor, Department of Psychology, and Professor, Department of Obstetrics and Gynecology, McGill University, Montreal, Canada; *Dominique C. Toran-Allerand*, M.D., Professor of Anatomy and Cell Biology, Center for Neurobiology and Behavior, and Center for Reproductive Sciences, Columbia University College of Physicians and Surgeons, NY; *Wulf H. Utian*, M.D./Ph.D., Honorary Founding President and Executive Director, North American Menopause Society, Professor and Chairman, Reproductive Biology, Case Western Reserve University, and Director, Department of Obstetrics and Gynecology, University Hospitals of Cleveland; *Robert A. Wild*, M.D., Professor and Chief, Section of Research and Education in Women's Health, Department of Obstetrics and Gynecology, and Adjunct Professor of Medicine (Cardiology), Oklahoma University Health Sciences Center; *Nancy Fugate Woods*, Ph.D., R.N., Director, Center for Women's Health Research, and Professor, University of Washington, Seattle

PREGNANCY AND DELIVERY CHAPTER

Raul Artal, M.D., Professor and Chair, Department of Obstetrics and Gynecology, SUNY Health Science Center at Syracuse, primary author, American College of Obstetrics and Gynecology guidelines on exercise and pregnancy; *Richard H. Aubry*, M.D., M.P.H., Director of Obstetrics, and Professor of Obstetrics and Gynecology, SUNY Health Science Center, Syracuse, NY; *Marcia Biel*, Ph.D., Psychologist in Private Practice, on boards of Postpartum Support International and Adjustments after Delivery, Kansas City, MO; *Constance J. Bohon*, M.D., Chief of Gynecology, Columbia Hospital for Women, and private practitioner, Women Physicians Associates, Washington, DC; *Robert C. Cefalo*, M.D./Ph.D., Director, Maternal Fetal Division, and Professor, Department of Obstetrics and Gynecology, University of North Carolina School of Medicine; *James F. Clapp, III*, M.D., Director of Research, Department of Obstetrics and Gynecology, MetroHealth Medical Center, and Professor of Reproductive Biology, Case Western Reserve University; *Diane D. Courney*, M.S.N., R.N.C., O.G.N.P., Assistant Professor, University of Texas Health Science Center at San Antonio School of Nursing; *Donald R. Coustan*, M.D., Chief, Department of Obstetrics and Gynecology, Women and Infants' Hospital at Brown University, and Chairman, Department of Obstetrics and Gynecology, Brown University School of Medicine; *Warren M. Crosby*, M.D., Clinical Professor of Obstetrics and Gynecology, University of Oklahoma Health Science Center; *Julia K. Dennis*, L.C.S.W., Social Worker in Private Practice, and Founder, Memphis area Depression After Delivery Support Group; *Ann L. Dunnewold*, Ph.D., licenced psychologist, President-Elect, Postpartum Support International; *Sherman Elias*, M.D., Professor, Department of Obstetrics and Gynecology, and Professor, Department of Molecular and Human Genetics in the Division of Reproductive Genetics, Baylor College of Medicine; *Palmer C. Evans*, M.D., Chairman, Tuscon Medical Center Foundation, and in practice at Ironwood Medical Associates; *Mary Anna Friederich*, M.D., obstetrician/gynecologist at Maricopa Medical Center, AZ; *Raphael S. Good*, M.D., Clinical Professor of Psychiatry and Obstetrics, University of Miami School of Medicine; *Barbara Hughes*, C.N.M., M.S., Clinical Director of Nurse Midwifery Practice at University Hopsital, Denver, CO; *Richard B. Johnston, Jr.*, M.D., Medical Director, March of Dimes Birth Defects Foundation; Chief, Section of Immunology, and Adjunct Professor of Pediatrics, Yale University School of Medicine; *Polly Russell Kornblith*, Ed. M., Co-Founder, Massachusetts Depression After Delivery; *Minda S. Lazarov*, M.D., R.D., Research Associate, Vanderbilt University School of Nursing, and Coordinator, Baby Friendly Hospital Initiative, U.S. Committee for Unicef/World Health Organization; *Richard L. Lowensohn*, M.D., Chief of Obstetrics, and Associate Professor, Oregon Health Sciences University; *Teresa Marsico*, C.N.M., President, American College of Nurse-Midwives; *Deborah McCarter*, R.N., B.S.N., Clinical Nurse 4, International Board Certified Lactation Consultant, Certified Childbirth Educator, Beth Israel Hospital; *Jill Blum Millis*, M.S.W., L.I.C.S.W., Clinical Social Worker in Private Practice, West Newton, MA; *Joyce A. Nettleton*, D.Sc., R.D., Director of Science Communications, Institute of Food Technologists; *Jennifer R. Niebyl*, M.D., Professor and Head, Department of Obstetrics and Gynecology, University of Iowa College of Medicine; *Mary Frances Picciano*, Ph.D., Professor of Nutrition, Department of Nutrition, Penn State University; *Fay O. Redwine*, M.D., M.S., Director, Perinatal Center, St. Mary's Hospital, Richmond, VA; *Bruce D. Shephard*, M.D., Clinical Associate Professor of Obstetrics and Gynecology, University of South Florida School of Medicine; *Joe Leigh Simpson*, M.D., Ernst W. Bertner Chairman, Department of Obstetrics and Gynecology, and Professor, Department of Molecular and Human Genetics, Baylor College of Medicine; *Robert Sokol*, M.D., Dean, School of Medicine, Wayne State University; *Gwendolyn V. Spears*, C.N.M., M.S.N., Director, Nurse-Midwifery Education Program, Charles R. Drew University of Medicine and Science, and Chief, Nurse-Midwifery, King/Drew Medical Center, Los Angeles

INFERTILITY CAUSES AND TREATMENT CHAPTER

Sandra Allenson, R.N.C., Certified in Infertility and Reproductive Endocrinology Nursing, and Coordinator, Northern Nevada Fertility Center, Reno; *Arnold Belker*, M.D., Clinical Professor of Surgery, Division of Urology, University of Louisville School of Medicine, KY; *Sidney Bundy*, M.A., licensed marriage and family therapist, psychotherapist; *Linda Hammer Burns*, Ph.D., Assistant Professor, University of Minnesota Department of Obstetrics and Gynecology, Psychologist Specializing in Infertility; *Maria Bustillo*, M.D., Director, Assisted Reproductive Technology, Mt. Sinai Hospital NY, and Immediate Past President, Society for Assisted Reproductive Technology; *Michael P. Diamond*, M.D., Director, Reproductive Endocrinology, Hutzel Hospital, Detroit; *Barbara E. Eck*, B.S.N., M.S.N., M.P.H., author, Infertility: A Guide for the Childless Couple; *Kathryn J. Go*, Ph.D., Laboratory Director, Pennsylvania Reproductive Associates, and Laboratory Director, IVF and GIFT programs, Pennsylvania Hospital, Philadelphia; *Alvin F. Goldfarb*, M.D., Professor of Obstetrics and Gynecology, Jefferson Medical College, and Director, the North American Society for Pediatric and Adolescent Gynecology; *Dorothy Greenfeld*, M.S.W., C.I.S.W., Director of Psychological Services, Yale Center for Reproductive Medicine, and Clinical Instructor in Obstetrics and Gynecology, Yale University School of Medicine; *George P. Henry*, M.D., President and Director, Reproductive Genetics Center and Reproductive Genetics In Vitro, Denver, CO; *Victor K. Knutzen*, M.D., Medical Director, Northern Nevada Fertility Center, and Associate Professor, University of Nevada-Reno Medical School, and President-Elect, Society for Assisted Reproductive Technology; *Virginia S. Lang*, Professor, Chief, Department of Obstetrics and Gynecology, The Jewish Hospital of St. Louis, Division of Reproductive Endocrinology, Washington University School of Medicine; *L. Russell Malinak*, M.D., Professor, Vice Chairman for Clinical Affairs, and Director, Residency Program, Baylor College of Medicine, Houston, TX; *Deborah L. Manzi*, M.D., Director, Reproductive Endocrinology and Infertility Division, and Assistant Professor of Obstetrics and Gynecology, Creighton Women's Health Center, Creighton University Medical Center, Omaha, NE; *Christopher R. Newton*, Ph.D., Clinical Psychologist, University Hospital, London, Ontario; *Miles J. Novy*, M.D., Scientist in Reproductive Sciences, Oregon Regional Primate Research Center, and Professor of Obstetrics and Gynecology, Oregon Health Sciences University; *Mary Lake Polan*, M.D./Ph.D., Professor and Chairman, Department of Gynecology and Obstetrics, Stanford University School of Medicine; *Miriam B. Rosenthal*, M.D., Division Chief, Behavioral Medicine, Department of Obstetrics and Gynecology, University MacDonald Women's Hospital, University Hospitals of Cleveland, and Associate Professor of Psychiatry and Reproductive Biology, Case Western Reserve University School of Medicine; *Zev Rosenwaks*, M.D., Director, The Center for Reproductive Medicine and Infertility, and Professor, Obstetrics and Gynecology, Cornell University Medical College and The NY Hospital/Cornell Medical Center; *Kaylen M. Silverberg*, M.D., Clinical Assistant Professor, Department of Obstetrics and Gynecology, Division of Reproductive Endocrinology and Infertility, University of Texas Health Science Center, San Antonio; *Ronald C. Strickler*, M.D.; *Anne Colston Wentz*, M.D., Special Assistant, Contraceptive Development Branch, National Institute of Child Health and Human Development, National Institutes of Health, and Former President, Society for Assisted Reproductive Technology

ABORTION CHAPTER

E. Hakim-Elahi, M.D., Medical Director, Planned Parenthood NYC, Medical Director and Director of Obstetrics and Gynecology, Laguardia Hospital in Queens, NY; *Richard U. Hausknecht*, M.D., Associate Clinical Professor of Obstetrics and Gynecology, Mt. Sinai

School of Medicine; *Robin L. Herstand*, M.S.N., Director of Social Services, Margaret Sanger Center, Planned Parenthood of New York City; *Joan Mogal-Garrity*, independent trainer and consultant in health care issues; *William K. Rashbaum*, M.D., Associate Professor of Obstetrics and Gynecology, Albert Einstein College of Medicine, and Member, Affiliate Medical Committee, Planned Parenthood of NYC and Rockland and Westchester Counties

MENTAL HEALTH CHAPTER

William J. Apfeldorf, M.D./Ph.D., Assistant Professor of Psychiatry, Cornell University Medical College; *Paula J. Caplan*, Ph.D., Clinical and Research Psychologist, University of Toronto, and Visiting Scholar, Brown University, and author, May '95 release, "They Say You're Crazy: How the World's Most Powerful Psychiatrists Decide Who's Normal"; *Margaret A. Chesney*, Ph.D., Professor, Department of Epidemiology, School of Medicine, U.C.S.F.; *Margaret F. Jensvold*, M.D., Psychiatrist and Director, Institute for Research on Women's Health, Washington, DC; *Karen Johnson*, M.D., Clinical Scholar in Women's Health, Stanford University, and Assistant Clinical Professor of Psychiatry, University of California-San Francisco; *Marilyn G. Karmason*, M.D., Clinical Associate Professor of Psychiatry, Payne Whitney Clinic, The New York Hospital/Cornell Medical Center; *Gwendolyn Puryear Keita*, Ph.D., Associate Executive Director, Public Interest, and Director, Women's Programs, American Psychological Association; *Carol Landau*, Clinical Professor of Psychiatry and Human Behavior, Brown University School of Medicine, and Director of Psychological Services, Women's Health Associates at Rhode Island Hospital; *Hannah Lerman*, Ph.D., Psychologist in Private Practice, Specializing in Women's Issues and Feminist Therapy, Los Angeles, CA; *Ellen McGrath*, chair of the American Psychological Association national task force on women's depression, author of "When Feeling Bad is Good," executive director of the psychology center in Laguna Beach, CA; *Jean Baker Miller*, M.D., Clinical Prof. of Psychiatry, Boston University School of Medicine, and Director of Education, Stone Center for Developmental Services and Studies, Wellesley College; *Susan Nolen-Hoeksema*, Ph.D., Associate Professor of Psychology at Stanford University, and author, "Sex Differences in Depression"; *Kelley L. Phillips*, M.D., M.P.H., Policy Director, Institute for Research on Women's Health, Washington, DC, and Associate Medical Director, Empire Mental Health Choice; *Nada L. Stotland*, M.D., Associate Professor, Departments of Psychiatry and Obstetrics and Gynecology, University of Chicago, and President, Caucus of Women Psychiatrists, American Psychiatric Association; *Thomas W. Uhde*, M.D. Professor and Chairman, Department of Psychiatry and Behavioral Neurosciences, Wayne State University School of Medicine; *Aline P. Zoldbrod*, Ph.D., Licensed Psychologist and Certified Sex Therapist in private practice, Boston

SLEEP AND FATIGUE CHAPTER

Dedra S. Buchwald, M.D., Associate Professor of Medicine, University of Washington, Seattle; *Mary A. Carskadon*, Ph.D., Director of Chronobiology, E.P. Bradley Hospital, and Professor of Psychiatry and Human Behavior, Brown University School of Medicine; *Rochelle Goldberg*, M.D., Assistant Professor of Internal Medicine and Neurology, and Cardiopulmonary Clinical Director, Sleep Center, Medical College of Pennsylvania; *James Krueger*, Ph.D., Professor of Physiology, University of Tennessee, Memphis; *Alison C. Mawle*, Ph.D., Research Biologist, Division of Viral and Rickettsial Diseases, Centers for Disease Control and Prevention; *Patricia N. Prinz*, Ph.D., Professor, Department of Psychiatry and Behavioral

Sciences, and Director, Sleep and Aging Program, University of Washington, Seattle; *Susan Redline*, M.D., M.P.H., Associate Professor of Medicine, Case Western Reserve University Department of Medicine, and Co-Director, Sleep Disorders Center, Cleveland VA Medical Center; *Quentin R. Regestein*, M.D., Director, Sleep Clinic, Brigham and Women's Hospital, Boston; *Thomas Roth*, Ph.D., Chief, Division of Sleep Disorders and Research, Henry Ford Hospital, Detroit, and Clinical Professor of Psychiatry, University of Michigan School of Medicine, Ann Arbor; *W. Shain Schley*, M.D., Chairman, Department of Otorhinolaryngology, and Associate Professor of Otolaryngology, Cornell University Medical College, and Otolaryngologist-in-Chief, The New York Hospital/Cornell Medical Center; *Stephen E. Straus*, M.D., Chief, Laboratory of Clinical Investigation, National Institute of Allergy and Infectious Diseases, National Institutes of Health

HEART DISEASE, HEART HEALTH CHAPTER

Vera A. Bittner, M.D., Associate Professor of Medicine, Division of Cardiovascular Disease, University of Alabama, Birmingham; *W. Virgil Brown*, M.D., Director, Division of Arteriosclerosis and Lipid Metabolism, and Charles Howard Candler Professor of Internal Medicine, Emory University School of Medicine, Past President, American Heart Association; *Trudy L. Bush*, Ph.D., Professor, Department of Epidemiology and Preventive Medicine, University of Maryland at Baltimore School of Medicine; *William P. Castelli*, M.D., Director, Framingham Heart Study; Lecturer, Preventive Medicine and Clinical Epidemiology, Harvard Medical School; and Adjunct Associate Professor of Medicine, Boston University School of Medicine; *James I. Cleeman*, M.D., Coordinator, National Cholesterol Education Program, National Heart, Lung, and Blood Institute, National Institutes of Health; *Graham A. Colditz*, M.D., Dr.P.H., Epidemiologist, Associate Professor of Medicine, Harvard Medical School, and Co-Investigator, Nurses Health Study; *Patricia Lena Cole*, M.D., Assistant Professor of Medicine, Division of Cardiology, Washington University School of Medicine, St. Louis; *Delos M. Cosgrove*, M.D., Chairman, Department of Thoracic and Cardiovascular Surgery, The Cleveland Clinic Foundation; *Susan M. Czajkowski*, Ph.D., Social Science Analyst, Behavior Medicine Branch, National Heart, Lung, and Blood Institute, National Institutes of Health; *Katherine M. Detre*, M.D., Ph.D., Professor of Epidemiology, University of Pittsburgh Graduate School of Public Health; *Richard B. Devereux*, M.D., Director, Echocardiography Laboratory, The N.Y. Hospital/Cornell Medical Center, and Professor of Medicine, Cornell University Medical College; *Pamela S. Douglas*, M.D., Director, Non-Invasive Cardiology, Beth Israel Hospital, Boston, Associate Professor of Medicine, Harvard Medical School, and Editor, "Cardiovascular Health and Disease in Women"; *Debra S. Echt*, M.D., Director, Cardiac Arrhythmia Section, and Associate Professor of Medicine, Vanderbilt University School of Medicine; *Kenneth R. Epstein*, M.D., Associate Director, Division of Internal Medicine, and Clinical Assistant Professor of Medicine, Jefferson Medical College, Philadelphia; *Sylvia K. Fields*, Ed.D., R.N., Coordinator, Primary Care and Community Programs, Office of Academic Affairs, Jefferson Medical College; *Thomas B. Graboys*, M.D., Director, Lown Cardiovascular Center, Boston, and Associate Professor of Medicine, Harvard Medical School, Brigham and Women's Hospital; *William L. Haskell*, Ph.D., Professor of Medicine, Stanford Center for Research in Disease Prevention, Stanford University School of Medicine; *Suzanne Haynes*, Ph.D., Chief, Health Education Section, National Cancer Institute; *Charles H. Hennekens*, M.D., Chief, Preventive Medicine, Brigham and Women's Hospital, Boston, and John Snow Professor of Medicine, Harvard Medical School, Co-Principal Investigator, Cardiovascular Component, Nurses' Health Study; *Paula A. Johnson*, cardiologist, Brigham and Women's Hospital, instructor in medicine, Harvard Medical School; *Frederick E. Kuhn*, M.D., Director, Preventive Cardiology, St. Agnes Hosptial, Baltimore; *John H. Laragh*, M.D., Director, Cardiovascular Center and Hypertension Center, Chief, Cardiology Division, Department of Medicine, and Hilda Altschul Master Professor of Medicine, The New York Hospital/Cornell Medical Center; *John C. LaRosa*, M.D., Chancellor, Tulane Medical Center, and Professor of Medicine, Tulane University School of Medicine; *Claude Lenfant*, M.D., Director, National Heart, Lung, and Blood Institute, National Institutes of Health; *Marian C. Limacher*, M.D., Associate Professor of Medicine, Division of Cardiovascular Medicine, University of Florida College of Medicine, Gainesville; *Joanne Manson*, M.D., Dr. PH, Co-Director, Women's Health, Brigham and Women's Hospital/Harvard Medical School, Associate Professor of Medicine, Harvard Medical School, Principal Investigator, Diabetes Component, Nurses' Health Study; *Suzanne Oparil*, M.D., President, American Heart Association, Director, Vascular Biology and Hypertension Program of the Division of Cardiovascular Disease, and Professor of Medicine, University of Alabama at Birmingham; *Dean Ornish*, M.D., President and Director, Preventive Medicine Research Institute, Sausalito, CA, author, "Eat More, Weigh Less" and "Dr. Dean Ornish's Program for Reversing Heart Disease"; *Mary L. O'Toole*, Ph.D., Director, Human Performance Laboratory, and Associate Professor of Medicine, University of Tennessee, Memphis; *Basil M. Rifkind*, M.D., Senior Scientific Advisor, Vascular Research Program, Division of Heart and Vascular Diseases, National Heart, Lung, and Blood Institute, National Institutes of Health; *Marie A. Savard*, M.D., Director, Center for Women's Health, and Clinical Assistant Professor of Medicine, Medical College of Pennsylvania; *Herbert J. Semler*, M.D., former head of the cardiology section at St. Vincent's Hospital, Portland, OR, founder of the Semler Cardiology Clinic; *Meir J. Stampfer*, M.D., Dr. P.H., Professor of Epidemiology and Nutrition, Harvard School of Public Health, co-investigator, Nurses Health Study; *Sandra P. Thomas*, Ph.D., R.N., Director, Ph.D., Program in College of Nursing, University of Tennessee, Knoxville; *Carl E. Thoresen*, Ph.D., Director, Health Psychology Graduate Program, and Professor of Education and Psychology, Stanford University; *Nanette K. Wenger*, M.D., Director, Cardiac Clinics, Grady Memorial Hospital, Atlanta, GA, and Professor of Medicine, Division of Cardiology, Emory University School of Medicine; *M. Donna Younger*, M.D., Assistant Medical Director, Joslin Diabetes Center, and Assistant Clinical Professor, Harvard Medical School

PROBLEMS WITH SEX CHAPTER

Edward O. Laumann, Ph.D., Professor of Sociology, University of Chicago; *C. Libbey Livingston*, Ph.D., A.N.R.P., Co-Director, Seattle Sexual Health Center; *William H. Masters*, M.D., Director, Masters and Johnson Institute, St. Louis, MO; *Beatrice (Bean) E. Robinson*, Ph.D., Assistant Professor, licensed Psychologist, licensed marriage and family Therapist, the Program in Human Sexuality, Department of Family Practice and Community Health, University of Minnesota Medical School; *Judith A. Seifer*, Ph.D., R.N., President, American Association of Sex Educators and Counsellors, and private practitioner, Sex Therapy, Lewisburg, West Virginia; *Shirley Zussman*, Ed.D., Director, Association for Male Sexual Function, New York City, and editor, "Sex Over 40" newsletter

SEXUALLY TRANSMITTED DISEASES CHAPTER

Sevgi O. Aral, Ph.D., Associate Director for Science, Centers for Disease Control and Prevention; *Karl R. Beutner,* M.D./Ph.D., Clinical Assistant Professor of Dermatology, UCSF, Member, Human Papillomavirus Advisory Board, American Social Health Association; *Peggy Clarke,* M.P.H., President and Chief Executive Officer, American Social Health Association; *Deborah J. Cotton,* M.D., Assistant Professor of Medicine, Harvard Medical School, and Infectious Disease Specialist, Massachusetts General Hospital, Boston; *Anthony S. Fauci,* M.D., Director, National Institute of Allergy and Infectious Diseases, and Chief, Laboratory of Immunoregulation, National Institutes of Health; *Penelope J. Hitchcock,* D.V.M., M.S., Chief, Sexually Transmitted Diseases Branch, Division of Microbiology and Infectious Diseases, National Institute of Allergy and Infectious Diseases, National Institutes of Health; *Richard P. Keeling,* M.D., Director, University Health Services and Professor of Medicine, University of Wisconsin, Madison; *William Schaffner,* M.D., Professor and Chairman, Department of Preventive Medicine, and Professor of Medicine (Infectious Diseases), Vanderbilt University School of Medicine, Nashville, TN; *Thomas Sedlacek,* M.D., Chairman, Department of Gynecology, Graduate Hospital, Philadelphia; *Judith N. Wasserheit,* M.D., M.P.H., Director, Division of STD/HIV Prevention, Centers for Disease Control and Prevention

CONTRACEPTION CHAPTER

Willard Cates, Jr., M.D., M.P.H., Former Director, Division of Training, Centers for Disease Control and Prevention, Corporate Director, Medical Affairs, Family Health International, Research Triangle Park, NC; *Jacqueline Darroach Forrest,* Ph.D., President for Research, Alan Guttmacher Institute, New York City; *Robert Hatcher,* M.D., M.P.H., professor of OBGYN at the Emory U. School of Medicine, and director of family planning at Grady Memorial Hospital; *Deborah Kowal,* M.A., President, Contraceptive Technology Communications, and Co-Author, Contraceptive Technology, and Adjunct Faculty, Emory University School of Public Health; *Anita L. Nelson,* M.D., Associate Professor of Obstetrics and Gynecology, Harbor-UCLA Medical Center; *Edward Robson Newton,* M.D., Associate Professor of Obstetrics and Gynecology, Division of Maternal-Fetal Medicine, University of Texas Health Science Center, San Antonio; *Michael S. Policar,* M.D., M.P.H., Medical Director, Solano Partnership Health Plan, and former national medical director for Planned Parenthood Federation of America; *Phillip G. Stubblefield,* M.D., Chairman, department of obgyn at Maine Medical Center; *James Trussell,* Ph.D., Professor of Economics and Public Affairs, and Associate Dean, Woodrow Wilson School of Public and International Affairs, and Director, Office of Population Research, Princeton University

Index